LASIK

Surgical Techniques and Complications

Lucio Buratto, MD
Stephen Brint, MD
Medical Illustrations by Massimiliano Crespi

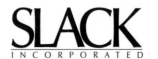

INCORPORATED

6900 Grove Road • Thorofare, NJ • 08086

Publisher: John H. Bond
Editorial Director: Amy E. Drummond
Associate Editor: Jennifer L. Stewart

LASIK: Surgical Techniques and Complications/[edited by] Lucio Buratto, Stephen Brint--2nd ed.
     p. ; cm.
Rev. ed. of: LASIK: principles and techniques. c1998.
Includes bibliographical references and index.
ISBN 1-55642-432-9 (alk. paper).
1. LASIK (Eye surgery) I. Buratto, Lucio. II. Brint, Stephen. [DNLM: 1. Keratectomy, Photorefractive, Excimer Laser--methods. 2. Cornea--surgery. 3. Refractive Errors--surgery. WW 220 L3446 1999]
RE336 .L28 1999
617.7'19059--dc21

99-046441

Printed in the United States of America.
Published by: SLACK Incorporated
     6900 Grove Road
     Thorofare, NJ 08086-9447 USA
     Telephone: 856-848-1000
     Fax: 856-853-5991
     www.slackbooks.com

DEDICATION

Life is a tough journey made easier with the right companion.
To Marie, my travelmate.
Lucio Buratto, MD

To those who have brought LASIK to my life:
Lucio Buratto, my first teacher; Steve Slade, my surgeon who let me throw away my glasses;
and Mark Brown, my friend and greatest supporter throughout the entire writing of this text.
Stephen Brint, MD

CONTENTS

Contents

EXPANDED CONTENTS

Section Two
*Lasers, Microkeratomes, Techniques, Complex
Cases, and Complications Management*

ACKNOWLEDGMENTS

Writing a book is a huge undertaking. It takes an enormous amount of time and calls for considerable sacrifice. The authors—surgeons in their primary role—are simultaneously dedicated to their professions, have congress commitments, and have their staff and business to manage. They also have a family.

Writing a book involves careful examination of all the existing literature on the specific subject and learning a large number of theories. It requires practice of all the surgical techniques and their variations in order to be able to describe them properly.

Then, the text has to be written, corrected, edited, rewritten, and modified a countless number of times. It requires thousands of photographs to be taken and films to be made, drawings have to be devised, processed, and produced with the help of a professional artist.

And that's not all. It must be translated, which complicates matters somewhat, as a good scientific translator is required; the English then has to be reviewed to ensure that it is suitable and will be easily understood by international readers. Even at this point the book still has not reached completion.

All the material has to be delivered to the publisher in an appropriate format, within the terms of the contract; the drafts have to be reread at least once or twice; we have to battle with the computers used to process the text and to scan the drawings, the text must be stored in a manner that can be easily retrieved by the publisher and used in the software needed to create the final product.

Writing a book is a very exhausting business. There is an incredible amount of work involved. All this would not have been possible without the smooth-running organization and help of a number of people that I would now like to thank personally:

First, I would like to thank Marco Moncalvi for his valuable and scrupulous work that was essential for completion of this job.

I would like to thank Claudio Genisi, Giuseppe Perone, Mario Perossini, and Francesco Carones for their useful suggestions.

I would like to thank Massimiliano Crespi for his beautiful drawings and particularly for his ability to transfer my thoughts onto paper.

I would like to thank Fiona Johnston for the translation of the Italian text.

Thanks also to Patrizia Arienti who managed the administration of the book.

My warmest thanks to all the contributors who took part in this project. They were invited to participate because they are experts in their field, because they have renowned professional competence, but also because of their inherent ability to write with clarity and to transmit all their professional knowledge to their colleagues with enthusiasm.

I would also like to thank Steve Brint for the important scientific contribution he gave to this book; I appreciate his patience, his availability, and I would like to thank him especially for his uplifting good humor in the darkest moments of the project.

And finally, my warmest thanks go to Marie Canel who directed every aspect of the enterprise—all things computerized, organizational, and editorial—with enthusiasm, with love, and above all with superhuman patience.

—*Lucio Buratto, MD*

CHAPTER CONTRIBUTING AUTHORS

Jorge L. Alió, MD, PhD
Alicante, Spain

Maria Clara Arbelaez, MD
Muscat, Oman

Carlos J. Argento, MD
Buenos Aires, Argentina

Walid H. Attia, MD
Alicante, Spain

Carmen C. Barraquer, MD
Santa Fe de Bogota, Colombia

Rafael I. Barraquer, MD
Barcelona, Spain

Perry S. Binder, MD
San Diego, California

Stephen Brint, MD
New Orleans, Louisiana

Lucio Buratto, MD
Milan, Italy

Cesar E. Carriazo, MD
Santa Fe de Bogota, Colombia

J. Charles Casebeer, MD
Scottsdale, Arizona

Joseph Colin, MD
Brest, France

María José Cosentino, MD
Buenos Aires, Argentina

Jonathan M. Davidorf, MD
West Hills, California

John F. Doane, MD
Kansas City, Missouri

Dan Durrie, MD
Overland Park, Kansas

Alexander Dybbs, PhD
Cleveland, Ohio

Miles Friedlander, MD, FACS
New Orleans, Louisiana

Eugene I. Gordon, PhD
Edison, NJ

Michael Gordon, MD
San Diego, California

José L. Güell, MD, PhD
Barcelona, Spain

Angela M. Gutierrez, MD
Santa Fe de Bogota, Colombia

David R. Hardten, MD
Minneapolis, Minnesota

Stephen D. Klyce, PhD
New Orleans, Louisiana

Michael C. Knorz, MD
Mannheim, Germany

Richard L. Lindstrom, MD
Minneapolis, Minnesota

Eric J. Linebarger, MD
Minneapolis, Minnesota

John T. LiVecchi, MD, FACS
Scranton, Pennsylvania

Jeffery J. Machat, MD
Windsor, Ontario

Heriberto Marotta, MD
Quilmes, Argentina

Susana Oscherow, MD
West Hills, California

Giuseppe Perone, MD
Appiano-Gentile, Italy

Louis E. Probst, V, MD
Windsor, Ontario

Jeffrey B. Robin, MD
Cleveland, Ohio

Fernando Rodríguez-Mier, MD
Alicante, Spain

Stephen G. Slade, MD
Houston, Texas

Enrique Suárez, MD
Caracas, Venezuela

Mercedes Vázquez, MD
Barcelona, Spain

Mark Walker, MD
Seattle, Washington

Steven E. Wilson, MD
Seattle, Washington

Roberto Zaldivar, MD
Mendoza, Argentina

CASE STUDY CONTRIBUTING AUTHORS

Cathy Albou-Ganem, MD
Paris, France

Till Anschütz, MD
Gaggeneau, Germany

Jean-Louis Arné, MD
Toulouse, France

M. Farooq Ashraf, MD
Baltimore, Maryland

Gordon Balazsi, MD
Montreal, Quebec

Arun Brahma, MB, FRCOphth
Dundee, Scotland

Lucio Buratto, MD
Milan, Italy

Francesco Carones, MD
Milan, Italy

Arturo Chayet, MD
Chula Vista, California

Melania Cigales, MD
Barcelona, Spain

Juan Alvarez de Toledo, MD
Barcelona, Spain

Klaus Ditzen, MD
Weinheim, Germany

Claudio Genisi, MD
Venice, Italy

Oscar D. Ghilino, MD
Buenos Aires, Argentina

José L. Güell, MD, PhD
Barcelona, Spain

Jack T. Holladay, MD
Bellaire, Texas

Jairo E. Hoyos, MD, PhD
Barcelona, Spain

Thomas Kohnen, MD
Frankfurt, Germany

Michiel S. Kritzinger, MD
Cresta, South Africa

Chan Wing Kwong, MD
Singapore

Daniel A. Lebuisson, MD
Neuilly, France

Laurence Lesuer, MD
Toulouse, France

Arturo Maldonado-Bas, MD
Cordoba, Argentina

Antonio Marinho, MD
Porto, Portugal

Heriberto Marotta, MD
Quilmes, Argentina

Marguerite B. McDonald, MD, FACS
New Orleans, Louisiana

Charles McGhee, MB, FRCOphth, PhD
Dundee, Scotland

Francesco Molfino, MD
Milan, Italy

Andreu Coret Moreno, MD
Barcelona, Spain

Marc Mullie, MD
Montreal, Quebec

Dominique Pietrini, MD
Neuilly, France

Mihai Pop, MD
Montreal, Quebec

Paolo Rama, MD
Venice, Italy

Jeffrey B. Robin, MD
Cleveland, Ohio

Luis Antonio Ruiz, MD
Santa Fe de Bogota, Colombia

Olivia Serdarevic, MD
New York, New York

Charalambos S. Siganos, MD
Athens, Greece

Dimitrios S. Siganos, MD
Athens, Greece

Walter J. Stark, MD
Baltimore, Maryland

Ron Stasiuk, MD
Melbourne, Australia

Roger F. Steinert, MD
Boston, Massachusetts

Peter Stewart, MD
Old Sydney, Australia

Jerry Tan, MBBS, FRCS Ed, FRCOphth, FAMS
Singapore

Renato Valeri, MD
Milan, Italy

Mercedes Vázquez, MD
Barcelona, Spain

Paolo Vinciguerra, MD
Milan, Italy

Keith Williams, FRCSC, FACS, FRCOphth
London, England

INTRODUCTION

My life as an ophthalmologist has changed dramatically ever since I made my first journey to Milan, Italy in 1990 to see the excimer laser being used in a way that it had never been used before. It continues to change almost monthly as what has come to be known as LASIK continues to evolve, taking new directions in instrumentation, techniques, and our enhanced knowledge of how to deal with problems, new and old, that are inherent in any surgical procedure

When Lucio Buratto and I coauthored *LASIK: Principles and Techniques* with the help of our many friends and colleagues 2 years ago, there was no definitive textbook on the subject. Subsequently, LASIK has blossomed into the most accepted form of refractive surgery by both physicians and patients alike. Presently, there seems to be no end to the ability of this procedure to evolve, through better, different microkeratomes, more accurate lasers, improved knowledge of wound healing, and increased understanding of both the importance and mechanisms of the quality of vision following LASIK.

This new textbook, *LASIK: Surgical Techniques and Complications*, attempts to cover a little of basic LASIK knowledge already established at the time of writing the first textbook, but more importantly to bring the reader up to the present state of the knowledge of this field as well as glimpse into the future.

Microkeratomes, lasers, instruments, and techniques that were not even dreamed of 2 years ago are now reality and finding their way into general use. The pioneers of these new techniques share the state of the art of their knowledge in this new text.

Complications, such as diffuse interlamellar keratitis, that were unnamed and barely recognized 2 years ago are discussed by several authors, both as to diagnosis as well as management. New and better ways of managing complications like decentered ablations and poor quality of vision following otherwise successful LASIK are now better understood and discussed.

As other modalities of refractive surgery, such as refractive IOLs, corneal rings and implants, and thermal keratoplasty have simultaneously evolved, LASIK is being used to complement the results of those procedures, as well as come to the rescue when complications arise.

This new textbook attempts to bring the reader—both novice as well as experienced refractive surgeon—up to date with the state of worldwide knowledge of these topics at the time of its publication. We hope that it provides joy in reading as well as well as improvements in the quality of vision that we try to provide for our patients.

—*Stephen Brint, MD*
October 1999

SECTION ONE

Evolution, Personal Techniques, and Complications Management

FROM KERATOMILEUSIS TO LASIK

Lucio Buratto, MD and Stephen Brint, MD

1

INTRODUCTION

The word *keratomileusis* is derived from the Greek word keratos, which means "cornea," and mileusis, which means "carving"—literally carving of the cornea. It is a procedure that attempts to change the refractive power of the cornea (ie, to reduce or eliminate myopic, hyperopic, or astigmatic refractive errors).

Myopic keratomileusis (MKM) is an operation that flattens the central cornea by increasing the radius of curvature of the anterior cornea by removing a specific amount of stromal tissue with a specific optic zone.

Barraquer's classical technique obtained this result in two surgical steps:

1. A lamellar cut using a microkeratome. The surgeon removes a corneal disc with parallel faces, about 300 to 360 microns thick and 7.0 to 8.5 mm in diameter.

2. A refractive cut with a cryolathe. The surgeon removes tissue from the stromal side of the frozen primary corneal disc in order to transform it into a refractive lenticle, which can correct the myopic or hyperopic refractive error.

Apart from its final refractive objectives, keratomileusis is truly a unique operation in the evolution of surgery in general, and ophthalmic surgery in particular. It was the first operation in which a piece of an organ was removed, modified, and replaced in its original position. A computer was used for the first time to determine the amount of surgery required.

For many years, one of the main problems of keratomileusis was the ability to find a suitable, safe way to fixate the corneal disc, allowing the surgeon to perform the refractive cut.

In Barraquer's original procedure, fixation of the disc to the die of the cryolathe was done by freezing, but it was technically difficult and extremely unreliable. At the time, the refractive cut was performed using a lathe for contact lenses.

Krumeich and Swinger developed the technique of fixing the corneal disc to the surface of the die without freezing by suction of the epithelial surface to the appropriately selected die; but again, the procedure was tedious and still not suitable for allowing an optimal refractive cut. The possibility of working in situ (the refractive cut being performed on the residual corneal bed instead of the resected disc), subsequently developed by Ruiz, overcame the problem of fixing the lamellar disc, which was common to the previous techniques. The procedure, however, also proved to be frequently inaccurate and difficult to perform because it required the refractive cut to be performed with the microkeratome, which lacked predictable precision.

Buratto first conceived of improving the refractive cut with a technique using the excimer laser. This procedure allowed the refractive resection to be performed with greater precision by optic zones, that could be modified depending on the clinical needs of the individual cases, and with predictability and repeatability far superior to previous techniques. Moreover, the laser procedure could be performed either in situ or on the stromal side of the corneal disc.

It is the use of the laser on corneal tissue that allowed the technical evolution of keratomileusis and marked its current acceptance and use.

This chapter will briefly describe the classical techniques of keratomileusis (ie, those developed prior to the advent of the excimer laser). It will also give a more detailed description of the advanced or "modern" techniques.

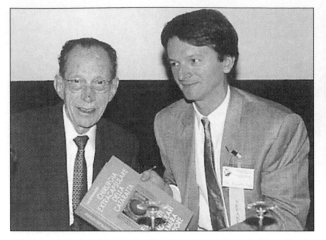

Figure 1-1. José Ignacio Barraquer and Lucio Buratto in Milan, Italy during the First International Symposium of the European Society of Refractive Surgery May 29-31, 1987.

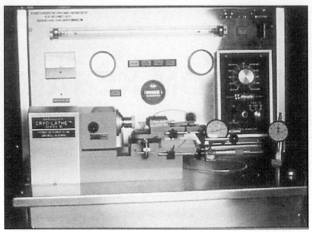

Figure 1-2. Barraquer's cryolathe: front view of the digital instrument.

THE HISTORY OF KERATOMILEUSIS

In 1949, Jose Ignacio Barraquer, MD, in his clinic in Bogota, Colombia, refined his ideas of performing a lamellar keratoplasty for refractive purposes to correct spherical ametropia. The initial procedure involved manual dissection of a lamella to about half the corneal thickness; this manual procedure made use of a corneal dissector or Paufique knife.

In 1958, Barraquer performed the first resection in situ following the removal of a corneal disc using a prototype microkeratome, which ran along a ring without guides. The cutting angle was 0°.

During that same year, Barraquer created human myopic and hyperopic lenticles from donor corneas through a planar cut and freeze techniques. This allowed him to create lenticles with optical power, which were required for the initial intrastromal implants.

In about 1962, Barraquer began using a more accurate microkeratome; it had a cutting angle of 26° (compared to 0° of the first prototype). In the same year, Barraquer invented the suction ring, dovetail guides between the ring, as well as the microkeratome, applanation tonometer, and first intraoperative keratoscope. Next, the cryolathe was invented, along with all the algorithms required for its development and function. Computer calculations for use of the cryolathe were used during surgery for the first time. The refractive resection of the primary corneal disc was performed on a lathe used for contact lenses—the main difficulty was good fixation of the disc.

Following numerous trials, Barraquer conceived of

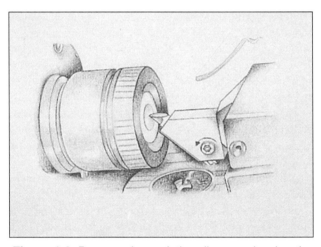

Figure 1-3. Barraquer's cryolathe: diagram showing the tip of the blade during the refractive resection.

freezing the lamella, which allowed it to be fixed then lathed in a subsequent step.

In 1964, the cryolathe was modified to try to simplify the device, but above all to ensure greater predictability (automatic computerized cryolathe).

In 1977, Richard Troutman, MD introduced keratomileusis in the United States, and the very first course on refractive surgery was organized at the Instituto Barraquer de America.

Between 1976 and 1986, a number of surgeons made their mark in the development of keratomileusis, among them Derek Ainslie, Lee T. Mordan, Martin Fallor, and Jorg H. Krumeich.

Between 1980 and 1983, Krumeich, Swinger, and Barraquer developed a new instrument, the BKS 1000, for a nonfreeze refractive cut. The difference was the corneal lamella was "fresh" (nonfreeze or BKS technique). Conceptually, this was an enormous step for-

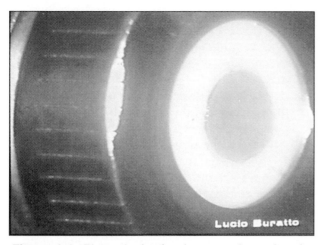

Figure 1-4. Phase I of refractive resection using the blade of the Barraquer lathe.

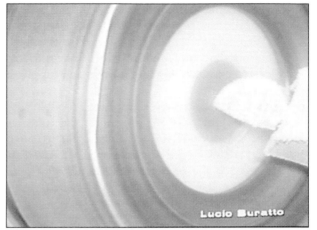

Figure 1-5. Phase II of refractive resection using the blade of the Barraquer lathe.

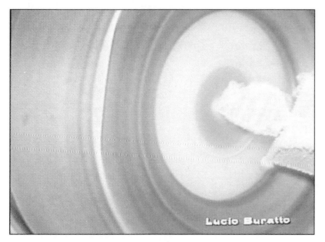

Figure 1-6. Phase III of refractive resection using the blade of the Barraquer lathe.

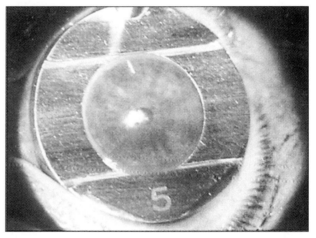

Figure 1-7. BKS 1000: the suction ring.

ward. Because the lamella was not frozen, the keratocytes were not damaged, giving obvious anatomical and functional rehabilitation advantages. There were, however, still a number of problems with good fixation of the lamella for the corneal refractive cut.

To try to overcome this problem, between 1983 and 1986, Luis Ruiz advanced in situ keratomileusis, which involved two superimposed parallel keratectomies using a microkeratome (a technique that was subsequently introduced in the United States by Leo Bores at the end of 1987).

One advantage was that tissue fixation was unnecessary (because the refractive cut was not being performed on the lamella but in situ on the corneal bed) and in the reduction of surgical time. Nevertheless, the procedure was still problematic because it was difficult to perform the two corneal cuts correctly with the microkeratome, and it was not easy to perform them exactly over the

visual axis. The centration over the pupil of the first non-refractive resection (cap) had to be perfect because the suction ring would always find its way to the same spot for the more important second refractive resection. Additionally, the thickness of the second refractive cut was not always as desired, despite having a complete set of plates designed to allow various resection thicknesses.

In 1983, Trokel explored the possibility of using photoablation with an excimer laser to perform refractive incisions and corneal ablation. In 1988, McDonald and Kaufman performed trials and the first surgical applications.

In 1989, encouraged by the work started in 1983 by Trokel, Marshall, and Seiler using the excimer laser in refractive techniques, Buratto presented the technique of intrastromal keratomileusis using the excimer laser, or photokeratomileusis. He suggested performing the refractive cut with laser ablation on either the flap (cap)

5

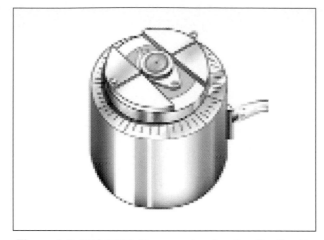

Figure 1-8. BKS 1000: Diagram showing the disc fixed to the work bench and die.

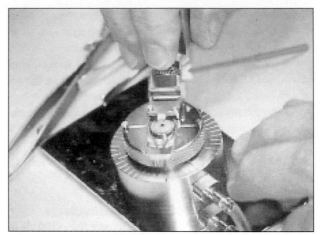

Figure 1-9. BKS 1000: Refractive cut. The disc is fixed to the die by a toothed ring and suction.

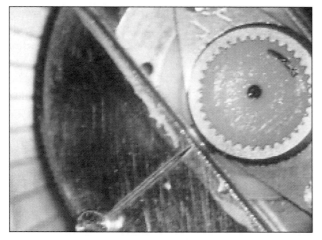

Figure 1-10. Lamellar disc on the bench after the refractive cut.

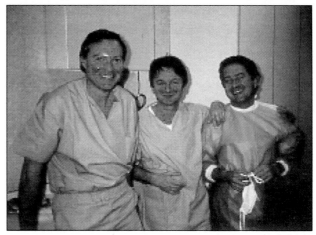

Figure 1-11. From left: Drs. Brint, Buratto, and Genisi in Milan, Italy in 1990 after an ELISK (excimer laser intrastromal keratomileusis) operation.

or in situ (excimer laser intrastromal keratomileusis [ELISK] on the cap or in situ).

This technique takes advantage of the excimer laser's submicron precision and lack of adjacent tissue trauma. The operation can be planned for the desired refractive correction with good repeatability and predictability. It is a procedure that can be performed both on the lamella (cap) or the cornea in situ (bed).

When the ablation is performed on the cap, the keratomileusis technique is much simpler and safer because mechanical fixation of the corneal disc is not required.

The surgeon is able to perform ablations on discs that have diameters, shapes, and thicknesses that do not have to perfectly correspond to the intended measurements. Moreover, it makes the technique accessible to a greater number of surgeons.

Between 1990 and 1991, Pallikaris pursued a previ-

ous idea developed by Barraquer and Pureskin and presented the concept of the nasal corneal hinge. This new surgical modification involved performing a partial primary keratectomy (ie, the surgeon did not remove a corneal disc but left a small amount of uncut tissue nasally, which formed a corneal hinge). The surgeon could then lift the tissue flap and perform an in-situ refractive procedure on the underlying stroma; the flap could then be repositioned in its original site. The variation was a major improvement in keratomileusis techniques, making it faster and simpler in many ways.

In 1991, Guillermo Avalos and Riccardo Guimaraes introduced the sutureless technique. They used filtered air or oxygen to partially dehydrate the stromal surface of the corneal bed and the refractive lenticle, facilitating good adhesion between the two surfaces and eliminating the need for sutures at the end of the operation. This

Table 1-1

MILESTONES IN THE HISTORY OF KERATOMILEUSIS: THE PIONEERS

1949—Barraquer: The first work on lamellar refractive keratoplasty, which is the basis of today's keratomileusis and LASIK.

1958—Barraquer: Experiments on the flap technique; creation of positive and negative lenticles following freezing and the planar cut using a prototype of the microkeratome. First intrastromal implants of corneal lenticles.

1962—Barraquer: The creation of the microkeratome with a 26° cutting angle, the pneumatic (suction) ring and track, the applanation tonometer, and the first intraoperative keratoscope. Invention of the first cryolathe and its algorithms. The use of the first computer in surgery.

1964—Barraquer: A computerized system replaces the electronic calculator. Invention of a more innovative cryolathe.

1977—Troutman: Introduces keratomileusis to the United States. Barraquer organizes the first course of refractive surgery at the Instituto Barraquer de America.

1980-83—Krumeich: Along with Swinger and Barraquer, he introduced the BKS 1000 for the nonfreeze technique (BKS technique); this was the beginning of innovative development of keratomileusis.

1983-86—Ruiz: Invention of the keratomileusis technique in situ (introduced to the United States by Leo Bores in 1987).

1983—Trokel: The first corneal application of the excimer laser followed by the first surgical application by Seiler (incisional), McDonald, and Kaufman (PRK).

1989—Buratto: The first application of the excimer laser to normally sighted human eyes, used in the stromal photoablation of a free corneal flap or in situ photoablation on the exposed stromal bed. First clinical results on fully functional human eyes (LASIK on the flap or LASIK in situ).

1990-91—Pallikaris: Advancement of the hinge technique with the creation of a corneal flap based on Barraquer's work (the hinge technique). First experimental application of photoablation in situ following partial keratectomy and creation of a corneal flap.

1991—Avalos, Guimaraes: Development of the sutureless technique for keratomileusis.

1991—Brint: First LASIK performed in the United States.

1992-96—Slade, Casebeer, Ruiz: All make their contribution to the study, development, and teaching of modern keratomileusis techniques in United States. Organization of practical courses throughout the world dealing with LASIK and ALK.

1996—Buratto: First applications of down-up LASIK with the lamellar cut from inferior to superior "down-up" direction (superior hinge technique or top hinge LASIK).

Table 1-2

CLASSICAL KERATOMILEUSIS TECHNIQUES

Barraquer: Refractive cut using a cryolathe on the stroma of the frozen lamellar disc.

Krumeich: Refractive cut using a microkeratome on the stroma of the fresh, nonfrozen lamellar disc, fixed mechanically to a die that is fitted to a workbench.

Ruiz: Refractive cut using a microkeratome performed on the stroma in situ following a superficial lamellar cut (superimposed double keratectomy).

technique was immediately applied to the flap technique with the nasal hinge.

These additional developments improved the technique, both as "restitutio ad intergrum" of tissue and the functional recovery of the patient. It also significantly decreased the amount of irregular astigmatism induced postoperatively.

Along with improvements in the technique itself, there were improvements in microkeratomes with automated movement allowing a lamellar cut, less dependent on the manual dexterity of the surgeon.

Brint then performed the first LASIK in the United States in June 1991. Slade, Casebeer, and Ruiz all contributed to the advancement of LASIK in the United States. Ruiz's original nomograms were constantly modified and new algorithms for myopia, astigmatism, and hyperopia evolved because of their commitment to the procedure.

In 1996, Buratto again modified the LASIK technique, performing the cut vertically (ie, from below upward as opposed to horizontally). The technique, called down-up LASIK (as compared to the classical technique), appears to be more physiologic, though at that time it could only be used when good globe exposure was achieved. The expanded use of the Chiron (Bausch & Lomb, Claremont, Calif, USA) Hansatome, which creates superior hinges, has allowed this technique to be more widely used.

This flap orientation follows the natural dynamic movements of the eyelid and provides better adhesion to the underlying surface, with a reduced possibility of the flap becoming displaced or developing striae in the immediate postoperative period.

The evolution of keratomileusis into LASIK has found its niche and is attracting the interest of surgeons and manufacturers alike. The race for additional improvements has begun. Further evolution of the procedure will almost certainly mean that this procedure will become a routine technique for correcting the majority of refractive errors—myopic, astigmatic, or hyperopic.

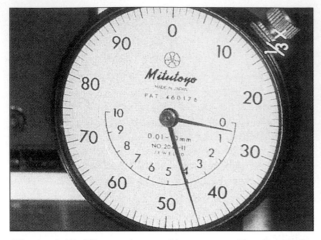

Figure 1-12. Micrometer used to measure the disc thickness in all free cap techniques.

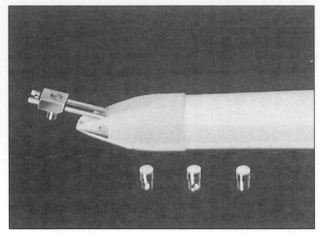

1-13. The first microkeratome model: 0° blade based on Castroviejo's electrokeratome (used with permission from C. Barraquer).

CLASSICAL KERATOMILEUSIS TECHNIQUES

The Evolution

When we refer to classical techniques, we mean all those procedures that over the years have involved laboratory research and clinical investigation, leading to keratomileusis techniques as we know them today.

At the time of this writing, these techniques are considered obsolete and are of a purely historical importance. Nevertheless, they have made an important contribution to the development of modern techniques, with valid references to the ideological and theoretical principles of the past.

Following is a brief description of each before moving on the more advanced, current techniques.

Common Procedural Aspects

The technique originally developed by Barraquer and the subsequent improvements by Krumeich and Ruiz have two main components in common: the lamellar cut and the refractive cut. However, depending on the individual technique, they require different instruments, nomograms, and operating steps.

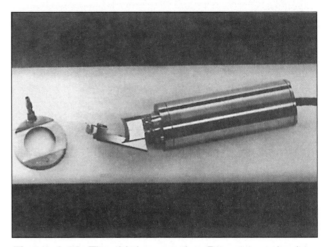

Figure 1-14. The third generation Barraquer microkeratome with a pneumatic ring (used with permission from C. Barraquer).

The primary lamellar cut allows the total or partial removal of a corneal disc with a predefined diameter and thickness. The surgeon can therefore expose the underlying stromal layers and perform the refractive resection.

The primary lamellar cut thus has no refractive power. We will now summarize the main surgical steps.

Table 1-3

CLASSICAL KERATOMILEUSIS TECHNIQUES
MKM Freeze: Barraquer Technique

Inventor: José Ignacio Barraquer (1960)

Definition: This keratomileusis technique uses a cryolathe, contact lens lathe, modified and combined with a freezing system.

Lamellar cut: A disc 300 to 360 microns thick with a diameter of 7.0 to 7.5 mm is desired.

Refractive procedure:

- The lathe is preset
- The corneal disc is placed on the die of the lathe
- The lathe and lamellar disc are frozen
- The stromal portion of the primary corneal disc is carved
- The refractive corneal cap is thawed and replaced in its position on the stromal bed
- Single or double antitorque sutures are used

Advantages: This was the very beginning of lamellar procedures and keratomileusis in particular. The work that led to this procedure still forms the basis of modern keratomileusis techniques.

Disadvantages:

- The technique is now obsolete
- Problems associated with size and complexity of an instrument such as a cryolathe
- Freeze damage to keratocytes that changes the structure of the tissue
- Prolonged healing times (the time needed for revitalization of the disc)
- The procedure requires a primary cut to provide a disc of adequate diameter and thickness for fixation and an accurate refractive cut. In addition, the cut must be well centered and of high quality, or the operation should be aborted

Intraoperative complications: There is a real possibility of total or partial damage to the primary corneal disc during the phases of freezing and/or processing at the lathe due to miscalculation of the refractive resection, mechanical malfunction, or human error.

The cut may be inadequate and/or decentered even if the freezing process is adequate. Or if there is incomplete adhesion or fixation of the lamellar disc, it may detach from the lathe's support plate.

There may be incomplete freezing of the corneal disc that may result in an irregular refractive cut, a disc with altered thickness, or a situation in which the surgeon cannot continue with the operation.

Postoperative complications: Freezing causes the majority of keratocytes to be killed. Replacement of the refractive corneal lenticle on its original corneal bed involves a very slow repair process and lengthy histological, anatomical, refractive, and functional recovery. This frequently causes poor re-epithelialization or filamentary keratitis, lengthy visual rehabilitation from slow cellular repopulation of the corneal lenticle, and a high amount of postoperative irregular astigmatism secondary to irregularities on the stromal surface of the corneal disc, or to microtraction forces between the lathed cap and underlying corneal bed.

Comments: Barraquer's technique marked the beginning of a new surgical era. The genius of its inventor opened the road to a completely new type of surgery and techniques that were revolutionary compared to traditional techniques used in eye surgery. The idea of removing tissue from the cornea, then performing the refractive procedure and replacing the modified tissue to its original site, was an extraordinary innovation that marked the very beginning of refractive surgery as we know it today. But, as with all innovative techniques, considerable evolution, research, and development were required. Inevitably, this meant that there were complications, poor results, and problems associated with the unreliability of the prototype instruments. Because this was groundbreaking research, it was impossible to compare it to any similar techniques, as there were no papers, references, or statistics on the subject. This technique is special because it allowed surgeons to study the cornea from a refractive aspect, which encouraged the development of the methods and instruments available today.

Table 1-4

CLASSICAL KERATOMILEUSIS TECHNIQUES
Krumeich-Swinger Planar Nonfreeze MKM Technique

Inventors: Jorg Krumeich & Casimer Swinger (1983)

Definition: Keratomileusis with a primary cut followed by the refractive resection on a "fresh" (nonfrozen) disc using a microkeratome with mechanical fixation of the corneal disc.

Lamellar cut: Corneal disc with thickness of 300 to 360 microns and a diameter of 8.0 to 8.5 mm.

Refractive procedure: The BKS 1000 instrument (Barraquer-Krumeich-Swinger) is used in this technique. The instrument was perfected by Krumeich and consists of a microkeratome that performs the lamellar cut and a bench for the refractive cut. The bench allows the corneal disc to be fixed stromal side up to a device (the die) during the refractive cut using the microkeratome. Fixation of the corneal disc on the surface of the chosen die is done by two means:

- Mechanically with a toothed ring that locks the peripheral portion of the disc to the peripheral surfaces of the die
- By aspiration, which creates suction to the epithelial surface of the disc through numerous microperforations on the die itself. Depending on their shape, the die or molds allow the surgeon to obtain the desired dioptric correction through the refractive cut with the microkeratome. The instrument therefore includes several dies for various hyperopic and myopic corrections

Advantages: From a clinical point of view, the fact that keratocytes are not frozen allows for more rapid tissue repair and faster functional recovery, which is qualitatively better than Barraquer's technique.

From a technical point of view, the equipment is easier to use than the Barraquer cryolathe. Moreover, most of the components are easily sterilized and the machine is compact in size.

Disadvantages:

- The instrument lacks the details and refinements that would make it even easier to use (eg, it is difficult to fix the corneal disc to the bench. Calibration and fixation of some of the screw-gauge components are not technically easy)
- The lamellar cut must produce a disc with a thickness, diameter, and shape suitable for good fixation, which will therefore give a good refractive cut
- Variations in disc thickness through drying during the maneuvers of centering and fixing on the die will have an adverse effect on the refractive outcome
- There may be mechanical microtrauma to the corneal disc during the refractive resection due to fixation with the mechanical ring, particularly in the paracentral and peripheral portions
- Nomograms are difficult to interpret

Intraoperative complications: The cut may be irregular, decentered, or have an incorrect thickness due to poor fixation of the primary corneal disc to the die of the bench, dehydration, or decentration. In this technique, controlled and rapid speed of all phases—resection, fixation, and refractive cut—is necessary, or dehydration will significantly alter the nomogram.

Postoperative complications:

- Insufficient refractive predictability
- Frequently unsatisfactory visual results (probably linked to poor quality of the refractive cut)

Comments: This technique was another important advance from the freeze technique because it removed the damaging freeze step. For many years, the BKS 1000 was the most popular instrument used in keratomileusis. Only a handful of surgeons, however, actually used the BKS 1000 routinely in refractive surgery, probably discouraged by the technical and instrumental difficulties that are inherent with this device.

Table 1-5

CLASSICAL KERATOMILEUSIS TECHNIQUES
Ruiz MKM in situ Technique

Inventor: Luis Ruiz (1986)

Definition: This keratomileusis technique involves two complete, free keratectomies with the microkeratome. They are parallel and superimposed. The diameter and thickness of the second resection (the second corneal disc is discarded) determine the preset refractive correction.

Refractive procedure: This is performed through a second stromal resection with the microkeratome. First, the surgeon cuts a 360° keratectomy (diameter 7.0 to 7.2 mm, thickness 130 to 160 microns). Second, another 360° refractive keratectomy is performed (diameter 3.5 to 5.0 mm with thickness depending on the dioptric amount to be corrected).

Advantages:
- The instruments are simple and easy to transport (even with a large number of rings and plates)
- Quick operating time

Disadvantages:
- The suction ring is normally replaced between the two keratectomies with resultant possible loss of suction
- Centration over the pupil and the two superimposed keratectomies can be difficult but is mandatory

Intraoperative complications:
- It may be difficult to obtain refractive corneal discs with a diameter and thickness that correspond to the surgical nomogram
- The primary or secondary cut may be decentered with respect to the patient's visual axis, or it can be an irregular shape and/or thickness. In the event of complications in deeper portions of the stroma, further operations are fraught with great difficulty

Postoperative complications:
- There is a significant percentage of both regular and irregular induced astigmatism
- Predictable, standardized refractive outcomes are difficult
- Loss of uncorrected and best-corrected vision is possible

Comments: With this technique, the difficulty of being able to calibrate, standardize, and have the surgeon correctly control microkeratome advancement is magnified because the surgeon has to perform two keratectomies. One of these (the refractive cut) is in the deep layers of the stroma, which does not leave a wide margin for error in the event of complications, leaving penetrating keratoplasty as a last resort. Moreover, the difficulty with centration between the two keratectomies over the patient's visual axis puts this procedure in the group of classical techniques now rarely used.

Table 1-6

CLASSICAL KERATOMILEUSIS TECHNIQUES
Step 1: Primary Lamellar Resection

1. Check the blade edge for quality under the microscope prior to inserting it in the blade holder; make sure the blade is securely in place, the edge is not damaged during placement, and the blade holder moves freely.
2. Meticulously assemble the microkeratome.
3. Insert the plate and make sure it "snaps" completely into position.
4. Perform a "dry run" of the microkeratome's performance, allowing it to move smoothly forward and backward in the suction ring stabilized on the side table (pay attention to the noise the machine makes—it must be a constant buzzing sound).
5. Administer anesthesia.
6. Position the patient under the microscope.
7. Carefully mark the visual and pararadial axis to ensure proper realignment of the cap and correct orientation (not upside down).
8. Check the suction ring by covering the ring with the thumb to ensure suction is working properly.
9. Activate suction.
10. Perform tonometry to check adequate IOP, which should be 65 mm Hg.
11. Check the applanation lens to ensure adequate diameter of resection.
12. Wet the guides of the ring and track.
13. Wet the exposed corneal dome.
14. Position the microkeratome at the beginning of the ring's dovetail guides.
15. Once again, check the correct insertion of the plate in the head of the microkeratome.
16. Activate the microkeratome motor.
17. Perform the primary keratectomy.
18. Deactivate suction and motor at the end of the pass.
19. Remove the disc.
20. Measure disc thickness with the micrometer.
21. Measure disc diameter using the reticule on the applanation lens.
22. Store the corneal disc in an antidesiccation chamber, epithelial side down, until needed for the refractive cut.

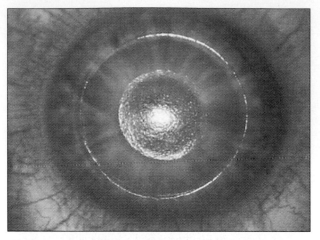

Figure 1-15. In situ keratomileusis. Note the wide lamellar cut and smaller refractive cut.

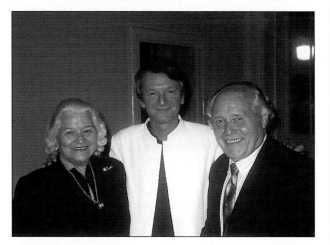

Figure 1-16. Buratto with Hans Hellenkamp and wife. Hans developed the Hansatome.

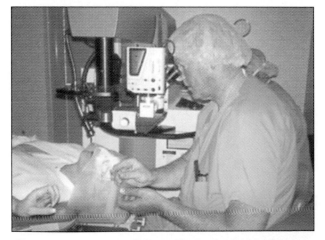

Figure 1-17. Stephen Brint performs the first LASIK procedure in the United States with the Summit laser.

CLASSICAL KERATOMILEUSIS TECHNIQUES
Step 2: Refractive Cut

In the classical techniques, the refractive cut is performed with instruments and methods that differ depending on the technique used.

The refractive cut allows the surgeon to remove a predetermined amount of stromal tissue of diameter and thickness that will vary according to the technique and refraction.

In all myopic procedures, tissue removal is deeper centrally and less so peripherally, except in Ruiz's original in-situ technique in which the second keratectomy is also planar but smaller than the primary keratectomy, allowing the corneal surface to drape into the resection and thereby flatten the cornea.

With the refractive cut, the dioptric power of the cornea is permanently changed based on the nomogram of a particular technique in order to obtain the desired refractive result.

Comments: The classical techniques, at the time of this writing, are of historical interest but are the basis of more advanced procedures that will be covered in following chapters.

The classical techniques have been mentioned here along with a short description of each because they give the reader a broader vision of the evolution of keratomileusis.

The unpredictability and poor degree of standardization of the refractive result added to the unacceptable incidence of complications, which restricted widespread acceptance of the classical techniques. However, it should be noted that when they are used in expert hands, they can still provide satisfactory results.

Beginning surgeons should be familiar with these theoretical complications and problems though they are rarely encountered.

Table 1-8

CLASSICAL TECHNIQUES
Primary Cut with the Microkeratome, Possible Complications, and Solutions

Complication	Most frequent cause	Possible available solutions
Corneal perforation	Due to the absence of incomplete seating of the microkeratome head.	Stop at first sign of aqueous—may be able to repair laceration with sutures if surgeon can stop quickly enough. If not, reconstruct as necessary—lens extraction with IOL, vitrectomy if necessary, resuture.
Thin or incomplete keratectomy	Poor suction and grasp of the suction ring to the conjunctival-scleral plane. Cut in which microkeratome advancement was too fast.	With a thin keratectomy, in situ photo-ablation may be possible if the stromal bed is well exposed. Close with or without sutures and re-operate 3 to 4 months later.
Keratectomy with irregular thickness one).	Poor adhesion between the suction ring and sclera. Inadequate suction during the cut.	Close with or without sutures and re-operate 3 to 4 months later (with a kera-tectomy deeper than the previous
Incomplete keratectomy Close	Surgeon error (released footpedal). Electrical failure. Obstruction of the progression of the microkeratome (speculum, lashes, drape, etc).	Manual keratectomy (if the cut has already passed the optic zone). with or without sutures and re-operate 6 months later.
Decentered keratectomy	Incorrect centering of the ring on the precorneal pupillary center. Poor grasp of the ring on the scleral plane	In situ photoablation well-centered over the pupil on the stromal bed if possible. Close with or without sutures and re-operate 6 months later if there is marked decentration, that does not allow for a complete centered photoablation.
Keratectomy with irregular surfaces	Irregular progression of the microkeratome. Dull blade. Irregular cutting speed. Obstruction of blade advancement due to poor globe exposure, speculum or drapes positioned poorly, a loss of power or suction. Low blade oscillation speed compared to the advancing speed.	Close with or without sutures and re-operate after 6 months.

		Table 1-9		
		CLASSICAL TECHNIQUES		
		Serious Complications During the Refractive Cut		
Technique	Main complication	Primary cause	Result	Possible available solutions
Barraquer	Destruction of or damage to the disc	Insufficient freezing of the lamellar disc prior to the lathing phase. Release of the lamellar disc from the base of the die. Air between the base of the die and the lamellar disc. Calculation or technical error	If the disc cannot be salvaged, use an alternate disc (homoplastic)	Use homoplastic tissue
Krumeich-Swinger	Damage to the disc	Incorrect assembly of the bench. Incorrect calibration of the zero value. Incorrect position of the die. Blade edges not sharp.	A donor disc must be used	Use homoplastic tissue
Ruiz	Imperfect centration of the primary cut and intrastromal refractive cut	Surgeon error. Poor centration and/or grasp by the suction ring on the stroma exposed by the first cut. The refractive disc is either too big or too small.	Irregular astigmatism. Poor functional visual recovery. Glare, diplopia, blurring, and halos.	Homoplastic keratomileusis with resection deeper than the cut obtained during the first operation. PKP in those cases that were not successful with the previous surgical solution.

PREPARATION FOR SURGERY

Lucio Buratto, MD and Stephen Brint, MD

2

PREOPERATIVE CONSULTATION

The preoperative consultation with a patient who is considering laser-assisted in situ keratomileusis (LASIK) does not differ greatly from patient consultations for other forms of refractive surgery. The patient not only should be informed of both the risks and benefits of the procedure, but the surgeon should evaluate what the patient's expectations are and determine if they are realistic.

The surgeon should describe the procedure to the patient, relating both the expected outcome and problems the patient may expect if complications are encountered.

This exam will also allow the surgeon to understand why the patient has chosen LASIK over other available refractive procedures and discuss potential results.

As part of the informed consent, the patient must be made aware of:
- Risks
- Benefits
- Reasonable expectations
- How the surgical procedure will be performed
- Other surgical alternatives

The patient should be allowed to view brochures and videos that summarize the risks and benefits of this technique. The surgeon should point out that the major advantages of LASIK include extremely rapid visual recovery and near total absence of pain both during and after the procedure.

This surgical procedure requires the active cooperation of the patient, and well-informed patients who know what to expect are better able to remain calm and cooperative during the procedure. Most patients are highly motivated in this respect.

It is important to explain that LASIK is a procedure composed of many steps, with each step requiring the successful completion of the previous. Any step that is not successful will necessitate aborting the procedure. This may be disappointing to the patient, but it makes the likelihood of serious complications rare. This information stimulates the patient to fully cooperate during the various steps of the procedure.

The patient should be advised that his or her vision may be blurry immediately postoperatively, especially at near, and that he or she may notice fluctuations in visual acuity through the day. The patient may also experience either over- or undercorrection, which in some circumstances (eg, driving a car) may necessitate the occasional use of corrective eyewear or an enhancement procedure to correct residual refractive error. This is especially true for patients with extreme corrections (myopia in excess of 10 diopters [D] or astigmatism in excess of 5 to 6 D).

The final objective of the preoperative consultation is to determine why the patient has decided to opt for surgery: whether it be freedom from spectacles or contact lenses, reasons associated with leisure activities, professional, or cosmetic reasons. By knowing these reasons, the surgeon gains a better understanding of the personality of the patient—if expectations are too high, if the patient demands perfection, if he or she finds it difficult to accept potential risks (this type of patient should be counseled on what can realistically be expected and perhaps may be rejected for surgery). Finally, the surgeon should always ask and document if there are any questions or concerns that have not already been addressed.

PREOPERATIVE EXAMINATION

This examination is the same for all refractive surgeries; it must be complete and should include the following:
- General medical history
- Ocular history
- Examination of the ocular adnexa

Table 2-1

PREOPERATIVE CONSULTATION

Initial interview with the patient (brochure, video)
Objectives include:

- Technique (how the surgical procedure will be performed)
- Limitations (reasonable expectations)
- Possible complications
- Potential postoperative problems
- Best possible outcome
- Worst possible outcome
- Risks/benefits
- Other surgical alternatives, if any
- Possible need for an enhancement procedure
- Understanding patient motivation:
     Independence from spectacles
     Independence from contact lenses
     Leisure activity
     Professional reasons
     Cosmetic considerations
- Job considerations or requirements (the patient must ensure that having LASIK will not become a disqualifying factor in the career he or she wishes to pursue, such as military, aviation, etc)

- Anterior segment slit lamp examination
- Quantitative and qualitative evaluations of lachrimal function
- Contact lens history
- Evaluation of the blink reflex
- Dilated fundus examination
- Intraocular pressure (by tonometry)
- Keratometry
- Computerized corneal topography
- Visual acuity
- Manifest and cycloplegic refraction
- Biometry
- Mesopic, scotopic, and photopic pupil diameter
- Pachymetry
- Specular microscopy of the endothelium
- Determination of the dominant eye
- Orthoptic examination
- Contrast sensitivity testing
- Ray tracing analysis
- Corneal sensitivity testing

GENERAL MEDICAL HISTORY

The patient's general medical history is helpful in identifying systemic pathologies that may be an absolute or relative contraindication to the LASIK procedure. In particular:

Diabetes. Generally speaking, diabetes does not affect the success of the LASIK procedure. However, in poorly controlled insulin-dependent patients, the disease can cause a few problems.

Refraction is often unstable in these patients; high blood sugar levels will cause the eye to become more myopic, making determination of the amount of "true" refractive myopia difficult. The risk of over- or under-correction is increased.

Cataracts usually appear earlier in diabetic patients. A careful preoperative slit lamp examination, even in a young patient, should help the surgeon determine if any lens opacity is dense enough to prove a contraindication to LASIK. The diabetic patient should also be warned of the possibility of precocious cataract formation and the possibility of a need for cataract extraction surgery sooner than expected in the general population.

In diabetic patients, the surgical wound may take longer to heal, with a corresponding increase in the risk of infection. Surgery is not recommended in diabetic patients with diabetic retinopathy, nephropathy, neuropathy, or a history of difficult wound healing.

Pregnancy/breast-feeding. These conditions could be considered a contraindication to surgery due to the fluctuation in refractive error that is often associated with pregnancy and breast-feeding. Moreover, the healing response following laser ablation may also be altered.

Tissue reaction is particularly important in photorefractive keratectomy (PRK), in which healing times are longer; also, PRK may require systemic drug therapy in the postoperative period (analgesics), which may be contraindicated in pregnancy or while breast-feeding.

Fluctuations in refractive error during pregnancy are temporary. Pre-pregnancy refractive information may be used when performing LASIK during pregnancy.

Any persistent deterioration of myopia during pregnancy or breast-feeding can be considered independent of the patient's condition and due to progression of myopia. Similar situations are observed with any hormone therapy (eg, contraceptive pills, estrogen for menopause).

LASIK is contraindicated during pregnancy and breast-feeding, as it may be necessary to prescribe medication for infection, severe pain (loss of the flap), or Sands of the Sahara syndrome. It is understood that drugs should not be administered during pregnancy or while breast-feeding if at all avoidable. Many pharmaceuticals have not been fully evaluated for their effects on the developing fetus or nursing infant.

Autoimmune/connective tissue diseases. Rheumatoid arthritis, systemic lupus erythematosis, scleroderma, nodular panarteritis, etc are conditions that can affect connective tissue, resulting in an abnormal and unpredictable reaction of the tissue to the laser ablation; they may also encourage stromal melting. These pathologies are absolute contraindications for PRK, but when LASIK is used, they are considered contraindications only if they are active or regularly recur. With LASIK, the exposure of stromal tissue is greatly reduced. It should be remembered that these conditions may require chronic use of steroids, which can delay wound healing and encourage infections.

Clinically significant atopia.

Immunodepressed patients. These patients are at high risk for infection.

Systemic pathologies that slow wound healing. These include psoriasis, diabetes mellitus (as previously discussed), Marfan's syndrome, Ehlers-Danlos syndrome, and other nonautoimmune/connective tissues diseases.

Allergies. The surgeon should keep in mind that drug therapy is used in the pre- and postoperative period, even though postoperative drug therapy requirements are greater for PRK than LASIK. LASIK normally does not involve pain; as a result, nonsteroidal anti-inflammatory drugs (NSAIDs), analgesics, or sedatives are generally not required.

Systemic infections (HIV or tuberculosis).

Drug therapy. The surgeon should determine if the patient is taking any therapeutic or nontherapeutic medicines. Some drugs may delay healing of the corneal wound. These include:

- Adenine arabinoside
- Azathioprine
- Steroids
- Cocaine
- Iodine solutions
- Sulfonamides such as sulfamethizole and sulfisoxazole
- Thiotepa

OCULAR HISTORY

A complete ocular history alerts the surgeon to conditions that may be contraindications to LASIK or that may require a delay in surgery.

LASIK should not be performed on a one-eyed patient. Surgery should also be avoided in recurrent herpetic keratitis, herpetic keratouveitis, or a history of ophthalmic herpes zoster. In the latter case, the surgeon should check for a mydriatic pupil. If the surgeon decides to proceed with LASIK on a patient with a history of herpes, general and topical administration of antiherpetic agents should be considered.

The patient with a history of blepharitis or blepharoconjunctivitis should be carefully monitored. If blepharitis is active, preoperative treatment is necessary. Blepharitis can increase the risk of infection and may play a roll in the development of Sands of the Sahara syndrome, as well as the risk that loose eyelashes and debris from the lids could interfere with the microkeratome pass.

A history of dry eye syndrome is also of considerable importance. This can complicate healing of the surgical wound and increase the risk of infection. Moreover, compromised epithelium, which is common in patients with dry eyes, can make flap manipulation more complicated and increase the risk of epithelial defects following the microkeratome pass.

Even in the absence of a history of dry eyes, lachrimal function should be evaluated preoperatively.

The patient should be questioned about allergies to systemic medications and any history of adverse reaction to eyedrops or contact lens solutions. Products that the patient is allergic to or that have caused an adverse reaction should be avoided. A comprehensive list of current medications (both prescription and over-the-counter) should be reviewed by the surgeon, as some systemic medications can cause pupil dilation (cortisone, antidepressives, antispastics).

History of retinal detachment surgery, vitrectomy, or cataract removal may make it difficult to position the suction ring and achieve adequate intraocular pressure (IOP) during the operation. A patient with a diagnosis of retinitis pigmentosa should be made aware that LASIK may further deteriorate night-time vision and create more of a risk for optic nerve damage (and subsequent vision loss) due to the elevation of IOP during the keratectomy. Retinitis pigmentosa is characterized by a poorly functioning or nonfunctional peripheral retina. As a result, vision in dim lighting is greatly decreased. Night-time glare and reduced contrast sensitivity that can result from LASIK may further decrease visual function at night.

Patients with glaucoma can have a number of problems. Postoperative use of topical steroids may increase IOP, however, since their use rarely exceeds 1 week, risk is minimal.

It is important to keep in mind that during the operation, IOP can reach levels in excess of 60 to 65 mm Hg (usually for less than 1 minute). There is a risk that this rise in IOP, however short, could cause further optic nerve damage. A rise in IOP also creates a theoretical risk of vascular occlusion.

A glaucoma patient with a history of trabeculectomy risks a poor flap resulting from inadequate suction due to scleral irregularity or possibly rupture of the bleb. This greatly increases the risk of infection (worst scenario being endophthalmitis). If the trabeculectomy bleb is flat, it is unlikely to create problems.

Previous radial keratotomy (RK) may cause the flap to be fragmented, particularly if the number of cuts exceeds eight and if the cuts are thin and/or small.

The surgeon should pay close attention to patients who relate symptoms characteristic of recurrent corneal erosion. Loosely adherent epithelium can increase the chance that the microkeratome pass will create defects. The surgeon should also be aware of any problems the patient may have related to contact lens wear: abrasions, oily tear film, fragile epithelium. About 5% of patients with a history of contact lens wear will have very fragile epithelium. Some corneal pathologies are characterized by corneal erosions not linked to trauma.

Patients who wear contact lenses should discontinue wear prior to preoperative testing (the length of time will be dependent upon the type of contact worn). If lens wear is resumed after the initial exam, it should be discontinued again prior to surgery (again, the length of time will depend on the type of contacts worn).

If the patient has a corneal graft, the surgeon must consider the risk to the endothelium and possibility of rejection.

The strength of the wound should also be considered as well as the possibility of inducing wound rupture.

A patient who has progressive myopia should not undergo LASIK, at least until a stable refractive error can be demonstrated.

Some patients are under the impression that the procedure not only corrects existing myopia, but prevents further progression. The surgeon should clearly explain that this is not the case. The patient should also be informed that the operation will not restore visual acuity lost to ocular or systemic disease.

EXAMINATION OF THE OCULAR ADNEXA

Globe position in relation to the eyelids and orbit must be examined. Anatomically, the conjunctiva is an adjoining structure, which will be discussed in the chapter on the anterior segment.

There are several factors that can hinder adequate globe exposure. The surgeon should note preoperatively if a patient has a prominent brow, small palpebral fissure, or deep-set eyes, and be prepared to alter technique and instrumentation to obtain sufficient exposure in placing the suction ring and making the microkeratome pass. Inexperienced surgeons should avoid patients with fea-

Table 2-2
GENERAL MEDICAL AND OCULAR HISTORY

General Medical History
  Diabetes
    Increased risk of infection
    Creates fragility of the corneal epithelium
    Possible refractive instability
  Pregnancy/breast-feeding
    Instability of refraction
    Problems with prolonged therapy
  Pathologies of connective tissue
    Dry eyes
    Uveitis/scleritis
  Autoimmune pathologies
    Dry eyes
    Uveitis/scleritis
  Atopia
  Allergies
    To antibiotics used in LASIK
    NSAIDS used in LASIK
    Analgesics used in LASIK
  General infections
    Pathologies that alter wound healing
Medical History of the Eye
  Previous history of eye surgery
    Problems with the suction ring/eye pressure
    Retinal detachment
    Vitrectomy
    Cataract surgery
    Filtering blebs
  Monocularity
  Retinitis pigmentosa
    Problems with night vision
    Damage to the optic nerve because of eye pressure during LASIK
  Glaucoma
    Filtering blebs
    Risk of changes in eye pressure during LASIK
  Previous refractive surgery
  Family history of retinal detachment

tures that will make adequate exposure difficult. These patients are better managed by experienced surgeons.

When the eye is deep-set, it is sometimes possible to perform a retrobulbar injection by proptosing the globe sufficiently enough to place the suction ring, though this is not always advisable. In some cases, despite the surgeon's best efforts, the shape of the orbit and adnexa prevent LASIK from being performed. If there is doubt, a speculum can be placed and the suction ring applied as a "test" during the preoperative exam.

In eyes with narrow palpebral fissures, a lateral can-

Table 2-3

ANATOMICAL FACTORS INFLUENCING GLOBE EXPOSURE

Extremely sunken eyes
- Relative: prominent brow
- Absolute: endophthalmos
- Cause: Old fracture of the orbit floor
  - Atrophy of orbit fat
  - Atrophy of orbit tissue
  - History of orbital tumor removal
  - History of orbital hematoma
  - Metastatic adenocarcinoma
  - Progressive facial hemiatrophy
  - Horner's syndrome
  - Parinaud's syndrome

Small palpebral fissure

Blepharophimosis
- Congenital
- Acquired
- Senile
- Spastic (contraction of the orbicular muscle at the eyelid canthals)
- Scars: trachoma, pemphigus, ulcerative blepharitis

Anchyloblepharon
- Congenital
- Acquired
- Adhesion between the free edges of the superior and inferior eyelids due to:
  - Trauma
  - Chemical burn
  - Thermal burn
  - Trachoma
    - Long-standing tarsorrhaphy
    - Diphtheritic conjunctivitis

Symblepharon
- Scar adhesion between the palpebral and the bulbar conjunctiva or cornea due to loss of the epithelial layer

thotomy may be necessary (following local infiltration anesthesia). The patient should be informed in advance if you suspect the possible need for this procedure.

It is important to observe whether there is evidence of active blepharitis. If present, it should be treated prior to surgery. There are a number of reasons for this: it has been suggested that secretions from the meibomian glands may in some way be responsible for Sands of the Sahara syndrome; it increases the risk for postoperative infection. An excessively oily tear film can interfere with the uniformity of the ablation, and loose eyelashes or debris from the lids could interfere with the passage of the microkeratome.

EXAMINATION OF THE ANTERIOR SEGMENT

The slit lamp allows detailed examination of corneal scars, corneal neovascularization, kerato-conjunctivitis sicca, superficial corneal dystrophy, keratoconus, pterygium, pterygoid, irregular epithelium, evidence of recurrent corneal erosion, filtering blebs, redundant conjunctiva, anterior uveitis, keratitis, and others. It is also important to examine the crystalline lens for any sign of cataract.

Generally speaking, LASIK is contraindicated in patients with keratoconus, although some surgeons advocate this. Treatment of patients with keratoconus can give very unpredictable results. The surgeon must be sure that the refraction is stable and the patient has sufficient corneal thickness. Obviously, the procedure should not be attempted on a severely deformed and thin cornea. The procedure can be successful in cases of very mild myopia or astigmatism in which the amount of tissue removed is minimal, but in cases of extreme refractive error there may be insufficient corneal thickness to achieve the desired correction. The surgeon must consider the preoperative corneal thickness, location of the cone (if it is centrally located it is easier to achieve an acceptable refractive result), and if there are corneal opacities.

The patient's age should also be taken into consideration. Normally, keratoconus is more progressive during the second and third decades of life, after which it tends to stabilize, making the outcome of LASIK more predictable. In any case, the patient should be informed that results may not be optimal, and that keratoconus can progress and require a corneal transplant in the future.

Corneal neovascularization is frequently observed in long-term contact lens wearers and is commonly seen at the superior limbus. This may result in intraoperative hemorrhage when the vessels are cut by the microkeratome. These hemorrhages are usually small and do not affect the outcome of surgery. The surgeon simply uses a Merocel sponge (Solan Ophthalmics, Jacksonville, Fla, USA) to remove any blood. In rare cases, the hemorrhage can be considerable, and if uncontrollable, the procedure may have to be aborted. All blood must be removed from the stromal bed prior to delivery of the refractive ablation. If blood seeps into the ablation zone during delivery, the laser should be stopped and continued only when the blood has been removed. It is important to maintain uniform hydration of the stromal bed.

Postoperatively, blood may seep into the interface.

This can interfere with visual function depending on the amount and location of the red blood cells (RBCs). Finally, an intraoperative hemorrhage may cause the patient to be overly anxious postoperatively.

Active anterior uveitis or active keratitis are also contraindications to LASIK. The same applies to any active ocular infection.

Corneal scars, filtering blebs, pterygium, pterygoid, and conjunctival cysts can make positioning the suction ring and achieving adequate IOP difficult. If there are any corneal scars, the surgeon must be sure they are stable.

Dry eyes tend to have fragile epithelium, which can cause the microkeratome pass to create epithelial defects. This increases the risk of postoperative infection and prolongs recovery. Evaluation of lacrimal function preoperatively is important and will be covered later in a separate section.

History of recurrent corneal erosion, basement membrane dystrophy, and any irregularity in the epithelial surface can have the same consequences as dry eye syndrome. Epithelial defects increase the incidence of epithelial ingrowth. Evidence of previous corneal erosion can be seen at the slit lamp with retroillumination as small vacuoles observed between the epithelium and Bowman's membrane. There are also hereditary forms of superficial corneal dystrophy. Of the corneal dystrophies that can lead to recurrent erosion of the cornea, they are:

- Cogan's microcystic dystrophy, which may be associated with dot-map-fingerprint dystrophy or Bietti's lacunar dystrophy
- Macular and granular corneal dystrophy
- Haab-Dimmer reticulum dystrophy
- Reis-Bucklers dystrophy

Bilateral or unilateral recurrent erosion in the absence of trauma should alert the surgeon to consider a diagnosis of corneal dystrophy, especially in young patients. Corneal erosion is also seen with bullous keratopathy, aphakia, anterior chamber IOLs, diabetes mellitus, and contact lens wear. Patients should be advised to use nonpreserved artificial tears in the postoperative period.

Redundant or loose conjunctiva can occlude the aspiration port of the suction ring and create pseudosuction. The microkeratome console indicates that vacuum is sufficient, but the IOP is not truly elevated.

Endothelial dystrophies, guttata, and ruptures in Descemet's membrane are contraindications to performing an intrastromal laser ablation.

Generally, a history of herpes simplex keratitis is a contraindication to LASIK; however, if attempted, topical and/or systemic antiviral prophylactic treatment

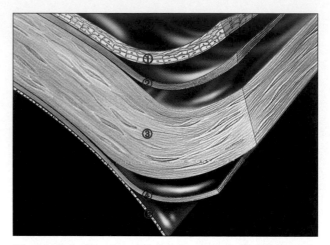

Figure 2-1. Structure of the cornea: 1. Epithelium. 2. Bowman's layer. 3. Stroma. 4. Descemet's membrane. 5. Endothelium.

should be used with the therapy, continuing into the postoperative period. These patients should have surgery on one eye at a time, with a reasonable period between procedures to monitor for recurrence. LASIK is absolutely contraindicated in patients with reduced corneal sensitivity due to herpetic keratitis. Intraocular pressure should be measured to rule out undiagnosed glaucoma. We will discuss how postoperative IOP is often lower than preoperative measurements in Chapter 9 .

LACRIMAL FUNCTION TEST

There are a number of tests used to evaluate lacrimal function.

Evaluation of the Tear Lake

Normally, tears pool at the posterior edge of the superior and inferior eyelids. The reflective surface of the inferior tear lake can be clearly seen with the slit lamp. This tear lake is in simultaneous contact with the eyelid and bulbar conjunctiva. The tear lake should be evaluated early in the slit lamp exam when its normal appearance can be observed. This observation should be made prior to any manipulation of the eyelids, which can express the meibomian glands, and with the slit lamp illumination low to prevent photophobia-induced tearing.

Interpretation

Qualitative: the tear lake may present with dappled superficial reflections due to excess lipids. This is often observed with blepharitis or excess meibomian secretions. There may be debris from make-up, mucous due to bacterial conjunctivitis, or globules of fat from ophthalmic ointments.

Table 2-4

TEAR LAKE EVALUATION

Instrument: Slit lamp
Technique:
- Position the patient using 10x or 16x magnification.
- The light beam of the slit lamp must be in the narrow slit position.
- The beam should be at a temporal angle of 60°.
- The illumination level should be set on low.
- The width of the slit should be 1.0 to 2.0 mm, the height of the slit maximized.
- The slit beam is focused on the inferior tear lake at the lateral canthus.
- The tear lake is examined by moving the slit beam nasally.
- At any given time, the slit beam can be used to optically section the tear lake for determination of depth.

Quantitative: the tear lake should be 1.0 mm wide.

In a patient with dry eye, the size of the tear lake is reduced due to reduction in the aqueous component—mucous filaments or pieces of debris may be observed.

TEAR (Break-Up Time)

The tear lake is colored with sodium fluorescein and observed under the slit lamp to evaluate the integrity of the tear film. An insufficient lipid or mucous layer causes evaporation with the formation of dry spots in the precorneal lachrimal film. These dry spots appear as dark areas or lines visible within an area of uniformly green (because of the fluorescein) tear film. A reduction in the aqueous component will also produce dry spots. The time between a full blink and the appearance of dry spots is know as the tear break-up time (BUT).

Normal tear film will demonstrate a BUT that corresponds with the normal blink rate (every 15 to 30 seconds), with the blink redistributing intact tear film over the cornea. In reality, the examination is difficult to repeat and is not very reliable; but a very short BUT indicates dry eyes. The examination must be performed prior to instilling topical anesthesia, which may reduce the BUT. If the patient finds it difficult to stop blinking, the surgeon should keep the eyelids open with his or her fingers.

Schirmer Test

This test gives a rough estimation of the aqueous volume of the tears (quantity). In association with other examinations and a detailed clinical history, it can provide information on decreased tear production. It also serves to document pseudoepiphora or excess lacrimation caused by irritation due to dry eyes.

Table 2-5

BUT EXAMINATION

Instruments: Slit lamp, sterile fluorescein strips, sterile saline solution
Technique:
- The surgeon wets one end of a sterile fluorescein strip with sterile saline solution. The patient is asked to look upward while gently pulling down the lower eyelid and inserting the fluorescein strip into the inferior fornix.
- The patient is positioned at the slit lamp; the slit beam is positioned obliquely.
- The patient is asked to look straight ahead with the slit positioned at 60°, the cobalt filter placed in the beam path, and magnification at 6x or 10x with maximum illumination. The slit beam should be 3.0 to 4.0 mm wide and at a maximum height.
- The patient is asked to fully blink one time and then keep the eyes open until told to blink again.
- The surgeon starts a mental countdown while observing the precorneal tear film. The count is stopped when one or more dry spots appear.

Interpretation:
There are no decisive values. Some consider 10 to 15 seconds or more to be a normal value; others allow 20 to 30 seconds. However, a value less than 10 seconds is considered to be pathological and may indicate a dry eye.

Initial dark focal areas that persist even after repeated blinking probably represent areas of negative coloration due to raised epithelium, as opposed to a break-up of the lacrimal film.

Sterile paper strips are used, measuring 5.0 mm x 40 mm (Whatman filter paper No. 41).

The strips are positioned in the inferior fornix; the capillary action will wet them with tears. The length of the strip that has been wet by the tears in a given time period is an indirect indicator of tear production.

Strips marked with a millimetric grid and unmarked strips with a millimeter scale are available. There are a number of Schirmer tests.

Schirmer Type I

- Measures reflex lacrimation and basal secretion; anesthesia is not used.
- Test for basic lacrimal secretion (or the Jones test).
- This is a type I test performed following instillation of topical anesthesia. It is useful in patients who find the test strips irritating and patients who wet the entire strip even though having dry eye symptoms.

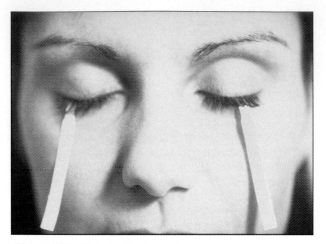

Figure 2-2. Bilateral Schirmer test.

Schirmer Type II

- Measures lacrimal reflex.
- Topical anesthesia is instilled and the nonanesthetized nasal mucosa is irritated using a cotton tip.
- This is done only on rare occasions because the lack of reflex in general does not produce signs or symptoms of dry eye. It is done mainly to evaluate the function of the cranial nerves.

Interpretation of Results

In the Schirmer type I and basal test, normal measurements are between 10 and 30 mm. Measurements between 5.0 and 10 mm are considered borderline and should be rechecked; results below 5.0 mm indicate dry eyes. Some interpret measurements between 10 mm and 15 mm as borderline, with pathological values being below 10 mm.

If the results of the type I test are abnormal, the basal test is unnecessary. If the results of the type I test are normal and the basal test is abnormal, dry eyes or a pseudoepiphora may be suspected. If the type II test produces results that are below 15 mm, anesthesia may have altered the result. If the type II test result is greater than the basal, the reflex is intact.

Diagnostic Dyes

In order to examine the ocular surface, staining with dyes is sometimes necessary. In ophthalmology, there are a number of dying agents available: fluorescein, macromolecular fluorescein (often used in fitting soft contact lenses), rose bengal, methylene blue, gentian violet (pyoctanin), and bromthymol blue.

Rose Bengal

Rose bengal acts differently from fluorescein. It

Table 2-6
SCHIRMER TEST

Technique:
- The sterile paper strip is folded while still in its packaging. The packaging is then opened and the folded end of the strip is placed about one-third of the way into the inferior fornix.
- The room lights are lowered to increase the patient's comfort. The patient's eyes can be kept closed or the patient can blink lightly. The surgeon waits 5 minutes or until the strips are completely wet.
- If they are not completely wet, the surgeon checks the degree of wetness (against a millimeter scale for unmarked strips).

The Basal Test:
This is performed as described above following instillation of topical anesthesia. The surgeon waits 3 to 4 minutes and then inserts the strips.

Schirmer Test Type II:
Three to 4 minutes after anesthetic instillation, the strips are inserted. The surgeon irritates one nostril and then the other with a cotton tip for about 10 to 15 seconds. The strips are left in position for about 2 minutes.

stains the zones that are covered with mucous, not just the deepithelialized areas; it also stains intact necrotic tissue.

Prior to being used, it is advisable to instill fluorescein to highlight any defects in the corneal epithelium. This is important, as rose bengal is extremely irritating if there are corneal abrasions present. This dye is very useful for highlighting keratitis sicca. Staining of the cornea and inferior bulbar conjunctiva is indicative of Sjogren's syndrome.

The test is performed at the slit lamp with the beam at 60°, 3.0 to 4.0 mm wide, and at maximum height. The illumination is moderate and no filters are used. Magnification of 6x or 10x should be used.

There are a number of systemic pathologies associated with surface ocular pathology such as dry eye, for example:

- Sjogren's syndrome
- Scleroderma
- Rheumatoid arthritis
- Lupus erythematosis
- Mixed connective tissue disease
- Dermatomyositis
- Polymyositis
- Chronic immune hepatitis
- Hashimoto's thyroiditis

Some systemic drugs may also cause dry eye, such as:
- Antidepressants
- Neuroleptics

Table 2-7

DIAGNOSTIC DYES I

Fluorescein:
- Yellow-green when in solution
- Yellow-green under blue light
- Yellow under yellow light
- Fluorescent if exposed to blue light
- Concentration 1% to 2%
- Colors liquid on contact

Indications:
- Evaluation of the integrity of the conjunctival-corneal epithelium
- Used in fitting contact lenses and evaluating tear BUT, etc
- Seidel test

Macromolecular fluorescein:
- Similar characteristics to fluorescein
- Molecular weight 710 instead of 376
- Brown in white light

Indications:
- Similar to fluorescein (preferable with soft contact lenses)
- Stains degenerated or dead cells (if rose bengal is not available)

Rose bengal: (a derivative of fluorescein)
- Concentration 1% to 2%
- Stains normal or pathological mucous
- Stains damaged epithelial cells
- Extremely irritating if used in the presence of a corneal abrasion

Indications:
- Evaluation of the moisture in the conjunctival-corneal epithelium
- Sjogren's syndrome
- Contact lens fitting
- Dilution test for Norn's lacrimal pool (along with fluorescein)

Table 2-8

DIAGNOSTIC DYES II

Mercurichrome:
- 1% to 2% aqueous solution
- Very poor staining power (a yellow filter increases visibility)
- Fluorescent under blue light

Indications:
- Stains deepithelialized areas and mucous

Methylene blue:
- Concentration 0.5% and 1%
- Changes on exposure to air (supplied in unit-dose packs)

Indications:
- Identification of the lacrimal sac during surgery
- Stains the corneal nervous plexus
- Stains the lymphatic vessels of the conjunctiva (with a subconjunctival injection)
- Stains degenerated or dead cells
- Stains corneal abrasions

Gentian violet:
- Concentration 1%
- Stains a dark purple-bluish color

Indications:
- Stains degenerated or dead cells
- Stains mucous
- Diagnosing Sjogren's syndrome (if rose bengal is unavailable)

Bromthymol blue:
- 0.2% aqueous solution
- Observations must be made immediately after instillation (position the patient at the slit lamp prior to instillation); observation is made after exactly 5 seconds
- Keep the tear ducts under pressure (punctal occlusion)
- Ask the patient to reduce blinking to a minimum

Indications:
- Determination of the pH of the tear film (eg, in fitting contact lenses)
- Stains degenerated or dead cells
- Stains mucous

- Benzodiazepines
- Antiemetics
- Betablockers
- Antihistamines
- Anti-Parkinson drugs
- Anti-arrhythmics

CORNEAL AESTHESIOMETRY

Corneal aesthesiometry measures sensitivity of the cornea. An empirical measurement can be made by placing a thread of cotton in contact with the cornea, causing blepharospasm. The absence or slowness of the reflex indicates corneal aesthesia or hypoesthesia. There are specific instruments (keratoesthesiometers) that actually quantify corneal anesthesia. The corneal aesthesiometer is an instrument fitted at one end with a thin, extendible nylon filament (Cochet-Bonnet model) or alternately the hair of an animal (Frey's model). The Cochet-Bonnet model is better known and more widely used.

The nylon filament protrudes at varying lengths from the glass container—the shorter the filament, the more rigid it will be, and the greater the pressure it will exert on the cornea.

The center of the cornea is more sensitive than the peripheral areas; the filament should perceived by the central cornea when it exerts a pressure of 10 to 12 mg/mm^2, and by the peripheral cornea when it exerts pressure of 16 to 18 mg/mm^2.

Table 2-9

CAUSES OF CORNEAL HYPOANESTHESIA

Related to the eye:
- Long-term contact lens wear
- Herpetic keratitis
- Ophthalmic herpes zoster
- Dense corneal scars
- Neurotrophic keratitis
- Keratoconus
- Trachoma
- Glaucoma
- Corneal dystrophy
    - Granular
    - Reticular
    - Macular
- Previous ocular surgery:
    - Cataract
    - Keratoplasty
    - Retinal detachment (scleral buckle): months or years after surgery
- Extensive electrocoagulation for glaucoma

The reduction of corneal esthesia in the event of keratoconus, disciform keratitis, interstitial keratitis, and vascularized scars (thermal burns, chemical burns, trachoma, pemphigoid) is usually mild.

Systemic causes:
- Diabetes
- Radiation damage
- Neurological pathologies that involve the trigeminal nerve or Gasserian ganglion
- Surgery of the Gasserian ganglion
- Psoriasis
- Temporal arteritis
- Myasthenia syndrome
- Other

It should be kept in mind that contact lenses will reduce corneal sensitivity. Patients who wear contact lenses should be asked to remove them several hours prior to the test.

Corneal hypoesthesia or anesthesia often results in dry eye syndrome. The hypoesthetic cornea is subject to all the complications associated with dry eyes, both pre- and postoperatively.

CONTACT LENSES AND LASIK

A contact lens is a foreign body placed on the cornea. It is tolerated only because it is supported by the tear film. The tear film must:
- Be stable
- Have an appropriate thickness
- Be osmotically adequate
- Undergo continual exchange
- Have an appropriate protein and electrolyte composition

All these factors allow the contact lens to be biocompatible with the eye.

The contact lens has several negative effects on the eye, and complications can result for a number of reasons, such as:
- Lens material
- Storage and cleaning solutions
- Poor fit
- Overwear
- Anatomical or pathological conditions of the eye

Physiologic changes resulting from contact lens wear include:
1. Alterations of the tear film
    a. Tear flow is increased (normal volume is 1 microliter/minute)
    b. Frequency of blinking (three to seven times/minute)
        - Increases in excellent contact lens wearers
          Blinking may be incomplete or decrease in frequency in patients who do not tolerate lenses well. This causes:
            - Decrease in tear volume due to evaporation
            - Reduced oxygen supply to the cornea
    c. The contact lens induces the formation of a lacrimal meniscus. This meniscus draws fluid from the remaining corneal surface by modifying the forces that regulate tension of the tear film, thus creating thin areas.
    d. Lacrimal osmolarity is increased by contact lens wear as well as increased evaporation of tear film. Normally, the increase in osmolarity secondary to evaporation is compensated for by increased secretion of isotonic fluid from the tear glands, changes in the lipid layer, and increased mucous production, which are also associated with contact lens wear.
2. Changes in the corneal surface include:
    a. Corneal abrasions. Occur frequently, particularly with semirigid contact lenses.
    b. Epithelial fragility. There is the possibility of developing recurrent epithelial erosions. These are due to poor adhesion of the epithelium to the basement membrane. Fragility is often seen in areas of previous corneal abrasion.
    c. Epithelial microcysts. Actually, this is a microbullous pathology of the epithelium and not microcystic, as the name suggests. It is probably caused by premature necrosis of the

epithelial cells when they migrate toward the surface. Important factors in the microbullous formation are:

- Prolonged lack of oxygen supply
- Mechanical irritation from the contact lens
- Chronic suppression of the epithelial metabolism
- Effects of toxic byproducts of metabolism that are kept in contact with the cornea by the lens

The microbubbles can be ruptured in the morning when the patient wakes. This painful occurrence is caused when reduced nocturnal lacrimal secretion allows the eyelids to adhere to the cornea and tear off areas of loose epithelium when first opened in the morning.

d. Corneal infiltrates
e. Neovascularization
f. Reduced sensitivity through adaptation to chronic mechanical stimulus or as the result of reduced oxygen supply to the corneal surface
g. Generalized epithelial edema, which can be observed approximately 1 hour following removal of the contact lens. It appears to be due to an accumulation of fluid between the cells

The low surface tension of precorneal tear film may induce epithelial edema. This factor is important at the beginning when reflex tearing is greater and reduces surface tension. Reduced oxygen flow causes an accumulation of lactate in the stroma, inducing an osmotic gradient across the epithelium.

3. Changes to the deep layers of the cornea include:
a. Stromal edema
b. Stromal thinning
c. Endothelial polymorphism and polymegatism

The corneal endothelium is essential in the prevention of corneal edema. This is a single layer of hexagonal cells of uniform size; these cells do no replicate. Contact lenses can cause several changes to the endothelium, such as:

- Bleb response. Endothelial edema caused by variations in pH is likely to produce recurrent episodes causing permanent damage.
- Polymegatism, which is a variation in endothelial cell size. This allows a more rapid onset of edema compared to normal endothelium and is slower in returning to normal.
- Polymorphism, which is a change in the hexagonal shape of the cell. With polymor-

phism, postsurgical edema easily develops, regardless of the endothelial cell density. It also tends to make the cells more unstable and fragile.

4. Corneal warpage syndrome. A change in the corneal curvature not due to corneal edema. It is a mechanical reshaping of the cornea by the contact lens. It usually appears as corneal flattening

Table 2-10
PREOPERATIVE EXAMINATIONS

Examination of surrounding eye structures
Relationship between the globe, eyelids, and orbit
  Sunken globe
  Narrow palpebral fissure
Blepharitis
  Risk of infection
  Interference with the microkeratome
  Sands of the Sahara syndrome
Examination of the anterior segment
Keratoconus
  Relative contraindication
Corneal neovascularization
  Caution during the lamellar cut
Dry eye
  Caution when manipulating the flap
  Caution during the lamellar cut
  Healing is more difficult
  Postoperative lubricants for a long period of time
Recurrent corneal erosion
  Caution when manipulating the flap
  Caution during the lamellar cut
  Healing is more difficult
  Postoperative lubricants for a long period of time
Corneoconjunctival alterations
  Possible difficulty with the suction ring
  Caution during the lamellar cut
Eye pressure
Examination of lacrimal function
  Test of the lacrimal meniscus
  Break-up time of the tear film
  Schirmer test I
  Basal secretion test (Jones test)
  Schirmer test II
  Rose bengal staining
Corneal aesthesiometry
  Cotton tip
  Cochet-Bonnet aesthesiometer
Evaluation of contact lens wearers
  Following an adequate period of discontinuation
  Pachymetry
  Refraction
  Corneal topography
Evaluation of blinking

and irregular astigmatism. Sometimes there are deep stromal striae and areas of opacity. The corneal curvature returns to normal once the contact lens has been removed, but this may take weeks or even months when rigid or semirigid contact lenses are worn.

5. Changes to ocular structures include:
   a. Giant papillary conjunctivitis
   b. Allergic keratoconjunctivitis
   c. Superior limbal keratoconjunctivitis
       Corneal warpage due to contact lens wear must be taken into account when preparing a patient for LASIK. Contact lenses should be discontinued for a period of weeks and serial refractions performed until stability is demonstrated.

Corneal topography may reveal the following:
- Irregular central astigmatism
- Loss of radial symmetry
- Inversion of the normal topographical shape
- Images similar to keratoconus

Pachymetry measurements reveal:
- Corneal thinning
- Thickening of the cornea due to edema from reduced oxygen supply (edema is not considered to be part of the corneal warpage syndrome).

Abnormal topography and pachymetry can be indications of corneal warpage and edema.

Generally speaking, soft contact lenses should be discontinued 2 weeks prior to preoperative testing and rigid lenses 1 month prior to the exam. This allows for baseline information to be gathered.

Actually, it has been observed that the changes induced by contact lenses often persist for much longer. Clinical studies have shown that the changes created by soft lenses persist for 4 to 10 weeks and rigid lenses for 8 to 16 weeks.

Corneal topography, refraction, and pachymetry should be repeated at intervals until stable. Generally, after patients discontinue soft contact lens wear, a reduction in myopia and increase in corneal thickness will be observed. In wearers of semirigid contact lenses, one usually sees an increase in myopia and increase in the corneal thickness. The surgeon should also remember to:
- Perform a careful examination of the corneal endothelium preoperatively
- Note the amount and location of any corneal neovascularization
- Be especially gentle so as not to damage fragile epithelium during the microkeratome pass and in manipulating the flap. The postoperative condi-

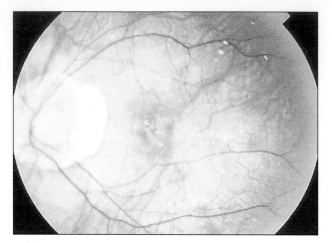

Figure 2-3. Fundus photo of myopic choroidal changes at the posterior pole.

tion of the epithelium should be considered in making management decisions
- Use lubricants for a few weeks in the postoperative period, especially in long-term contact lens wearers

BLINKING

Normal blinking occurs at a frequency of three to seven times per minute. Frequency is influenced by a number of factors; for example, anxiety will increase the frequency, whereas boredom will reduce it. It would appear to be a contradiction, but intense concentration will also reduce the blinking rate. This is clearly seen in people who work at a video monitor for many hours or people who watch a lot of television. In these cases, particularly in dry conditions, it may lead to dry eye symptoms and patients may find it increasingly difficult to tolerate contact lenses.

Complete and regular blinking is essential for preserving the architecture and function of the tear film.

Blinking has a protective role in moistening the cornea and keeping it clean. The blinking movement also assists in drainage of tears and occurs as a protective reflex.

The frequency of blinking is reduced in patients affected by Grave's disease, Parkinson's disease, as well as following alcohol consumption and in contact lens wearers, particularly if the lenses are not well-tolerated. Reduced blinking encourages evaporation of tears and increases dry eye symptoms.

Infrequent or incomplete blinking causes:
- Break up of the structure in the tear film secondary to evaporation
- Corneal hypoxia with contact lens use

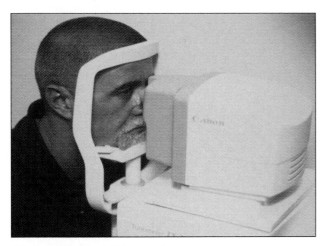

Figure 2-4. Air puff tonometry.

DILATED FUNDUS EXAM

Examination of the posterior segment can reveal pathology that may make the operation difficult. Vitreal syneresis, for example, may make it difficult to achieve an adequate elevation of IOP.

Careful evaluation of the retina allows for the diagnosis of any myopic choriretinopathy that may prevent best-corrected visual acuity from reaching 20/20. Some patients expect to have better vision following LASIK than they had with their glasses or contact lenses and need to be informed that this is not possible and that we are eliminating refractive error and cannot restore vision lost to retinal defect or disease.

One must also thoroughly check the peripheral retina for any lesions, holes, or tears (rhegmatogenic or retinal rupture) that will need treatment prior to LASIK. The appearance of a retinal abnormality should be carefully documented and the patient informed of preoperative presence. The same applies to maculopathies. It may be useful to have preoperative photography and angiography. With alterations to the posterior pole—statistically more frequent in subjects with severe myopia (involving the macular region) compared to those with slight or moderate myopia—it is advisable to perform angiography for a number of reasons: it provides a record of the preoperative condition of the central retina and evaluates to what degree these retinal defects affect the patient's visual potential.

All patients, especially those with degenerative retinal changes associated with myopia, should be informed that the operation only corrects refractive error and will not prevent the progression or development of retinal problems. The importance of a yearly dilated fundus exam should be stressed. This examination may also discover previously undiagnosed retinitis pigmentosa.

Finally, it should be mentioned that the high pressure that the eye is subjected to during the keratectomy may result in occlusion of the central retinal artery. This is a rare occurrence, however the surgeon should be aware of its possibility. The preoperative fundus exam should therefore evaluate and describe the integrity and condition of the chorioretinal blood vessels. This can provide a comparative clinical record if required at a later stage.

TONOMETRY

This measurement is performed to rule out glaucoma or other pathology that may cause abnormal IOP. Abnormal findings should be evaluated and treated prior to preceding with LASIK.

Glaucoma with a decreased visual field should motivate the surgeon to reduce the period of elevated IOP as much as possible during the LASIK procedure. There have been some recent publications that show that IOP is reduced following LASIK for myopia and hyperopia. This may be an artifact.

There is little information available regarding accuracy of IOP measurements following LASIK, but there appears to be little difference between applanation tonometry and the noncontact version.

If a very low IOP is observed, this should alert the surgeon that there may be problems achieving suitable IOP for the operation (65 mm Hg).

EVALUATION OF PUPIL SIZE

Pupil size should be evaluated under photopic and mesopic lighting conditions. Following refractive surgery, visual quality can be significantly affected by the size of the pupil. An ablation zone that is smaller than the pupil diameter will create glare and reduce contrast sensitivity.

Problems with night vision are often due to spherical aberrations created when the pupil diameter is larger than the effective optic zone (this is a prismatic effect due to the aspheric shape of the cornea and cannot be corrected). Normally, this occurs when the pupil is relatively large (ie, in low-light conditions). One way of avoiding this problem is to enlarge the optic zone. This carries with it the risk of central island formation if a broadbeam laser is used; moreover, the more the ablation zone is enlarged, the greater the amount of tissue removed. Leaving inadequate residual stromal tissue increases the risk of corneal ectasia.

The best solution may be to use a multizone technique. This allows for a larger effective optic zone and reduces the amount of tissue removed. Flying spot lasers can modulate the ablation very gradually and avoid the abrupt transition from the ablated to nonablated zones, solving this problem very nicely.

The multizone techniques, or the techniques that allow creation of transition zones, blend the area between the untreated and treated cornea. As a result, phenomena such as halos, glare, and monocular diplopia are less intense and less frequent as compared to single-zone ablations.

These disturbances tend to be more serious when a greater refractive error is corrected because the variation induced between ablated and unablated areas proportionately increases. In a myopic patient, a residual refractive error will further aggravate the situation.

In general, younger patients have larger pupils, therefore some surgeons tend to correct these myopes later in life, waiting until the patient is at least 25 years old. However, in reality, pupil constriction due to age occurs very slowly, even taking decades, so waiting until the patient is 25 years old makes little sense.

Patients with large pupils (as a general rule greater than 5.0 mm under scotopic light) and particularly patients treated with optic zones considerably smaller than the pupil diameter under scotopic light (at least 1 mm smaller) should be warned that there is a possibility of glare, halos, or difficulty with night driving following LASIK. A pupillometer can be used to measure pupil size. The problems with pupillometry are linked to the fact that the pupil must be regular and static. It is not always easy to distinguish the pupil from the iris stroma, and measurements can be influenced by the refractive indices of the anterior segment of the eye.

There are several measuring methods:
- Direct comparison: a strip with holes of increasing size is placed in front of the pupil until one of the holes corresponds to the pupil (a Morton's pupillometer). A tangential or transparency comparison can also be performed (Schloesser's pupillometer).
- Projection: an image of the pupil is projected onto a graduated grid (Magnani's pupillometer) under normal lighting conditions.
- Infrared: involves an infrared photograph taken in the dark. A true scotopic pupil diameter is possible to obtain, as the pupil does not constrict when exposed to light in the infrared spectrum.
- Topography: the topographical examination also measures pupil diameter; however, the light intensity required for this test produces results that cannot be compared to conditions in the real world.
- Light amplification pupillometer (Colvard's

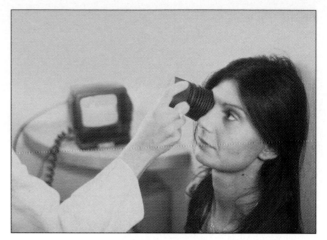

Figure 2-5. Pupillometry with the Buratto pupillometer (note: the photo was taken in daylight for clarity but the test is actually done in the dark).

pupillometer): this pupillometer allows an evaluation of the pupil under low light intensity. The instrument can therefore reproduce conditions similar to those of night driving. This simulation is not possible with all methods. For example, the direct comparison method cannot be performed if the light intensity in the examination room is not adequate enough to see the pupil.

Colvard's pupillometer works easily. Low levels of light enter the instrument, stimulating a photocathode, which excites the electrons. The electrons hit a phosphorescent screen, resulting in intensification of the image. The instrument is used much like a direct ophthalmoscope: a lens system inside the instrument brings the anterior segment into focus. A graduated grid is projected onto the image by the instrument and allows the pupil diameter to be measured.

In initial studies performed with this new type of pupillometer, the measured diameters have been between 1.0 and 3.0 mm greater than those measured with other pupillometers that cannot be used under dim lighting conditions.

This problem is complicated further by Lee Nordan and Jack Singer, who suggested that the functional optic zone decreases with an increase in the degree of refractive correction. The aspheric corneal surface created by the surgical procedure reduces the diameter of the functional optic zone because of a lack of focalization of light. Given that the transition zone between the treated and untreated cornea is steeper with the greater the refractive correction, the quantity of unfocused light increases and the functional optic zone is reduced. It is thus possible that there is a relationship between the amount of correction and the optimal pupil diameter. In effect, the real diameter of the ablation is much smaller than the maximum ablation zone. This means that even if the maximum ablation diameter is 6.5 mm in the transition zone, 80% of our treatment is found within a diameter of 4.5 mm.

If we examine postoperative topography, we see a much smaller ablation area than we expected.

Finally, it is important to consider a concept by Peyman, et al in reference to the entrance pupil (ie, the projection of the pupil on the cornea). Ideally, this is an area that should be totally covered by the refractive ablation in order to prevent any problems with quality of vision. The projection of the pupil onto the cornea (or the entrance pupil) is always larger than the actual pupil size.

This has greater significance in eyes with a deep anterior chamber. The large distance between the iris and anterior corneal surface makes the entrance pupil quite large in severe myopes.

KERATOMETRY

Keratometry is necessary but more useful when compared to and validated by computerized corneal topography. However, keratometric measurements alone provide us with important information regarding the shape of the cornea.

If the keratometric value indicates a flat cornea (less than 41 D), there is a high risk for a free cap; the surgeon can then attempt to reduce this risk as much as possible while being prepared to deal with a free cap if it occurs. A flat cornea protrudes less through the suction ring than a curved cornea. As a result, the portion of cornea that is presented to the microkeratome blade is small and the corneal flap is more likely to be completely severed before the microkeratome stops.

An excessively steep cornea (greater than 47 D) can result in a buttonhole flap. However, the mechanism is not clear. The following suggestion has been made: the progression of the plate pushes on the central apex of the steep cornea, creating a small dip. When the blade reaches the apex of the cornea, it cuts around this dip and perforates the flap centrally. (This theory is disputed by the fact that there are no superior or inferior perforations in cases of keratoconus).

Keratometry can also estimate mild irregular astigmatism in the visual axis. Finally, a discrepancy between the keratometric values and the subjective refractive values may indicate lenticular astigmatism of which the patient should be made aware.

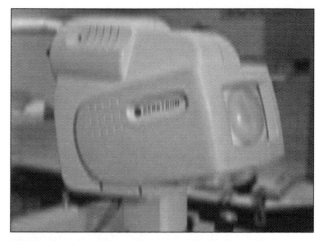

Figure 2-6. Corneal topography: the Optikon Keratron.

COMPUTERIZED CORNEAL TOPOGRAPHY

This test presents a precise and detailed mapping of the corneal surface. The information provided is useful both diagnostically and in management of the postoperative cornea. The instrument provides the surgeon with indepth information on the entire corneal surface and allows study of the more significant parameters, such as keratometric measurements, the dioptric power, and allows comparison between the preoperative and postoperative cornea.

The shape of the anterior surface of the cornea is very important because it determines the quality of the retinal image.

Videokeratography was developed specifically to evaluate the cornea topographically. In comparison to keratometry, videokeratography can provide accurate keratometric readings of the paracentral cornea. It provides information on the peripheral cornea and gives indices that measure irregular astigmatism and correlate to potential visual acuity.

This test is useful not only for planning surgery, but is indispensable for identifying preoperative pathologies that may otherwise pass unnoticed, such as subclinical keratoconus. In the pre-operative evaluation of the LASIK patient, this diagnostic tool takes on a fundamental and clinically essential role. The preoperative maps should be obtained prior to any instillation of drops. In contact lens wearers, it is advisable to perform computerized corneal topography (CCT) only after the lenses have been discontinued for at least 15 days (soft lenses) or 30 days (hard or semirigid lenses). In practice, it may take two or three times this long to obtain accurate topographic data. A contact lens that is too tight will flatten the cornea; a contact lens that is too large will reduce the oxygen supply to the cornea and result in an increase in corneal thickness. In contact lens wearers, the corneal map should be repeated several times at appropriate intervals until stability is demonstrated. Two consecutive maps that are similar indicate that the cornea has stabilized. A differential map can be produced by comparing two similar maps to highlight any areas of differences.

One of the latest developments now being used more frequently is LASIK assisted by topography (topography-assisted LASIK), or topolink. This new technique should allow LASIK to be used in patients with abnormal or irregular corneal surfaces.

At present, LASIK and PRK treatments are based on models of symmetrical ablation for refractive correction. It is presumed that the corneal surface and laser beam used are symmetrical.

If an asymmetrical surface is treated with a symmetrical beam, it stands to reason that the same asymmetry will remain on the new surface; in other words, in the deeper layers of the corneal stromal, the same asymmetry originally seen on the surface will be reproduced. As a result, the vision obtained following laser correction will at most be equal to that obtained with spectacle correction.

The treatment does not take into account the individual corneal surface but is based on an "average" or typical structure. If the cornea is irregular, vision obtained using contact lenses is superior to that obtained with spectacles because the irregularities are masked by the tear film that acts as the interface with the contact lens. In practice, a large number of corneas are irregular. By using LASIK and PRK assisted by topography, the individual structure of the specific cornea defined by topography becomes the basis of the ablative laser correction. This is particularly useful in specific situations, such as:
- Irregular astigmatism
- Nonorthogonal astigmatism
- Asymmetric astigmatism
- Irregular corneal surfaces resulting from previous refractive surgery
- Irregular corneal surfaces due to trauma, etc

There are some hardware and software requirements for topography assisted LASIK.
- A flying spot excimer laser system.
- A system that can perform off-axis scanning (ie, the laser pulse can be positioned at every corneal area in any order).

- It is important that the laser provides excellent correlation between the laser frequency and the diameter of the spot. The smaller the spot, the higher the frequency of the laser beam so that the treatment will be completed within a reasonable period of time.
- The laser cavity must be reliable and extremely stable (like the ceramic laser head) and provide a homogeneous energy flow during the entire laser treatment. This is extremely important because the number of laser pulses required for these treatments is higher than a standard treatment for myopia.
- An active eye-tracking system. The laser impulse must be exactly positioned to correct the corneal irregularities, otherwise it will be very difficult to perform topolink treatments.
- Feedback scanner control. This checks the correct position of the scanning mirror prior to the activation of the laser impulse.

Topography requirements: the measurements of curvature and smoothing algorithms must be extremely precise; they must be able to measure the corneal curvature between a minimum of 30 D and a maximum of 60 D to span all the typical dioptric powers seen on irregular corneal surfaces. The power of the corneal curvature is given in diopters; this measurement must be converted into height or elevation. Only in this way can it be used to calculate the exact profile of the ablation. The surgeon must have measurements of height and of spherical and astigmatic refraction; at this point, the topography-assisted laser treatment is determined by defining the desired postoperative keratometric power. The postoperative topography is simulated and the laser ablation is calculated.

Topography-assisted laser ablations can be calculated by either using the desired postoperative keratometric power or by making manual adjustments. Additionally, these options can be combined to produce an optimal treatment for each specific patient. As a result, the surgeon is in a position to plan the postoperative corneal profile.

With this new technique, a truly personalized treatment will become reality. This treatment not only corrects the refractive error but can also improve the patient's visual acuity given that irregularities in the cornea can be eliminated and the surgeon can produce a smooth, regular corneal surface.

At the time of this writing, laser ablations directed by real-time topography are not possible because topography requires a reflective corneal surface. There is the possibility of alternative topography for use in LASIK. It is called the Orbscan. It is a slit scan corneal topography/pachymetry system, produced by ORBTEK, Inc (Salt Lake City, Utah, USA).

In normal topography, concentric rings are projected onto the tear film; 256 points on 25 to 30 rings are used to produce the topographic map. A reflected image and shape of the corneal surface are obtained by calculating the amount of distortion from the "normal" model.

With the Orbscan, a series of luminous cleavers are projected—20 from left to right and 20 from right to left. An image is acquired for every projection, and edge detection is used to obtain the curvature of the anterior and posterior curvature of the corneal surface. This system calculates the best spherical form (ie, a sphere that contains the most corneal surface). The dots in this sphere are green. Those below it are blue through purple, and those above it are yellow through red.

This is an important test because it also examines the posterior surface of the cornea. As a result, rapid diagnosis of corneal ectasia is possible. Pachymetry values can also be obtained. Another important feature is that in order to acquire data, the system does not depend on a reflective surface; therefore, this test can be performed immediately after the ablation.

REFRACTION/VISUAL ACUITY

It is useful to have a measurement of the uncorrected visual acuity at distance, and particularly in older myopic patients, uncorrected near vision. Myopic patients, who are 45 to 50 years of age need to understand the implications of opting for full-distance correction with LASIK. The presbyopic myope is often able to read well without correction and needs to understand how losing this will affect his or her lifestyle. The patient that comprehends this and knows that reading glasses will be necessary following surgery will not be unpleasantly surprised.

Uncorrected visual acuity is always useful for evaluating the efficacy and predictability of the procedure.

Best-corrected visual acuity (BCVA) is determined by both subjective and cycloplegic refraction. BCVA is the benchmark that serves to evaluate the safety of the procedure. If the refractive procedure improves uncorrected visual acuity but best-corrected visual acuity actually decreases, the surgery has caused an important aspect of the patient's vision to become worse. If this reduction in BCVA increases with higher levels of correction, the surgical procedure cannot be considered safe in those ranges and should not be used clinically. The US Food and Drug Administration (FDA) evaluates this when approving a refractive procedure. Clinically, the success of a refractive procedure is judged by this as well

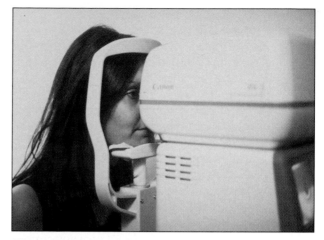

Figure 2-7. Autorefractometry.

as whether the refractive error is totally or partially corrected, allowing the patient to eliminate or reduce his or her dependence on spectacles or contact lenses.

The greater the precision of the correction (100% correction), the greater the predictability of the operation. With predictability, the operation achieves validity and patient satisfaction.

The most important factor is safety of the procedure. Independent of the refractive result, it is essential that BCVA is maintained at its preoperative level.

An improvement is frequently seen in patients with severe myopia. The visual acuity may improve because the minification effect of strong myopic lenses is reduced following surgery; however, this type of improvement is not considered a "real" increase in BCVA.

The important thing is that there is no reduction of BCVA, or if there is a reduction, it is minimal. The FDA closely scrutinizes the amount of lost lines of BCVA in evaluating a refractive procedure.

Patients who have less than perfect preoperative BCVA may encounter serious problems if they lose a line (eg, not being able to obtain a driver's license).

Subjective refraction should be performed at a 12-mm vertex distance. This must be considered, as vertex distance becomes increasingly important as the amount of myopia increases. Laser software calculates the corneal plane refractive ablation that it will deliver based on the vertex distance entered during treatment programming.

A cycloplegic refraction must also be performed to rule out error secondary to accommodation. In some cases, severe myopic ametropia associated with alterations of the posterior pole (myopic staphyloma) makes retinoscopy difficult. Cycloplegia is induced by instilling one drop of cyclopentolate three times (at 10-minute intervals). A cycloplegic refraction is performed 30 minutes after the last drop is instilled.

Alternately, 1% tropicamide can be instilled at least three times (again, at 10-minute intervals) and refraction performed 15 minutes after the last dose. If the cycloplegic refractive error is less than the manifest, it is probably due to accommodation and indicates that the manifest refraction overcorrected the patient. When this occurs, the patient should be re-refracted using a fogging technique. If this confirms the cycloplegic refraction, it indicates the difference was due to accommodation and that the degree of myopia to be corrected should be based on the less minus refraction. If the fogging technique does not confirm the cycloplegic result, one should consider the age of the patient and decide on a compromise of the two refractions, generally choosing less minus. It is always better to undercorrect than overcorrect. Enhancement of undercorrection is easier than that of overcorrection.

In order to avoid error in refraction, we recommend a contact lens over-refraction for myopes greater than 10 D. The refraction should be performed over a high-power disposable contact lens that also refers the refraction to the corneal plane.

For accurate surgery, the best refraction allows calculation at the corneal plane, which is where the refractive ablation will occur. This is also valid for evaluating high hyperopia (> 4.0 D) and high astigmatism.

Almost all excimer lasers require the refraction be entered at the spectacle plane and the vertex distance entered. However, most allow entry with a zero VD (corneal plane). If 20/20 corrected vision is not possible, it may indicate other problems: early keratoconus, irregular astigmatism, or corneal warpage syndrome (from contact lenses).

The refraction must be stable for at least 2 years—some feel 18 months. This is important, as an eye that has progressive refractive changes should not be considered for surgery. In the case of myopia, progression after surgery could totally or partially eliminate the effects of the surgery; with hyperopia, improvement would simulate overcorrection.

BIOMETRY

Biometry is used to obtain the axial length of the eye and help define stability. It is not always easy to obtain accurate biometry because of the posterior pole in moderate to severe myopes. Axial length is a purely indicative value that should be considered as confirmatory to other measurements of refractive error.

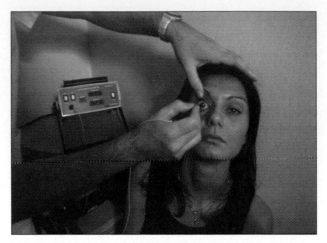

Figure 2-8. Ultrasound pachymetry.

Biometry may prove to be important postoperatively in monitoring the progression of myopia.

If there is regression postoperatively, there are two possibilities:
1. The ablative effect was not permanent but has regressed.
2. The myopia has progressed, indicating that it had not completely stabilized prior to surgery.

Biometry can define whether the cornea has changed or whether the axial length has increased.

PACHYMETRY

This measurement is essential any time a lamellar corneal cut is planned. Types of pachymetry include:
- Optical: independent of or part of the endothelial cell count (Haag Streit optical pachymetry is mounted on the slit lamp)
- Ultrasound
- With a scanning laser

The most common method of pachymetry is ultrasound, but there has been renewed interest in the optical method. This is combined with an endothelial cell count. It is inexpensive and has the advantage of being extremely comfortable for the patient. The instrument is noncontact, thus anesthetic is not required (anesthetic may increase corneal thickness) and the test can be performed immediately postoperatively.

Ultrasonic pachymeters provide highly repeatable results with minimal variations between observers. However, different measurements occur between different models of pachymeters and from central to peripheral measurements (a difference of up to 50 microns centrally and paracentrally, and up to 150 microns at the periphery). It is an important test because preoperative

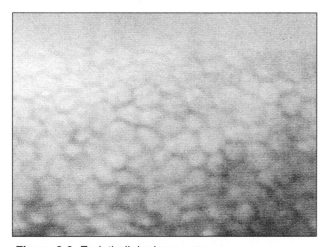

Figure 2-9. Endothelial microscopy.

corneal thickness affects the ability to perform the refractive procedure, especially if the preoperative cornea is excessively thin.

It is even more important in high refractive errors requiring deeper ablations. With LASIK, a few cardinal rules must be followed in planning the surgery. They all refer to the maximum amount of stromal tissue that can safely be removed. The greatest risk is there may be too little residual tissue after surgery, which carries the risk of corneal ectasia.

One rule suggests leaving at least 200 to 250 microns of residual stroma; the final total corneal thickness will be at least 360 to 410 microns (assuming the flap to have a thickness of 160 microns). Another suggestion is that the corneal flap and ablation depth together total at most 50% of the total corneal thickness. It is advisable to measure the central and paracentral corneal thickness at 3.0 mm, 5.0 mm, and 7.0 mm from the center of the cornea. Normally, the surgeon should use the thinnest of the four to eight measurements.

Some surgeons prefer to do pachymetry during surgery just before the suction ring is applied. Care should be taken in disinfection of the pachymetry probe if this method is used. Some surgeons have noticed a significant difference between the preoperative measurements and the actual measurements obtained intraoperatively, suggesting that the depth plate used in surgery should be selected on the basis of its actual cutting depth as demonstrated by intraoperative pachymetry.

If there is any opacity or other alteration of the cornea, optical pachymetry is recommended, as it will give further indication of the thickness of the central, paracentral, and peripheral corneal regions. This measurement is essential in patients with keratoconus, as it gives an evaluation of the corneal thickness if the surgeon elects to operate. Recently, papers have been pub-

lished that address the issue of performing LASIK on eyes with keratoconus: LASIK appears to improve vision and does not interfere with penetrating keratoplasty if required in the future. The tissue reaction is similar to the reaction of a normal cornea. LASIK does not seem to stimulate the progression of keratoconus. Obtaining a good cut and choosing the ablation that should be used with keratoconus still remains a problem.

Some factors may influence pachymetry, making the result totally unpredictable, including:
- Chronic contact lens wearers have an apparently reduced corneal thickness.
- The pachymetry of an excessively wet cornea may be artificially thick, while that of a dry cornea due to prolonged exposure to air or the light of the operating microscope may be artificially thin.
- Topical anesthesia tends to increase the thickness of corneal tissue because of edema formation.
- Similarly, there is an increase in the thickness of the cornea because of corneal markings.

Postoperatively, pachymetry may be important for evaluating whether there is sufficient residual thickness to avoid corneal ectasia. It is also important to determine whether further surgery is possible (for undercorrection or regression) using LASIK.

SPECULAR MICROSCOPY

Presently, there have been no reports in literature of any alterations to the endothelium or cell loss as a result of LASIK. Specular microscopy evaluates the endothelium both qualitatively and quantitatively. Specular microscopy allows both cell density (number of cells per mm^2) as well as shape of the cells (they should be hexagonal) to be examined. Most surgeons report no difference between preoperative and postoperative counts after 6 months. Others have actually seen improvement. In chronic contact lens wearers, the contact lenses disturb the endothelium. Once these are no longer worn following LASIK, the endothelium is restored to its natural condition. Pallikaris, et al reported an 8% loss in endothelial cell count over 12 months. This figure probably increases in proportion to the amount of correction. According to Pallikaris, loss of endothelial cells is inevitable, considering the shockwave from laser ablation and corneal manipulation. There are a number of other factors that may create endothelial changes:
- An increase in temperature
- Postoperative inflammatory reaction
- Flipping over the flap
- Topical drug therapy

Normally, there is a reduction in cell count in the central area of the cornea with an increase in the diameter of the cells peripherally. An endothelial cell count is essential in eyes following penetrating keratoplasty and in eyes with endothelial pathology, such as Fuch's dystrophy or endothelial trauma. This examination allows diagnosis of guttata and other endothelial pathologies.

DETERMINING THE DOMINANT EYE

When a patient is not having bilateral simultaneous surgery, the nondominant eye should always be treated first. The surgeon may avoid problems associated with anisometropia between surgery on the first and second eye.

The patient is asked which is his or her "camera," or "shooting" eye. This will normally be the dominant eye. There is a more accurate technique for identifying the dominant eye: the patient is asked to fixate on an object a few meters away; he or she is asked to place a finger in front of his or her nose at arm's length as a reference point; the patient is then asked to close one eye and then the other. On closing one eye, the object will not move from the position perceived in binocular vision (this is the dominant eye). The nondominant eye normally is the more ametropic eye or the eye with poorer corrected visual acuity. This is, however, not always the case, so it is sometimes more logical to correct the dominant eye first if it has the higher refractive error with poorer corrected or uncorrected visual acuity.

There are other reasons for operating on the dominant eye first:

- This eye is normally less tolerant of contact lenses than the nondominant eye.
- Surgery on the fellow (nondominant) eye is expected to be delayed for a long time.

ORTHOPTIC EXAMINATION

Particularly in patients with anisometropia or severe ametropia, this examination is useful for evaluating ocular motility and binocular vision. The examination evaluates BSV (binocular single vision), whether there is phoria (well-compensated or not). If there is tropia, orthopic examination also evaluates whether there is stereopsis, suppression, or muscle weakness. The purpose is the evaluation of potential post-surgical diplopia. A phoria can be well-compensated only through optical correction and therefore decompensates when surgery eliminates the need for correction. If there is any doubt about BSV, particularly in severe anisometropes who

Table 2-11

PATIENT SELECTION FOR LASIK

Indications
- Patient must be at least 18 years of age (with rare exceptions)
- Refraction must be stable for at least 18 months, evaluated in cycloplegia (retinoscopy or refraction after having applied one drop of 1% cyclopentolate eyedrops every 10 minutes for three applications, the final application at least 30 minutes prior to refraction)
- Myopia: range of spherical equivalent between -1 and -14 D (many surgeons restrict the range of LASIK to 12 D but others extend it to 16 to 18 D; some will implant a refractive IOL when myopia exceeds 10 D and others will combine LASIK with the implantation of an IOL in a phakic eye for higher myopia)
- Hyperopia from mild to moderate: +2 to +6 D
- Astigmatism from mild to severe: 2 to 7 D
- Central corneal thickness in excess of 500 to 550 microns for mild and moderate myopia (less than 10 D) and above 550 microns for severe myopia (above 10 D)
- Corneas that are not excessively flat (mean keratometric value in excess of 39.24 D = 8.6 mm)
- Corneas that are not excessively steep (mean keratometric value in excess of 47.0 D = 7.81 mm)

Patients not suitable for PRK
- Tend to form keloids
- Drug intolerance
- Poor compliance to treatment regimens
- Desire rapid visual recovery
- Steroid responders

have never been corrected or who have not been corrected for some time, a trial of contact lens wear is advised. The surgeon should wait 1 to 2 weeks following use of the lens, and then the orthoptic examination is repeated.

The orthoptic examination should include the following:

- Cover/uncover test
- Suppression test (biprism)
- Worth four-dot test
- Lang's test
- Hess-Lancaster test

CONTRAST SENSITIVITY

Over the years, significant improvements have occurred in diagnosis and treatment of refractive errors. Surgeons acknowledge that Snellen visual acuity alone is not sufficient. Contrast sensitivity testing is more accurate in measuring true quality of vision. It consists of the measurement of visual acuity with different degrees of contrast (low, moderate, and high). Frequently following an apparently successful LASIK procedure producing excellent uncorrected visual acuity, the patient may still complain of problems associated with low lighting (the classical example is night driving). Halos, glare, and visual disturbances at night may depend on negative clearance. This is caused by physiologic pupillary dilation that is larger than the optic zone obtained with ablation. Here, a spherical aberration occurs that may reduce contrast sensitivity. To avoid this aberration, positive clearance must be obtained (the size of the pupil must be equal to or smaller than the optic zone). In order to measure clearance, the pupil diameter must be measured under scotopic light conditions, as discussed in the chapter on pupil measurement. Pupil measurement with the topography unit is inadequate because of the luminance of the placido disk.

A patient with excessively large pupils under scotopic light should be warned of the risks of difficulty when night driving or should be advised about other types of surgery. Alternately, the surgeon may be able to enlarge the ablation zone. However, even with positive clearance, the patient may still complain of night glare.

Contrast Sensitivity Testing

Contrast sensitivity was developed in the 1950s; it was adopted in the 1980s in clinical practice to evaluate visual function in the presence of cataract. The surgeon looks for the minimum level of contrast that the patient is able to perceive. This is the threshold value and varies as a function of spatial frequency.

For this test, the patient looks at a screen with a striped pattern; the degree of contrast is reduced to the point that the patient can no longer distinguish the striped pattern; this is considered to be the threshold of the patient's contrast sensitivity. Patterns with different spatial frequencies are used for this test in order to examine different aspects of vision. In this test, four to five different spatial frequencies may be used.

The instruments used for this test may include plastic test patterns or computerized systems displayed on a monitor. The paper/plastic test patterns have symbols shown in varying shades of gray on a background, which is evenly illuminated. These test patterns must be protected from dust and deterioration from sunlight, as this can alter the background and value of the contrast. With the computerized display, calibration systems must be used regularly to check that contrast remains standardized. In order to evaluate contrast sensitivity, the examination must be performed under conditions that will not affect the pupil diameter. The examination should be performed under dim lighting conditions. The surgeon

should also consider that the evaluation of the pupil diameter may be false because of ambient lighting.

The Horizon contrast sensitivity chart (Vector Vision, Dayton, Ohio, USA) appears to maximize the "naturalness" of the pupil. It reduces the illumination necessary for the examination to a minimum so that normal mesopic pupil diameters will be measured. The results are presented as a curve on special graph paper.

The abscissa shows the values of spatial frequency and the ordinate value of the minimal contrast perceived in relation to various spatial frequencies. It is also possible to indicate the inverse value on the ordinate, which is the contrast sensitivity.

Contrast (C) is the percentage difference in brightness between different points of stimulation; sensitivity to contrast (S) is the inverse of C (1/C). In order to facilitate comprehension and use the test clinically, it is measured on a logarithmic scale similar to the visual field. A relationship is based between the mean logarithmic threshold value of the population and the logarithmic threshold result of the tested patient. If the patient's result is equal to the mean value for the population, the value will be 1.0. If better, it will be higher than 1.0; if worse, it will be less than 1.0.

The clinical result may be normal or subnormal. There are four types of alterations:

- Overall reduction in sensitivity
- Reduction in sensitivity at low spatial frequencies
- Reduction in sensitivity at moderate spatial frequencies
- Reduction in sensitivity at high spatial frequencies (eg, macular pathology)

The Role of Contrast Sensitivity Testing

The test should be used in all routine clinical exams, not only for refractive surgery. For example, the fact that a highly myopic patient sees better when wearing contact lenses rather than spectacles—even though the visual acuity is the same—depends partly on distortion and minification of the image induced by spectacles. It is also secondary to the low contrast with spectacles or barely within the lower limits of normal.

The same thing occurs in patients following LASIK. In refractive surgery, this test is not used to determine whether or not to perform refractive surgery. It is used to provide better understanding of various patient visual complaints that are difficult to evaluate. This is one of the reasons why a preoperative baseline is needed. Contrast sensitivity allows the surgeon to distinguish problems of visual function related to the retina from problems associated with optical media. In order to do perform this, a source of glare (a small lightbulb, for example) is placed above the test pattern or monitor screen. With normal media, patients see this light source as concentrated light; if the patient has any media opacities, he or she will perceive a halo, which will reduce contrast sensitivity. The test is done with and without the glare source.

RAY-TRACING ANALYSIS TO TEST VISUAL FUNCTION

This is an objective method for evaluating visual function; it was developed for the videokeratography unit Technomed C-Scan.

This method uses a tracing ray and the pupil diameter to determine the potential corneal visual acuity using the videokeratographic map as a starting point. The tracing ray module of the C-Scan works by giving a graphic representation of the image quality of two points at the object plane. These are projected through the videokeratographic map on the plane of the better image shape. In other words, the two imaged points at the examination plane are represented by two peaks of intensity that must be resolved spatially to discriminate them as separate entities.

Because visual acuity is defined as the ability to separate two isolated points, it is possible to make an objective determination of best visual acuity using the tracing ray of the corneal maps.

The power of resolution of the cornea depends not only on the corneal surface but also on the depth of the anterior chamber and pupil diameter, so information is also required on corneal shape, pupil diameter, and anterior chamber depth.

Distortion of the peak, distance of the peak, and peak separation are three parameters that have been defined to help us understand when these two peaks have separated. Peak separation is the most useful of these parameters. The spatial resolution (ie, visual acuity) is best defined when this value equals 100%.

The potential visual acuity of the cornea can be determined by the tracing ray analysis of two separate spots through the videokeratographic map: the depth of the anterior chamber and pupil entrance on the analysis plane that determines the spatial distance necessary to discriminate these two spots as separate entities.

The tracing ray screen presumes an anterior chamber depth of 3.0 mm (however, this parameter can be modified) and calculates the pupil diameter from the image of the pupil during videokeratography. This pupil, which is measured under the luminance of videokeratography (25.5 cd/m^2), is automatically integrated in the tracing ray analysis with the videokeratographic map that determines the potential corneal visual acuity.

Given that discrimination of two points (visual acuity) is linear (unidimensional), the potential corneal visual acuity is automatically calculated along the flat axis of the corneal astigmatism on the keratographic map. It can also be calculated on the more curved axis. This will give a two-dimensional estimate of the potential corneal visual acuity, which can be better correlated to the two-dimensional characteristics of the videokeratographic map.

Role of Ray-Tracing Analysis as a Test of Visual Function

The smoothness and uniformity of the cornea is essential for good vision. Some refractive patients with excellent final outcome may have vision disturbances with night driving, for example. This is not seen with normal tests of visual function but may be identified by means of this analysis.

DIGITAL RETROILLUMINATION

During LASIK, retroillumination allows the surgeon to study the interface (ie, the surface cut by the microkeratome and ablated stromal surface). Irregularities on these surfaces may create disturbances of visual function.

Retroillumination is obtained by illuminating the fundus and using the light reflected from it toward the "bleached" cornea—naturally if the other refractive structures are transparent.

This examination is very important because it provides a picture of the optic quality of the cornea.

This may be altered by:
- Opacity in the tissues
- Surface irregularities
- Alteration of the refractive index

In LASIK, the latter may be a consequence of nonuniform thickness or interstitial formation between the flap and the stroma. It occurs if the margin of the ablated surface is sharp (ie, with no transition zone because the flap cannot completely mirror the stromal surface).

The most common reason for alterations in visual function is a surface that has been poorly cut by the microkeratome or poorly ablated by the laser, or without a transition zone. Other reasons may include epithelial ingrowth or stromal hypertrophy.

Digital retroillumination is obtained using an instrument produced by Nidek (Birmingham, Ala, USA): the Nidek EAS 1000 system.

During the examination, it may prove useful to test different patient positions in order to obtain the best possible image of the area under examination.

Table 2-12

PREOPERATIVE EXAMINATIONS

Examination of the posterior segment

Vitreal syneresis
    Problems with the suction ring
    Difficulty obtaining adequate pressure for the lamellar cut
Retinopathies (diabetic, myopic, dystrophies, etc)
    Inform the patient
    Problems with suction in severe myopia
    Problems with pressure in severe myopia
Keratometry
    Irregular astigmatism
    Keratoconus
    Flat cornea
    Excessively steep cornea
Computerized corneal topography
    Keratoconus
    Irregular astigmatism
Examination of the refraction/visual acuity
    Subjective
    Cycloplegic
    Autorefraction
Biometry
Examination of pupil size
    Warn the patient in advance about possible problems with night vision
    Discuss other types of surgery
    May contraindicate refractive surgery
Pachymetry
    Following an appropriate period of suspension of contact lenses
Specular endothelial microscopy
    Cell count
    Cell shape

The instrument's light tone can be inverted so that the diffracted light provides a dark image in which there is no diffraction, then the image will be pale. Vinciguerra has created an evaluation scale for the ablated surfaces; this is based on the nonuniformity observed according to the image obtained with retroillumination.

V0 = unobservable nonuniformity
V1 = slight nonuniformity
V2 = severe nonuniformity

Clinical Use

Digital retroillumination can be used preoperatively as well as both early and late postoperatively. It can also be used in PRK.

In LASIK, light diffraction is examined at the interface. As mentioned previously, this is the only means available for studying the interface.

The examination is very useful, for example, when a patient has visual disturbances even though the corneal map and slit lamp measurements are normal.

In this case, retroillumination that can highlight slight or important nonuniform surfaces may provide a feasible explanation for these phenomena. At this point, it is possible to retreat the patient and achieve a smooth interface surface.

This examination can also be used intraoperatively to allow immediate correction of any ablated surface irregularities.

SCHEIMPFLUG CAMERA AND LASIK

The Scheimpflug camera (ESA 1000, Nidek) is an instrument based on Scheimpflug's principle. On the basis of this principle, the surgeon can obtain a clear image of a sloping plane on the condition that the plane of the eyepiece, the object, and the film cut the same point and that the angles are the same.

The instrument and examination procedure were developed during the late 1960s.

Initially (in the late 1970s and early 1980s), they were used to study the crystalline lens and its cataractous evolution. It provides linear densitometry. The difference in darkening the photosensitive film corresponds to variations in the density of the crystalline lens opacity.

In refractive surgery, the Scheimpflug camera functions in a similar manner to computerized videokeratography—it serves to evaluate the extension and uniformity of the ablated corneal zones.

Two types of images are obtained: one in a sagittal section, the other in retroillumination.

By using the software available for the images, in sagittal section it is possible to calculate:

- The radius of posterior and anterior corneal curvature
- The characteristics of any opacity: degree, depth, area, and volume

From the images in retroillumination, it is possible to obtain:

- Alterations of stromal transparency
- Lines of tension or striae
- Uneven refraction

The software can calculate the area affected by treatment. It is possible to display the different images obtained with the various examinations (preoperatively and postoperatively).

BILATERAL OPERATION

Simultaneous or Sequential?

In ocular surgery, surgeons are generally skeptical about operating on both eyes simultaneously because of the risk of serious bilateral complications that may irreparably damage visual function, for example, an uncontrollable postoperative infection.

The situation is not so problematic where LASIK is concerned. Let us take a look at some aspects of a simultaneous operation:

- First, if a complication appears in the first eye, the surgeon must avoid treating the second eye at the same session.
- Postoperative complications, such as over- or undercorrection or a decentered or nonuniform ablation, are detected in the later postoperative period and cannot be considered in the decision of whether or not to operate on the second eye.
- Infection is the most serious problem.

Other risks (eg, dislocation of the flap, striae, etc) are not reported to increase with simultaneous bilateral surgery when compared to sequential surgery. Infection appears to be the only increased risk, as it can be transferred from one eye to the other.

Disruption of the corneal epithelium facilitates the onset of infection, but this is not related to the simultaneous operation; however, infection from a badly sterilized operating field or microkeratome is very likely to affect both eyes. The bilateral infection will be facilitated if the patient does not follow the postoperative antibiotic treatment or routine hygiene norms, such as avoiding swimming during the first 2 weeks.

Blepharitis is also a predisposing factor for bilateral infection. However, post-LASIK infection has rarely been reported in literature, even following simultaneous bilateral surgery.

Surgeons should therefore consider simultaneous operation to be a high-risk procedure in patients with predisposing factors or patients considered to be unreliable with their eyedrops.

Most patients are normally not at risk, as sterilization of the operating field and instruments is rarely an issue. However, many surgeons are still not comfortable with simultaneous bilateral operation.

Patients undergoing simultaneous bilateral operation must be kept under close observation so that any infection may be rapidly identified.

Operating on the second eye days or weeks after the first allows the surgeon to observe whether there have been any intraoperative or postoperative complications,

Table 2-13
CONTRAINDICATIONS TO LASIK

Absolute contraindications

- Keratoconus (observed by topography and pachymetry)
- Ophthalmic herpes zoster
- Active inflammation of the anterior or posterior segments (eg, herpetic keratitis)
- Patients with particularly sunken globes or small palpebral fissures that may make suction ring application and microkeratome progression difficult
- Thin corneas with pathological thickness
  Instrument: pachymetry values below the standard safety values (less than 450 to 500 microns)
  Clinical: ectatic areas visible at the biomicroscope and/or corneal topography (eg, early keratoconus) or areas of abnormal thinning (remains of an ulcer, etc)
- Marked pupil decentration
- Large diameter pupil (greater than 7.0 mm under mesopic light) with high ametropia
- Pregnancy

Relative contraindications to LASIK

- Mild keratoconus
- Endothelial dystrophy (cell count of less than 1500 or 1000)
- Monocular patient
- Anterior basement membrane dystrophy
- Abnormal closure of the eyelids
- Active connective tissue pathology
- Systemic vasculitis
- Thin cornea
- Dry eye syndrome, which can be identified with routine clinical tests (Schirmer I and II, BUT, etc) or incomplete blinking
- Glaucoma with previous filtering surgery
- Patients with diabetic retinopathy who require laser photocoagulation

Situations that require special care when performing LASIK

- Flat corneas: it is easy to have a free cap. A thin or perforated flap may also occur
- Small orbit: it may be difficult to insert the suction ring
- Post-RK: risk of having the incisions open, also epithelial ingrowth
- Post-PKP: the cornea may have an irregular curvature or thickness
- Post-antiglaucomatous filtrating surgery: there is a risk that suction will not be adequate and/or there may be damage to the filtering blebs

whether the treatment was centered correctly, whether the desired refractive has been achieved, etc. However, patients prefer and often demand bilateral surgery, requiring the surgeon to perform bilateral surgery on the

Table 2-14

SIMULTANEOUS BILATERAL SURGERY

Disadvantages
- Bilateral complications
  Infection
  Bilateral overcorrection
  Bilateral undercorrection
- Inability to change the nomogram for the second eye on the basis of the inappropriate refractive result in the first eye (this often has little correlation anyway)
- Impossibility of immediate knowledge of decentered or nonuniform ablation
- Bilateral enhancement treatment necessary (in the event of undercorrection)

Advantages
- Simultaneous bilateral correction of the refractive error
- Visual equilibrium restored more rapidly (absence of postoperative anisometropia)
- Night glare is reduced more rapidly; the patient perceives this disturbance to a lesser degree because he or she is not comparing the result with a nonoperated eye
- BCVA improves more rapidly
- There is a reduction in visual disturbances correlated to
  Night glare
  Ansiometropia
  Aniseikonia
- The patient's anxiety level is reduced as the interval between the two operations has been eliminated
- The double-dose of psychological and emotional trauma linked to the two separate operations is eliminated

Economic and time-saving benefits:
- Only one interruption of the patient's professional life
- Only one interruption of the patient's private life
- Reduction in functional and anatomical healing times
- Fewer postoperative visits are necessary

same day. Simultaneous surgery is desirable to the patient, as the entire surgical process for visual correction can be completed in a single session.

There are a number of advantages to bilateral surgery. First, there is greater visual equilibrium (ie, there is no functional difference between one eye and the other) in terms of refraction, vision quality, and disturbances. Secondly, there is simultaneous bilateral correction of the refractive error with greater all-round visual comfort. There are also functional advantages through a reduction of correlative visual abberations.

The bilateral operation also avoids monocular vision during the interval between the first and second operation; the patient does not have to use monolens spectacles (the patient cannot wear contact lenses because of the upcoming second operation). The patient's anxiety level is also reduced; the anxious wait between one operation and the next, and the double-dose of emotional stress inherent to the operation, are eliminated.

There are economic and time-saving benefits as well. The patient interrupts his or her normal routine, professional or otherwise, on just one occasion.

The number of postoperative visits is reduced. The time required for ocular rehabilitation is also reduced. The bilateral operation also prevents the patient from comparing the quality of his or her vision between the operated and nonoperated eye.

However, there are also disadvantages associated with a bilateral operation. As mentioned, it is not possible to have an immediate check of postoperative complications, such as decentered or a nonuniform ablations. Any residual error in the first eye, such as over- or undercorrection, cannot be calculated for the operation on the fellow eye.

Recently, Gimbel completed a retrospective analysis of a group of patients that had undergone simultaneous bilateral surgery, comparing them with patients operated on sequentially. The results of the study showed no statistically significant differences between the two groups. The results from LASIK performed simultaneously were similar to the results of the sequential operation in terms of refractive and visual outcomes, frequency of enhancement operations, and frequency of complications.

This study has been duplicated with similar results by Waring and coworkers. We agree that bilateral simultaneous surgery is safe, and we routinely perform it using a completely new operating set-up, new sterile microkeratome, blade, drapes, etc for the second eye.

LASIK and Contrast Sensitivity

Jean-Louis Arné, MD

Preoperative and postoperative evaluation of quality of vision is of major importance in the consideration of a refractive surgical procedure. Contrast sensitivity testing is currently considered the most reliable way of evaluation of the quality of vision.

In Perez-Santoja, et al, an initial decrease of contrast sensitivity 1 month after surgery followed by a rapid recovery was reported on 14 operated eyes; Wang, et al reported similar results in 137 eyes. Both studies evaluated subjects using the CVS 1000 E and FACT 101 chart, which are very popular tests and easy to use but have relatively poor sensitivity.

Our study consisted of 50 eyes (29 patients) who underwent LASIK to correct myopia ranging from -5.3 to -13 D. Contrast sensitivity was tested preoperatively with contact lenses, then 1, 3, 6, and 12 months postoperatively using two different tests: CVS 1000 (Vector Vision) and Gradual (Opsia). The Gradual (Opsia) test is commercially available and allows the exploration of contrast sensitivity at three levels of luminance:

- 5 cd/m^2, which corresponds to scotopic conditions
- 85 cd/m^2, which reproduces the condition of normal indoor artificial illumination
- 700 cd/m^2, which corresponds to the luminance of outdoor sunshine

Ten spatial frequencies are explored at each level of luminance, three of which are particularly demonstrative:

3, 12, and 24 cycles per degree. Independent of the testing method of evaluation, we noted a decrease in contrast sensitivity at all spatial frequencies at 1 month postoperatively.

At 3 months, scores using CVS 1000 testing had returned to their preoperative values.

Gradual testing showed that the recovery of normal values occurred only at 12 months after surgery and took a particularly long time under low luminance conditions.

A precise evaluation of contrast sensitivity after refractive surgical procedures requires excellent patient cooperation and understanding during execution.

Each clinic's LASIK informed consent form should inform patients that their recovery to normal visual contrast in conditions of reduced illumination may be extended well into the postoperative period. Return to the preoperative level of contrast evaluation is illustrated in the table below.

REFERENCES

1. Perez Santoja JJ, Sakla HF, Alio JL. Contrast sensitivity after laser in situ keratomileusis. *J Cataract Refract Surg.* 1998; 24(2):183-189.
2. Wang Z, Chen J, Yang B. Comparison of laser in situ keratomileusis and photorefractive keratectomy to correct myopia from -1.25 to -6.00 D. *Journal of Refractive Surgery.* 1997;13(6):528-534.

Table 2A-1

EVOLUTION OF CONTRAST SENSITIVITY (GRADUAL)

Luminance	5 cd/m^2			85 cd/m^2			700 cd/m^2		
Spatial frequency	3.0	12.0	24.0	3.0	12.0	24.0	3.0	12.0	24.0
Preoperative	8.8	4.5	2.2	9.0	5.4	3.6	9.5	6.9	5.4
1 month	7.8	3.5	1.4	7.8	4.8	2.7	8.9	6.3	4.3
3 months	7.8	3.4	1.5	8.0	4.6	2.5	9.0	6.0	4.3
6 months	8.0	3.6	1.7	7.9	4.8	3.0	8.8	6.6	5.3
12 months	8.6	4.1	1.9	8.9	5.4	3.4	9.6	6.9	5.6

Contrast Sensitivity and LASIK

Jack T. Holladay, MD

Standard Snellen visual acuity following LASIK is excellent, with some patients actually achieving 20/10. Although this is certainly not the norm, high contrast visual acuity in good lighting conditions is excellent. Functional vision, however, includes more than high contrast visual acuity. What about a patient's vision in low light levels when the pupil is large or in conditions in which the objects are not high contrast, such as faded newspaper print?

One additional measure of visual function is contrast sensitivity—the sensitivity of a patient's vision to changes in contrast. Two different optotypes are currently available: those that use standard Snellen letters and those that use gradings (sinusoidal and square wave). Old and more recent studies have shown that letters are much more reproducible, sensitive and specific than sinusoidal gradings. Tests that are familiar to the clinician include the Pelli-Robison chart, which keeps the letter size constant while decreasing the contrast on each successive line. Regan charts, which come in varying contrasts (98%, 11%, and 2%) keep the contrast of the letters constant on each chart and decrease the letter size in LogMar steps to conform to the worldwide standards for letter acuity charts.

Recent studies demonstrate that as the pupil increases in size with increasing darkness, there is a corresponding decrease in the contrast sensitivity, particularly at the lower contrast. The mean decrease has been approximately one line of acuity in darkness with contrasts less than 13%. The clinical significance of this decrease is difficult to assess because it depends on the patient's lifestyle and visual needs. To put these values in perspective, however, this decrease is very similar in magnitude to the change many contact lens wearers experience.

The explanation for this contrast sensitivity loss in darkness is due to the increasing size of the pupil and the shape of the cornea following current excimer ablation.

The cornea is changed from a prolate surface (steeper centrally) to an oblate surface (flatter centrally). An oblate surface is worse than a sphere optically because it exhibits more spherical aberration. Spherical aberration simply means the paracentral and peripheral light rays are refracted too strongly, causing them to reduce the contrast of the central rays forming the foveal image. Because the contrast of the retinal image is reduced, contrast sensitivity is reduced. The problem increases with pupil size because more and more paracentral and peripheral rays are allowed onto the retina as the pupil increases.

It is possible to make the shape of the optical zone prolate following LASIK, but approximately 25% more tissue removal is necessary. Laser companies are currently working on changing the ablation profile to obtain a prolate optical zone, which should be available within the next year. The reduction in scotopic contrast sensitivity should be eliminated, or at least reduced, and the patient's visual function should be comparable to preoperative values. In a specific patient with a large correction, relatively thin cornea, and a large pupil, the perfect prolate surface may not be obtainable without breaking the 250-micron remaining posterior stromal thickness. However, by considering the amount of correction, pupil size, corneal thickness, and desired asphericity, an optimal result for each patient may be obtained. For example, a patient with a 600-micron central corneal thickness, 4 D of myopia, and a maximum pupil size of 6.0 mm in darkness can have the perfect prolate shape. In contrast, a patient with a 480-micron thickness, 10 D of myopia, and a 10 mm pupil size in darkness may still require a slight oblate shape. As our knowledge of visual outcomes increases with additional visual performance studies, visual results will continue to improve a procedure that is already very successful.

Preoperative Pupillometry in LASIK

Renato Valeri, MD

Achieving uncorrected 20/20 vision following a LASIK operation is undoubtedly a very important objective; however, the quality of vision under different light intensities is an equally important consideration.

Some patients with an excellent visual result in daylight complain of a dramatic reduction in vision under poor lighting conditions to such a degree that night driving may be compromised because of halos, monocular diplopia, clouding, and glare.

In order to provide a good refractive and visual outcome under all light intensities, it is necessary to perform an ablation with an optic zone proportional to the pupil

Table 2C-1	
PUPIL SIZE BY AGE	
Age	**Pupillometry**
< 25	5.68 mm
26 to 35	5.43 mm
36 to 45	5.18 mm
> 46	4.89 mm

Table 2C-2	
PUPIL SIZE BY REFRACTION	
Ametropia	**Pupillometry**
> -16.00 D	5.45 mm
-10.00 to -16.00 D	5.26 mm
-5.00 to -9.00 D	5.41 mm
0.00 to -4.00 D	5.34 mm
+3.00 to 0.00 D	4.94 mm
+9.00 to +4.00 D	4.68 mm

diameter. As a result, the preoperative measurement of the pupil diameter under scotopic light is very important.

Pupil diameter can be measured by a number of methods:

- The Rosenbaum pupil caliper: this does not provide accurate evaluation; under low levels of environmental light (3.0 lumen) necessary to simulate the conditions of nighttime driving on a suburban street (0.5 to 6.0 lumen), the pupil edge cannot be distinguished, especially if the patient's iris is very dark.
- Some modern autorefractometers: keratometers such as the Canon RK-5 record pupil diameter using an infrared television camera; these are very handy instruments. However, its fixation target stimulates accommodation and it is impossible to standardize the instrument's luminosity, making these measurements less precise and difficult to reproduce.
- Pupillometer with luminous amplification: one designed by Colvard (Oasis) is proving to be a relatively accurate device and is easy to use. The machine has several limitations—it is difficult to focus because of the small image size, the procedure must be performed with a moving eye, and the results cannot be recorded. The absence of an integrated low lighting system necessitates the use of a room with standardized light intensity.
- A better option is to use an instrument with an infrared television camera connected to a monitor, where it is possible to measure the pupil diameter and have a permanent record of the results (a prototype presented by Buratto and produced by Micromed). With this prototype, the designers attempted to standardize the pupil measurement

by another actinic light source to provide a background of 3 lux, inserted inside the fold that isolates the eye from the outside. Results can be printed out, allowing the surgeon to check the measurements and perform sequential measurements as well as having printed documentation.

The important factor to keep in mind with any pupillometry method is standardization of the examination conditions: controlled environmental lighting of 3 lux, examination performed after the patient has been in the room for at least 30 seconds, fellow eye kept open. Despite these precautions, the pupil measurement is not always repeatable because it is affected by the physical/neural conditions of the patient and the physiological spasm of the iris.

In order to analyze the pupillometry variations under various degrees of ametropia, we examined 1500 consecutive patients under standard conditions with no preexisting ocular pathology. Table 2C-1 shows the pupillometry in relation to age: the findings confirm that with increase in age, scotopic dilatation decreases. Table 2C-2 shows the pupillometry in relation to ametropia: from these findings there appears to be no difference between various groups of myopia.

There appears to be a difference between the myopic and hyperopic groups (5.3 mm versus 4.7 mm), but as the mean age of the groups differ (35 years for the myopic group and 41 years for the hyperopic group), it is possible that a proportion of the pupillometry variations between the groups may be due to age difference.

In 10% of our patients, the scotopic pupillometry was greater than or equal to 7.0 mm; "blindly" performing an operation on these patients may therefore be disadvantageous for both the patient and the surgeon.

Preoperative Pachymetry in LASIK

Renato Valeri, MD

All refractive surgery techniques that utilize the excimer laser modify the curvature of the cornea and its refractive power by tissue photoablation.

With the LASIK technique, there are four basic measurements that must be considered and carefully monitored in order to ensure the resistance of the cornea and its stability over time, but which also must allow for excellent quality of vision. These measurements are:

- Flap/cap thickness
- Residual corneal stromal thickness
- Diameter of the ablation (the optic zone)
- Ablation depth

These parameters combined provide a good picture of the corneal thickness, which is mandatory for a good outcome.

Past experience with lamellar surgery demonstrates that in order to preserve corneal integrity and avoid postoperative corneal ectasia, at least 250 microns of residual stromal tissue must remain at the end of the treatment. The majority of surgeons would avoid a refractive ablation in eyes with thin corneas where the residual stromal thickness would be less than 250 microns after the flap has been lifted (the flap usually measures about 160 microns); others suggest that the residual stroma when the 160-micron flap amount of tissue removed by the ablation must not be less than 50% of the initial corneal thickness.

Generally speaking, large optic zones are preferred, as they reduce the incidence of halos, glare, and night-time haze. Because this involves more tissue ablation, the amount increases in proportion to the degree of myopia. It is mandatory to perform precise pachymetry, as even with less than severe myopia this critical 250 micron limit is sometimes approached.

In clinical practice, we use four types of pachymetry:

- Optical
- Orbscan-type optical
- Ultrasonic
- Specular microscope-obtained

However, there are variations in measurements and repeatability between the various methods.

The Orbscan system has the advantage of combining two fundamental measurements (pachymetry and computerized corneal topography) and also offers a pachymetry measurement of the entire cornea. This makes the instrument of great interest to surgeons. Measurements generally exceed the ultrasound pachymetry values by about 20 to 30 microns. The instrument is not always easy to use, particularly in uncooperative patients. The fact that the Orbscan unit is likely to become the reference instrument in topography-linked ablations may encourage greater interest.

Ultrasonic pachymeters are easy to use, provide accurate measurements, and supply highly repeatable results. The only limitation is that the ultrasound waves propagate at different speeds depending on the degree of corneal hydration; variations in hydration, seen for example in contact lens wearers, can result in inaccurate measurements.

Haag Streit-type pachymeters are not very accurate and require a learning curve. This means that the measurements are not very repeatable. While they are relatively inexpensive, they should not be the technique of choice for the refractive surgeon. They should be considered only for back-up or comparison.

Measurements using specular microscopes are largely dependent on the model used. Our experience is based on three different models. The values obtained were 10 to 20 microns lower compared to values obtained with ultrasound pachymetry. As the specular microscope is not required for LASIK and is very expensive, it is rarely used. Moreover, with this instrument, it is difficult to take measurements outside the central or paracentral cornea.

Normally, the patient is asked to discontinue wearing contact lenses at least 7 days prior to the pachymetry measurement for refractive surgery. In the past, when we took measurements in contact lens patients without keratoconus, we observed significant variations in the corneal thickness and the topographic appearance of the eye even 2 to 4 months following discontinuation of the contact lenses.

It is still not clear whether ultrasound pachymetry is affected by the interface following LASIK. This is suggested by postoperative evaluation of corneal thickness (1-month postoperatively), which is often greater than expected despite the fact that the desired refractive correction was obtained.

Total awareness of and analysis of the pre-, intra-, and postoperative pachymetry values will make a further contribution to the full understanding and predictability of results obtained from all LASIK techniques.

Why Unilateral Surgery?

Francesco Carones, MD

Although simultaneous bilateral surgery is very attractive to both the surgeon and patient, I will outline my reasons for performing and recommending unilateral surgery. This approach seems safer to me, and if we reduce the time interval for treatment between the two eyes to a few hours, it may also be very satisfactory and acceptable for the patient.

The option of performing simultaneous bilateral surgery is very attractive to the patient as well to the surgeon, because it enhances the "wow" effect of LASIK surgery. The patient's request to restore binocular vision in the fastest way without many office visits is certainly one of the major reasons for considering bilateral surgery. However, like all other refractive surgical procedures, LASIK must also respect one of the fundamental criterion of this surgery: safety. In fact, as we focus on the patient's need to restore vision in the fastest and most comfortable way, we must also take into account the need for safety.

I routinely perform and suggest unilateral LASIK for two reasons: first, I consider this approach safer than bilateral simultaneous surgery; second, I believe this is not too troublesome for the patient, especially when we reduce the time interval between the two eyes to a few hours.

Safety is the rationale to this approach and may be summarized as follows. When I approach a surgical procedure, I cannot exclude the possibility of a complication. It is certainly possible to change the surgical program and postpone the second eye treatment when a complication occurs during the treatment of the first eye. But in some cases, it is impossible to detect or foresee a certain complication intraoperatively, and some complications may not only be disturbing to the patient, but also potentially dangerous when the second eye has been treated simultaneously. Among these complications, infectious problems are obviously the most dreadful, but other situations, like Sands of the Sahara (SOS) syndrome, may bring early unsatisfactory results, making the patient consider the surgery unsuccessful. Some of these complications may be transmitted to the second eye (infections) or replicated during the treatment of the second eye. These examples are typical complications that are not detectable while performing surgery but are detectable the day after. Because of this, unilateral surgery seems safer to me.

Let us now consider a second approach. As I mentioned above, most of the patients want and need rapid recovery and restored binocular vision, and certainly LASIK usually provides these features. Regardless of the type of surgery, a postoperative visit is mandatory on the first postoperative day. I believe most surgeons prefer to perform this exam themselves before sending the patient to his or her referring ophthalmologist. Patients are happy to have their eye checked by the surgeon as well. I consider the first postoperative day visit as one of the most important—refraction, uncorrected and best spectacle-corrected visual acuity, and anterior biomicroscopy are all evaluated criteria. At this time, it is possible to assess the success of the procedure and the absence of complications: the epithelium is usually completely healed, the presence of flap folds or interface problems may be detected and managed, and vision is usually satisfactory.

On the first postoperative day, once having assessed the first eye surgery as uneventful, I recommend performing surgery on the fellow eye. Patients usually accept this approach with great enthusiasm, because they have the chance to evaluate the results of the surgery on their first eye; at the same time, they do not have to wait long to have their binocular vision restored. It is my opinion that compared to simultaneous surgery, this approach causes only a 24-hour delay in vision recovery. On the other hand, it gives surgery a higher safety level with less risk of unexpected surprises.

In my practice there are a few exceptions to this approach. In very few cases, I treat both eyes at the same time when a patient strongly opposes waiting for 24 hours and accepts the theoretical additional risks of bilateral surgery, once explained. Apart from those cases presenting with complications, I frequently postpone the second eye treatment when vision recovery in the first eye is slower than usual, like in the correction of hyperopia or hyperopic astigmatism.

Why Bilateral LASIK?

Jeffrey B. Robin, MD

During the last 5 years, refractive surgery has undergone an amazing evolution from the periphery to the mainstream of eye care. There are many reasons for this, primarily because of the transition from incisional to laser refractive procedures, with the intended improvement in accuracy, reduction in side effects, and expansion of indications. As its popularity increased, refractive surgery was no longer reserved mostly for those individuals who had specific vocational or avocational needs, but became a viable first-line option for nearly any individual who required corrective eyewear for distance visual needs.

Although restricted by government regulatory agencies, the growth in popularity of refractive surgery has been most dramatic in the United States. For the first 2 years following US Food and Drug Administration (FDA) premarket approval of the excimer laser for PRK, the American public was inundated with physician, societal, and commercial educational and marketing efforts for this procedure. Interestingly, it is estimated that PRK surgical volumes during this time were no greater than those for RK in the year prior to FDA approval. Only in 1997 (3 years after FDA approval) did laser refractive surgical volumes begin to increase and, since then, the annual increase has been estimated as greater than 100%. A careful inspection of these volume estimates indicates that the number of LASIK procedures performed in the United States began to rise dramatically in 1997 and have continued to increase to the point that LASIK is by far the predominant refractive surgical procedure performed on the American public. It is estimated that nearly 1 million laser refractive procedures will be performed in the United States in 1999 and more than 75% of those procedures will be LASIK.

What are the reasons for LASIK's immense popularity? Certainly, for the majority of potential refractive surgery patients, LASIK offers no tangible benefit in accuracy or final visual acuity over PRK; in fact, some studies have documented slightly better visual functioning in PRK patients. It is also well recognized that the flap presents a potential source of vision-threatening complications for LASIK patients. Therefore, it is likely that the popularity of LASIK is due primarily to convenience for the patient. Uncomplicated LASIK procedures offer the probability of minimal postoperative discomfort and rapid visual recovery. Looking at this issue more closely, one can postulate that the potential discomfort issue is probably not that significant. It has been well documented that the combined use of topical nonsteroidal anti-inflammatory agents and therapeutic soft contact lenses eliminates most acute postoperative discomfort in PRK patients. Thus, one can assume that the speed of visual recovery is likely to be the predominant factor behind the explosion of public interest in laser refractive surgery in the United States.

Rapid visual recovery following LASIK enabled refractive surgeons to offer the possibility of having bilateral surgery at the same session, as opposed to the traditional practice (dictated by the inevitable delayed visual recovery) of unilateral sequential surgery, which was the standard for PRK in most parts of the world. It is likely that the prospect of bilateral same-session LASIK with rapid vision recovery has been a major stimulating factor in the explosive growth of laser refractive surgery in the United States. Several studies (Waring GO, personal communication; Hardten D, personal communication) over the last 3 years have documented that patients prefer bilateral same-session LASIK as opposed to the unilateral sequential approach; and properly applied, the increased risk of bilateral same-session LASIK appears to be more theoretical than factual.

WHY BILATERAL SURGERY?

The major benefits of bilateral same-session LASIK include avoidance of anisometropia and minimal disruption of patients' lives. The inevitability of anisometropia is a significant issue because most patients have sufficiently large refractive errors, making it difficult to tolerate spectacles after unilateral surgery. Other anisometropia-related concerns with unilateral surgery include contact lens intolerance and also the plight of rigid contact lens wearers: rigid contact lens wearers cannot wear their lens in the unoperated eye for fear of possibly inducing curvature changes preoperatively. A significant percentage of patients seeking refractive surgery are contact lens intolerant. Therefore, the prospect of simply putting a patient in a contact lens in their unoperated eye is not always feasible; in these individuals, anisometropia may become a serious functional concern. Furthermore, although difficult to precisely gauge, prospective LASIK patients place great value on being able to have surgery in one session, thus minimizing disruption to their busy professional and personal lives.

WHY NOT BILATERAL SURGERY?

Certainly, no procedure—including LASIK—is risk free. Bilateral same-session surgery, by definition, bears greater potential risks than the unilateral sequential approach. In reality, the operative questions are how much is the risk increased and, in a practical world, whether the benefits of bilateral same-session surgery justify this approach. Opponents of bilateral same-session LASIK cite several reasons for avoiding this. The most prominent of these reasons include:

1. The avoidance of bilateral catastrophic complications.
2. The ability to minimize side effects such as night glare and halos.
3. The ability to modify surgical technique and/or laser settings based on response of the first eye.

Let us address each of these objections.

Potentially catastrophic complications following LASIK include serious flap creation problems (eg, intraocular penetration, distorted flaps, buttonholes), infections, flap viability problems (eg, melting and perforation), and visually significant scarring. The likelihood of serious flap creation problems occurring in both eyes of a LASIK patient is minimal because if these occurred on the first eye, most surgeons would not proceed with surgery on the second eye. The incidence of infection following LASIK is estimated at less than 1 in 5000. Avoiding bilateral same-session surgery at this low risk level would be tantamount to only fitting soft contact lenses in one eye because they are a well-documented risk factor for corneal infection. Postoperative flap viability problems usually occur several days, weeks, or longer following surgery; if one were to use this as a sentinel reason for performing only unilateral surgery, the exact timing of when it would be safe to perform surgery on the second eye would stretch into weeks or months. Visually significant interface scarring following LASIK is extremely rare, although the author has personally observed two cases, both of which responded well to topical corticosteroids with no permanent sequelae. Less dramatic interface haze scenarios, such as those that can occur with noninfectious keratitis (Sands of the Sahara syndrome), can conceivably affect vision, although they usually respond well to rapid diagnosis and aggressive therapy.

Concerns regarding the potential of LASIK causing serious visual symptoms, such as disabling night glare, can be minimized by careful patient selection (avoiding patients with large scotopic pupil diameters and higher degrees of correction) and good operative technique. With the recent introduction of scanning excimer lasers with larger potential beam diameters, as well as tracking mechanisms for maximal centration, it is likely that even in this patient population the risk of serious postoperative visual symptoms will be minimal.

The final objection to bilateral same-session surgery—the ability to modify surgical technique for the second eye based on results of the first—is really an historical hold-over from the era of incisional surgery in which significant under- or overresponses from expected corrections were a common phenomenon. For the majority of PRK or LASIK patients, the incidence of final corrections being within 1 D of target is greater than 90%. One exception is that of high ametropes, in which a greater incidence of undercorrections and overcorrections has been documented.

PERSONAL EXPERIENCE

The author has been performing refractive surgery since 1983 and began performing bilateral same-session incisional refractive surgery in 1992 (the author's wife was his first bilateral RK patient). The convincing factor enabling the offering of bilateral same-session RK was rapid visual recovery. It was clear that, even with the problems associated with RK, patients having bilateral same-session surgery were more enthusiastic and satisfied than those who had unilateral sequential procedures. The author began performing PRK in 1990 and, because of the delayed visual recovery, the vast majority of these procedures have been unilateral sequential. Concerns noted above regarding anisometropia and contact lens intolerance were common factors in the author's PRK experience. The author began performing LASIK in 1994 and was impressed by the procedure's RK-like rapid visual recovery but with greater accuracy and fewer side effects. Although regulatory issues limited the author's initial LASIK experience to unilateral procedures, by 1996 he began offering bilateral same-session LASIK.

In the last 1000 LASIK procedures performed, 90% have been bilateral same session and the incidence of complications has not differed significantly between this group and the initial unilateral only group. Like incisional patients, the author has observed the bilateral same-session LASIK patients to be much more enthusiastic and much more satisfied with their experience. In the author's experience, no patient has been adversely affected by having bilateral same-session surgery.

IS BILATERAL LASIK FOR EVERYONE?

No patient should be coerced or otherwise convinced to have bilateral same-session surgery. Even if bilateral same-session surgery is common in a particular practice, the refractive surgeon and staff should emphasize the availability of the unilateral sequential approach to prospective LASIK patients. The informed consent process should clearly note that, even though the additional risk is minimal, bilateral same-session surgery does involve greater risk than unilateral sequential surgery.

Bilateral same-session surgery appears to be an appropriate option for patients who are likely to have predictable and rapid visual recovery with minimal chance for significant under- or overcorrection. For LASIK patients, this includes low and moderate myopes (less than 10 D spherical equivalent), low astigmats (less than 3 D), and low hyperopes (less than 4 D). Obviously, with continued improvements in laser technology and software, as well as continued adjustments to nomograms, the incidence of significant deviations from target corrections should continue to decrease.

Surgeons should approach bilateral same-session surgery much more cautiously in LASIK patients with ocular or systemic conditions that could adversely affect (or be adversely affected by) the procedure. A good rule of thumb is if the surgeon cannot be supremely confident of an accurate and safe result, the patient should have unilateral sequential surgery (in addition, of course, to a thorough informed consent).

LASIK SURGICAL INSTRUMENTS AND ACCESSORIES

3

Lucio Buratto, MD and Stephen Brint, MD

INTRODUCTION

Laser-assisted in situ keratomileusis (LASIK) is considered a surgical procedure based on the use of two instruments:
- A microkeratome
- An excimer laser

As part of correct operating procedure, the eye must be carefully prepared:
- The eyelids must be suitably retracted to provide good exposure of the globe
- The cornea must be marked correctly
- The flap must be raised appropriately
- The hinge must be well-protected
- The interface must be carefully washed with balanced salt solution (BSS)
- The flap must be repositioned accurately

This is why some specific surgical instruments are required for the correct completion of a LASIK procedure.

SUPPLIES AND EQUIPMENT FOR LASIK

Drugs

Topical Anesthesia
Proparacaine 0.5% or oxybuprocaine: instill one drop two to three times beginning 5 minutes prior to surgery.

Alternatively, 4% lidocaine: instill one to two drops 5 minutes prior to surgery, with one drop immediately prior to placing the suction ring.

Antibiotics
Ofloxacin (Ocuflox, Allergan, Irvine, Calif, USA) or Ciloxin (Alcon, Fort Worth, Tex, USA): one to two drops 30 minutes prior to surgery.

Nonsteroidal Anti-Inflammatory Drug
Diclofenac (Voltaren, CIBA, Atlanta, Ga, USA): instill two drops both 30 minutes and 5 minutes prior to surgery.

Surgical Preparation
- Betadine or other disinfectant for periocular skin preparation
- Adhesive aperture drape or Steristrips (3M, St. Paul, Minn, USA)

Surgical Attire for Operating Room Staff
- Mask
- Cap
- Sterile powder-free gloves

Instruments and Equipment
- Assorted lid speculums
- Corneal marker prepared with gentian violet
- Spatula or smooth-angled forceps for lifting the flap
- Flap and hinge protectors (metal or Merocel sponges)
- Irrigation cannula
- Barraquer tonometer
- BSS
- Merocel sponges
- Fully assembled microkeratome
- Ultrasonic pachymeter
- Excimer laser

Back Table Supplies and Instruments
These items are seldom needed in routine procedures but should always be readily available in the laser suite in case they are needed:
- Beaver blades and holder
- Assorted forceps for flap/cap manipulation
- Tying forceps

- Needle holder
- 10-0 nylon sutures
- Fine scissors
- Antidesiccation chamber
- Fenestrated corneal spatula
- Bandage contact lenses

SURGICAL DRAPE

Isolation of the surgical field (the lids and lashes) is accomplished by using a plastic, self-adhesive aperture drape. These are available in a variety of styles, ranging from a simple 16 x 16 aperture drape to drapes that perforate into two parts and are designed specifically for LASIK.

The drape should be applied using an aseptic technique; manipulating the drape as little as possible will help prevent contamination. Care must be taken when applying the drape to prevent the adhesive areas from accidentally sticking to nonsterile areas or to itself. Once applied, if the drape does not adequately isolate the lashes and retract the lids, begin again with a new drape. Attempting to reposition a drape seldom produces satisfactory results.

Plastic drapes do not bring foreign material or debris into the surgical field. They are also nonreflective, antistatic, water-repellent, hypoallergenic, and can be easily removed.

3M makes several Steridrape models that can be used for LASIK (1020, 1021, 1024, 1030, 1060, 1062). Alcon's Eye Packs drape is also recommended (circular aperture/103020, oval aperture/103120). Drapes designed with a lateral pocket for collecting irrigating fluid may be useful (3M 1024).

Advantages of disposable adhesive drapes:
- Readily available
- Competitively priced
- Easy application

Disadvantages:
- Disposable plastics contribute to the ecological problems associated with disposal of non-biodegradable waste.
- A build-up of static electricity in a dry environment can make these drapes hard to handle.
- Some surgeons do not use drapes, preferring to isolate the lashes with Steristrips. These hypoallergenic microporous tapes, made from nylon and polyester, are backed with acrylic adhesive.

SPECULUM

The speculum must provide adequate exposure of

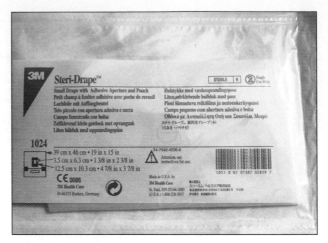

Figure 3-1. Drape (3M) with a central oval opening and a bag for fluid collection.

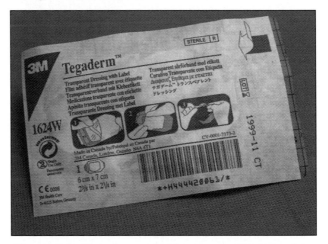

Figure 3-2. Tegaderm adhesive drape, which must be cut into two parts: one for the upper eyelid and one for the lower.

Table 3-1
THE SURGICAL DRAPE
• Isolates the surgical field
• Made from plastic (polyester) with a self-adhesive aperture
• Not a potential source of lint or debris
• Nonreflective
• Antistatic
• Water-repellent
• Hypoallergenic
• Easy to remove
• Equipped with a lateral pocket to collect fluids
• Maintains an aseptic surgical field
Advantages of disposable adhesive drapes
• Readily available
• Competitively priced
• Easy application
Disadvantages
• Environmental impact in terms of waste disposal

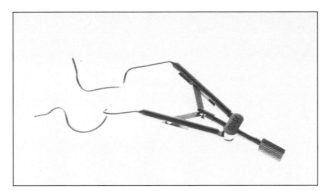

Figure 3-3. Buratto-Machat speculum.

the globe without creating excessive discomfort for the patient. It should be lightweight with a compact design. It must lock and be strong enough to prevent forceful blinking by the patient, while not interfering with placement of the suction ring or microkeratome pass.

The surgeon should evaluate exposure after the drape and speculum are in place. The intercanthal space must be large enough to correctly position the suction ring and allow for the microkeratome to pass without obstruction. If the microkeratome comes into even minimal contact with the speculum during the pass, the quality of the cut can be affected (irregular flap). If the microkeratome is completely blocked by the speculum, an incomplete flap results and the procedure will have to be aborted. Both the surgeon and the assistant should check for possible obstructions to the microkeratome pass prior to advancing the instrument.

A screw adjustable speculum is preferable, as it allows for maximum exposure. The speculum should be opened slowly to avoid causing the patient undue discomfort. However, the patient should be warned that the speculum will have to be opened widely and that some discomfort may be felt.

When the speculum has been opened the arms are parallel, creating a wide operating field that is large enough to accommodate the suction ring. The eyelids and drape should be retracted completely away from the path of the microkeratome. The speculum should be designed so that the adjustable hinge rests comfortably on the temporal side of the orbit. The hinge should be angled down so that it remains stable and does not interfere with engaging the microkeratome into the suction ring.

Finally, the speculum must be designed to allow both a temporal and superior surgical approach.

The Buratto-Machat speculum (Asico, Westmont, Ill, USA) with adjustment screws works well for this purpose.

Aspirating Speculums

Aspirating speculums allow the attachment of suction to the speculum. They can be very useful for LASIK.

Aspirating speculums serve to remove fluid from the conjunctival fornices along with any debris present, and prevent the reflux of irrigating fluid and debris under the flap. The aspiration device attached to the speculum should be switched off during placement of the suction ring and the microkeratome pass. The noise produced by aspiration could give the surgeon the impression that the suction ring is not correctly placed. Moreover, if suction is lost, the surgeon may mistake the sound for the aspirating speculum.

The disadvantage of aspirating speculums is that they tend to be thicker and less manageable.

Application of the Speculum

The blades of the speculum are widened slightly using the adjustment screw; the inferior arm is gently introduced under the edge of the lower lid, then the superior arm is positioned under the upper lid. Contact with the cornea should be avoided. Ensure that the drape isolates the eyelids and eyelashes from the surgical field. Center the speculum in the interpalpebral space and open the arms to provide optimal retraction of the eyelids, allowing for placement of the suction ring and the microkeratome pass. The speculum must be positioned so that it does not slide or become decentered during the procedure.

Removal of the Speculum

When removing the speculum, great care must be taken to prevent the blades from coming in contact with the cornea, displacing the flap. Partially close the blades, then gently remove the inferior blade while the assistant retracts the lower lid; remove the superior blade while retracting the upper lid.

Other Types of Speculums

The Liebermann adjustable wire speculum provides good exposure and locks to resist forceful blinking. The adjustment screw is positioned temporally and angled at 45°, following the shape of the face. This allows either a temporal or superior approach.

The Buratto-Machat adjustable speculum is a variation of Liebermann's design. The blades are more steeply angled to increase exposure and the adjustment screw lies against the side of the face, clear of the microkeratome. The ability to adjust and lock the speculum is important when patients have a narrow palpebral fissure or blepharospasm.

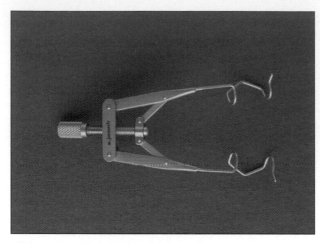

Figure 3-4. Buratto speculum (Janach).

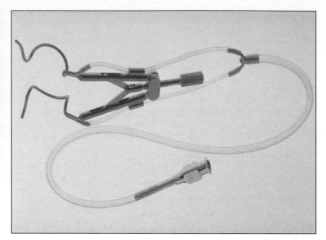

Figure 3-5. Slade speculum with aspiration.

Table 3-2
AVAILABLE SPECULUMS

Nonaspirating
- The Liebermann adjustable wire speculum
- The Buratto-Machat adjustable speculum
- The Slade adjustable speculum
- The Bansal nasal speculum
- The Manche speculum
- The Güell speculum
- The Kraff adjustable nasal speculum with solid arms

Aspirating
- The Machat-Buratto adjustable speculum
- The Liebermann speculum
- The Slade speculum
- The Bansal speculum
- The Pannu-Barraquer speculum
- The Pannu-Kratz-Barraquer speculum
- The Barraquer wire speculum

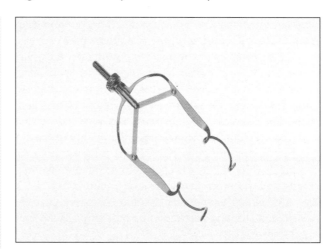

Figure 3-6. Buratto speculum (Duckworth and Kent).

The Slade adjustable LASIK speculum is also based on the Leibermann design. It has been modified to maximize exposure and allow easier positioning of the suction ring, as well as good clearance for the microkeratome pass.

The Murdoch speculum has fenestrated blades and automatically locks to provide maximum exposure. It is also used for photorefractive keratectomy (PRK).

The Bansal nasal LASIK speculum is designed to facilitate the microkeratome pass. The blades are solid, minimizing interference and contamination by eyelashes. To remove the speculum after surgery, the arms are squeezed closed and gently removed, minimizing the possibility of flap displacement.

The Manche LASIK speculum was designed specifically for down-up LASIK. The elongated, angled arms follow the temporal profile of the face.

The Güell speculum is especially useful when the microkeratome pass is made from 6 to 12 o'clock. Temporal access is also good for microkeratomes that approach laterally.

The Kraff adjustable nasal speculum has solid blades. This design can be used in both nasal and superior hinge procedures, but is ideally suited to microkeratomes with temporal insertion. A screw mechanism allows easy adjustment. The solid blades minimize interference and contamination from eyelashes.

Aspirating Speculums

The Machat-Buratto adjustable aspirating speculum can be used for both nasal and superior hinge techniques. It is ideal for narrow palpebral fissures or with blepharospasm. It provides maximum exposure for placement of the suction ring and the microkeratome pass. The hinge is angled to lie against the side of the face. Ports in the blades allow for continual aspiration.

The Liebermann aspirating speculum is designed like

Table 3-3

THE SPECULUM

The speculum should be:
- Lightweight
- Compact
- Strong enough to prevent forceful blinking
- Retract the lids sufficiently
- Allow both a temporal and superior surgical approach
- Have a locking, adjustable screw device
- Be hinged on the temporal side of the orbit
- Have the hinge angled down so as not to interfere with the microkeratome

Types of speculums:
- Simple wire adjustable
- Disposable
- Fitted with aspiration

the original with the addition of six aspiration ports in each blade. It is supplied with silicone tubing and a connector.

The Slade adjustable aspirating LASIK speculum (Asico) provides continual aspiration through multiple ports.

The Bansal aspirating speculum is designed to maximize exposure and aspirate irrigating fluids, preventing reflux of debris and secretions into the interface.

The Pannu-Barraquer aspirating speculum provides continuous aspiration to prevent the accumulation of fluid in the surgical field. The speculum hinge is angled to lie against the side of the face, allowing easy insertion and movement of the microkeratome.

The Pannu-Kratz-Barraquer speculum has six ports on each blade to provide continuous aspiration. The speculum hinge is angled to allow free movement of the microkeratome.

The Kratz aspirating speculum is adjustable. Six ports on each blade allow for aspiration of fluid. It is supplied with silicone tubing and a connector.

Disposable Speculums (With and Without Aspiration)

The Barraquer wire speculum has an automatic locking device. The aspirating system consists of a luminescent ring attached to the speculum, which is attached to the globe via a vacuum. It has been designed so that the suction ring can be placed inside and outside the operating field. The system is also made up of a spring-loaded 3-cc syringe is attached to supply vacuum to the luminescent ring.

THE CORNEAL MARKER

Before the keratectomy is performed, the cornea should be marked to provide reference points that will allow the correct repositioning of the corneal flap, especially in the case of a free cap.

Many surgeons use a gentian violet pen to mark the cornea with a pararadial line; the technique consists of marking the prepupillary cornea and then drawing a line from a paracentral point to the limbus. When the flap is repositioned, the point where the pararadial line crosses the incision acts as a reference for alignment. This technique is simple and effective, but not optimal. It was refined by Ruiz, who designed a marker that was very popular for a number of years. It consists of two concentric circles—the inner circle is 3.0 mm in diameter, and the outer circle is 10.5 mm. A pararadial segment joins the two circles. The smaller circle is centered over the visual axis, identifying the central cornea for the keratectomy. The outer circle helps in centering the suction ring. The central opening of the ring roughly corresponds to the circular marking. The pararadial line has two main objectives: to orient the corneal flap/disc correctly and to prevent a free cap from being replaced upside down (epithelium down). Only when the cap is correctly positioned will the pararadial line be straight.

Modern LASIK techniques (nasal or superior hinge) require a change in marking methods. LASIK is now performed without intentionally creating a free cap; a hinge of tissue is left, creating a flap. Large diameter lamellar cuts no longer have to be perfectly centered, making central and peripheral markings unnecessary. However, it is extremely important that the flap is repositioned correctly. This is why radial and/or pararadial markings are necessary. Use of toxic dyes should be keep to a minimum. The marking of three radii—two radial and one pararadial—is sufficient. All three aid in repositioning the flap. The pararadial mark also allows the correct orientation of a free cap. The Buratto marker is designed to avoid the central 4.0 mm of the cornea, the radii extend from 6.0 mm to 11 mm. These segments are thin, leaving a precise but blunt line to avoid causing epithelial damage. The radial markings allow the flap to be correctly realigned; the pararadial marking allows correct orientation of a free cap.

Marking in Case of a Free Cap

When a free cap occurs, the surgeon becomes immediately aware of the importance of corneal marks prior to

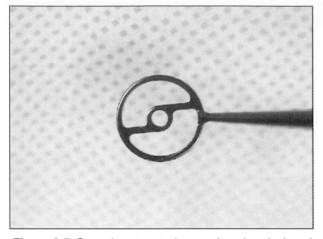

Figure 3-7. Central-paracentral corneal marker designed by Ruiz (note the pararadial segments).

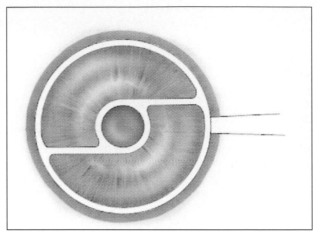

Figure 3-8. How to use the central-paracentral corneal marker designed by Ruiz.

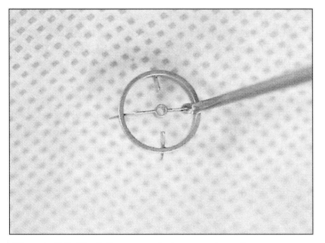

Figure 3-9. Radial-paracentral corneal marker.

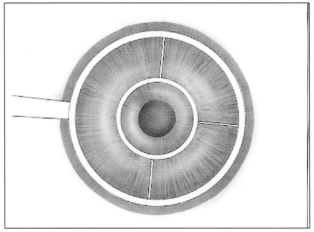

Figure 3-10. Central-paracentral corneal marker with three radial segments.

performing the keratectomy. The free cap is gently removed from the microkeratome and placed in an anti-desiccation chamber, epithelial side down.

If the lamellar cut is sufficiently large and well centered, the refractive ablation can be performed. The flap is then replaced on the stromal bed with a fenestrated spatula. The free cap must be repositioned precisely with the corneal markings serving as reference points to correct orientation. The pararadial distinguishes the epithelial surface and prevents inversion (the pararadial line will be continuous only if positioned epithelial side up).

Marking Technique

The segments of the marker that will contact the cornea are stained with gentian violet. The marker is applied to a dry cornea so that the marks are clearly visible and dispersion of dye is avoided. The marker is firmly and evenly applied to leave three radii marked on the surface. In the nasal hinge technique, these should be inferior, superior, and temporal. In the superior hinge technique, the radii should be inferior, nasal, and temporal. The unmarked quadrant corresponds to the hinge. After the marker is applied, irrigate the cornea to remove any residual dye and dry the conjunctival sac with Merocel sponges. Proceed with the keratectomy and refractive ablation. After the flap has been correctly positioned, the markings will coincide exactly with those on the peripheral cornea.

A number of markers are available:

The Machat marker consists of two intersecting circles (3.25 mm and 3.75 mm) positioned on the peripheral temporal cornea. The keratectomy incision crosses the circles, providing four alignment points. The different diameters of the circles prevent the free cap from being repositioned upside-down. Machat's LASIK marker has the two circles positioned separately on the cornea.

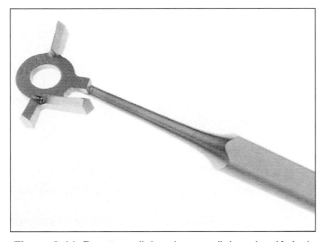

Figure 3-11. Buratto radial and pararadial marker (Asico).

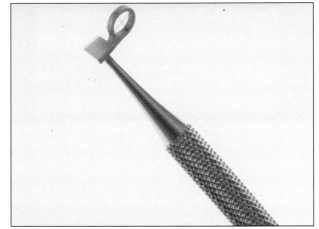

Figure 3-12. Slade marker (Asico).

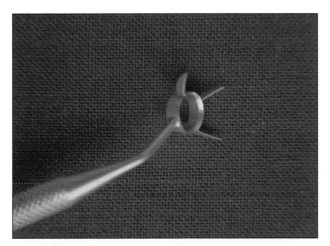

Figure 3-13. Buratto three-radius marker (Janach).

Table 3-4
CORNEAL MARKERS
• Buratto marker: 3.0 mm no-contact optic zone. Two radial and one pararadial mark extend from 6.0 to 11 mm. Allows realignment of the flap and prevents upside-down positioning of a free cap.
• The Ruiz marker
• The Machat marker
• The Kritzinger-Updegraff marker
• The Duckworth and Kent marker
• The Manche marker
• The Christenbury marker
• The Bansal marker
• The Slade marker

The Kritzinger and Updegraff marker uses seven radial markers and one pararadial marker. The radii are very short, reducing the amount of dye contacting the cornea. The markings on the peripheral cornea can be used to center the laser ablation, aligning them with the grid on the laser microscope. By centering the marker over the visual axis, the laser ablation can be centered very accurately. The concentric circular markings of the Kritzinger and Updegraff marker aid in centering the suction ring. Once the lamellar cut has been completed and the flap flipped over, the peripheral markings can be used as reference points for the alignment of the grid.

According to Pallikaris, good marking must include at least three points on the corneal surface, the center of the pupil, and two points on the peripheral cornea. The Pallikaris marker is designed to provide these three marks and allow precise repositioning in the event of a free cap.

The Duckworth and Kent marker is arch-shaped. It

has a diameter of 10 mm and supports two straight segments. One measures 5.0 mm and extends radially from the periphery to the center; the other measures 3.0 mm and is eccentric, situated on the edge of the arc at a right angle to the radial segment.

The Manche marker has a 4.0 mm no-contact optic zone. Two radial markings and a pararadial mark extent from 6.0 to 12 mm.

The Christenbury marker has a 3.0 mm no-contact optic zone with a centering element. The radial markings extend from 6.0 to 12 mm.

The Bansal marker has two pararadial and three radial marks, providing five points for repositioning the flap. The 6.0 mm no-contact optic zone allows centering without disturbing the central cornea. The asymmetric markings prevent the flap from being repositioned upside-down in the event of a free cap.

The Slade marker has a 3.0 mm no-contact zone for centering and pararadial markings extend from 6.0 to 12 mm.

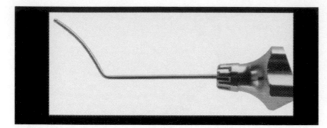

Figure 3-14. Curved cannula for irrigating the interface.

The Machat marker, designed for superior-hinge LASIK, marks two intersecting circles (3.25 and 3.75 mm) on the inferior cornea (9.5 mm) The no-contact optic zone is 3.0 mm in diameter. The two circles produce four points for realignment of the flap and prevent inversion of the flap in the event of a free cap.

IRRIGATION CANNULAS

BSS or other liquid must be used at least six times during a LASIK operation.

The first irrigation is mainly to remove conjunctival secretions. Once the speculum has been engaged and prior to marking, the cornea and conjunctival sac are washed with BSS. Merocel sponges are then used to remove the residual fluid and any secretions that may be present. The corneal surface is then dried carefully before marking.

The second irrigation begins once the corneal marking has been done. The cornea and conjunctiva are irrigated as above and then dried and cleaned with Merocel sponges. This is used to remove dye residue from the cornea and conjunctiva.

The third irrigation begins once the suction ring has been applied and a few seconds prior to the lamellar cut. The corneal surface must be wet with two to three drops of BSS or Ophthaine, which will facilitate the microkeratome pass along the corneal surface, making the completion of a good cut easier. If the cornea is dry, the cut surface may be uneven and the epithelium abraded. When using instruments with tracks, it is useful to apply a drop of liquid on each of the suction ring tracks to facilitate the microkeratome pass. Most microkeratome manufacturers suggest using distilled water. In the instruction guide for the Hansatome (Bausch & Lomb Surgical, Claremont, Calif, USA) recommends avoiding BSS prior to the keratectomy because the salt solution may damage the Hansatome microkeratome; salt-free solutions should be used.

Slade uses a salt-free, glycerin-based anesthetic (Ophthaine). It has a balanced pH and contains glycerin;

Table 3-5
USE OF THE CANNULA

Irrigation
- To remove conjunctival secretions
- To remove residual dye from the cornea
- To wet the cornea and facilitate the pass of the microkeratome along the track
- To create a lake on the stromal bed
- To clean the interface
- To wet the central epithelium following drying of the flap
- To flip back and reposition the flap at the end of the ablation
- To "massage" the flap after irrigation of the interface in order to squeeze out any liquid trapped at the interface

as a result, it lubricates (without being an oxidant) in addition to providing anesthesia.

The fourth irrigation requires two to three drops of BSS applied to the stromal bed at the end of the ablation, prior to repositioning the flap. BSS is applied uniformly on the in-situ stromal tissue using the back of a cannula. The liquid forms a lake, which allows the flap to distend easily and evenly over the underlying corneal bed and return to its original position. The flap is repositioned by inserting the cannula under the epithelial side of the flap, close to the hinge. The flap is then pulled toward the center of the cornea until it has returned to its original position.

The fifth irrigation requires the most important use of the irrigation cannula: cleaning the interface, which is performed following flap repositioning. This step is used to remove epithelial cells and debris from the interface so that postoperatively the cornea is perfectly clear and transparent without epithelial ingrowth. Irrigation also facilitates spontaneous repositioning of the flap on the bed with perfect centration. The BSS irrigation cannula for LASIK must be able to perform this maneuver correctly; that is, it must be designed to provide the best result with minimal trauma.

The sixth application of irrigation consists of another drop of liquid placed on the central corneal surface once the flap has been replaced and dried. This protects the central cornea. Many cannulas are suitable for this maneuver. The Buratto cannula works well. This instrument was designed specifically for irrigating the interface but is also useful in the other intraoperative steps.

The three-holed cannula (one hole is in the tip and the others on the sides) allows an even irrigation flow in three directions. It is long enough to irrigate the entire surface of the interface and is curved to follow the

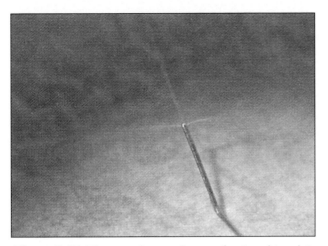

Figure 3-15. Three-port cannula: one front and two lateral for irrigating the interface.

corneal curvature. It is thin (25 gauge) and the tip is flat, which facilitates its insertion under the corneal flap without dragging epithelial cells into the interface. It is available in a right-handed or left-handed version for surgeon comfort and for optimization of the procedure. The shape of the cannula is very useful for repositioning the flap at the end of surgery and for distending it correctly with a smoothing movement that starts from the hinge and moves in the opposite direction. The same cannula is available with five holes.

The irrigation cannula can be attached to a filter, such as a hydrophilic 0.22 micron sterile filter, which will filter the liquid prior to irrigation under the flap.

Other available cannulas include:

The Slade LASIK cannula. This is a 26-gauge cannula designed exclusively for the LASIK procedure. It has a spatula tip for easy insertion below the flap. The cross-shaped section of the cannula allows the surgeon to introduce it laterally below the flap without dragging epithelial cells into the interface.

The Bansal cannula/spatula for LASIK: this is a single instrument used to lift the flap and irrigate the corneal bed. The smooth blunt anterior surface engages and lifts the flap with minor epithelial trauma. The curvature is the same as the corneal curvature, which conforms nicely to the flap. There is also a 25-gauge cannula for irrigating the flap and stromal bed.

The Kritzinger-Updegraff irrigation cannula. This has been designed to be connected to the bottle of BSS and provide a slow, continuous, controlled flow of BSS under the flap to clean the interface.

The Microtech Inc cannula. This is a dual-purpose cannula with two irrigation holes on both arms. It is used to manipulate and reposition the cap. It is also available with three irrigation holes.

Table 3-6
OTHER CANNULAS

Buratto cannula with three to five holes
The three-holed version (one at the tip and the other two on the sides) produces an equal irrigation flow in three directions; it is long enough to irrigate the entire surface of the interface; this thin cannula (25-gauge) is curved to follow the corneal contour. It has a flattened tip to facilitate its insertion under the corneal flap without dragging epithelial cells into the interface. The five holes of this cannula are distributed as follows: one hole in the tip, two on the front of the shaft, and two on the back.

Models specific for right and left eyes are available for use in down-up LASIK
- Slade LASIK cannula
- Bansal cannula/spatula for LASIK
- Pallikaris irrigation/aspiration cannula
- Kritzinger-Updegraff irrigation cannula
- LASIK cannula by Microtech, Inc
- Kritzinger-Updegraff aspiration cannula

The Pallikaris irrigation/aspiration cannula: the frontal extremity of this cannula is slightly curved and consists of an aspiration tube with a cutting edge. This tube also incorporates an even smaller, deeper one for irrigation. The latter has a blunt edge with an internal diameter that is slightly larger (by about one-third) than the diameter of the irrigation tube. The irrigation amount should never exceed the amount of aspiration when both tubes are being used. The tips of the cannula can be exposed or covered by a silicone sheath.

The Rubinstein irrigating cannula. This is used for initial lifting and repositioning of the flap and for irrigating below it. It is also used in enhancement treatments. It is sufficiently rigid to exert pressure on the flap to smooth the folds and remove any fluid from the interface. It has five holes.

The Dishler cannula (30-gauge). Its small size allows the cannula to pass easily below the flap. Its curvature follows the natural curvature of the cornea. Its blunt tip will not damage stromal tissue; this is particularly useful in enhancement, as the stroma is more fragile. It is useful for repositioning the flap and can be used to remove excess fluid from the interface. It has four irrigation holes. It is a available as 7.0 mm and 9.0 mm, and either disposable or reusable.

The Manche cannula. This is characterized by a solid extremity that facilitates the cannula's insertion under the flap without damaging the edge and epithelium. It is also used to reposition the flap. It has three holes—one on the inferior surface and the other two on the sides.

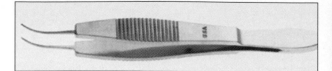

Figure 3-16. Buratto LASIK forceps (Asico).

The Güell cannula. This has seven irrigation holes distributed as three holes on each side and one on the front of the tip.

Kritzinger-Updegraff's aspiration cannula for LASIK. This has a number of holes and is held in the fornix to aspirate the excess irrigation fluid. The large number of holes prevents the needle becoming occluded by the conjunctiva and ensures continuous aspiration with BSS.

Cannulas can also be used for a number of different maneuvers:

- To flip the flap over at the end of surgery and reposition it on the stromal bed
- To massage the corneal surface once the interface has been irrigated to evacuate any liquid or air remaining underneath
- To compress a damp microsponge against the cornea when the stromal bed and stromal surface of the flap are being cleaned
- To aspirate fluids from the operating field

FORCEPS

Forceps are used to lift and reflect the flap nasally, replace the flap during the primary procedure, and dissect and lift the flap during an enhancement procedure.

Forceps should be smooth (nontoothed), as any indentation may damage the fragile flap or epithelium. A long or flat, wide grip will increase the grasp the forceps have on the flap.

Following the microkeratome cut, the flap must be elevated to expose the stroma for ablation. At the end of the ablation, the flap must be repositioned. Similarly, during enhancement procedures the flap must be dissected and lifted from the underlying stroma. The flap can be elevated with a number of instruments; however, an appropriate forceps will do the job better than any other instrument (spatulas, cannulas, etc).

The surface between the forceps arms must be slightly rough to allow a grasp of the tissue that is being manipulated. The Buratto forceps have been designed for this specific purpose.

Some surgeons use a spatula to lift the flap, but this maneuver may drag epithelial cells into the interface and encourage postoperative epithelial ingrowth. The Buratto

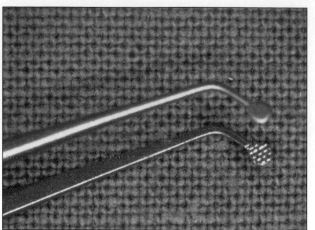

Figure 3-17. Buratto flap forceps (Janach).

Table 3-7
FORCEPS

Required for:
- Reflecting the flap nasally
- Replacing the flap during a primary procedure
- Lifting the flap during an enhancement procedure
- Buratto forceps: no teeth and slightly curved arms with finely sanded tips. This instrument is ideal for lifting the flap. The curve of the forceps corresponds to the edge of the corneal flap
- Bansal forceps
- Hersh forceps
- Pierse forceps
- Manche forceps

forceps have slightly curved arms with finely sanded tips, allowing easy flap lifting. The curved shape of the forceps conforms to the edge of the corneal flap.

The Bansal forceps are curved and used to lift the flap from the corneal bed. They correspond to the corneal curvature to allow easy insertion under the flap. Smooth, rounded tips minimize epithelial trauma.

Pierse-type forceps are particularly suitable for detaching the flap in an enhancement procedure.

Hersh forceps have a double-grip design to prevent the flap from being folded and facilitates flap lifting.

The Manche forceps are designed to be used in a primary LASIK procedure, in an enhancement, and in a case of a free cap. The tip is oval shaped.

FLAP POSITIONER

Once the microkeratome cut has been completed, the flap must be lifted and positioned nasally using the nasal hinge technique or superiorly using the down-up proce-

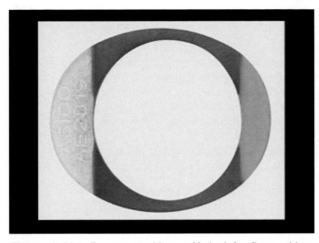

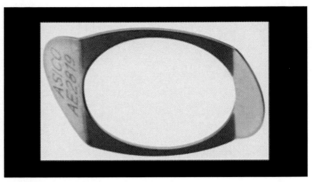

Figure 3-18b. Buratto positioner (Asico): lateral view.

Figure 3-18a. Buratto positioner (Asico) for flaps with a nasal or superior hinge: front view.

dure. Contact between the flap and conjunctiva must be avoided, as this may contaminate the stromal surface with secretions or debris.

The flap should not be excessively wet. If this happens, the stroma or epithelium will swell and an edematous flap will have a decreased ability to spontaneously adhere.

The flap should not be allowed to fold over or roll over on itself. To achieve this, the surgeon should have a specific instrument available on which to lay the flap. It may have a number of shapes. The flap positioner designed by Buratto consists of two half-moon shaped devices—one is convex and the other is concave. By rotating the device, it may be used for both the right and left eyes. A metal wire that gives good balance to the instrument joins the two half-moons.

The concave surface collects the flap during ablation. To reposition the flap at the end of the ablation, the irrigation cannula must be passed under the flap, which may require irrigation from the flap positioner. The flap is then flipped back to its original position.

FLAP STABILIZER

The stabilizer is used to immobilize the flap during enhancement procedures in which various materials (epithelium, debris, etc) must be removed from the stromal side of the flap. The forceps designed by Pallikaris are ideal for this purpose. The tip is curved at 45° with respect to the handle.

The instrument consists of a solid plate that has the same shape as a hinged flap and a metal wire ring measuring 6.0 mm in diameter. When the instrument is closed, the ring rests gently on the plate. The flap is positioned on the plate and held by the ring. In this way, the instru-

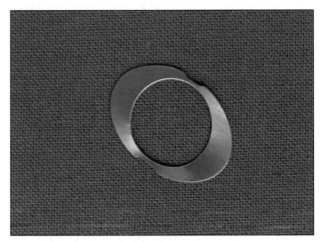

Figure 3-19. Buratto flap positioner (Janach).

ment can hold the flap firmly with minimal or no damage to the cut corneal tissue.

SPATULAS

Spatulas are used in a number of different situations during the LASIK procedure and are specifically designed for that purpose.

A. Spatulas for Raising and Repositioning

1. They must be thin, narrow, and flat to penetrate the interface. They must also be at least as long as the flap diameter and curved to adapt to the corneal surface. They are used in both the primary operation and enhancement treatments.
2. There are also spatulas used to spread the liquid formed during the ablation.

B. Spatulas to Protect the Hinge

They must be thin and broad to protect the flap stroma. They must also be short in order to cover the central portion of the hinge, where tissue is more likely to be involved in the ablation. These spatulas can also be used to retract the flap so that a greater amount of space is left for the ablation.

C. Test Spatulas

They are used to perform the striae test. They must have blunt ends and be atraumatic: mushroom and olive-tipped spatulas are preferable.

D. Fenestrated Spatulas

They are used for maneuvering or reapplying the disks of tissue. There are also spatulas for raising and repositioning the flap.

A. SPATULAS FOR LIFTING AND REPOSITIONING

After the microkeratome cut, many surgeons raise the flap using toothless forceps. Others prefer to use a fine spatula. This type of spatula may be useful at the end of the ablation for distending the flap. For this reason, it is inserted under the flap close to the hinge to flip the flap over on the corneal bed. It can be used once the interface has been washed to massage the cornea to remove any residual liquid if the surgeon suspects that some liquid remains at the interface.

Slade's enhancement spatula has a semi-cutting edge to raise the flap and separate the epithelium.

Slade's enhancement spatula type II has a finely serrated and semi-sharp edge to raise and separate the epithelium for an efficacious enhancement treatment. The fine serrations are efficacious for dissecting the edge of the corneal flap where adhesion is greatest: along the cut edge of Bowman's layer.

Machat's enhancement spatula has a double tip. One semi-cutting angled tip has been created to dissect the edge of the corneal flap where adhesion is at a maximum: along the cut edge of Bowman's layer. This short tip is used to dissect, with excessive insertion, under the flap, which may dislocate epithelial cells and result in epithelial growth at the interface. At the other end, there is a fine spatula that helps detach all the adhesions of the corneal flap from the stromal bed. It has a semi-cutting edge that efficaciously raises the flap and separates the epithelium.

It is ideal for opening and closing the corneal flap.

Kritzinger-Updegraff's spatula for raising and manipulating the flap has a flap elevator. This spatula was designed to slide underneath the flap and cut the adhesions cleanly through the epithelium without detaching them. The flap is then raised. This elevator leaves a smooth cut surface and facilitates repositioning

Table 3-8
USE OF SPATULAS

- Spatulas for raising/removing or spreading the liquid formed during the ablation
- Spatulas to protect the hinge
- Test spatulas (striae tests)
- Fenestrated spatulas for maneuvering or reapplying the disks of tissue
- Spatulas for positioning the drape

of the flap following the laser ablation.

Herzig's enhancement elevator/spatula has two tips. A wider oval semicutting tip is used to cut the epithelium and fibrosis formation at the edge of the flap. The instrument's design allows a smooth, continuous movement of the spatula tip along the entire flap circumference. Following release of the flap edge, the smaller extremity is used to gently separate the stromal surface from the stromal bed and can be used to rotate the flap.

Rothchild's double-tipped spatula is two-tipped. One tip of this spatula is slightly pointed while the other is rounded to begin the dissection.

Probst's tape/ribbon spatulas an example of a spatula used to position the drape. It is used to insert the surgical drape painlessly into the fornices to provide maximum exposure of the bulb with isolation of the interpalpebral opening from eyelashes and the Meibomian gland ducts.

The spatula can also be used to improve distention of the flap at the end of surgery, when distention is not optimal. It is used if fine lines are observed or the edges of the flap are tucked in following positioning by passing the spatula gently and firmly over the cornea several times, the surgeon can distend the flap correctly.

The spatula can also be used during the ablation to provide uniform distribution of any liquid formed during the ablation or to avoid or reduce the risk of central island formation.

It can also be used during surface or intrastromal phototherapeutic keratectomy (PTK). With certain types of lasers that have an ablation process that does not provide total uniformity of the surfaces, some surgeons perform PTK of the ablated stroma using a liquid that is suitable for that purpose. The spatula can distend this liquid during the smoothing process. The drying action is often performed using Merocel sponges.

This type of spatula can be used in enhancement procedures to detach, raise, and reposition the flap. Of the spatulas available for raising and positioning the flap during the primary operation, we feel that the following deserve mention:

Buratto's spatula. This is fine, long, and curved so that it adapts to the corneal surface. It is flat and pointed

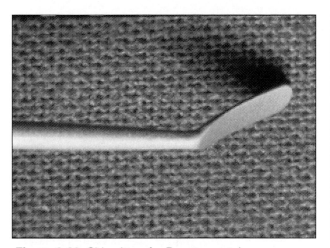

Figure 3-20. Side view of a Buratto spatula.

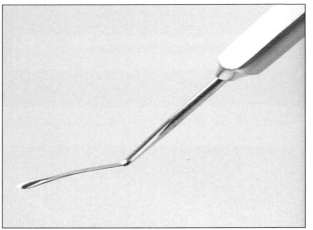

Figure 3-21. Slade spatula (Asico).

to easily penetrate under the flap. It is blunt so that it can be used without damaging the tissues.

Zaldivar's LASIK spatula. This spatula is designed to raise the flap from the stromal bed and reposition it following laser treatment. It can also be used as a squeegee to remove any folds from the flap.

Maloney's flap flipper/squeegee. This has a flat, 1.0 mm tip that facilitates raising and repositioning the flap. The rounded part of the spatula serves to remove folds and excess fluid from under the flap.

Lindstrom's LASIK marker and spatula. This is double-tipped with a spatulate tip to raise the flap and another tip to mark it.

Lindstrom's PRK/LASIK spatula. One tip has a semi-cutting spatulate edge designed specifically for the efficacious removal of epithelium in PRK. The other extremity has a special curvature and is used to raise and position the LASIK flap.

Bangji's spatula for primary LASIK and enhancement. This is used to overturn the cap or flap of the stromal bed during primary LASIK. It is also used to remove epithelium during enhancement and flap repositioning.

Enhancement spatula. A number of models are commercially available.

B. FLAP PROTECTOR AND RETRACTOR

During the refractive ablation, the surgeon must be careful to prevent the stromal part closest to the hinge from being included in the laser ablation; if this happens, irregular astigmatism may result. In any case, the final refractive result will change. The flap must be protected every time the lamella cut has a small diameter and/or the planned ablation is wide (myopic ablations with wide transition zones, astigmatic ablations, particularly when the axis of the astigmatism coincides with the hinge axis, hyperopic ablations).

The stromal part of the flap close to the hinge must be protected. A number of spatulas have been designed to cover and protect the stromal portion of the flap above the hinge.

In actual fact, commercially available spatulas are not really suitable for this purpose because the design is not appropriate. The part that protects the hinge must be straight and the part that covers the flap must be semi-circular. Moreover, the flap must be retracted as far as possible toward the hinge to provide the laser with a wide area on the in-situ stroma, particularly with those lasers that perform the treatment on large optic zones, or with peripheral transition zones; and particularly when the diameter is reduced or the hinge is large.

Buratto's spatula is ideal for both protection and retraction. This spatula is wide enough to protect the flap stroma, both close to the hinge and toward the center. It is fitted with a small tooth that runs along its entire length; this tooth is inserted into the hinge and is highly efficacious in retracting the flap and providing maximum exposure of the in-situ stroma to the ablation.

The instrument is angled for comfortable use in both the right and left eyes, with both the nasal and superior hinge techniques. Other spatulas include:

Slade's flap spatula. This is used to retain the flap below the hinge to allow maximum exposure of the stromal bed and to protect the flap during the laser ablation.

Buratto's superior flap holder/retainer. This was specifically designed for the down-up LASIK technique. It is positioned prior to raising the flap and used to retain the flap during the laser ablation, exposing the stromal bed to a maximum and protecting the superior hinge. It prevents the flap from coming into contact with the con-

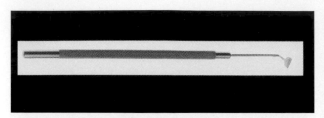

Figure 3-22. Buratto flap retractor and protector (Asico).

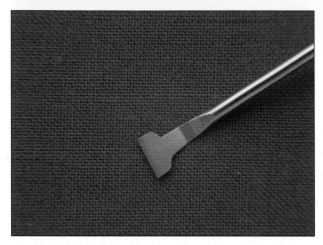

Figure 3-24. Buratto flap retractor and protector—close-up (Asico).

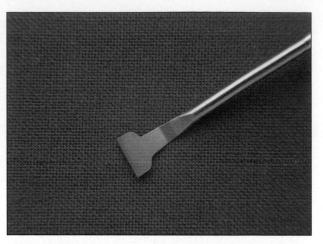

Figure 3-23. Buratto flap retractor (Janach).

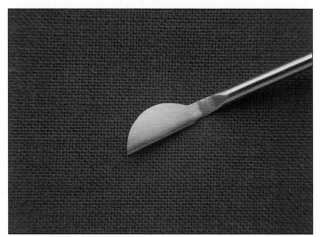

Figure 3-25. Another model of a Buratto flap retractor (Duckworth & Kent).

junctiva, eyelashes, eyelids, and Meibomian gland secretions.

Some surgeons use flap shields in paper, silicone, or plastic, which are cut to shape using scissors. A flap-shaped mask is obtained. This is used to cover and protect the stromal surface of the flap and prevent it from being accidentally involved in the laser ablation.

C. TEST SPATULAS

Test spatulas are used at the end of the operation to check that the flap has correctly adhered to the underlying surface (ie, the striae test).

The olive-tipped spatula for Slade's striae test is used to check whether the flap has adhered correctly to the underlying cornea. This test involves exerting gentle pressure at about 1.0 mm outside the incision. Fine folds must form and run toward the center of the flap; if this occurs, we can assume that the adhesion of the flap to the underlying cornea is optimal. Pressure is localized and must be gentle to avoid trauma to the epithelium. A dry sponge, the tip of forceps, or an olive-tipped spatula can be used for this purpose. The spatula works best. Buratto's spatula has a blunt tip. It is smooth, half-moon shaped, and ideal for this purpose.

Prior to positioning the spatula on the eye, the sur-

geon should tell the patient what is about to happen, otherwise the patient may move suddenly (through the discomfort created by contact) and the flap may dislocate.

Striae Test

Following flap repositioning, a damp Merocel sponge is gently rubbed from the hinge toward the opposite part of the flap: the cut line is gently dried. Finally, the cornea is left to dry spontaneously for 30 to 60 seconds with the eyelids open between the arms of the speculum.

The adhesion test is performed. This involves exerting pressure on the external edge of the keratectomy using an olive-tipped spatula; folds will be observed on the flap (striae test) and the surgeon will see that the edge of the cut has correctly adhered to the underlying bed.

The test is performed in at least three quadrants of the cut area (it is unnecessary in the area corresponding to the hinge). Then, under high magnification, the surgeon

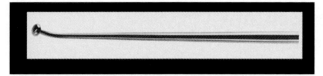

Figure 3-26. Buratto blunt spatula for the striae test (Asico).

checks that the flap has been perfectly repositioned in its original site and is perfectly distended. The edges of the flap and the portion of the underlying stroma corresponding to the keratectomy must perfectly match without showing signs of shrinkage or dehiscence; the same applies to the markings. If any anomalies are observed, it is better to raise the flap and repeat repositioning and the adhesion steps.

D. FENESTRATED SPATULAS

A fenestrated spatula is used to reposition free caps (360° cuts) following the refractive procedure. It must have a concave shape in addition to being fenestrated to provide an adequate resting surface for the flap, which must be free from any liquid retention. The concave shape is suitable for resting the flap (which is convex) on the cornea when necessary.

NEEDLE HOLDERS

Generally speaking, LASIK is a technique that does not require sutures. In some cases, for example when the free cap does not adhere sufficiently, sutures may be needed. A microsurgery needle holder and nylon 10/0 thread will be needed.

Table 3-9

SPATULAS

Spatulas for initial flap lifting and repositioning
- Buratto spatula
- Zaldivar LASIK spatula for the flap
- Maloney flap flipper/squeegee for the flap
- Lindstrom flap spatula for PRK/LASIK
- Lindstrom spatula and marker for LASIK: double-ended with both spatula and marker

Enhancement spatulas
- Slade enhancement spatulas type I and II
- Machat enhancement spatula
- Kritzinger-Updegraff elevator/manipulator spatula
- Herzig lifting spatula for retreatment

Protector and retractor spatulas
- Buratto spatula for protection and retraction. It is large to protect as well as retract the stromal part of the flap, encouraging maximum exposure of the in situ stroma for the ablation. The instrument is angled to allow comfortable use for both the right and left eyes in both nasal and superior hinge techniques

Olive-tipped spatula for the striae test
Fenestrated spatula for a free cap
Spatula to position the drape

The Lid Speculum

Chan Wing Kwong, MD

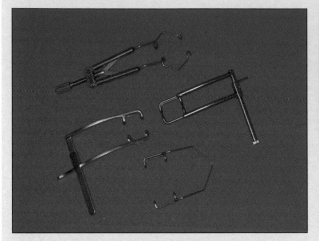

Figure 3A-1. Examples of lid speculums commonly used for LASIK surgery. Clockwise from top: Liebermann speculum, Murdoch speculum, Barraquer speculum, and Preori speculum.

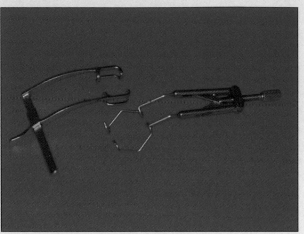

Figure 3A-2. Two examples of locking speculums recommended for LASIK. Preori speculum, which locks by friction (left), and Liebermann speculum, which locks with a screw mechanism (right).

Selection of an appropriate lid speculum is an essential step in performing LASIK surgery. Lid speculums serve three important functions in LASIK surgery:

1. Exposure of the eye. Adequate exposure of the eye with good retraction of the eyelids is essential for effective and safe LASIK. Lid speculums provide globe exposure, which allows room for the placement of the vacuum suction ring and consequent achievement of the desired intraocular pressure necessary for the lamellar keratectomy.

2. Protection of eyelids and lashes. Lid speculums keep the eyelid margins and eyelashes away from the path of the advancing microkeratome head. This helps to prevent jamming of the microkeratome head and inadvertent injury to the patient's eyelid margin or eyelashes.

3. Aspiration of fluid. Some speculums have aspiration ports built into the blades. When connected via silicone tubing to a suction pump, these speculums allow fluid in the conjunctival cul-de-sac to be constantly aspirated. It is thought that constant removal of irrigation fluid and tear secretions from the eye may minimize the likelihood of postoperative diffuse lamellar keratitis (Sands of the Sahara syndrome).

Several different types of lid speculums are commonly used for LASIK (Figure 3A-1). The choice of a speculum is very much dependent upon the individual surgeon's preference. However, some specific recommendations can be suggested:

1. Locking speculum. Use a speculum that has a locking device. This will ensure adequate retraction of the eyelids that cannot be overcome by the blepharospasm of a nervous patient. Excessive blepharospasm has been known to break the vacuum of the microkeratome suction ring, resulting in incomplete or free corneal flaps. Locking speculums will also allow for better retraction of the eyelids, which will aid in exposing the eye of patients with narrow palpebral apertures (Figure 3A-2).

2. Length of the speculum blades. Different speculums have varying blade lengths. In eyes with a small palpebral aperture where it is difficult to obtain good exposure of the globe, as in some Asian eyes, it is recommended that the surgeon select a speculum with short blades, such as a Murdoch or Preori speculum, rather than one with long blades like a Liebermann speculum (Figure 3A-2). Using speculums with short blades will provide a larger opening of the palpebral aperture, allowing successful application of the microkeratome suction ring.

With the appropriate choice of a lid speculum for LASIK, the surgeon will be assured of adequate exposure of the eye for application of the suction ring, resulting in the creation of a perfect corneal flap for LASIK in every case.

GENERAL LASIK SURGICAL TECHNIQUE 4

Lucio Buratto, MD and Stephen Brint, MD

INTRODUCTION

This chapter will describe the basic steps in a LASIK (laser-assisted in situ keratomileusis or laser intrastromal keratomileusis) procedure using any of the currently available microkeratomes and lasers. In other chapters, we will describe the technique using two of the more commonly used microkeratomes—the ACS (Automated Corneal Shaper, Bausch & Lomb, Claremont, Calif, USA) and the Hansatome, both used with the Technolas laser. LASIK is currently the most sophisticated evolution of the keratomileusis procedure developed by Barraquer.

The primary lamellar cut may be performed using any type of microkeratome, either manual or automated. The cut is performed either:

1. With a hinge, that is with a subtotal resection of the corneal disc leaving a small peripheral portion connected to the stroma either nasally (nasal hinge) or superiorly (down-up technique). With the hinge, the ablation can only be done in situ, or is on the stromal bed. The hinge technique is currently the preferred technique, with the number of procedures performed in this manner beginning to approach the popularity of the classical nasal hinge. The choice of techniques is largely dependent on the surgeon's availability and choice of microkeratomes.

2. Without a hinge, that is with a complete resection of the corneal flap. This was the original technique of laser intrastromal keratomileusis, as described by Buratto in 1989, in which the operation was performed on the stromal side of a 250 to 300-micron disc that was then replaced with or without sutures. If the free cap was too thin, the ablation was performed in situ, as is now done in a free cap situation. Presently, techniques that do not have a hinge are rarely used and usually are for therapeutic modalities.

GENERAL COMMENTS ABOUT LASIK WITH A CORNEAL HINGE

The refractive ablation of the corneal stroma with the excimer laser following a complete lamellar cut with the microkeratome was initially performed, as described by Buratto, with the ablation on the stromal surface of the disc following a 360° lamellar cut. Pallikaris proposed a hinge that allowed a flap connected to the residual cornea, an idea previously suggested by Barraquer. Surgeons now prefer performing the ablation on the corneal stroma in situ.

The technique involved using a microkeratome fitted with a device that would limit the excursion, thus avoiding a complete cut. In this way, a portion of the corneal disc was not cut and approximately 1.0 mm of disc remained attached to the underlying tissue. This creates a sort of hinge between the stromal bed and the so-called corneal flap (thus the name "hinge technique"). Classically, the hinge both in automated lamellar keratoplasty (ALK) and then in LASIK was located nasally. More recently, as a result of Buratto's idea that a superior hinge is more physiologic, there has been development of microkeratomes that perform the cut from down upward. The development of these new microkeratomes has also made it possible to create larger flaps, in excess of 10 mm diameter, with advantages for the large ablations required in hyperopia and astigmatism.

MICROKERATOME FOR LASIK WITH A NASAL HINGE

This technique can be performed with a number of different microkeratomes.

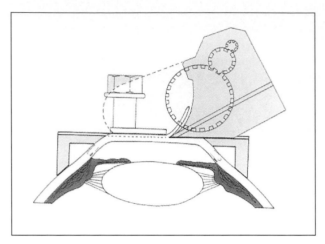

Figure 4-1. The cutting phase: creation of the corneal flap in relation to the ring, plate, blade, and corneal surface.

Automated Microkeratome

The ACS microkeratome is the machine that has been widely available and most frequently used for LASIK, despite no longer being the most modern. It has the following characteristics:

- Electromechanical movement of the metal blade (8000 oscillations per minute).
- Automated forward and reverse movement on the suction ring track (double run direction).
- Stopping the microkeratome pass at a preset point, with an adjustable stop device added to and integrated with the instrument. The flap is thus formed with a hinge. The flap is lifted and placed nasally to expose the underlying stromal tissue for refractive ablation.
- The depth plate can be removed and interchanged. For LASIK, a 160-micron plate is normally used, but 130 or 180 and 200-micron plates are also available for use, as tailored to the flap thickness versus ablation depth, or for enhancements.

In the first generation model, the length of the pass was obtained by adjusting a calibrated micrometric screw on the stop device mounted to the posterior portion of the head. In the later generation of this microkeratome, the stop device is fixed and requires no adjustment. In the earlier model with an adjustable stop, by adjusting the micrometric screw it was possible to move the stopping point forward or backward and identify where the microkeratome pass will be stopped and how large the hinge will be. As the microkeratome moves along the toothed track, it reaches the preset stopping point, and the cut is stopped. At this point, the other footpedal is pressed and the direction is reversed, leaving an intended nasal hinge.

SCMD Microkeratome

Movement of the SCMD metal blade is activated by a turbine fueled by nitrogen protoxide, with an oscillation of 15,000 revolutions per minute (RPM). The advancement of the microkeratome is manual. It is fitted with a stop device that allows the creation of a hinge. Multiple suction rings allow for various flap sizes, and four stop rings are provided to create various hinge sizes. One hundred and thirty and 150 fixed plate microkeratome heads are available.

LKS Moria Microkeratome

A turbine fueled by nitrogen protoxide activates the LKS Moria microkeratome. The blade is metal and oscillates at 14,000 RPM. Advancement of the instrument is manual. The instrument is fitted with an adjustable stop device, and the precalibrated fixed plate heads are available in 130, 160, and 180 microns (see Chapter 18 for more information about this microkeratome).

BKS 1000 Microkeratome

The BKS 1000 is electromechanical using a metal blade. It is fitted with a stop device that restricts the pass of the microkeratome on the ring. The depth plates are interchangeable. Movement is manual.

Clear Corneal Molder

The Clear Corneal Molder microkeratome has an electromechanical movement. A diamond blade with angulation of 0°, as developed by Drs. Nascimento and Guimarres of Brazil, allows the surgeon to observe the cutting. Measurement of the plate varies from 50 to 350 microns and is surgeon controlled.

Phoenix-Universal Keratome

This microkeratome has a piezoelectrical movement of the blade at a high oscillation rate: 14,000 RPM. The Phoenix-Universal was designed for the hinge technique. The plate and ring are fixed. The blade operates parallel to the cut tissue, at 0° angulation. The instrument has a computerized control to regulate resistance and cut speed on the cornea, making it unique compared to the other microkeratomes. It was recently withdrawn from the market.

Eye Technology Microprecision (MKS) Microkeratome

The MKS is activated by turbine propulsion of the blade. It uses a steel blade that oscillates at a very high rate (20,000 RPM) with a 9° attack angle. Advancement s manual. The stop mechanism allows calibration of the hinge technique.

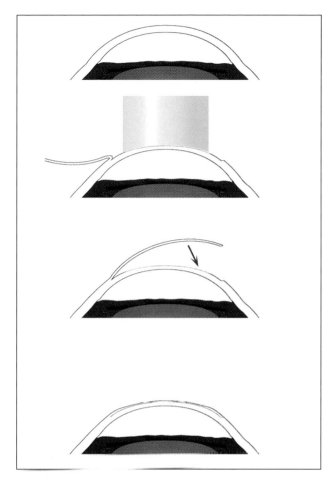

Figure 4-2. Myopic LASIK: basic steps of the operation.

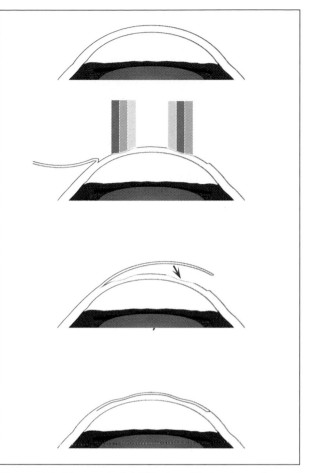

Figure 4-3. Hyperopic LASIK: the ablation is performed largely in the peripheral stroma.

Innovatome Microkeratome

The Innovatome is an automated microkeratome with an electromechanical movement. It is unique in that both blade movement and advancement are cable driven, allowing for a lightweight head. The blade is metal. It has a very high oscillation rate: 12,000 to 15,000 RPM. The fixed plate head is available as 130, 160, or 190 microns.

Summit Krumeich-Barraquer Microkeratome (SKBM)

The SKBM is an electromechanical device with surgeon control of cutting and advancement speeds, which are then automated. Four suction rings to select flap diameter and adjustable hinge size. Fixed 160- and 180-micron heads are available. Multiple suction ports in rings and advancement is disabled if poor suction occurs.

MICROKERATOMES FOR THE SUPERIOR HINGE TECHNIQUE

The Hansatome Microkeratome

This has a completely new design. The motor is placed vertically with respect to the suction ring; the head is one-piece with a fixed plate. The ring has a single track and a pin. The microkeratome is positioned on the suction ring using the pin. It is designed specifically for the superior hinge technique, with simple assembly. An internal control system checks the calibration of the unit prior to each operation. Safety features include a device that will not allow the cut to begin until appropriate levels of vacuum are reached. The cut will be interrupted if vacuum falls below this threshold level. Fixed heads of 160 and 180 microns are available.

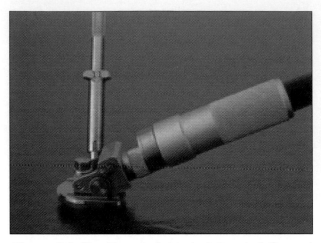

Figure 4-4. The Bausch & Lomb Automated Corneal Shaper.

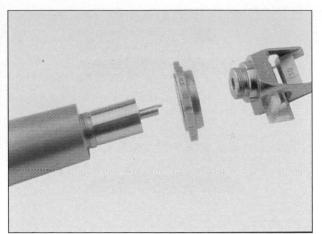

Figure 4-5. Moria's LSK One.

Carriazo Barraquer Microkeratome

This new microkeratome was designed to create a hinge located according to the surgeon's needs. It can therefore produce a superior or nasal hinge, or the hinge can be placed at any location. It uses heads with fixed plates of 130, 160, and 180 microns. It may be used with a manual (turbine) or automated (electrical) movement. The instrument uses the same console as the LKS, the other microkeratome produced by Moria. The blade oscillates at a speed of 14,000 RPM. The head is a single piece and does not require assembly. The head locks into the ring automatically through a bayonet pin (see Chapter 19 for more information about this microkeratome).

CHECKLIST FOR ALL MICROKERATOMES

In order to avoid complications and less than optimal results, it is of fundamental importance to follow a checklist of all the important steps to which every surgeon, even the most expert, must adhere. The surgeon who is just beginning to perform LASIK should pay particular attention to the checklist. It should be easily visible to both surgeon and assistant to facilitate memorization of the steps. Presurgical checks, reduction of lost time, and increased safety are enhanced by following the checklist. Each instrument's checklist will vary slightly.

Microkeratome Checklist

1. The voltage supplied must be appropriate to the machine.
2. Insert connectors and plugs into the appropriate receptacles.

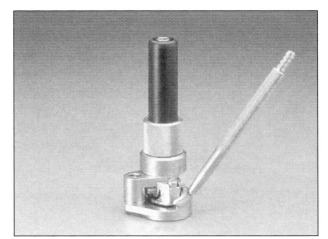

Figure 4-6. Chiron Hansatome for the superior hinge.

3. Connect pedals to the motor and suction console as appropriate.
4. Examine the head of the microkeratome in the open position.
5. Connect the cable of the microkeratome to the power supply.
6. Examine the blade carefully under high magnification and discard if poor.
7. Check that the blade holder moves freely in its groove if the blade holder is a part of the instrument, and that the blade/blade holder moves smoothly if they are a single unit.
8. Attach the blade to the blade holder correctly.
9. Check that the blade and plate have been inserted correctly where applicable and are secure.
10. Apply the stop device and fix it correctly in position (in current models this system is fixed).
11. On a test run, check for smooth movement of the

blade and advancing system that propels movement of the microkeratome.

12. Check that the stop has been calibrated in the appropriate manner on the older models (not necessary on the current models).
13. Connect the motor to the power supply cable.
14. Insert the head into the handle or motor of the microkeratome.
15. Activate the motor and listen to the noise it produces. It should create a buzz or hum that is constant, uniform, with even intensity.
16. Insert the head of the microkeratome in the ring and simulate the forward and backward pass. The movement must be constant and smooth until the head reaches the stop.
17. Ensure the handle is firmly attached to the ring.
18. Connect the suction tubing to the end of the handle.
19. Activate suction and check the value on the display, with and without occlusion.
20. Under the microscope, check the integrity of the tracks and absence of foreign bodies and/or debris that may interfere with correct movement of the microkeratome.

LASERS FOR LASIK

Many lasers are now available worldwide. These include:

Technolas Model 117C and 217

This is a scanning/flying spot laser. It has a fluence of 130 mJ/cm^2 and a pulse frequency of between 20 to 50 Hz. It has an active eye tracker. For myopia, it uses a spiral/random scanning spot; for hyperopia, it uses an annular scanning spot beam; for astigmatism, it is meridional.

Technolas Model 116

This is a broadbeam laser. It has a fluence of 130 mJ/cm^2 and a pulse frequency of between 10 to 40 Hz. The optic zone has a maximum diameter of 7.0 mm. It does not have an eye-tracking system. For myopia, it uses an iris diaphragm; for hyperopia, it uses an annular scanning spot beam; for astigmatism, it is linear.

Nidek

The Nidek laser is a scanning slit-beam laser. It has a fluence of 130 mJ/cm^2 and a pulse frequency of 30 Hz but may reach 46 Hz. The eye tracker is passive. For myopia, it may use an iris diaphragm or a scanning slit rotated through a 120° pass. For hyperopia, it uses an annular scanning slit beam. For astigmatism, it is rotatable.

Meditec

This laser uses a scanning slit beam. It has a fluence of 250 mJ/cm^2 and a frequency of 20 Hz. It does not have eye tracking. For myopia, it uses a rotating shield; for hyperopia, it uses an inverse rotating eye mask; for astigmatism, a variable rotating eye mask is used.

LaserSight

This is a scanning/flying spot laser. Fluence is 160 to 300 mJ/cm^2 and pulse frequency is 100 Hz. The eye tracker is active. For myopia, it uses a linear rotating scanning spot; for hyperopia, it uses an annular scanning spot beam; for astigmatism, it is meridional.

Summit Technology

Summit is a broadbeam laser. Fluence is 180 mJ/cm^2; it has a pulse frequency of 10 Hz. The ablation has a maximum diameter of 6.5 mm, extending to 9.5 mm if using the Axicon lens for hyperopia. It has no eye tracker. For myopia, it uses an iris diaphragm or erodable laser disc; for hyperopia and astigmatism, it uses an erodable laser disc.

Autonomous Tech

This is a scanning/flying spot laser. It has fluence of 180 mJ/cm^2 and pulse frequency of 100 Hz. The eye tracker is active. For myopia, it uses a spiral scanning program; for hyperopia, it uses an annular scanning slit beam; for astigmatism, it is meridional.

VISX

VISX (Santa Clara, Calif, USA) is a broadbeam laser. It has fluence of 160 mJ/cm^2 and a pulse frequency of 5 to 6 Hz that can be increased to 10 Hz. It does not use eye tracking. For myopia, it uses an iris diaphragm; for hyperopia, it uses a rotating scanning slit beam; for astigmatism, it uses sequential and elliptical programs, iris diaphragm, and rotatable slit.

PREOPERATIVE LASER CHECK

Below is a typical laser checklist. The surgeon must check:
- The optical system of the laser for correct functioning
- Fluence testing
- Homogeneity of the beam
- Patient data inserted in the computer is correct and appropriate for the surgical operation and the surgeon's nomogram adjustment (these findings should be checked again by the laser technician, and then checked by the surgeon)

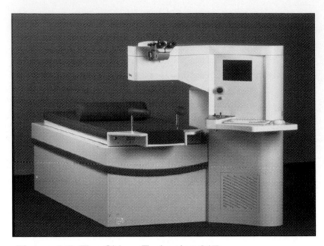

Figure 4-7. The Chiron Technolas 217.

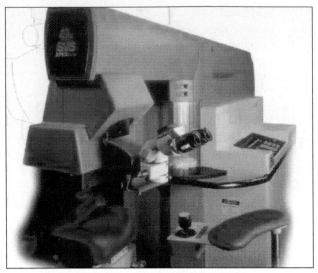

Figure 4-8. The Summit Apex Plus Model B.

- Alignment beams and reticules are concentric with the test ablation
- The refractive cut is correct on the test plates
- Eye tracking if appropriate
- Any necessary gases are flowing at the correct pounds per square inch (psi)

Each laser is subject to a number of steps that must be followed in order to obtain an appropriate calibration. Evaluation must be quantitative (check the fluence) and qualitative (check the homogeneity). The outcome of LASIK requires each pulse to have specific energy and homogeneity. Given that the emission from the laser can vary from time to time and optics degrade, this must be checked at every operating session or between cases, depending on the laser. The software is programmed to deliver a specific number of pulses of a specific shape for each diopter to be corrected; there is an internal monitoring system for fluence; however, an external check is always necessary.

Calibration

Calibration (test for fluence and homogeneity) is similar for every type of laser. Each laser has a target (plate, sheet, block, filter, etc) to ablate, which acts as the parameter to evaluate fluence and uniformity. This target is normally made from polymethylmethacrylate (PMMA) or mylar.

For checking fluence, the surgeon must evaluate whether the number of laser pulses for ablating the target falls within the laser manufacturer's approved range. If the number of pulses for ablating the target is greater than desired, the fluence is low; if the number is less than desired, fluence is high. The surgeon must always allow only a minimum of variability with respect to the desired level. There are two factors that control fluence: voltage and gas. If the fluence is too low, the voltage must be

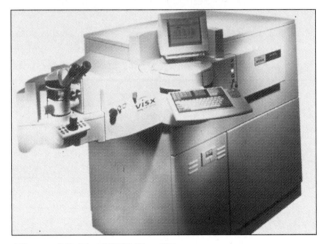

Figure 4-9. The VISX Star S2.

increased; if this is not enough to create an increase in energy emission, the gas must be refreshed/replaced. If this is still not sufficient, it means that there are other problems along the optical pathway of the laser. A technician must be called and the procedure postponed. If an increase in voltage is always required each time the gas is changed to match this desired fluence, it means there is a deterioration of one of the optical components of the laser. The component must be replaced. If the fluence is excessively high, voltage must be reduced. In order to evaluate the beam homogeneity (ie, how evenly the energy is distributed), the surgeon must check the appearance of the ablation is obtained on the target used for the fluence test.

Homogeneity must be evaluated two ways:
- Microuniformity. Any alteration in the microuniformity will appear as localized irregularity of the energy.

- Macrouniformity. Any alteration in the macrouniformity will appear as an irregularity in the pattern of the ablation, which will neither be symmetrical nor asymmetrical. For example, one quadrant is ablated to a greater degree than the others, or alternately, the central ablation is less than the peripheral ablation. Generally speaking, alterations of uniformity are secondary to the deterioration of laser optics.

OUTPATIENT SURGICAL CENTER

LASIK surgery is typically performed in a free-standing laser center, surgery center, or physician's office under topical anesthesia. Rarely, local infiltration anesthesia is used. The patient is at the surgical center for the time necessary for the operation, including preoperative preparation and for 30 to 60 minutes after the operation, at which time the patient can be discharged.

A typical flow pattern for the LASIK procedure could be:

Area 1:
- Reception area for welcoming the patient
- Waiting area where the patient completes the informed consent and other paperwork

Area 2:
- Preoperative area; once the patient has removed his or her jacket, he or she is given a cap, shoes or shoe covers, and, if necessary, a disposable gown, which need not be sterile.

Area 3:
- Laser operating room; it should be equipped to the same standard as a typical surgical room because the entire procedure must be performed in an environment as sterile as possible. The temperature and humidity levels must be constant and appropriate. Generally, the values recommended by the excimer laser manufacturers should be followed. Humidity must be between 20% to 50%; and must never exceed 50%. The temperature must normally be between 18° to 22°C. The operating room must be sterile and the air must be circulated through HEPA filters. It would be advantageous to have an independent electricity source in the event of power failure. Some of the newer microkeratomes have a back-up power source, and laser manufacturers suggest an uninterruptible power supply.
- A scrub area for the surgeon and assistant.
- A room for cleaning and sterilizing instruments.

Area 4:
- Post-procedure area; once the surgery is complet-

Table 4-1

CURRENT LASIK PROCEDURE

The current, normal operation can be summarized as follows:

1. Administer preoperative medication: sedation and preoperative antibiotic and NSAID drops.
2. Administer anesthesia.
3. Position the patient's head parallel to the floor with the cornea perpendicular to the laser beam.
4. Prepare the lids and operating field.
5. Drape the lashes and lid margins.
6. Insert the speculum.
7. Irrigate the cornea and conjunctival cul-de-sac, removing any debris or mucous and check exposure.
8. Reassure the patient.
9. Mark the cornea.
10. Check the microkeratome and its performance in the track.
11. Position the suction ring and, when sure of proper placement, engage suction.
12. Check the IOP with a tonometer (Barraquer-type or pneumotonometer).
13. Moisten the cornea with BSS or a nonsaline solution (topical anesthetic). The amount of moisture depends on the type of microkeratome.
14. Insert/position the microkeratome; check that the depth plate is present and secure.
15. Forward and reverse microkeratome pass.
16. Turn suction off. Remove the ring and microkeratome.
17. Position a sponge or plate and lift the flap with a smooth cannula or spatula.
18. Gently dry the bed.
19. Protect the flap when needed.
20. Create centration according to the laser and engage the eye tracker.
21. Perform photoablation.
22. Wet the stroma.
23. Reposition the flap.
24. Irrigate the interface.
25. Stroke the surface of the flap, edges, and the cornea with a damp Merocel sponge.
26. Perform an adhesion test (eg, striae test).
27. Remove the speculum and drape.
28. Perform the blink test.
29. Medicate.

ed, the patient is asked to rest quietly for 20 to 30 minutes. During this period, the flap position is checked at the slit lamp initially and then again prior to discharge. Postoperative medications are instilled along with postoperative instructions. The patient is then discharged.

PREOPERATIVE MEDICATION

Thirty minutes prior to the operation, one or two drops of topical antibiotic are instilled as prevention against infection and an nonsteroidal anti-inflammatory drug (NSAID) is used to reduce inflammation and postoperative pain. We prefer ofloxacin (Ocuflox, Allergan, Irvine, Calif, USA) and sodium diclofenac.

ANESTHESIA

General anesthesia is currently used only by a handful of surgeons and only under very unusual conditions.

Infiltration anesthesia is also rarely needed. It is performed with a retrobulbar or peribulbar injection. If this induces conjunctival edema, it may be impossible to position the suction ring and achieve adequate suction.

Topical anesthesia made up of 4% lidocaine or 0.5% proparacaine + oxybuprocaine eyedrops—one drop of each 5 minutes prior to the operation and another drop prior to applying the suction ring, or 0.5% proparacaine alone. This is currently the most popular method of anesthesia. Instillation is started when the patient is positioned at the operating table and is followed by adding anesthetic to the conjunctival limbus by means of a sponge soaked in 4% lidocaine or 0.5% proparacaine. This avoids excessive instillation of anesthetic to the cornea, which has a certain degree of epithelial toxicity. If the epithelium is damaged, it may create problems during the lamellar cut, during manipulation of the flap, during short- and long-term wound healing.

POSITIONING THE PATIENT AND PREPARING THE EYE

The patient should be positioned on the operating chair/table in a comfortable position that will ensure a stable, immobile, and appropriate position for the entire operation. The patient should be advised to assume a comfortable and quiet position and to not move his or her arms and legs during the operation. The patient's head must be positioned so that the invisible line that unites the forehead and chin through the center of the nose is perpendicular to the operating microscope and laser beam and parallel to the floor. The head must not be rotated or inclined. The fellow eye is covered with an opaque plastic shield to prevent cross fixation and to prevent the drape from touching the lashes, inducing blinking and discomfort.

PREPARATION OF THE OPERATING FIELD

The periocular skin is cleaned with a solution of Betadine (Purdue Frederick, Norwalk, Conn), being careful not to allow it into the eye, as it is toxic to the epithelium. The skin is then dried with sterile gauze. Trimming the lashes is almost never necessary because of the use of adhesive plastic drapes. However, it may be useful to cut the more temporal eyelashes prior to the lamellar cut as they may interfere with correct passage of the microkeratome. If this is the case, it is better to cut them one by one, only if needed. A true trichotomy is not recommended because of itching that is generally perceived at the eyelid margin postoperatively, leading to rubbing, hence possible flap dislocation.

The eyelashes must be excluded from the operating field by a drape to increase sterility and because they may interfere with proper movement of the microkeratome. If necessary, Steristrips may be used to obtain greater retraction of the eyelids. The adhesive drape must be applied carefully in a way that both covers and retracts the lids. We recommend the 3M 1020 drape.

Steridrape

Application of the Drape

In order to cover the eyelashes and skin, a drape with a central fenestration is preferable; the patient is asked to open his or her eyes wide, then the drape is applied to the lower eyelid, including the eyelashes. The same procedure is performed on the upper eyelids. The drape must be sterile. Lateral pouches to collect residual liquid or other materials (sponges, etc) may be useful or gauze may be placed under the edge of the patient's cap over the ear. Alternately, the drape may be without a fenestration but fitted with an adhesive area. The central adhesive area of the sterile drape is applied while the patient keeps both eyes wide open. In this way the drape adheres well to the superior and inferior eyelashes; then the drape is cut in the intercanthal opening with scissors to expose the corneal surface (taking care not the damage the epithelial surface). When the speculum is positioned, both sides of the adhesive part will be folded under to exclude the superior and inferior eyelashes from the operating field.

Corneal exposure must be optimal and centered. The surgeon should be able to see an equal amount of sclera both inferiorly and superiorly to ensure that the head position is optimal and the cornea will be perpendicular to the laser beam.

Further Thoughts on Anesthesia

Lucio Buratto, MD

When the speculum has been positioned, additional drops of anesthetic are applied to the conjunctival fornix (avoid reaching the cornea). They are allowed to act for 30 to 40 seconds. This will contribute to a reduction in sensations caused by the speculum.

Two microsponges may be wet with abundant anesthetic; one is placed superiorly and the other is placed inferiorly. They are removed and wet again with anesthetic, then applied nasally and temporally and allowed to act for 30 to 40 seconds each time. This will contribute to reducing the irritation caused by the suction ring.

To the perilimbal conjunctiva, apply a sponge ring (Chayet type) soaked in anesthetic and allow it to remain for 30 to 40 seconds; during this time, the cornea can be wet and protected by one to two drops of monodose artificial tears. If the patient is unusually anxious, it may be useful to perform deeper conjunctival anesthesia. This is done by inserting two Merocel sponge fragments soaked in anesthetic into the superior and inferior fornix. The eyelids are then closed using Steristrips and an active eye pressure pad is applied for 10 to 15 minutes (the cornea is first protected with a drop of high density adhesive artificial tears). The eye pressure pad facilitates the spread of anesthetic to the deep globe conjunctiva and provides an excellent level of anesthesia comparable to subtenons. The applied pressure must be only moderate, otherwise when IOP is reduced there may be some difficulty in raising the pressure sufficiently when the suction ring is applied, which will create problems during the microkeratome cut. In the event of a significant drop in IOP, the suction must be allowed to engage for an extra 10 to 20 seconds prior to performing the microkeratome cut.

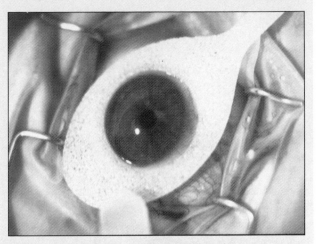

Figure 4A-1. Keracel sponge soaked in anesthetic is applied on the conjunctiva.

Particularly in these rare cases, intraoperative tonometry must be performed prior to performing the cut.

If the patient is hyperactive and has a tendency to blink or squeeze, eyelid akinesia may be necessary (van Lint technique); this may be followed by conjunctival anesthesia, as mentioned.

Peribulbar, retrobulbar, or subtenon's infiltration anesthesia should be avoided because it may create conjunctival edema, which in turn will make adhesion of the suction ring difficult. This form of anesthesia also makes it impossible for the patient to correctly fixate, making correct centration of the ablation less predictable. Rarely is an injection of BSS (containing some drops of anesthetic agent) necessary in order to proptose the globe when it is particularly enophthalmic or sunken in its orbit.

Placement of the Speculum

Lancaster, Buratto, or Liebermann-type speculums with a locking adjustment are most frequently used. The surgeon frees and opens the two arms of the speculum using the adjustment screw to adapt it to the patient's eyelid opening. The arms of the speculum are introduced individually under the edges of the eyelids, assisted by lid retraction and avoiding contact with the corneal surface. The instrument is centered within the interpalpebral space, and then the screw is turned until the arms sufficiently open the eyelids. The eyelids must be opened far enough to allow correct application of the suction ring and unobstructed use of the microkeratome. The speculum must not be too loose or too tight; perfect tension must provide centration and balance of the speculum. Incorrect adjustment may cause displacement, decentration, or loss of the speculum during the operation, sometimes with severe consequences.

It may be necessary to vary the type of speculum, for example, to use a pediatric type on patients with very small fissures. It is helpful to have several types of speculums available. The Barraquer wire type is helpful in small orbits and can be pushed backward with the placement of the suction ring on top of it to achieve exposure and suction. The patient must be strictly cautioned not to blink in this situation.

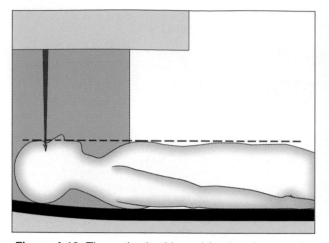

Figure 4-10. The patient's chin and forehead are on the same plane and the eye is positioned exactly below the laser.

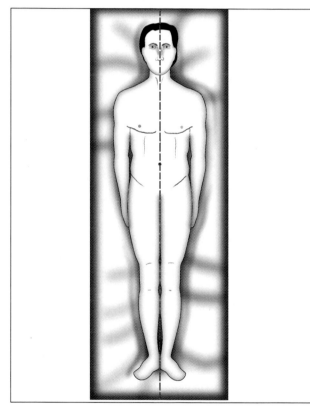

Figure 4-11. Correct positioning of the patient's head and body with respect to the laser.

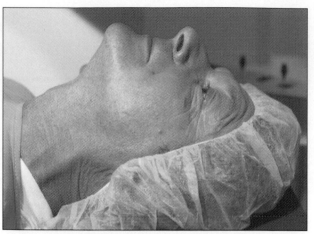

Figure 4-12. The patient's chin is too high and, as a result, the eye does not appropriately fixate on the laser fixation light.

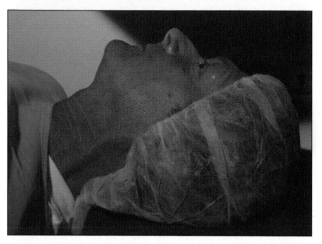

Figure 4-13. The head is rotated to the right and the chin is raised, which may lead to decentration and error of the axis.

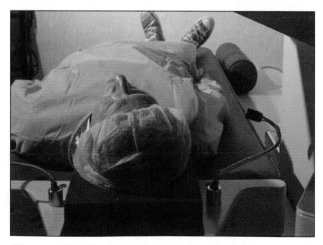

Figure 4-14. The head is rotated to the left; as a result the astigmatic ablation will be off-axis and the spherical ablation will be decentered. In addition, the patient position is not comfortable.

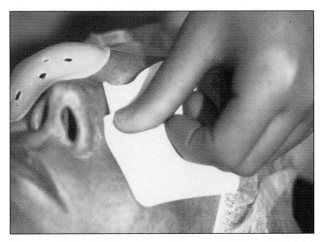

Figure 4-15. Lint-free drape in a synthetic material to clean the eyelids in preparation for the operation.

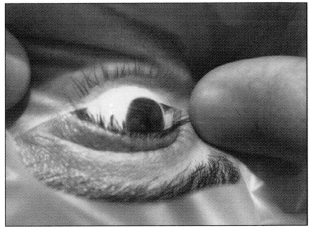

Figure 4-16. Positioning the sterile drape to exclude the eyelashes from the operating field. The same maneuver is used for the upper eyelid.

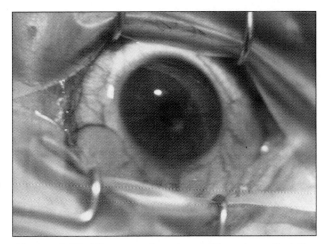

Figure 4-17. The speculum is positioned so that the drape covers the eyelashes and excludes them from the surgical field.

Irrigation of the Cornea and Conjunctival Sac and Maintaining Exposure

The exposed cornea and conjunctiva are irrigated using balanced salt solution (BSS), removing residual fluid, secretions, and debris using Merocel sponges. During this maneuver, the surgeon observes the patient's reaction to touch and manipulation. This gives the surgeon an idea of the patient's apprehension and ability to cooperate. If there is poor exposure, the first thing that must be done is try to create downward pressure on the suction ring in order to proptose the globe and improve exposure, then change the speculum (the Barraquer speculum is an alternative) If it is still not adequate, a retrobulbar injection of BSS or BSS and anesthetic may be necessary to increase the intrapalpebral space necessary for correct positioning of the instruments. This risk of injection in long myopic eyes greatly limits its use, as

well as the chance of inducing chemosis. Rarely, a lateral canthotomy may be necessary following adequate surface and deep infiltration lid anesthesia. Even more rarely, it may be necessary to proceed without the speculum, in which case the assistant keeps the patient's eyes open manually. However, only expert surgeons should treat cases of this type.

Paracentral Marking

In the past, the Ruiz paracentral marker was the most frequently used. Currently, the Buratto, Machat, and Slade markers are more popular. These are wiped with gentian violet and then applied to a dry cornea. These markers must be used on the portion of the cornea opposite the hinge. The marker must be applied carefully and gently (without damaging the epithelium) so that the marks are visible throughout the procedure. The corneal surface is then irrigated to remove excess dye, alcohol or dry residue and the conjunctiva is swabbed using Merocel sponges. If there is a significant degree of preoperative astigmatism associated with the ametropia, it may be useful to make the astigmatic axis using the Mendez ring positioned on the sclerocorneal plane. The keratometric and topographical reading and using preoperative marking with the patient at the slit lamp with identify this meridian. This may facilitate cylindrical ablation with the laser.

Patient Reassurance Prior to Suction Ring Application

Speak to the patient with a soothing, gentle voice and tell him or her that:
- The operation will be short
- He or she will feel slight pressure on the eye
- He or she will hear the vacuum pump

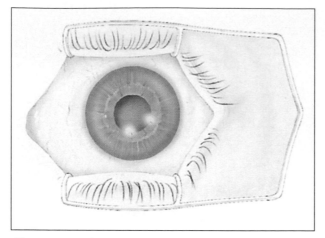

Figure 4-18. Correct position of the speculum: the two arms will produce a symmetrical opening of the eyelids and the cornea will be equidistant from both.

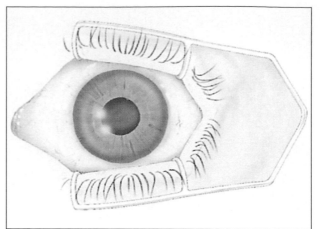

Figure 4-19. The arms of the speculum are positioned incorrectly creating a poor opening of the eyelids temporally.

- The fixation light of the laser may fade in and out for a few moments
- He or she will smell a burning hair-type odor
- He or she should relax and lie quietly with both eyes wide open
- During suction, there may be transitory amaurosis
- During the laser treatment, he or she should keep staring at the fixation light

If necessary, a member of the staff can hold the patient's hand for a few minutes during the procedure to calm and reassure.

Positioning the Suction Ring

The suction ring is applied and positioned on the eye. The ring is placed at the sclerocorneal plane and carefully centered on the basis of the previous paraperipheral epithelial marking, decentering it slightly either nasally or superiorly depending on the type of hinge to be created (nasal or superior). Also, placement should be based on the keratometry readings, with steeper corneas (> 44.00) producing larger flaps with larger hinges and requiring more decentration, and flatter corneas (< 42.00) producing smaller flaps with smaller hinges thus requiring more perfect centration. This allows the surgeon to perform the ablation, even with large zones, while protecting the underside of the overturned flap.

The suction ring should be firmly placed on the globe. Pushing on the appropriate pedal then activates suction. The surgeon ensures that the ring is well-adhered to the globe by simulating small displacements and observing the slight mydriasis induced by the suction itself. The surgeon should remember that redundant conjunctiva can produce the false sensation that the suction ring has adhered to the globe by obstructing the suction

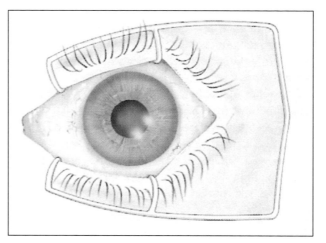

Figure 4-20. The arms of the speculum do not open the eyelids appropriately nasally.

orifice. If this is the case, intraocular pressure, as measured with the surgical tonometer, will be insufficient.

The Microkeratome

The surgeon should have checked, once again, that:
- The microkeratome is functioning correctly
- The plate has been inserted and seated correctly (if the machine has a removable plate)
- The microkeratome stop mechanism has been calibrated so that at least 1.0 to 1.2 mm of tissue remains uncut at the end of the microkeratome pass (if the instrument has an adjustable stop device)—this applies for both nasal and superior hinges
- If the surgeon hears any strange noises during microkeratome testing, the cause should be determined and corrected, or a different microkeratome used

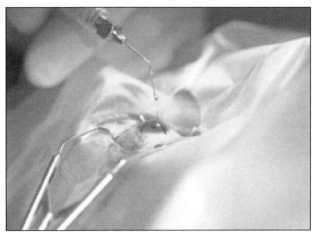

Figure 4-21. Once the speculum has been positioned, the corneal surface and conjunctiva should be irrigated.

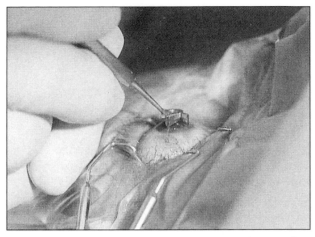

Figure 4-22. Epithelial marking with Asico's three-radius marker: the cornea is dried with a sponge tip prior to marking.

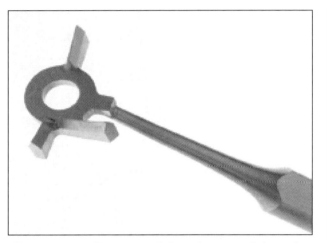

Figure 4-23. Buratto radial and pararadial marker (Asico).

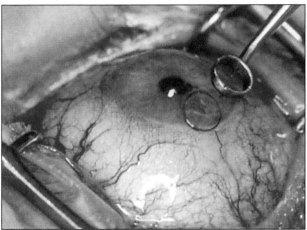

Figure 4-24. Temporal circular marking for the LASIK nasal hinge technique.

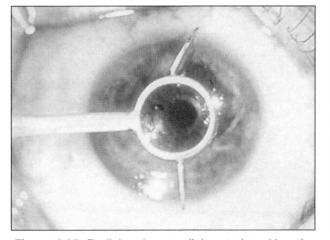

Figure 4-25. Radial and pararadial central marking: the latter was done to avoid the incorrect upside-down positioning of a free cap (epithelium below and the stroma above).

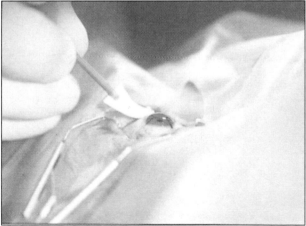

Figure 4-26. The fluid in the conjunctival sac is dried with a Merocel sponge tip, which also removes secretions and debris.

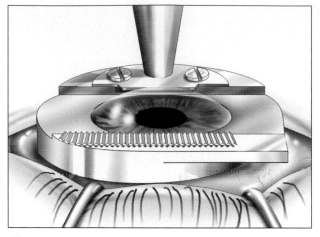

Figure 4-27. The suction ring is correctly positioned on the globe.

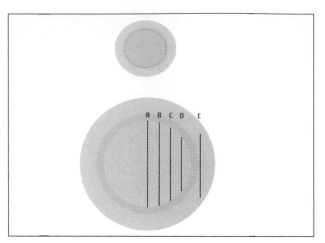

Figure 4-28. The stop device must be positioned in order to produce a proper hinge: position D is correct.

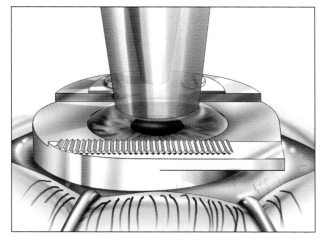

Figure 4-29. Tonometry: the cornea must be almost dry during the correct performance of this test.

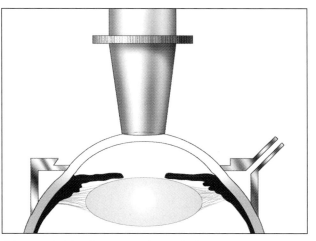

Figure 4-30. Cross-section of the tonometer. The tonometer must be exactly vertical with respect to the center of the corneal surface and positioned over the pupillary area.

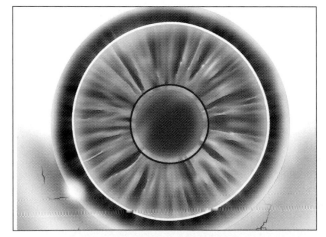

Figure 4-31. Tonometry: the applanated area has the correct diameter. It indicates that the pressure has reached required levels of about 65 mm Hg.

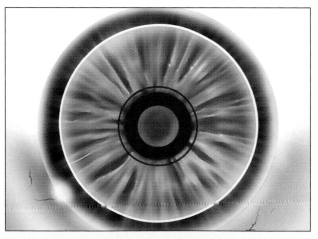

Figure 4-32. The applanated area is much smaller than the circumference in the lower part of the tonometer. The pressure is greater than necessary. One should keep suction on for a short time.

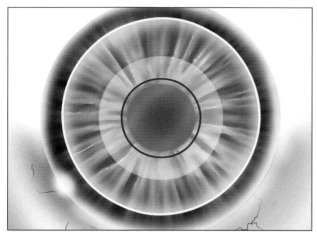

Figure 4-33. The applanated area is larger than the circumference of the tonometer. The pressure is lower than necessary—do not proceed with the cut.

Tonometry

Tonometry is performed using a Barraquer tonometer on a dry cornea or the pneumotonometer. It should indicate a value of at least 60 to 65 mm Hg, confirmed by the fact that the area of applanated cornea must lie well inside the circular grid on the applanating surface of the tonometer. Many expert surgeons no longer perform tonometry, relying on digital touch and pupil dilation with the patient reporting amaurosis. However, this step is indispensable for inexperienced surgeons for at least their first 200 cases. We feel that this step should always be performed, as good suction is critical to a good cut. In the latest generation microkeratomes, pressure is continually monitored using instrumentation incorporated into the machine. The vacuum values are displayed on the console. However, this measures pressure in the tubing, not ocular pressure. Redundant conjunctiva may give pseudosuction. Tonometry must be repeated if there is any manipulation of the eyelids, the drape, or the suction ring.

Wetting the Corneal Surfaces

The suction ring track is slightly moistened with distilled water or, better yet, topical glycerine-based anesthetic (proparacaine), to allow the microkeratome to advance more smoothly. The cornea is also wet to allow the plate to pass more smoothly over the epithelial surface. Excess fluid is removed using a Merocel sponge to prevent it from being thrown by the gears of the microkeratome onto the optics/mirrors of the laser, thus disturbing beam quality.

Placing the Microkeratome on the Suction Ring

The microkeratome is inserted in the track of the suction ring from a temporal direction for the nasal hinge technique. The gears should engage the teeth of the suction ring if this type of microkeratome is used. If a microkeratome for a superior hinge is used, its head must be inserted vertically on the pin of the suction ring. The surgeon should be comfortable when performing the cut and ensure that there are no obstructions in advancement of the instrument. The surgeon's arm may rest comfortably on the armrests of the surgical chair, adjusted to the appropriate height. The surgical gown, power cables, and suction tubing must be free and not interfering with the surgeon's arm movements. All the connection systems (cables, connection cords, and tubing) must be able to move freely. This also applies to the footpedal that controls microkeratome movement, which must be positioned comfortably to allow the surgeon to easily activate it.

Performing the Cut: Initial, Intermediate, and Final Steps, and Microkeratome Return

Prior to beginning the lamellar cut, the patient must be warned that he or she will hear noises and perceive vibrations. This helps prepare the patient and reduce anxiety and unexpected movement when the motor is activated. This noise should be demonstrated to the patient with a count down "1-2-3… buzz." The head of the microkeratome is brought into contact with the ring. The motor may be activated for 1 to 2 seconds, and the microkeratome is allowed to complete 1.0 to 2.0 mm of the pass. In this position, the microkeratome is ready to perform the cut. The surgeon ensures that the plate is firmly inserted in the head of the microkeratome if the instrument is fitted with removable plates. The footpedal, which activates forward progression of the microkeratome, is pushed and the cut is performed until the stop engages. If the instrument is manual, the surgeon smoothly moves the instrument with the surgeon's arm in a neutral position to reach the stop device.

Once the microkeratome has completed its pass, the reverse pedal is pushed to allow the return of the microkeratome to its starting position. Some microkeratomes have an automated return function. If the instrument is manual, the surgeon reverses it to its initial position.

Suction Ring and Microkeratome Removal

The suction pump is deactivated; the suction ring and

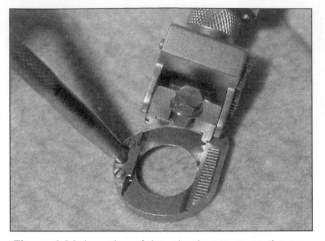

Figure 4-34. Insertion of the microkeratome on the suction ring: the microkeratome is tilted and inserted in the track on the toothed side.

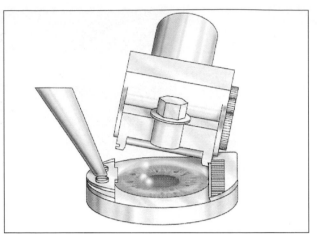

Figure 4-35. First, the surgeon inserts the part of the microkeratome where the gears are located; the head remains tilted.

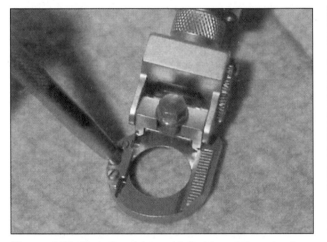

Figure 4-36. Both the right and left sides of the microkeratome rest on the suction ring.

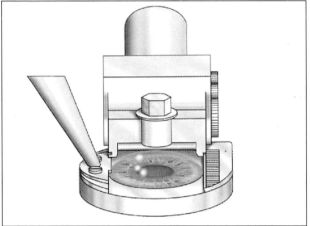

Figure 4-37. The head is then straightened and inserted in the track, allowing it to rest flat in the ring.

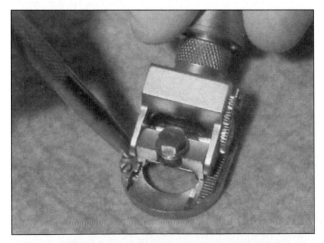

Figure 4-38. The microkeratome advances until the two lateral wings are correctly inserted on the ring.

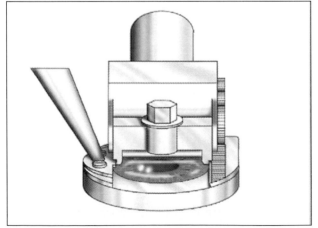

Figure 4-39. Finally, the head is moved forward along the track to insert the microkeratome gears on the teeth of the track.

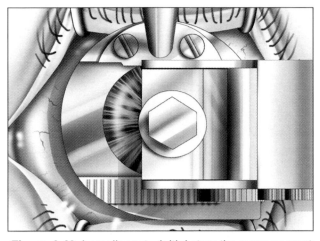

Figure 4-40. Lamellar cut—initial step: the surgeon must ensure that the microkeratome advances at a uniform speed and the pass is obstruction-free.

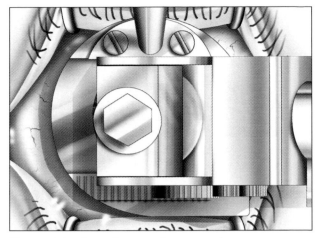

Figure 4-41. Lamellar cut—last step: the surgeon must have a reference point on the ring that will indicate the true stopping point.

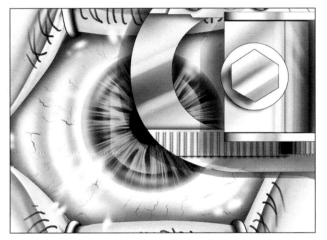

Figure 4-42. Removal of the microkeratome and the suction ring together; alternately, the microkeratome can be removed first, followed by the ring.

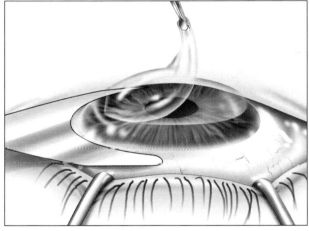

Figure 4-43. Lifting the flap with atraumatic nontoothed forceps.

microkeratome are removed carefully, usually as a unit. These are handed to the assistant, who will ensure they are disassembled, cleaned, and sterilized at the end of surgery.

LIFTING THE CORNEAL FLAP

At the end of the primary keratectomy, the corneal flap is overturned nasally onto the perilimbal conjunctival surface. A blunt smooth spatula or smooth open forceps, without grasping the flap, is used. The flap is reflected nasally onto the conjunctiva or a sponge. If the cut was done using the superior hinge (down-up technique), the flap will be reflected superiorly and retracted using a flap retractor. Some surgeons feel it is better not to allow the flap to rest on the conjunctiva. Some surgeons position the flap on a metal instrument with a half-

moon shape. This is to prevent the epithelial and stromal portions of the reflected flap from coming into contact with the conjunctiva, which can become contaminated with secretions or debris, increasing the chance of debris in the interface. Some surgeons keep the suction ring in position, deactivating or lowering suction (available with some microkeratomes) and positioning the flap nasally on the ring itself. This, however, requires one of the surgeon's hands to continue holding the ring, leaving it unavailable for other maneuvers. Some surgeons place a piece of Merocel sponge nasally and rest the flap on it; the problem with the sponge is that, by absorbing liquid, it will swell and may fold the flap and overhydrate it. It is important to avoid epithelial trauma to the flap surface or residual cornea. Postoperatively, this will create foreign body sensation and tearing and will make flap adhesion to the underlying bed more difficult.

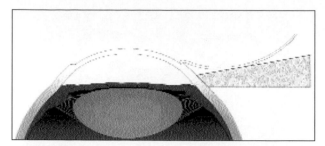

Figure 4-44. The flap is placed on a sponge. Initially this is fine.

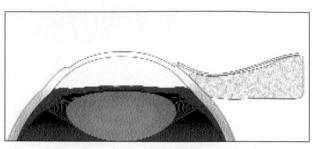

Figure 4-45. The sponge then absorbs liquid and swells, causing flap edema. This is not acceptable.

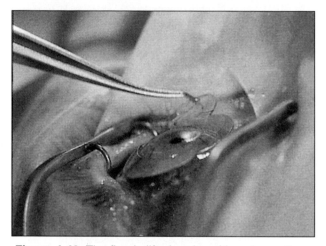

Figure 4-46. The flap is lifted and positioned nasally on a flap positioner.

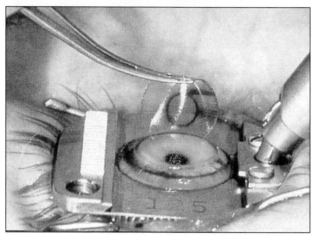

Figure 4-47. Lifting the flap and positioning it on the suction ring. In this case, the suction ring stays in position even during the ablation phase (without suction being active).

If the cut has created a free cap, the cap will be attached to the head of the microkeratome; in this case, it should be delicately removed and placed in an antidesiccation chamber until it is replaced. The transfer should be with a fenestrated spatula or toothless Buratto or similar forceps (Janach, Como, Italy; and Asico, Westmont, Ill).

The diameter of the obtained flap may be measured and the shape of the noted resection. This examination should be brief to avoid dehydration and excessive exposure.

DRYING THE IN SITU STROMAL SURFACE

The stromal surface is carefully, but quickly and evenly, dried with a Merocel sponge prior to performing the refractive cut (ie, the in-situ laser ablation). A damp stromal surface will reduce the ablative effect. During the ablation, fluid typically accumulates centrally with broadbeam lasers. This is the probable cause of central islands.

Another area where fluid not originating from the ablation accumulates is close to the hinge; again, it should be dried carefully. The desired correction, optic zone, and blend parameters have been input into the laser's computer and should once again be checked according to patient's chart or laser worksheet.

PROTECTING THE FLAP

During the ablation, particularly when a large optic zone or astigmatic ablation is performed, the surgeon must protect the internal surface of the corneal flap and hinge to avoid the ablation striking the area. There are some tips that may be helpful in doing this:

- Retract the flap with an appropriate instrument that will also protect the stromal surface (the Buratto or similar spatula).
- Retract and shield the flap with a Merocel sponge. The unwieldy shape, size, and swelling renders it somewhat unstable, thus it is not the technique of choice.

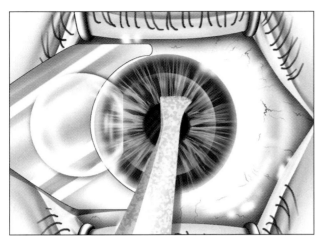

Figure 4-48. Prior to starting the ablation and in the interval between each ablation phase, the in-situ superficial stroma is carefully dried.

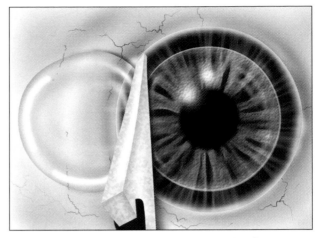

Figure 4-49. During the ablation phase, the flap stroma must be protected from the effects of the ablation. This can be done with a sponge or by means of a special instrument.

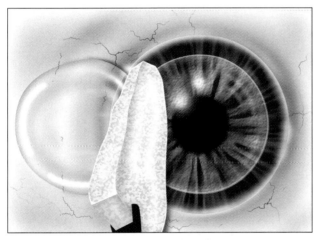

Figure 4-50. The sponge absorbs liquid and expands, reducing the ablation zone. Protecting the hinge with a sponge is therefore not the best technique.

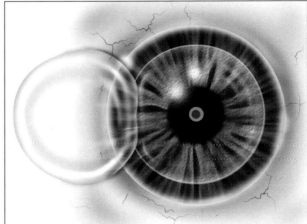

Figure 4-51. Prior to performing the ablation, the laser beam must be focused. The two focus targets must be superimposed.

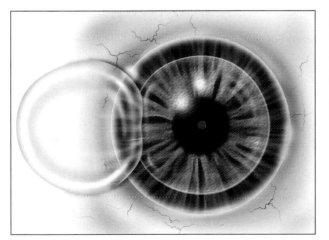

Figure 4-52. The aiming beam.

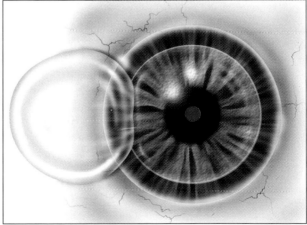

Figure 4-53. The two focus targets are turned off and the eye tracker light is turned on. When this is well-centered on the prepupillary area, the eye tracker will be fixed.

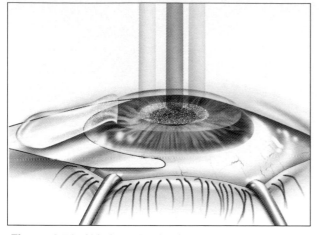

Figure 4-54. Ablation with the flying spot while the flap rests on the flap positioner without hinge protection.

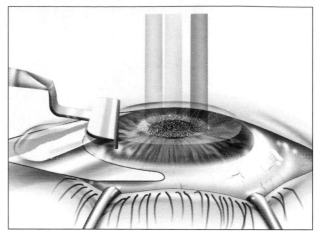

Figure 4-55. Protection of the flap with the Buratto retractor/protector.

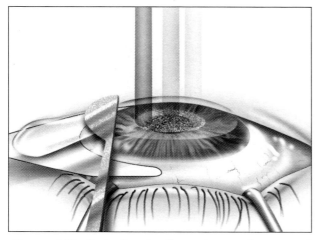

Figure 4-56. Protecting the flap using another type of Buratto spatula, randomized flying spot ablation.

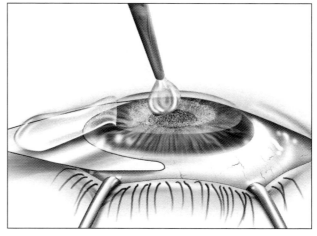

Figure 4-57. Following the ablation, one drop of BSS is applied to the stroma. It is spread evenly over the stromal surface.

PATIENT FIXATION

The patient must be able to see the fixation light and maintain fixation. He or she should be warned that the aiming beam will be blurred when the flap is elevated and may occasionally fade out. The laser aiming system must be centered on the center of the pupil. The magnification of the microscope is adjusted and brightness is set at the appropriate level to obtain good contrast on the stroma without creating too much glare for the patient, who must maintain good fixation. If the laser has an eye-tracking device, this is now adjusted and engaged. The eye tracker is a system of high-speed image sequences that tracks the center of the pupil and allows the laser treatment to be well-centered. Once the center has been identified, the eye tracker follows eye movements and adjusts the laser beam so that the laser shots will be directed on the most appropriate corneal zone.

PERFORMING THE ABLATION

To correct severe ametropias, in order to avoid an excessively deep ablation, many surgeons who use broadbeam lasers prefer to perform the ablation with two or more optic zones, which creates a gradual, more uniform ablation of the corneal tissue. Normally, a blend zone is created as the final transition zone to produce a more uniform ablation (6.0 to 7.0 mm). Alternately, an aspheric ablation may be used. With the scanning lasers (slit or spot), the beam scans the corneal surface, creating a more precise and smoother ablation profile compared to the multizone technique of broadbeam lasers. Moreover, scanning laser ablation is more homogeneous because this type of laser makes better use of the more homogeneous, small, central portion of the beam. With astigmatism associated with spherical treatment, by ablating one meridian more than the opposite, the pho-

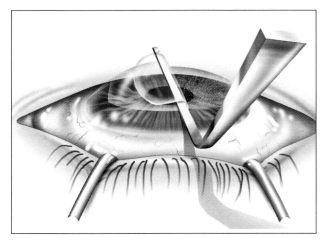

Figure 4-58. The flap is repositioned with the same cannula that was used to place a drop of BSS on the stroma or with an appropriate spatula.

toablation extends peripherally. The surgeon is thus advised to keep in mind the necessary measures to protect the nasal hinge and flap.

At completion of every ablation zone or ablation phase with lasers that sequence between zones, it is useful to gently wipe the surface with a sponge or spatula to remove the layer of fluid that may form. This helps prevent central islands (along with use of the pretreatment software).

Scanning lasers (slit or spot) have the advantage of not requiring pretreatment. Regardless, at the flap hinge there will be a tendency for fluid to accumulate and this must always dried.

WETTING THE STROMA

Once the ablation has been completed, most surgeons wet the stromal interface with a drop of BSS that is gently and evenly spread over the surface. This will encourage distention of the flap, allowing the flap to "float," easily and evenly on the stromal bed. The flap will automatically return to its original position. Alternately, a drop of BSS can be placed on the stromal bed prior to flipping it back; the flap will tend to reposition itself correctly on the cornea.

REPOSITIONING THE FLAP

Finally, the flap is gently raised and repositioned back to its original position using a specific spatula or closed forceps. The spatula is inserted under the flap on the epithelial surface close to the hinge. At this point, the flap is pulled toward the center of the cornea. The layer of liquid on the stroma facilitates its repositioning. Using the same spatula or a closed McPherson forceps, the flap is carefully distended with a repeat movement from the

hinge toward the opposite corneal bed. If the flap had been resting on a metal surface, it may have adhered to it during the time it was left in contact. The surgeon, in this situation, can pass an irrigating cannula under the flap to detach it from the flap positioner.

IRRIGATION OF THE INTERFACE

The surgeon now removes the metal plate or sponge that supported the flap. After repositioning the flap, the interface is irrigated to remove any debris or epithelial cells so that the cornea will be perfectly clear and transparent postoperatively and epithelial ingrowth is minimized. This irrigation also facilitates spontaneous repositioning of the flap on its bed, with perfect alignment. A special interface cannula is used for this type of irrigation, such as the Slade or Buratto. The same cannula may be used to gently massage the flap from the hinge toward the opposite side of the cornea in order to remove excess BSS from the interface. In addition to facilitating perfect realignment of the two stromal surfaces, this reduces postoperative flap edema and prevents fluid from becoming trapped in the interface.

DRYING THE FLAP SURFACES AND EDGES

Drying the Corneal Surface

Using a moistened, expanded Merocel sponge, the flap is then gently "painted" by performing a repetitive gentle movement, first from the hinge toward the opposite direction (up-down in the down-up technique; from nasal to temporal in the nasal hinge technique). After the flap is well-aligned and begins to adhere, the movement is changed to other radial directions. This contributes to obtaining a homogeneous and uniform distension of the flap in all directions with complete filling of the bed and a symmetrical, even gutter.

The surgeon must ensure that the flap adheres well to the underlying surface. A number of tests may be used to do this:
- The cornea is completely dehydrated by means of filtered low-power compressed air. This air flow is directed onto the epithelium until the tissue appears to be dry; while this method produces perfect adhesion of the flap to the underlying cornea, it also involves flap dehydration and shrinkage, which may lead to flap retraction; thus, we prefer to avoid this technique or use for only a few seconds.
- The cornea is allowed to dry spontaneously with

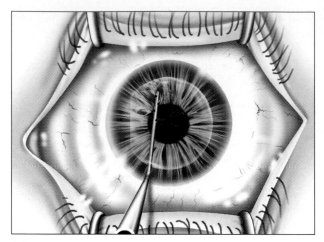

Figure 4-59. The interface is carefully washed with an irrigating multihole cannula.

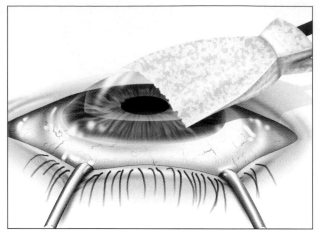

Figure 4-60. The corneal surface is gently dried and distended with a damp sponge to avoid any epithelial trauma.

the eyelids open for 1 to 5 minutes, with the speculum still in position. The cornea will dry spontaneously, allowing the flap to firmly and progressively adhere to the underlying stroma. The central cornea may be kept moist with a drop of BSS or methylcellulose.

- The amount of time required for adhesion varies depending on the site of the hinge, the size of the flap, its thickness, and the quality of the cut, whether the epithelium is intact or not, and the amount of flap edema. The time also varies from surgeon to surgeon, depending on personal experience and comfort. The minimum time required is 1 minute; the maximum is normally around 5 minutes. It may be shorter if the hinge is superior, the flap is large, when there is perfect alignment of the flap, when the flap has minimal edema, and when the epithelium is intact.

ADHESION TESTS

After about 2 minutes, the surgeon checks adhesion. This is performed by exerting pressure slightly peripheral to the edge of the keratectomy with a dry Merocel sponge, an olive-tipped spatula, or a closed McPherson forceps. If there is good adhesion of the flap, fine folds with radiate into the flap (striae test). Under high magnification, the surgeon checks that the flap is well repositioned perfectly aligned and distended. The edge of the flap and margin of resection at the edge of the bed match perfectly with the width being perfectly symmetrical (gutter test). If there is any doubt, the surgeon should lift the flap and repeat the steps of irrigation, repositioning, and smoothing/painting/distending the flap. All of the adhesion tests should be rechecked.

REMOVAL OF THE SPECULUM AND DRAPE

Speculum removal must be done very carefully; the surgeon's fingers must guide the arms of the instrument while the assistant retracts the eyelids, avoiding any contact with the cornea. It may be useful to ask the patient to look in the opposite direction of the removal. It is better to remove the lower arm first, and then the upper one, after tension on the locking screw is slowly released.

The drape must also be removed very carefully. It is helpful to remove if from nasal to temporal while keeping the patient's lids open with the thumb and forefinger of the opposite hand. Instruct patients not to squeeze, as they sometimes tend to do so as the drape is being removed.

BLINK TEST

Adhesion of the flap to the stromal bed is checked once again. The patient is asked to blink repeatedly, without squeezing. Watch for flap stability at this time. Some surgeons apply a plastic shield or dark glasses to protect the eye against involuntary trauma. Others will check the flap, ask the patient to rest with the eyes closed for 15 to 20 minutes, and then check the flap again before the patient is released.

MEDICATION

One to two drops of sterile broad-spectrum antibiotic eyedrops, a drop of corticosteroid, and a drop of NSAID are instilled at the conclusion of the procedure.

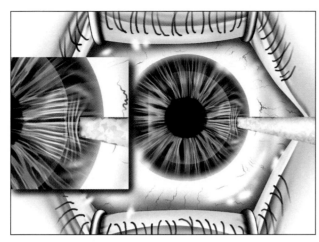

Figure 4-61. Slade striae test: the peripheral cornea is gently depressed and the radiating striae into the flap indicate adhesion.

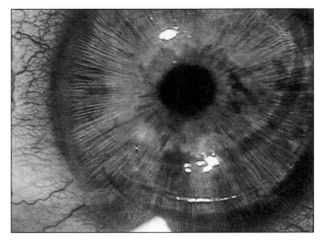

Figure 4-62. Striae test to check adhesion of the flap.

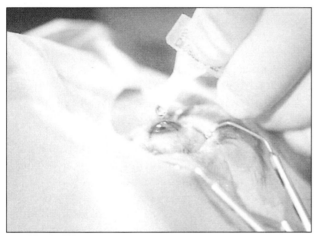

Figure 4-63. Medication with single-dose antibiotic eyedrops (ofloxacin) and an NSAID (Voltaren).

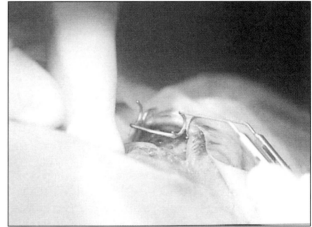

Figure 4-64. The speculum is gently removed, avoiding contact or displacement of the flap.

POSTOPERATIVE EXAM AND INSTRUCTIONS

At this point, the patient is transferred to the postoperative area. The flap may be checked, then the patient is asked to rest with the eyes closed. About 20 to 30 minutes later, the eye is examined at the slit lamp. If the flap is perfect and free of interface debris, the patient is discharged.

The patient is advised not to rub his or her eye. To avoid this happening, he or she is advised to wear dark glasses during the day and a protective shield at night for 4 to 7 days. The patient is also given medication instructions, including:

- Antibiotic eyedrops
- Corticosteroid eyedrops
- NSAID eyedrops if necessary

- Lubricating eyedrops are especially important during the first 2 weeks due to corneal denervation (particularly if the patient normally wears contact lenses)

Finally, the patient is advised to sleep for 3 to 4 hours after surgery. This will facilitate flap adhesion and allow re-epithelialization of the wound line. In the majority of cases, when the patient awakes, the wound will have already epithelialized and any burning and tearing will have stopped. The patient begins to see relatively well.

ASTIGMATISM CONSIDERATIONS

In treating corneal astigmatism, the axis of greatest astigmatism should be marked preoperatively at the slit lamp. With certain lasers, the surgeon may project onto the cornea the device that allows a check of the axis of astigmatic ablation. Moreover, during the ablation, treatment axis can be verified to the axis marked preoperatively. It is always advisable to protect the flap from the peripheral astigmatic ablation using the methods we described previously. This especially applies to with-the-rule myopic astigmatism in which the ablation is performed horizontally with the nasal hinge technique, and in against-the-rule astigmatism in which the ablation is performed vertically, potentially ablating a superior hinge. If the patient has incisional astigmatic surgery, a lamellar cut that is slightly deeper than the standard should be performed and the flap must be handled with special care and attention (a 180 to 200 micron plate will produce a cut thickness equal to or greater than 180 microns).

HYPEROPIC CONSIDERATIONS

Hyperopic correction may be performed as a primary procedure or as an enhancement in overcorrected eyes previously operated with incisional (radial keratotomy [RK]), surface (photorefractive keratectomy [PRK]), or lamellar (automated lamellar keratoplasty [ALK] or LASIK) techniques. This is performed similarly to myopic LASIK, the difference being a peripheral rather than central ablation that is almost totally uninvolved. Moreover, the ablated area is much larger than in myopic treatment. Thus, the surgeon must create a large flap/bed (compatible with the diameter of the cornea) and always protect the hinge and retract the flap. This allows the ablation to be more evenly distributed over the cornea, creating a better and more stable result. It also helps to avoid ablating the hinge and adjacent stroma; creating a double and irregular ablation.

COMMENTS

The last decade has been a time of tremendous change in lamellar refractive surgery. We have evolved from traditional keratomileusis, as conceived by the genius of Jose Louis Barraquer, to LASIK as it is performed today. LASIK continues Barraquer's concept of lamellar corneal surgery with the micron precision of excimer laser corneal tissue removal. Microkeratomes have evolved from the brilliant, though now outdated, manual Barraquar design to the automated current models that create large, smooth beds with both nasal and superior hinges. Improvements such as fixed plates and stops have added additional safety and quality to the cut. The fact that sutures are rarely needed allows the flap to be replaced to its natural position more regularly, with less induced astigmatism, distortion, and avoiding the need to manage and remove sutures. Functional recovery is greatly improved with increased patient satisfaction.

LASIK AND SUTURES

Lamellar refractive surgery should be performed with full respect of the anatomy of the flap/cap, both during the primary cut and during manipulation before and after the refractive ablation, until the flap is repositioned. The flap should be handled without damaging it through incorrect use of instruments that may penetrate, deform, compress, or alter it in any way. Blunt, toothless surgical forceps with relatively large tips should be used. The pressure exerted by forceps must be gentle—any compression or groove on the flap caused by improper use of forceps may influence the final outcome of the operation. Corneal hinges have largely minimized the issue of repositioning. Here, caution is needed in refloating, placing, and repositioning following the in-situ photoablation. The surgeon must be very careful when handling the flap, as it has a fragile 0.7 to 1.0 mm attachment. Any excessive traction, stretching, or compression may tear and disinsert the base of the flap from the underlying stromal bed. In the event of a free cap, when the cap is transported, a specially designed concave Barraquer fenestrated spatula should be used. Any necessary rotations or adjustments to the orientation of the flap should be performed using a Merocel tip. Respect for the anatomy must also be used if sutures are required. Only fine, sharp needles of excellent quality should be used. Prior to placing the suture, the flap must be correctly returned to its original position and gently handled to not disrupt position. Repositioning and suturing (when sutures are used) are manual surgical steps and, as such, cannot be standardized. Although sutures are rarely needed, the surgeon must be prepared with suture options for the free cap or flap.

Antitorque Sutures

If an antitorque suture is needed, four interrupted sutures (nylon 10/0) at the cardinal points are placed to center and stabilize the flap; the first is placed at 12 o'clock (the tip of the needle must enter at approximately 0.75 mm from the free edge of the flap). The second suture is placed at 6 o'clock, the third at 9 o'clock, and the fourth at 3 o'clock; it is then possible to begin a continual antitorque suture with eight passes.

Technique

10/0 nylon should always be used; this suture consists of eight passes positioned obliquely with respect to the peripheral portion of the flap. At the end of suturing, the pattern obtained should resemble four "M's" oriented toward the peripheral cornea. Suturing begins at 12 o'clock—a needle with an inclination of about 45° is used and is entered perpendicularly to the corneal flap at about 0.75 mm from the free edge. Once the needle has passed through the edge of the flap, it proceeds parallel to the iris plane, continuing at about half the depth of the peripheral cornea to return vertically at about 1.0 mm from the external edge of the cut. In order to ensure that the return pass of the suture has a greater vertical component and is less oblique, it is advisable to compress the corneal portion with the tip of forceps just in front of where the needle will exit. The second pass is performed with the same technique with the tip of the needle oriented parallel to the horizontal meridian (half past 1 o'clock). The third pass enters at 3 o'clock with the needle inclined at 45°; the fourth enters at the center of the inferior quadrant and passes parallel to the vertical meridian. This technique continues until all eight passes have been completed.

Once this suture has been completed, the four interrupted sutures at the cardinal points are removed. Each pass should be snugged with forceps to compensate for elasticity of the monofilament, without overstretching. During adjustment of the suture tension, the knot is buried in the peripheral parenchyma. Uniformity of the tension in the suture is confirmed using intraoperative keratoscopy.

It is most important that the eight-bite antitorque suture is even and uniform, with an equal distance between the various points to avoid irregular astigmatism and to speed quality visual recovery. The suture must be under moderate tension to compensate as edema of the flap begins to resolve.

The disadvantage of this type of suture consists primarily in its surgical difficulty, the learning curve, and judging the right tension in the various sectors. The time required for careful placement is another disadvantage, particularly when surgeons are inexperienced.

In Barraquer's original technique, following the application of the first antitorque suture, another is applied with pass points that lie in the middle of the first one. This allows a more homogeneous distribution of tension (double antitorque or double pass. This suture is also helpful as the final attempt to remove flap striae, which are long-standing and resistant to more typical stretching techniques.

External Compression Sutures

These consist of the placement of sutures that apply external pressure to the flap, passing through the peripheral uncut cornea so that the sutures overlie, compress, and stabilize the flap/cap without inducing any direct tissue trauma. These may be placed according to the technique designed by R. Guimaraes (Bra technique), or alternately, according to Buratto's single or double rectangular suture. All these sutures serve to compress and anchor the flap in position without inducing traction, creating suture-induced astigmatism, or producing compression-related refractive changes of the flap and underlying bed.

Technique

This involves passing the needle and suture (10/0 nylon) external to the flap at 11 o'clock (ie, through peripheral host tissue). The needle is then passed once again at 7 o'clock external to the flap, then at 5 o'clock, and again at 1 o'clock, where the knot is tied. The knot is rotated and buried. A rectangular-shaped suture is formed with four anchor points that pass at about 1.5 mm outside the flap. In order to exert the appropriate posterior compression force, the two vertical passes must be about 3.0 to 4.0 mm from each other and must be under the right tension regulated by the surgeon.

The suture may be removed on day 3. The same suture can also be used horizontally (double rectangular suture), but this may disturb the patient in that it creates more of a foreign-body sensation with blinking. This suture is useful for both a free cap and a dislodged flap technique. Containment and anchoring performed with this type of suture provide sufficient protection during the immediate postoperative period against dislocations or detachment of a free cap.

Free Cap and Sutureless Technique

In 1991, Avalos introduced the concept of the sutureless technique to various lamellar procedures with the then-used 360° cut. The cap is first removed from the antidesiccation chamber or microkeratome. The specific corneal surfaces (corneal bed and stromal side of cap) are carefully washed with BSS or sterile saline solution, and the cap is transferred and repositioned on its original corneal bed. The transfer maneuver has been performed using a Barraquer fenestrated spatula. The tissue is positioned with the epithelium facing upward, while trying to center it using a blunt anatomical forceps, or better yet, gentle manipulation with moist Merocel sponges with the cap floating on a drop of BSS. Avoid contact or traction in the optic zone. Using forceps or damp Merocel sponges, the flap is rotated to match the paracentral markings made at the beginning of the procedure, as well as keeping symmetrical gutter margins. For this maneuver, the epithelial cap should be kept dry and the interface wet to facilitate flap rotation. The surgeon may have to add an additional drop of BSS to the interface and repeat two, three, or four times to achieve perfect alignment.

After correct flap positioning and realignment to its original site, the entire circumference of the flap is carefully dried with a surgical sponge. In order to obtain correct firm adhesion between the corneal surfaces, following appropriate hydration and washing of the interface, it is advisable to smooth out the residual BSS from under the flap using a spatula or Merocel sponge on the surface of the flap itself. This will prevent formation of a liquid meniscus under the flap, which may even cause the flap to float on the liquid, a situation called "floating flap." This phenomenon will delay adhesion between the flap and stromal bed and is often the primary cause of dislocations and/or decentration of the flap in the immediate postoperative period. To allow the flap to adhere to the underlying bed, filtered compressed air can be minimally used to dry the corneal surface and edges of the keratectomy. Compressed air may be supplied from a cylinder or centralized source. Pressure must be reduced with a reduction valve—the air is also filtered using one or more millipore filters. It should be pointed out that filtered air is currently used by just a handful of surgeons, as it may cause the formation of folds and striae due to excessive dehydration of the flap/cap. It is better to use spontaneous and more physiological corneal dehydration of environmental natural air dehydration.

The speculum is carefully removed, the eyelids are gently returned to their natural position, and the eye is protected with a shield. Within a few hours, the epithelium will have covered the margin of the keratectomy, providing further adhesion and stability to the flap. The sutureless technique reduces the technical procedure time even though there is always the possibility of complications such as dislocation and/or loss of the flap immediately postoperatively even if the surgeon takes all the precautions recommended and described.

Accidental trauma and inadvertent rubbing of the eye favors this complication. In the event the flap is dislodged, the surgeon should repeat the repositioning procedure using the same corneal flap. With total loss of the flap, a second operation with the use of a homoplastic flap may be required.

The sutureless technique is therefore more indicated for LASIK flap techniques, providing the best results with lower degrees of risks. The flap is continuous with the underlying bed for a few millimeters, which maintains its anatomical relationship with the peripheral corneal tissue. Many surgeons feel that it is still better if the hinge is positioned superiorly. In the hinge technique, the edges of the incision must be smoothed and dried once the flap has been carefully distended. The surgeon should then wait between 1 and 5 minutes, according to his experience, leaving the eye exposed to allow the cornea to dry further and encourage a more physiological tissue adhesion. The corneal surface should have a drop of BSS or methylcellulose applied centrally to prevent epithelial desiccation during the drying period.

The Adjustable Suction Ring

Lucio Buratto, MD

ALK is a technique that uses the microkeratome not only for the lamellar cut but also to perform the refractive cut.

In the ALK technique, the ring is chosen on the basis of the diameter of the desired flap cut and on the basis of the radius of corneal curvature measured preoperatively (preoperative keratometry). The ring size is chosen according to the specific nomograms relative to the chosen surgical technique. In order to modify the flap diameter with this technique, it is necessary to replace the ring with another contained in the surgical set that will guarantee the preset measurement. Various interchangeable rings are much more useful for the refractive cut using the microkeratome.

As an alternative to the choice of rings, it is preferable to use an adjustable ring. This means having a single ring that can be adjusted according to the operating needs. By means of a micrometric adjustment system, the height of the cut plane and diameter of the cut can be regulated as needed. As previously mentioned, the diameter of the cut depends on the amount of corneal tissue exposed through the central opening of the ring itself. The first system, invented with an adjustable suction ring (developed by Ruiz), was the ACS unit (original Automated Corneal Shaper). The adjustable ring is made from stainless steel. There are three components: the first, which comes into contact with the patient's eye (geared ring or great ring) and adheres through suction from the suction pump; an intermediate section that is designed for the attachment of the handle (vacuum ring); and the superior portion, which is designed for passage of the microkeratome (track ring). The three ring components must be joined together to create a single unit. The geared ring is screwed in a clockwise direction onto the vacuum ring; since this has a smaller diameter, it locks into the inside of the first ring. Then the track ring is screwed on top of the two previous rings so that the track for the microkeratome run is in the superior position. To screw the track ring over the other two rings, the latter are placed on a special disk (the ring tool) that facilitates assembly of the three components. With a special clamp (tool knob), the parts are tightly screwed together to guarantee stability. The tracks on the superior portion of the ring act both as guides for the microkeratome pass

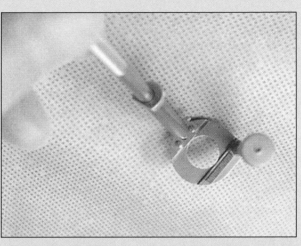

Figure 4B-1. The Chiron ACS: the adjustable ring with handle and adjustment wrench inserted.

and allow placement of the applanation disc to verify the diameter of the resection.

The adjustable ring has a micrometric thread ring that allows the operator to change the height of the superior portion without raising the ring from the sclerocorneal plane. If the superior ring is rotated in a counterclockwise direction, it is raised with respect to the inferior plane of the ring, reducing the tissue diameter that can be cut with the microkeratome; on the contrary, if the thread ring is rotated in a clockwise direction, the superior ring descends toward the sclerocorneal plane, exposing a greater quantity of corneal tissue through its central opening. The more the ring descends toward the sclerocorneal plane, the greater the diameter of the corneal disc resection.

With this adjustment, it is possible to reduce or increase the diameter of both the primary flap resection and the secondary keratectomy on the basis of parameters obtained from the nomogram, according to the desired refractive correction. Most importantly, the mechanism allows adjustment of the diameter of the optic zone of the cut.

The adjustable ring is used for ALK, but not for LASIK. In other words, it is used in the procedures that involve a refractive cut using the microkeratome. The nonadjustable LASIK ring gives a larger, more desirable flap to allow sufficient room for ablation.

Optical Zone, Pupil Diameter, and Requested Correction

Jean-Louis Arné, MD

It is commonly known that the occurrence of halos and night glare can arise from the optical properties governed by the size of the treatment zone and the pupil diameter in dim light conditions, presumably because the scotopic pupil dilates beyond the diameter of the optical surgical zone.

Seventy-two patients who underwent LASIK for myopia between -4.12 and -13.37 (mean -7.31) were questioned about the presence of halos postoperatively, as well as preoperatively, since some highly myopic patients naturally experience halos around light sources at night.

Using the Colvard infrared pupillometer, we measured scotopic pupil diameter. Corneal topographic examination was performed pre- and postoperatively including a Holladay diagnostic summary, with particular attention to the coefficient of asphericity.

The normal aspheric cornea has a negative asphericity, which means it becomes flatter than a sphere as we move toward the periphery. After treatment, there is a modification of anterior and posterior corneal curvature, and the peripheral cornea becomes steeper than its central part with a transition zone from untreated to treated corneas. For each eye, we determined the coefficient of "aspherization" as the difference between postoperative asphericity minus preoperative asphericity. There was a strong correlation between this coefficient of aspherization and the level of treated myopia.

Twenty-two percent of the patients complained of halos preoperatively and were excluded. Twenty-eight of the others complained of postoperative appearance of night halos. The frequency of halos was higher when the size of the treatment zone was smaller or when the scotopic diameter of the pupil was larger, but there was no statistically significant relationship. Mean preoperative asphericity was -0.13. Mean postoperative asphericity was +1.79.

We found a significant relationship between the rate of aspherization and the frequency of occurrence of postoperative halos in the eyes without preoperative halos.

Even though it is likely multifactorial, the primary determinant of halo effects after LASIK appears to be the change in corneal asphericity even if other factors (such as scotopic pupil dilatation or size of the optical zone) may also contribute to its occurrence.

As aspherization is correlated to the level of treated myopia, the diameter of the treatment zone is the only factor that the surgeon can modify in order to avoid postoperative halos and glare. The aspheric corneal surface created by LASIK decreases the diameter of the functional optical zone as a result of nonfocused light. A broad transition zone develops, resulting in halos and glare.

Ablation Zone, Pupil Diameter, and Requested Correction

Francesco Carones, MD

The issue of ablation zone diameter (sometimes improperly called "optic zone") is certainly crucial in planning LASIK treatment. The appropriate ablation diameter has to be decided, taking into account different parameters such as attempted dioptric correction, residual corneal thickness, and pupil diameter.

Ablation zone diameter, attempted correction, residual corneal thickness, and pupil diameter are closely related parameters when planning LASIK treatment. A satisfactory surgery often relies on the correct balance of these parameters, thus the relationship between them should be known in detail.

The general rule is theoretically, the ablation diameter should be as large as possible to reduce halo effects and night visual disturbances. This rule, however, often conflicts with another surgical parameter to take into account: the residual corneal thickness after LASIK. We know that for a certain correction, the larger the ablation diameter, the higher the amount of tissue removed and, consequently, the central ablation thickness. For low corrections there are no problems, but when attempting high myopic corrections using large ablation diameters, it may be problematic to respect what is considered the "safety" residual thickness (250 microns for the stromal bed). In these cases it is necessary to reduce the ablation diameter to a value that respects all safety features.

Pupil diameter is one of the issues to consider when planning treatment. Pupil diameter can easily be measured using infrared pupillometers (available on the market for a reasonable price). They provide pupil diameter

Table 4D-1

TREATMENT PARAMETERS

	Optimal conditions	Not optimal but could be performed	Never perform
Myopia up to –6 D	Pupil Ø: < 7.0 mm and Ablation Ø: > 5.5 (8.0) mm	Pupil Ø: 7.0 to 9.0 mm or Ablation Ø: 5.0 (6.5) to 5.5 (7.5) mm	Pupil Ø: > 9.0 mm and Ablation Ø: < 5.0 (6) mm
Myopia –6 to –8 D	Pupil Ø: < 6.5 mm and Ablation Ø: > 5.5 (8.0) mm	Pupil Ø: 6.5 to 8.5 mm or Ablation Ø: 5.0 (6.5) to 6.0 (8.0) mm	Pupil Ø: > 8.5 mm and Ablation Ø: < 5.0. (6) mm
Myopia > –8 D	Pupil Ø: < 6.0 mm and Ablation Ø: > 5.5 (8.0) mm	Pupil Ø: 6.0 to 7.0 mm or Ablation Ø: 5.0 (6.5) to 6.0 (8.0) mm	Pupil Ø: > 7.0 mm and Ablation Ø: < 5.0 (6.5) mm
Hyperopia (any amount)	Pupil Ø: < 6.5 mm and Ablation Ø: > 6.0 (9.5) mm	Pupil Ø: 6.5 to 7.5 mm or Ablation Ø: ³ 6.0 (9.0) mm	Pupil Ø: > 7.5 mm and Ablation Ø: < 6.0 (8.5) mm

measurement under scotopic conditions, which is the way pupillary diameter has to be measured, because of complaints by patients regarding night vision when the pupil dilates. As a general rule, pupils measuring 6.0 mm or less in diameter are very unlikely to have visual disturbances at night, at least for low to medium myopic corrections. Larger pupils require larger ablation diameters to avoid visual disturbances, and higher attempted corrections require the same because of the greater light scattering that occurs at the ablation edge. Thus, when we have a certain amount of correction to perform on an eye with a certain pupil diameter, the only parameter we have to change is ablation diameter.

Depending on the laser we use, this could be considered the central spherical ablation diameter as well as the overall diameter, including the transition-blend zone.

Table 4D-1 gives some guidelines on how to avoid night-vision side effects when correcting different errors. The ablation diameter is central spherical, with overall diameter in brackets. We can see that myopic and hyperopic corrections behave in a different manner. Basically, while for myopic corrections the ablation diameter can vary, hyperopic corrections always need an ablation zone as large as possible, depending on the laser system in use, regardless of the amount of correction to be made and the pupillary diameter. This is because the actual ablation diameter is usually smaller than attempted when correcting hyperopia, and patients may be disturbed by the multifocal effect of a small ablation diameter. Moreover, issues related to residual corneal thickness after hyperopic LASIK are almost meaningless, because of the deeper ablation in periphery rather than in the center of the cornea. By respecting the above guidelines, the LASIK surgeon can be confident he is doing the best that laser technology offers today in preserving optimal vision to the patients at night, though this may not be enough in some situations and patients may still complain of night vision troubles.

Flap Repositioning

Jack T. Holladay, MD

The variety of methods for repositioning the flap is as large as the number of surgeons performing the procedure. There are, however, some common parameters that appear to be present in most techniques. Avoiding folds in the flap and hydration during the ablation are common techniques to most surgeons. The stromal bed is usually irrigated, painted with a sponge, or scraped before the flap is replaced.

At this point, there is a significant divergence of techniques, with some surgeons repositioning the flap with a dry stromal bed or one drop at the hinge and others who use profuse irrigation with single or double cannulas to float the flap into place. Those who replace the flap on a dry bed usually irrigate under the flap to prevent debris or other contaminants. Interestingly, Sands of the Sahara (SOS) syndrome is believed to be seen more often with the dry techniques because contaminants (oil leak from the keratome motor, detergent in the gears, contaminated irrigation bottles, etc) are much more likely to remain.

In any case, once the flap is down, inspection of the

gutter gap is the most important parameter for proper alignment—even more important than the surgeon-placed alignment marks. Alignment marks are extremely important when a free cap occurs, but with the standard flap, the gutter gap is the critical alignment parameter. Most surgeons stroke or paint the flap along its axis with either a Merocel sponge or a soft artist's paint brush. Aggressive stroking can sometimes lead to striae along the axis of the flap, and in older patients, can result in rupture of the hemidesmosomes and epithelial folds, and even abrasion. Aggressive stroking in the axis of the flap may only result in the gutter gap being smaller opposite the hinge than on the sides. The flap has been stretched more along its axis than perpendicularly resulting in striae along the axis of the flap.

More recently, surgeons are beginning to stroke the flap in both directions so that the gutter gap is absolutely symmetrical at all points. Few surgeons use a convex compressor centrally to stretch the flap even more than possible by stroking. Whichever technique is used, the endpoint is always the same: the smallest possible symmetrical gutter gap. Some surgeons allow the flap to air dry for 1 to 5 minutes, while others use a quick burst of air or oxygen at the periphery to dry the gutter gap.

Surgeons who always use a soft contact lens leave the lens in place from 2 to 24 hours and claim slipped flaps never occur. The majority of surgeons simply have their patients rest with the eyes closed for an observation period (10 minutes to 2 hours), making sure the gutter gap remains symmetrical before discharging the patient. If a significant epithelial defect is present, a bandage soft contact lens is recommended to provide enhanced patient comfort and reduce the chance of flap slippage.

Compulsive inspection of the gutter gap at the end and shortly after surgery is a very important factor in avoiding microstriae in the flap. Ideally, the gutter gap should be almost absent, as well as symmetrical, before patient discharge. Although some epithelial remodeling occurs 1 year following LASIK, with commensurate improvement of visual acuity, proper repositioning of the flap can result in no microstriae and more rapid visual recovery.

Training the LASIK Surgeon

Daniel A. Lebuisson, MD and Dominique Pietrini, MD

LASIK has now become a quick and automated procedure. LASIK is no longer a new technique, however it requires well-established methods of education. More than surgical skill, LASIK requires meticulous training to minimize the learning curve, allowing easy handling of the microkeratome and laser, as well as explicit knowledge of all the steps of the procedure. As with flight lessons, training should be done with great care, time, and help of a trained surgeon. The success of a LASIK treatment depends on a large number of details, all of which have to be checked before starting the treatment. Respect for the procedure during the surgical phase is the key to success. Surgeon inexperience can result in a residual refractive error or a real tissue complication, which occurs far more rarely. A number of surgeons worldwide began performing refractive surgery with radial keratotomy and then with the excimer laser, but most were afraid to use the microkeratome. It was the development of an automated microkeratome (Barraquer-Ruiz) that was very important for beginning surgeons to feel secure with the critical keratectomy step.

THE LASER

The new LASIK surgeon, especially if he or she has no experience with PRK, must learn how the laser works for PRK and LASIK and should observe many live PRK and LASIK procedures with the laser he or she will use. It is also important to perform lamellar keratectomies not only during training sessions but also under the microscope of the laser to feel more comfortable in the operating situation.

Calibration and fluence must be checked before each treatment. Errors can occur at this step and a double check is strongly advised to avoid refractive errors and decentration.

THE MICROKERATOME

The new LASIK surgeon must understand perfectly how the microkeratome performs the lamellar cut and must be aware of all the potential problems of the procedure. The presence of an experienced surgeon for the first procedures is absolutely necessary.

The best way to learn the keratectomy is to first participate in training courses supervised by surgeons or authorized technicians. The first thing to learn is not only assembling and disassembling, but also cleaning the microkeratome. The novice surgeon will then perform as many keratectomies as possible on pig eyes. The technician will simulate laser failure, microkeratome blockage, and power switch off. Many types of technical hitches are reviewed during this "drill" training. The surgeon must learn how to manage all problems. The new surgeon must use a late-generation microkeratome, which is safer than the first-generation models. In our experience, the Hansatome (Bausch & Lomb) has the shortest learning curve and highest safety level and is especially suited for beginners.

For Gimbel and Marinho, the incidence of complications from LASIK is inversely related to the experience of the surgeon with the procedure. We agree with this assumption. In our first 100 cases (1996) with ALK-E and the Technolas 117, the rate of complications for one surgeon was 7%. All intraoperative incidents included free flap, blockage, buttonhole flap, and decentration greater than 1.0 mm. Postoperative complications related to poor surgical technique were noted in 5% (irregular astigmatism, interlamellar inflammation, flap folds, etc). During 1998, the rate of complications for 600 to 700 cases has dramatically dropped to 1% (these two cases exhibited no visual consequences).

The improvement of technique combined with sophisticated new microkeratomes allow beginners to avoid the problems innovators faced during 1992 to 1996. New surgeons are able to perform their first cases with confidence and safety. To follow the procedure step-by-step is more important than to improvise.

SELECT THE FIRST PATIENT

The orbital configuration and exposure of the eye are among the most important criteria for successful LASIK. It is difficult at the beginning of the learning curve to detect the "easy" or "difficult" eyes. Large, exophthalmic, and bulging eyes facilitate the placement of the suction ring and keratome and will lower the risk of poor suction or mechanical stopping of the keratome during the cut. Avoid dry eyes to lower the risk of epithelial defects during the surgery. Caution should be exercised when considering eyes with previous eye surgery (strabismus, pterygium, etc)

During the learning phase do not select eyes with large pupils. Centration must be perfect for these patients. The same comment is applicable for hypermetropic cases and astigmatic treatment. Start with moderate myopia (-4 to -10). This is the range of psychological safety for both beginners: patient and surgeon.

Select a right eye if you are right-handed, a left eye for those who are left-handed, so you will be able to comfortably insert the microkeratome in the suction ring. The patient should not be nervous and must have

confidence. Each patient must have a complete examination and a form should be maintained for retrospective analysis.

THE FIRST SURGERY: STEP BY STEP

Especially for the first procedure, eyelashes should be removed from the surgical field with a drape or strips to clear them from the suction ring and microkeratome blade and gears.

Anesthesia

Especially for the first treatments, which will probably be longer than a routine procedure, topical anesthesia should be applied as late as possible and not more than twice to avoid epithelial defects during the surgical maneuvers.

Eye Exposure and Marking

A wire speculum will provide the best exposure (Buratto-Machat or Liebermann). Pressure on the speculum also provides better exposure of the eye. Avoid excessive marking of the cornea because of the epithelial toxicity of ink and alcohol. Betadine is not necessary.

Patient position is verified by the assistant or nurse and by the surgeon. Many decentrations occur when the patient is not well-aligned or moves his or her head during the treatment. A drape can mask the displacement.

Lamellar Cut

Always try to perform large and thick flaps for the first cases, for example, with the Hansatome, use the 9.5 mm suction ring and the 180-micron plate, as the most important criteria for the flap are
- Large diameter
- Sufficient thickness (around 150 microns) provided by high IOP
- Good centration (easy to obtain with large rings)

An experienced surgeon should view the track of the microkeratome, as it is easier to detect potential obstacles with a lateral view outside of the microscope. We recommend examining the blade under the microscope immediately before cutting to ensure that the blade is not damaged during manufacturing or assembly.

IOP is usually checked manually by experienced surgeons, but during the learning curve it is absolutely necessary to check IOP with the tonometer on a wet cornea. High IOP is probably the most important factor of a successful keratectomy.

The fear of a free flap is exaggerated. With new microkeratomes (Hansatome, Carriazo, etc) the occurrence of such an event is very rare. If it does occur, the relaxed surgeon acts slowly under the microscope and gently moves the microkeratome. The flap is grasped with a smooth forceps and wet with a balanced physiologic solution. After the laser, the flap is put back in place and usually no suture or bandage contact lens is necessary. Free flaps occur when suction is insufficient or lost. Such flaps tend to be thin. Buttonhole or irregular flaps may be caused by blade imperfections or buckling of relatively steep corneas during the microkeratome pass.

Laser Ablation

After the lamellar cut, the refractive power of the cornea is unchanged and you have only prepared the stromal exposure. There are two crucial conditions for a good laser ablation:

- Perfect centration (easier with an active eye-tracking system). Pupil centration is the main concern.
- Dry stroma during the entire procedure. It is preferable to start LASIK with a new laser, which is very fast, and avoid the novice's prolonged procedure time.

For P. Dougherty, refractive and visual acuity outcomes after photorefractive keratectomy are influenced minimally by the refractive surgical experience of the surgeon. So, we can conclude that this is the same for LASIK. This is true only if all conditions are respected.

Cap Repositioning and Cleaning the Stromal Bed

In our opinion, the cap should be repositioned immediately at the end of the laser treatment and is best unrolled by its stromal side with a Merocel sponge to avoid epithelial contact with the stroma, which could lead to epithelial inoculation of the stromal bed. Irrigation of the interface should be performed only under protection of the flap to avoid the transport of particles from the conjunctiva. We feel that no irrigation is necessary in 90% of cases. Hydration increases the rate of flap folds. Replacing the flap is the best treatment of peripheral bleeding.

Wait a few minutes with the speculum in place and then after removing the speculum, observe blinking action on the flap: nothing must happen.

It is recommended for beginners to check the flap at the slit lamp just before the patient leaves the facility.

End of Procedure

We do not cover the eye with bandage contact lenses and we do not patch the eye. This could lead to secondary flap displacement. The patient is given protective eye shields for two or three nights.

Maintenance

Rigorous and meticulous maintenance of the equipment is necessary. Many microkeratome complications are due to not increasing the skills of nurse and surgeon. Blade, energy, mechanical device, laser system, etc, must be verified and maintained according to each company's rules and recommendations. The nurse must be trained in maintenance and assembly. All surgical procedures must be recorded in a data recording system and results must be analyzed periodically.

CONCLUSION

After 5 years of LASIK experience, we are still enthusiastic about it and still learning. The new LASIK surgeons have the opportunity to begin with high safety levels but still have to master their own learning curves. This learning process may today be short and safe. The participation of all surgeons' first patients provides a realistic likelihood of minimizing LASIK complications.

Draping the Eye in LASIK

Jeffrey B. Robin, MD

WHY DRAPE?

Since Pasteur and the recognition of microbial sources of infection, draping has been an integral part of surgical procedures. In modern surgery, draping generally serves several purposes, including:

- Easy identification of the area undergoing the procedure

- Isolation of the cleansed and prepared area from the remainder of the body
- Establishment of a sterile "field" surrounding the surgical area

In LASIK, identification of the target surgical field is not an issue. Draping, however, is important in this procedure in order to isolate the ocular surface from the surrounding eyelids, nose, and facial skin, as well as eyelashes. Additionally, given the surgeon's position in

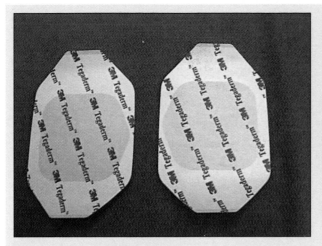

Figure 4G-1. Tegaderm adhesive.

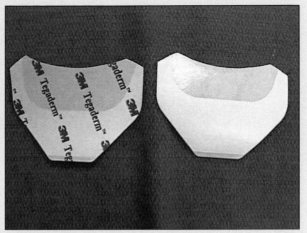

Figure 4G-2. Tegaderm trimmed to the curvature of the eyelid margin.

LASIK (behind the patient's head), draping can be used to establish a convenient sterile field on the patient's forehead and/or maxillary area.

In addition to the general goals of surgical field establishment and isolation, draping in LASIK can also serve critical mechanical purposes. Properly applied surgical drapes can help to retract the eyelids, enabling maximum exposure for flap creation and subsequent ablation. Furthermore, surgical drapes can be used to keep the eyelashes and eyelid skin out of the path of microkeratome translation during flap creation.

DRAPING TECHNIQUES

Draping techniques in LASIK vary widely among experienced surgeons around the world. Factors involved in determining preferences include individual surgeon experience, local regulations (hospital, surgical center, governmental), and availability of draping materials.

Corneal refractive surgical procedures have evolved over the last two decades so that, in most areas of the world, they are considered to be "clean" but not necessarily "sterile" endeavors. This probably has to do with the fact that these procedures are totally extraocular and do not carry the same degree of potential or sequelae for infection as do intraocular procedures. Many prominent and experienced corneal refractive surgeons do not even use sterile gloves for these procedures. Thus, there is less compunction in corneal refractive surgery to utilize full body or even full head and face draping, as is frequently used in intraocular surgery. Additionally, corneal refractive procedures require patients to fixate and thus be awake and relatively alert (no general anesthesia or heavy sedation); patients can become apprehensive or uncomfortable under full facial drapes. Therefore, most surgeons do not utilize full facial draping in corneal refractive procedures. However, there are many areas of the world where local practices and/or regulations, as well as surgeon preference, have dictated the continued use of full facial (and even full body) draping in corneal refractive procedures. In these situations, greater concern must be focused on patient comfort and apprehension and may require the use of additional items, such as external oxygen supplementation (nasal cannulae). During the last two decades, ophthalmologists world wide have amassed significant experience in corneal refractive surgery. Given the wide usage of the "clean" (versus "sterile") approach, combined with the extremely low infection rate and concerns for patient apprehension, it appears that it is reasonable not to use full body and full facial draping in these procedures (unless local regulations or standards dictate otherwise).

A Simple Draping Strategy for LASIK

It is possible to address the traditional goals of surgical draping, as well as the specific mechanical concerns outlined above, using a simple draping strategy for LASIK procedures. The core of this strategy is to use an adhesive drape that will isolate the ocular surface from the eyelids and surrounding face, as well as retract the lid margins and keep the eyelashes away from the microkeratome. The most prominent manufacturer of adhesive surgical drapes is the 3M Company (St. Paul, Minn, USA), which makes a variety of adhesive drapes for intraocular and extraocular ophthalmic surgery; there is even a model line for refractive surgery (a complete listing and description can be found at http://www.mmm.com). In order to address mechanical concerns of the eyelid and eyelashes, an adhesive drape without an aperture should be used. There are several

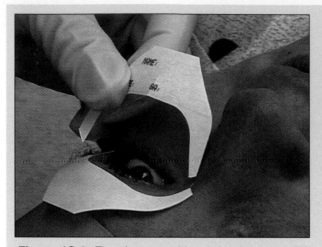

Figure 4G-3. Tegaderm provides a barrier to eyelid skin, eyelashes, and eyelids.

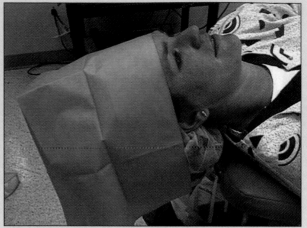

Figure 4G-4. A sterile drape applied to the forehead.

models, varying in size and accompanying drainage pouch.

The author has successfully used adhesive ophthalmic drapes without apertures for both incisional refractive procedures and photorefractive keratectomy. However, in these scenarios, it was the author's experience that keeping the eyelashes out of the surgical field was quite difficult; this became a critical problem with lamellar refractive procedures such as LASIK. Additionally, in using these adhesive ophthalmic drapes without apertures it became apparent that excess draping beyond the eyelid margins could interfere with microkeratome translation, flap retraction, and even laser ablation.

Recently, the author began using Tegaderm (3M), which is a small, transparent sterile adhesive dressing used primarily for protecting intravenous sites. The Tegaderm adhesive (Figure 4G-1) is approximately the size of the adult orbit and can be easily cut and trimmed (prior to its application) to approximate the curvature of the eyelid

margins (Figure 4G-2). While being very simple to apply, it is the author's impression that Tegaderm adhesive is much more tenacious than that used in ophthalmic adhesive drapes and its use provides an excellent barrier to eyelid skin, eyelashes, and eyelid margins (Figure 4G-3). Furthermore, there is rarely excess drape material that could interfere with the actual LASIK procedure.

In conclusion, although there is a great variety of draping techniques and products used by refractive surgeons, the author has found that the combination of a disposable (Figure 4G-4) or nondisposable sterile drape for the forehead with the use of the Tegaderm adhesive dressing provides a simple and effective draping system that will easily accomplish the sterility and mechanical goals for draping in LASIK.

The author has no financial or proprietary interest in any of the products or companies mentioned in this case study.

Drying the Edge

Luis Antonio Ruiz, MD

LASIK surgery has become the standard for refractive surgery, with excellent results in terms of accuracy, safety, short recovery time, and a minimum of postoperative symptoms.

Among the potential complications that could adversely affect some of the benefits by either defect or excess are inadequate drying techniques and ineffective drying.

For several years, we have been using and teaching

the drying technique using compressed filtered air and a variety of cannulas. The most effective cannula has been the shower head type, which provides excellent results. There are some concerns, however, about the exact drying time and the irregularities that may occur if the cannula is improperly used.

One of the most common techniques is to leave the eye open. With the compressed air at room temperature, the expected drying time is 4 to 7 minutes. This will

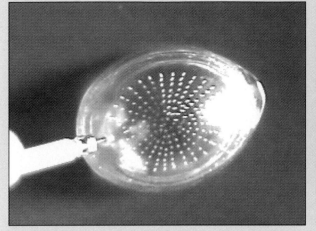

Figure 4H-1. View of the airflow chamber.

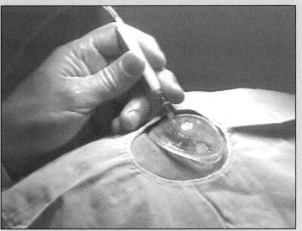

Figure 4H-2. Airflow chamber applied to the eye.

leave a very uniform flap, but for some surgeons, the concern is the length of drying time, which is sometimes longer than the actual surgery time.

To greatly reduce drying time, I have designed an air-flow chamber which, due to the air movement inside the chamber, reduces the drying time from 4 to 7 minutes to a remarkable 20 seconds. Once the ablation is finished and the flap is back to its original position, we check the borders with a Merocel sponge to ensure symmetry; then we proceed to place the air chamber over the eye for 20 seconds. At the end of this time we withdraw the cham-

ber and speculum, and, with the manual movement of the eyelid, we check the adherence of the flap. Then we finish the surgery.

The chamber is made up of two clear plastic shields. The lower one consists of holes to allow for a uniform air flow. There is a cavity between the shields that is connected to the air source.

In the presence of a free cap, once the cap is clean and replaced on the bed, the only difference in the drying technique is that now it will take between 60 and 90 seconds.

The Upper Limits of LASIK

Luis Antonio Ruiz, MD

One of the most controversial points in LASIK is the maximum limit for the correction in both myopia and hyperopia.

The four key elements that will determine the possibilities of performing a successful refractive correction are:

1. Corneal thickness. A key limitation due to the fact that presently there is no way to modify the corneal thickness.
2. Thickness of the residual layers of the cornea. Despite the fact that most surgeons look for a minimum of 250 microns for the thickness of the remaining posterior layers, we think that 230 microns is a very safe limit to avoid corneal ectasia. In the past, ectasia has not resulted by leaving even a 200-micron thickness. Therefore, when we analyze what is the maximum diopter power to be corrected with LASIK, we need to consider the

two surgical elements that can be modified. These are the thickness of the flap and the thickness of the resection or ablation.

3. Thickness of the flap. After many years of experience, we believe that is completely safe to lift a flap of 110 to 130 microns of thickness, which, depending on the case, will result in 30 to 50 microns more of potential ablation corresponding to between 4 and 6 more diopters.
4. Thickness of the resection or ablation with the laser. The thickness of the resection or the ablation is the other element that can be modified to favor the amount of correction. As shown in Figure 4I-1, we can see how for a -20 D correction with an optical zone of 6.0 mm using spheric ablation we need 264 microns, while for the same amount of correction with aspheric ablation, we need 54 microns less for the same opti-

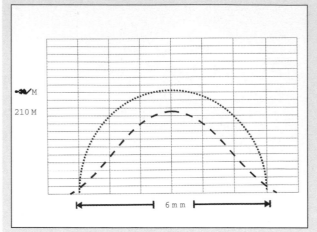

Figure 4I-1. 20 D of myopia.

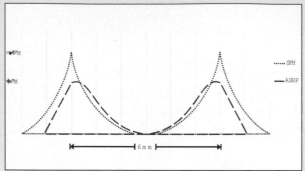

Figure 4I-2. 10 D of hyperopia.

cal zone, which is similar to what results in multizone ablations.

On the hyperopic Figure 4I-2, for corrections of 10 D there is a 50-micron difference in favor of the aspheric ablation. According to all of the previously considered points, we can effectively save tissue by lifting a flap of less thickness, and by using aspheric ablations, considerably increase the amount of diopters to be corrected within the same optical zones used for lower corrections.

Flap Lifting
Roger F. Steinert, MD

PRIMARY PROCEDURE

After withdrawal of the microkeratome and suction ring from the surgical field, the flap should be lying in its natural position. Reflection of the flap must be atraumatic to the edge. For this reason, I use a dry, solid, thin spatula with a tapered end that readily slides into the interface (Rhein Medical 8-16148). Irrigating spatulas or a spatula with adherent moisture must be avoided in order to avoid stromal hydration that will cause uneven laser tissue removal.

The spatula is slid into the interface about two-thirds to three-quarters of the distance away from the flap hinge, parallel to the hinge. The spatula is then swept toward the hinge, breaking the adhesive forces of the interface and smoothly elevating and reflecting the flap.

The reflected flap must not be allowed to lie wrinkled or folded. Also, the flap must not become contaminated with debris from the lashes, conjunctiva, tear film, or irrigating solution. A solution is the use of the Chayet sponge drain (Solan #400122 or Visitec #581098), which keeps the reflected flap elevated and isolated from debris. Alternatively, the surgeon may cut a thin piece of debris-free surgical sponge and place it at the limbus adjacent to the hinge.

RELIFTING A HEALED FLAP

Flap healing occurs primarily at the cut edge of Bowman's layer. Little adhesion develops within the interface itself, even after several years. A vascularized flap edge, or a very peripheral cut, may develop a dense scar that precludes relifting the original flap and requires recutting with the microkeratome. In most cases, however, where the flap edge is fully within clear cornea, a flap may be successfully relifted even years after the original procedure.

The healed flap edge is most easily seen at the slit lamp. One tip of an open, fine-pointed jeweler's forceps can readily break through the Bowman's layer scar and extend the break for about 1 hour. The patient is then prepared in the usual fashion under the excimer laser operating microscope. The microkeratome step is omitted. Instead, the tapered end of the flap spatula (Rhein Medical 8-16148) is directed circumferentially at the flap edge, extending the break that was begun at the slit lamp.

If a slit lamp is not available, the use of an oblique illuminating light and pressure on the peripheral cornea with the tip of an instrument, such as a Sinskey hook, will show a discontinuity in the light reflection, indicating the location of the flap edge. This technique is more difficult than beginning the procedure at the slit lamp, however.

The goal is to cleave the epithelium as cleanly as possible. Simply sweeping the blunt aspect of a spatula across the flap or lifting the flap without first cleaving the epithelium will result in large sheets of torn epithelium. These epithelial defects will increase postop-erative pain, delay healing, and increase the risk of epithelial implantation into the interface or melting of the flap edge.

After completing the circumferential opening of the flap edge, the dry spatula then reflects the flap in the same manner as a primary procedure.

LASIK WITH A NASAL HINGE USING THE ACS MICROKERATOME

5

Lucio Buratto, MD and Stephen Brint, MD

A. The Microkeratome

INTRODUCTION

For many years, the Chiron Automated Corneal Shaper (ACS) microkeratome has been the most popular and frequently used instrument in laser-assisted in situ keratomileusis (LASIK) procedures worldwide.

Initially, the lamellar cut was performed with manual advancement. The precision of the cut with a manual instrument depends not only on the quality of the instrument but also on the surgeon's skill.

There are numerous environmental, mechanical, and thermal factors that affect the quality of a manually cut corneal disc, such as the speed at which the microkeratome is advanced, the consistency of this movement, and the pressure exerted on the suction ring and microkeratome head.

In order to improve the quality of the cut, manufacturing companies began to create instruments that would advance automatically. One of the results of this research was the ACS. Originally, this microkeratome was designed by A. Ruiz to perform an in situ refractive cut using the microkeratome (automated lamellar keratoplasty [ALK] technique). More recently, it was adapted to perform the ELISK (excimer laser intrastromal keratomileusis) technique, and now to perform LASIK.

In addition to facilitating the technique, this instrument makes the keratectomy precise and standardized, simultaneously improving the quality and anatomical condition of the corneal flap and stromal bed.

THE ACS MICROKERATOME

The ACS has a system of gears located in the head of the microkeratome. When these come into contact with a toothed track on the suction ring, they advance the instrument forward and backward. Using this device, the movement of the microkeratome is regular and uniform, and automatically stops at the end of the pass.

The ACS instrument consists of the following:

- The microkeratome
- A suction ring, either adjustable or fixed (the LASIK ring)
- A series of applanation lenses and other accessories, including:
    - A Barraquer tonometer
    - A corneal marker
    - Forceps and spatulas
    - An Allen wrench
    - A hex wrench
    - A magnet for handling the blade
    - A testing tool to check the movement of the blade

THE CONSOLE

The console contains the power supply and suction pump. The pump produces a vacuum that is equivalent to 22 inches Hg. It transmits vacuum to the suction ring through plastic tubing.

On the front panel of the console, various functional parameters of the instrument are displayed. Both activation of the motor and suction pump are controlled by footpedals. This allows the surgeon to initiate both functions. One pedal controls the suction pump (press and release to activate, press and release again to deactivate). Another pedal controls the microkeratome motor and has two sides; one side activates blade oscillation and forward movement of the instrument (advancing the microkeratome head across the suction ring), the other side moves the instrument in the reverse direction. The cut is performed during the forward advance of the microkeratome. The reverse movement returns the microkeratome

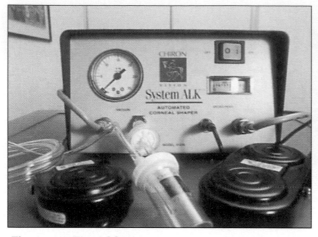

Figure 5-1. The ACS instrument console and foot switches: the double pedal controls the movements of the microkeratome. The single pedal activates suction.

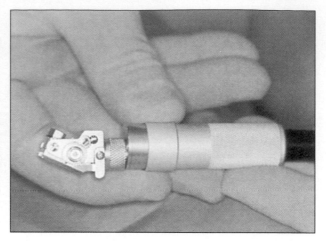

Figure 5-2. The ACS motor is contained in the handle of the microkeratome.

to its starting position, allowing the lamellar flap to be freed from the head and returned to the stromal bed.

THE MOTOR

The microkeratome motor is housed in a cylindrical handle. A protective Teflon cap covers the pin that drives blade oscillation and the threads that drive microkeratome movement (it is removed when the motor is attached to the head). The power supply cord is inserted into the appropriate receptacle on the console and is then clicked into place at the other end of the motor. When the pedal that activates the motor is pressed, the noise heard from the motor should be a uniform buzz, constant in both intensity and tone. This should be checked again after the head has been attached to the motor. If the sound is irregular, the surgeon should check that the eccentric is clean, the blade is free of defects, and if the head has been assembled correctly. Monitoring the voltage indicators on the control unit's console for a higher than normal reading can suggest that there is an increase in resistance.

THE HEAD

The head of the microkeratome consists of two portions attached by a central hinge. This allows the instrument to be opened (without separating the two parts). It allows easy insertion of the blade without risk of damaging the edge. The posterior aspect, as in Barraquer's original instrument, has an opening for the eccentric drive mechanism of the motor to be engaged and then screwed in. The clearly visible eccentric terminal is con-

nected to two larger gears that combine to form the core of the instrument's automated mechanism.

Once attached to the head, the motor activates this gear mechanism, making automated movement possible. The first gear transmits the rotary impulse to the two larger gears and produces the movement that drives the microkeratome. The motor used to power the microkeratome is a 12 volts (V) micromotor that provides a blade oscillation rate of 7500 to 8000 RPM. It is housed behind the eccentric, forming the cylindrical handle of the microkeratome. The eccentric creates the connection between the motor and the blade holder found in the microkeratome head.

THE STOP MECHANISM

The microkeratome's stop mechanism, which allows creation of a hinge, is fixed over the collar that is screwed onto the posterior end of the head. The stop mechanism is fixed to the microkeratome head and tightened securely by using an Allen wrench (supplied with the instrument). The stopping point of the microkeratome (or the length of its traverse across the cornea), and, therefore, the size of the hinge can be adjusted by means of a screw on the protruding portion of the stop. This is normally set to stop the instrument at the point that allows the largest hinge size (or the shortest traverse across the cornea) for all cases.

Once mounted, the protruding portion of the stop will come into contact with the peripheral portion of the suction ring during the forward cut, limiting the complete pass of the microkeratome along the track. This produces a partial keratectomy, the formation of the desired hinge, and a corneal flap.

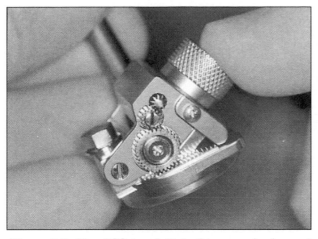

Figure 5-3. The ACS head. Note the gears for forward and reverse movement of the microkeratome on the ring and fixed stop mechanism.

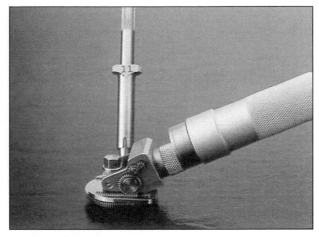

Figure 5-4. The ACS microkeratome is advanced on the ring to check the smoothness of the mechanism.

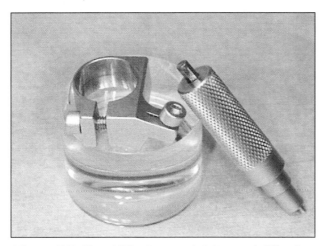

Figure 5-5. The ACS stop mechanism and Allen key used to tighten it on the head (these rest on an applanometer). The latest generation instruments have a stop mechanism incorporated in the head.

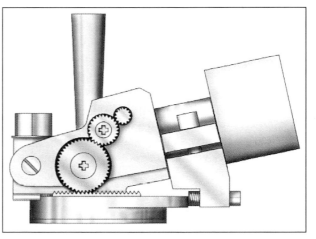

Figure 5-6. Side view of the ACS stop mechanism.

BLADE AND BLADE HOLDER

The blade is shaped on both sides. It is removed from its plastic container using a magnet, so there is no contact with the blade edge. Before the blade is inserted into the microkeratome head, it should be examined under high magnification. The surface and cutting edge should be carefully examined. Any irregularity on the surface will increase friction and slow the microkeratome pass. This will reduce blade oscillation during the cut and can stop advancement of the microkeratome.

The blade holder is inserted into the cavity in the bottom of the opened head of the microkeratome, with the deep groove on its side facing toward where the motor will be inserted. The blade is pressed into place on the top of the blade holder. The blade holder in newer instruments mirrors the shape of the opening in the blade (square on one side and round on the other), making

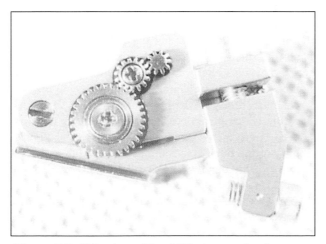

Figure 5-7. Side view of the ACS stop mechanism.

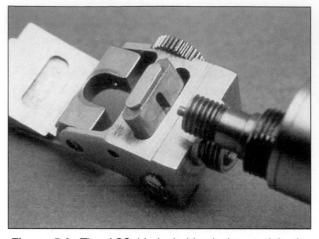

Figure 5-8. The ACS blade holder is inserted in the groove of the microkeratome head. The motor is positioned so that the eccentric, which will be inserted in the groove of the blade holder, can be seen.

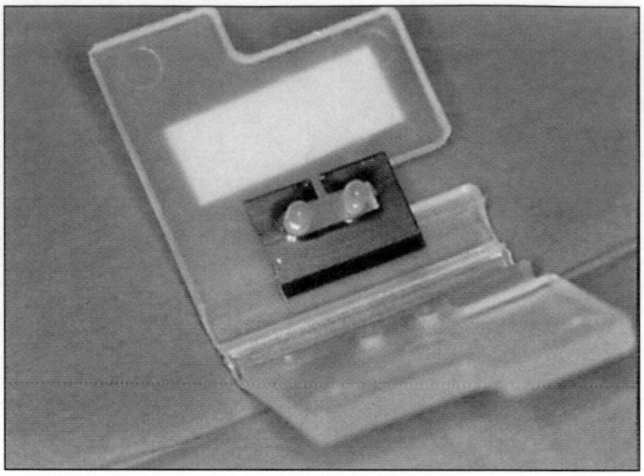

Figure 5-9. The ACS blade in its transparent plastic container.

incorrect placement of the blade impossible. In all cases, the rounded side of the blade opening should be on the side of the microkeratome where the gears are located. Correct assembly of blade and blade holder is verified by testing after assembly.

The posterior side of the blade holder has a groove to engage the eccentric mechanism of the motor. The eccentric allows the rotation of the motor to be transmitted to the blade and blade holder—this produces oscillation.

Once the blade has been inserted in the blade holder and the head of the microkeratome has been closed, the collar is screwed on and tightened (the smooth edge of the collar is placed toward the microkeratome head).

A testing tool is provided that simulates movement of the eccentric. The tool is inserted into the posterior opening of the microkeratome head (through the collar). By rotating the tool, the surgeon can check oscillation of the blade edge on the inferior face of the microkeratome. Blade movement must be free of any friction or resistance. If not, the head should be opened, the blade and blade holder removed, and the head cleaned before attempting reassembly. If friction persists, the blade should be replaced. The blade angle during the cut is 26° to the corneal plane.

THE DEPTH PLATE

Following assembly and testing of the blade movement, the depth plate is seated into its groove on the anterior edge of the microkeratome head. For LASIK, a plate that provides a thickness of 160 to 180 microns is used. Sometimes plates of 130 or 200 microns are used. These numbers represent the approximate thickness in microns of a resection resulting from the use of that specific plate.

The thinner the plate, the greater the thickness of the lamellar resection, because the space between the plate and blade will be larger and will, therefore, allow greater exposure of the corneal tissue to the microkeratome blade.

The resection thickness of each plate is indicated by the number etched on the front of the plate. An interesting detail of the ACS can be observed on the superior portion of the plate; it has a screw that locks into the groove on the anterior edge of the microkeratome head; this fixes the plate firmly to the microkeratome head, preventing alteration of the plate-blade relationship. This large superior screw head also allows absence of the plate to be immediately noticed by the surgeon (a very important factor).

In order to insert the plate in the groove on the microkeratome head, a special instrument is used (hex wrench), which is supplied with the ACS set.

The wrench is placed over the screw head to allow the surgeon to place his or her finger over the front of the plate (the side where the number is etched) and firmly seat the plate. A click can be heard and felt when positioning is correct. Tightening the screw by turning the wrench will firmly fix the plate into position. Verify that the front of the plate does not extend beyond the front portion of the microkeratome head. Incorrect plate positioning in the microkeratome head, in addition to total absence of the plate, will leave the blade exposed and cause a perforating keratectomy.

As with all the other components of the instrument, the plate must be meticulously clean. Debris on the plate can alter the expected depth and smoothness of the corneal resection.

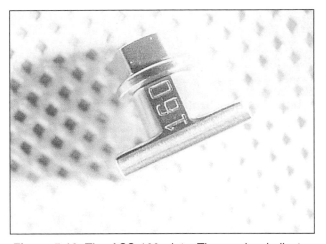

Figure 5-10. The ACS 160 plate. The number indicates thickness of the cut that will be obtained with this plate.

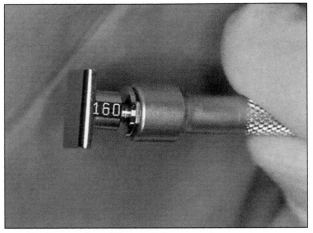

Figure 5-11. The ACS plate is supported prior to being assembled on the head of the special wrench.

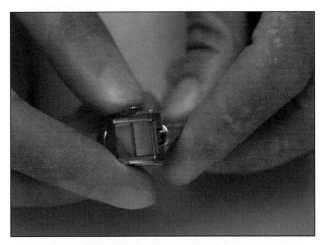

Figure 5-12. The plate has not been inserted completely. If the microkeratome is used with the plate in this position, serious complications are likely.

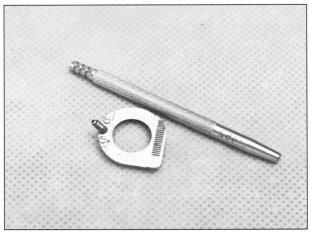

Figure 5-13. The ACS suction ring and handle.

THE SUCTION RING

The LASIK ring is fixed in diameter. The resection diameter is not adjustable but will vary depending on keratometry. For LASIK, a fixed ring is sufficient because the diameter of the lamellar flap is not an essential feature, as it was in procedures such as ALK, which were performed prior to excimer lasers. This ring produces a flap averaging 8.0 mm in diameter, sufficient to accommodate most ablations.

The two tracks of the ring are different sizes, in fact, one track is slightly shorter than the other (the longer providing a dovetailed connection to the shaper head). This facilitates insertion of the microkeratome into the ring.

To assemble, the handle is screwed to the ring and connected to the control unit of the ACS by suction tub-

ing. Suction is tested by occluding the bottom of the ring (with the thumb or on the palm of the hand) and pressing the suction pedal. The pressure indicator on the front panel of the console should read 24 or greater when the ring is occluded, and 15 when not occluded. If the vacuum pump is not functioning properly, the unit must not be used.

The head of the microkeratome (without the motor) is then inserted into the ring. Movement of the head in the ring must be smooth and without friction or resistance.

The head is now attached to the motor and connected to the console. The microkeratome is again inserted into the ring and advanced and retreated across the ring track. Ensuring that the large gear on the head of the microkeratome mates perfectly with the first tooth on the suction ring track, following this test will prevent binding and

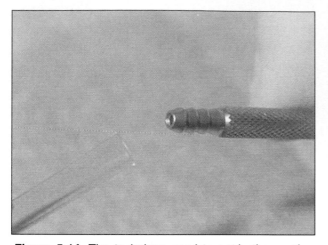

Figure 5-14. The technique used to apply the suction tube to the suction ring handle.

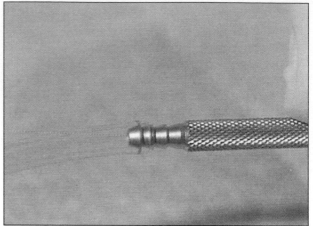

Figure 5-15. The tubing has been inserted incorrectly.

"false starts" when the keratectomy is performed. The ring and microkeratome are now ready to use.

Suction Ring Functions

1. Globe fixation. Inferiorly, it has a triangular chamber with curved edges that adapt to the curvature of the corneal and scleral surfaces. The patient's cornea protrudes through the central opening (about 11 mm).
2. It raises the intraocular pressure (IOP) to a value of 65 mm Hg (or greater) to firm and hold the globe for the resection.
3. It guides the progress of the automated microkeratome through the double-channel track, providing stability for the microkeratome.

THE CONTROL UNIT AND FOOTPEDALS

The control unit has two functions: to power the vacuum pump and the motor of the microkeratome.

A vacuum indicator shows the vacuum levels reached during suction (optimal value between 22 to 27 mm Hg). The vacuum is transmitted to the suction ring through plastic tubing.

A voltage meter on the front panel indicates the power delivered during the advancement or retreat of the microkeratome (optimal value is 12 V).

There are two footpedals:

1. The suction pedal. By depressing and releasing this pedal, suction is initiated and maintained. The pedal is once again depressed and released to disengage suction.
2. The power pedal. This is divided into two side-by-side parts, one that allows the surgeon to activate

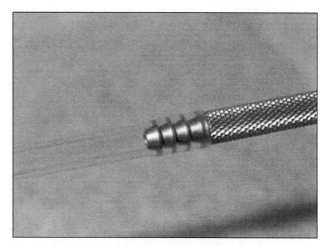

Figure 5-16. The tubing has been inserted correctly.

and advance the microkeratome, and the other allows the microkeratome to return to its original position once the cut has been completed.

We feel it advisable to keep the pedals on a table and have a technician operate them at the surgeon's command. Alternately, the surgeon activates the pedals on the floor. This avoids accidental activation/deactivation during the procedure.

ACCESSORIES

Applanation lenses: These allow the surgeon to check the intended resection diameter (used primarily in ALK techniques).

Applanation tonometer: Used to confirm that IOP is greater than 65 mm Hg prior to the microkeratome pass.

Antidesiccation chamber: Used for storing the corneal disc, epithelial side down, in the event of a free cap.

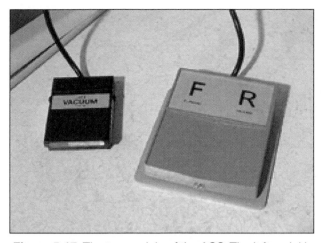

Figure 5-17. The two pedals of the ACS. The left pedal is used to activate suction. The right pedal is used for forward and reverse movement of the microkeratome.

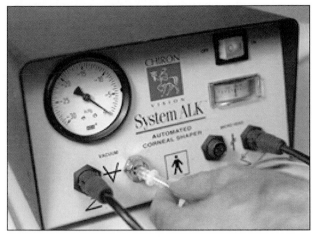

Figure 5-18. ACS control panel. The assistant connects the aspiration tubing to its attachment.

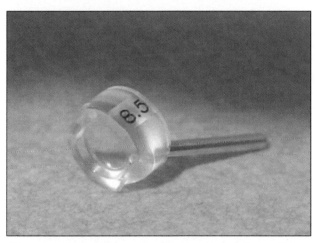

Figure 5-19. An 8.5 mm applanation lens. It is applied to the suction ring with suction activated and provides information on the diameter of the flap to be cut.

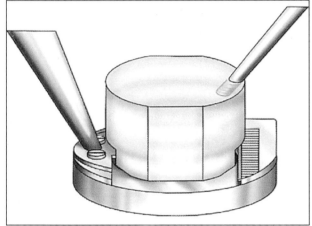

Figure 5-20. The drawing shows the applanation lens inserted correctly on the ring.

Fenestrated corneal spatula: Used to transfer the free cap of the cornea to the antidesiccation chamber and in replacing it on the stromal bed.

Corneal marker: Used to mark the cornea with a pararadial line so that a free cap can be replaced correctly on the corneal bed.

Hex wrench: This metal tool is used to insert and lock the plate into the microkeratome head.

Allen wrench: This tool is used to fix the stop device to the microkeratome head.

Magnet: Used to insert the blade onto the blade holder.

Testing tool: A metal shaft with an eccentric pinion like that of the motor, used to check the oscillatory movement of the blade, and located on the other end of the Allen wrench.

Instruments that are not included with the ACS but prove useful in lamellar surgery include:

Keratome scope: an instrument used in ALK to check the gap between the blade and depth plate in the microkeratome and to confirm the exact thickness of the refractive cut (second keratectomy).

Once the plate has been selected from the nomogram, the keratome scope is used to check the thickness of resection that will be achieved with that specific plate.

Ultrasound pachymetry: Permits intraoperative measurement of the thickness of the stromal bed, the flap, or the corneal disc removed during the refractive cut (during ALK). For example, if the thickness of the flap measured by pachymetry is greater than the desired value, the thickness of the refractive cut must be modified. This avoids complications arising from an excessively thin residual cornea. With LASIK, it is mandatory to know total corneal thickness to determine what the residual bed thickness will be following keratectomy and ablation.

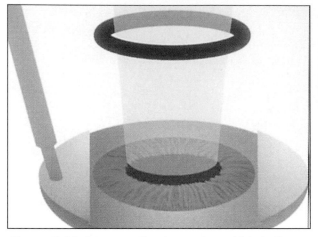

Figure 5-21. Intraoperative tonometry, which indicates whether the pressure is appropriate for the cut.

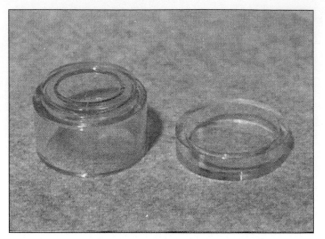

Figure 5-22. Antidesiccation chamber, which is used only in the case of a free cap.

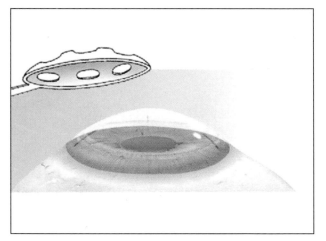

Figure 5-23. Fenestrated spatula for repositioning the lenticle in case of a free cap.

ACS CHECKLIST

1. Check that the available power supply is correct for the instrument.
2. Connect the power cable.
3. Connect the footpedals to the appropriate sockets.
4. Turn the unit on and confirm that the green light is illuminated.
5. Connect the microkeratome motor cable to the appropriate socket of the console.
6. Test motor function. push the pedal and listen for uniform buzzing in both the forward and backward directions. The voltage indicator should read 12 V for both directions when the microkeratome head is attached to the motor.

Table 5-1

COMPONENTS FOR ASSEMBLY OF THE ACS FOR STANDARD LASIK

- Shaper head
- Blade holder
- Disposable blade (sterile single-use)
- A magnetic blade-handling tool
- Collar ring
- 130, 160, 180, or 200-micron depth plate
- Combination blade-testing tool and Allen wrench
- A suction ring
- Suction ring handle
- Disposable sterile vacuum tubing (single-use)
- Motor power cord (disinfected, not steam autoclavable)
- ACS motor and protective cap (disinfected, not steam autoclavable)
- Power supply/vacuum console

7. Examine the microkeratome head when open and check that the blade holder is correctly positioned and moves freely inside its groove.
8. Check for perfectly smooth operation of the gears.
9. Carefully examine the blade under a high-magnification microscope.
10. Position the blade onto the blade holder using the magnetic tool.
11. Close the head and screw on the collar.
12. Insert the desired depth plate, pushing until a click is heard, then while holding it firmly in place, turn the wrench to tighten the screw.
13. Apply the stop device, firmly securing it (this applies to early-generation machines; the more modern ones have a fixed stop device).

14. Check that the adjustment screw on the stop device is correctly set.
15. Test the smooth, unrestricted movement of the blade with the testing tool.
16. Attach the handle to the suction ring.
17. Insert the microkeratome head (without the motor attached) into the suction ring and test for smooth, unrestricted movement.
18. Attach the head to the motor, activate the motor, and listen to the noise that it produces. There should be a uniform buzz, constant in both tone and intensity.
19. Insert the microkeratome head into the suction ring. Using the footpedals, advance and reverse the microkeratome (this takes about 7 seconds). The movement should be constant and regular, without indication of resistance.
20. Connect the suction tubing to the terminal portion of the handle.
21. Activate suction and check the value on the display; it must indicate a value of 15 (±3) without occlusion of suction.
22. With the thumb, occlude the bottom of the ring, the indicator should read 24 or greater.
23. Under the microscope, check the integrity of the tracks and for absence of foreign bodies and/or impurities that may interfere with the smooth movement of the microkeratome.

POWER SUPPLY AND SUCTION UNIT ASSEMBLY

The power supply and suction unit are placed a short distance from the laser. The main electric supply cable is connected to the back of the unit and should be plugged into an electrical outlet of appropriate voltage. The plug must be firmly inserted in the receptacle in the back of the unit. If necessary, adhesive tape can be used to fix the cable to the table, thus avoiding its detachment during a procedure.

The suction pedal and motor pedal are connected and within easy reach of the technician or surgeon who will operate them. The suction tubing is connected to the vacuum pump port. The microkeratome motor cable is connected to the console.

When the power switch on the front of the console is placed in the "on" position, the green light should be illuminated.

The motor is connected to the power cable and activated with the footpedal. The indicator should show a reading of 12 V in both directions. The pedal is pushed forward and backward for about 10 seconds each time,

and the surgeon checks that the noise emitted is constant and even.

When the head is attached to the motor, the surgeon should verify blade oscillation when the motor is activated.

ASSEMBLY OF THE ACS HEAD

- The microkeratome head consists of six parts:
- The head
- The blade holder
- The blade
- The posterior collar ring
- The depth plate
- The stop

Assembly of the ACS begins with the shaper head. Pick up the shaper head and turn the largest gear with your finger. The gears should move freely and smoothly in both directions.

If the movement is not smooth, the shaper head should be cleaned and re-autoclaved.

Remove the posterior collar and open the shaper head. Any residual moisture is dried using Merocel sponges. The head should be completely dry.

With the head of the ACS hinged open, an oval-shaped slot is visible, which houses the blade holder. The blade holder has a groove on one side that must face toward where the motor will be inserted. If the blade holder is not inserted correctly, the eccentric of the motor will not engage the slot of the blade holder, and the blade will not oscillate. Moreover, this could cause serious damage to the motor. Once the blade holder has been inserted, use your finger to check that the movement of the blade holder is smoothly in its slot. If not, remove the blade holder and check that the slot and holder are completely dry. If resistance is still felt, reclean the shaper head.

The blade is supplied in a plastic container with the manufacturer's logo embossed on one side. The container is placed on the table so that the logo faces up. The plastic container is fashioned with tabs attached to both top and bottom. Hold down the tab attached to the bottom of the container while gently lifting the tab attached to the top of the container. Examine the top surface of the blade under high magnification and verify that it is free of defects. Approach the blade with the magnetic blade handling tool by sliding it onto the noncutting side of the blade. This prevents the magnet from causing the blade to "jump" out of the holder, possibly causing damage to the cutting edge. Care should be taken to avoid any contact with the cutting edge of the blade. Now you can easily examine the bottom surface of the blade and cutting

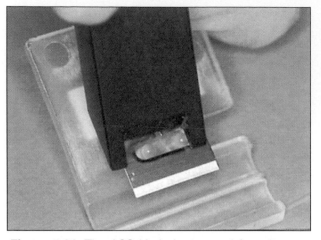

Figure 5-24. The ACS blade is removed from its container by means of a magnet.

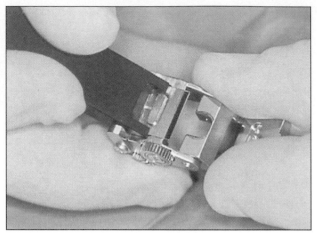

Figure 5-25. The ACS blade is inserted in the blade holder using a special magnet.

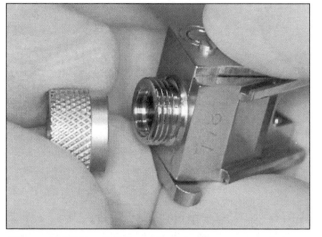

Figure 5-26. The ACS head is closed by means of a special collar.

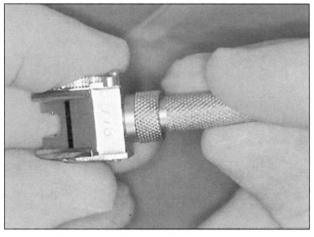

Figure 5-27. Smooth blade movement is checked using a special instrument.

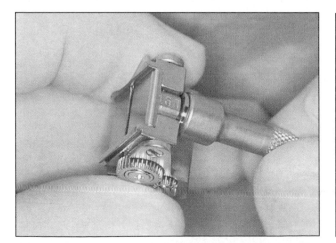

Figure 5-28. The plate is inserted in a groove on the head of the ACS.

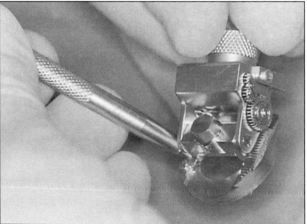

Figure 5-29. Checking the free movement of the ACS microkeratome on the suction ring.

edge under high magnification and verify that they are free of defects.

Both the blade and raised portion of the blade holder have a rounded and a squared edge. The blade can only be placed onto the blade holder when it is correctly oriented. The magnetic blade handling tool is used to firmly seat the blade onto the raised portion of the blade holder. Once the blade has been inserted, the head of the ACS is closed and the posterior collar is tightened, with the smooth part facing the ACS head. (Note that in some older instruments the raised portion of the blade holder has a rounded edge on both ends. In this case, verify that the blade holder is correctly oriented by peering into the orifice where the motor is inserted and confirming that you can see the deep groove where the eccentric will engage. The blade is then oriented onto the holder with the round end toward the gears of the head. Should the collar be tightened with the smooth part facing away from the ACS head, it will not be possible to screw the head onto the motor shaft.

The plate is inserted next (normally with a thickness of 160 or 180 microns).

On the front, there is a cylindrical protuberance or nut that coincides with a groove in the ACS head (the numbers are engraved here). The screw in the boss is loosened using the wrench. The plate is then inserted into the front of the ACS head. For ease of insertion, it is advisable to hold the wrench with the thumb and middle fingers using the index finger (placed over the numbers) to stabilize the plate during insertion. Care must also be taken to insert the plate parallel to the recess in the front of the ACS head. Should the plate tilt, it may contact the blade's cutting edge.

When insertion is correct, a click can be heard and felt as spring-loaded buttons click into place around the plate shaft. Once seated, continue holding the plate in correct position with the index finger while turning the wrench with the thumb and middle finger until the screw is tight. Visually check that the front of the plate is flush with the leading edge of the microkeratome head.

Next, blade movement is checked with the testing tool. The tool is inserted into the drive shaft opening and turned repeatedly in both directions. Blade action can be observed from the bottom of the head. The tool should turn smoothly, with no friction or resistance. Should the movement not be smooth, the ACS head should be dismantled, cleaned, and dried. If the action does not improve, a new blade should be inserted.

MOTOR ASSEMBLY

The white protective cover of the motor shaft is removed and the shaft is manually turned to check for resistance. If resistance is encountered, the motor must not be used and should be serviced. Then, the ACS head is screwed onto the exposed shaft of the motor. The power cable (already connected to the console) is plugged into the end of the motor.

SUCTION RING ASSEMBLY

The suction ring of the ACS LASIK set is assembled by firmly attaching the suction handle. The disposable tubing is then attached to the suction handle and the lock is snapped into the vacuum port of the console. Care must be taken to ensure than the suction tubing is firmly attached to the unit. Next, the suction is tested by depressing the suction foot switch. The suction gauge should show 15 when not occluded; the ring this then occluded with the thumb (or on the palm of the hand), and the gauge should indicate at least 24. This vacuum reading assumes that the unit is operated near sea level. Adjustments must be made to these values when used in extreme altitudes. The microkeratome is now assembled!

Prior to staring every procedure, we check that:

- The suction functions perfectly by occluding the ring with the thumb. The ring should attach firmly and not be dislodged by its own weight.
- The needle of the manometer on the console indicates suction has stabilized at 23.
- The progression and return of the microkeratome on the ring is correct.
- There is no debris in the microkeratome motor or inside the eccentric that could block or reduce rotation of the eccentric, stopping advancement of the microkeratome.
- The noise of the microkeratome is typical and the reading on the voltmeter is checked to ensure that the blade is meeting no resistance.
- The selected plate has been inserted correctly (180 for slight myopia, 160 for moderate myopia, and 130 for severe myopia).
- The blade has been inserted.
- The stop mechanism has been applied correctly.
- The plate is positioned and correctly inserted (final check)

MICROKERATOME MAINTENANCE

The ACS microkeratome is a very sophisticated instrument. It requires diligent maintenance and regular upkeep, even during periods when it is not being used. The ACS should be completely dismantled and cleaned immediately after every surgical procedure.

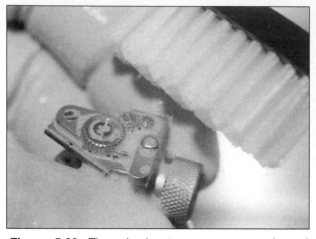

Figure 5-30. The microkeratome gears are cleaned using a toothbrush and diluted Palmolive soap.

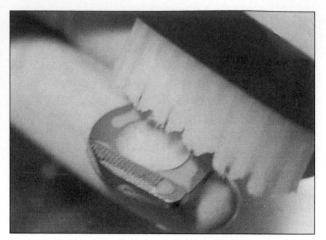

Figure 5-31. The suction ring is cleaned with a brush and Palmolive soap.

Bilateral simultaneous surgery can be considered one procedure. In this case, the external gears and surfaces of the head are dried with compressed air and smooth advancement of the instrument in the suction ring is rechecked between eyes (the same blade being used for both keratectomies).

Cleaning solution: A cleaning solution of two parts green Palmolive soap (Colgate-Palmolive, New York, NY, USA) (used to wash domestic tableware) to 100 parts warm water is used (in Italy, a neutral soap such as Last–mani delicati can be used). Palmolive is recommended, as it contains ingredients that allow good lubrication of the ACS gear mechanism.

All components of the head and suction ring are soaked in this solution for a few minutes, brushed well with a soft toothbrush, and rinsed completely with distilled water. Extra care is taken to remove any debris from the gears of the shaper head and from the track and grooves of the suction ring. The gears of the shaper head should be turned while immersed in the cleaning solution for about 1 minute to allow for distribution of the cleaning solution through the inside of the drive mechanism.

Alcohol is used only on metal parts (do not use it on any of the plastic components). Distilled water is used for rinsing, compressed air is used for drying, and a millipore filter can be attached to the air pipe to trap any particulate material.

Cleaning the head and blade holder of the ACS:
1. Remove the stop mechanism and depth plate.
2. Remove the collar, open the shaper head and remove the blade and blade holder (the magnetic blade handling tool should be used in handling used blades to prevent accidentally cutting oneself, and disposed of in a sharps container).

3. Clean the surfaces of all components using a soft toothbrush after soaking in warm Palmolive soap solution for a few minutes.
4. Turn the shaper head gears while immersed in the cleaning solution.
5. Rinse completely with distilled water.
6. Carefully dry the surfaces with compressed air.
7. Re-insert the blade holder in its slot.
8. Close the head once again and secure it with the collar.
9. Place the instrument in an autoclave for sterilization (dry all components completely following sterilization if the instrument is being stored).

Cleaning the suction ring:
1. Clean with warm Palmolive soap solution.
2. Brush all surfaces with a soft toothbrush, especially the teeth of the track.
3. Rinse with distilled water.
4. Dry the suction port on the ring and inside the handle with compressed air.
5. If the adjustable ring is being used, separate all components for cleaning, rinse completely, dry, and reassemble for autoclaving.
6. Sterilize in an autoclave.

Cleaning the depth plate:
1. Clean with warm Palmolive soap solution.
2. Rinse with distilled water.
3. Dry with compressed air.
4. Sterilize in an autoclave.

Cleaning the applanation lenses and tonometer (these acrylic components should not be soaked in alcohol or placed in an autoclave). Clean with warm Palmolive soap solution. They can be disinfected by soaking in Cidex or another alcohol-free chemical disinfecting product. Rinse with sterile distilled water. The

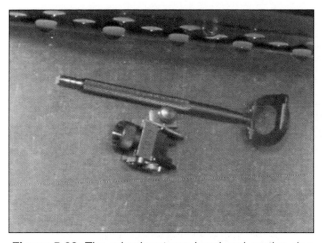

Figure 5-32. The microkeratome head and suction ring are subjected to the ultrasound and then washed with distilled water.

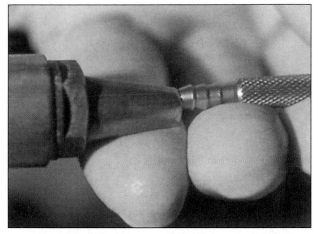

Figure 5-33. The suction ring and its handle are dried with compressed air.

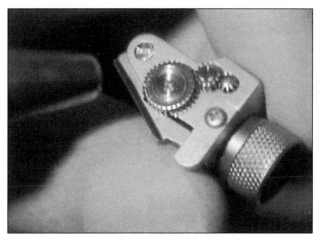

Figure 5-34. The microkeratome and gears are dried carefully and then sterilized.

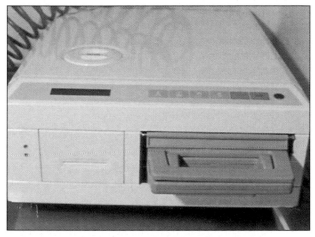

Figure 5-35. The autoclave uses distilled water and completes a sterilization cycle in just 6 minutes.

applanation lenses should be stored in their storage container.

Cleaning the corneal markers and spatulas:
1. Clean with warm Palmolive soap solution.
2. Brush all surfaces with a soft toothbrush to remove dye and debris.
3. Rinse with distilled water.
4. Dry with compressed air.
5. Sterilize in an autoclave.

Cleaning the ACS motor and power supply unit: the ACS motor can be disinfected by wiping with alcohol or another chemical disinfecting agent. At the end of the surgical session, the eccentric is gently brushed with a soft, dry toothbrush to dislodge any debris. Two to 3.0 mm of the eccentric is then held in a container of anhydrous alcohol and the motor activated for 10 seconds in each direction. Excess alcohol is then blotted from the eccentric with a lint-free dry instrument wipe and the motor allowed to run for 1 minute. The protective cap should always be placed on the motor when not actually in use and the motor should always be stored cap down to prevent moisture from running into the motor's mechanism. Use a soft damp cloth to clean the console housing. Do not use solvents.

The motor power supply cord can be disinfected by wiping with alcohol or another chemical disinfecting agent. The ends should never be immersed in liquid.

Never allow the suction ring or suction tubing to draw liquid into the vacuum pump. This will cause extensive damage to the unit.

Disposable accessories (supplied in a sterile pack): The system blade is supplied in a disposable sterile pack for single use. Vacuum tubing is supplied in a sterile pack for single use.

The following components can be sterilized in an autoclave:

Table 5-2
COMPONENTS OF THE ACS
• Power supply and vacuum pump console
• Electric supply cable (for connection to a standard wall outlet)
• Microkeratome motor power cable
• Disposable suction tubing
• Suction and motor footpedals
• Motor
• Shaper head and blade holder
• Disposable single-use blade
• Magnetic blade handling tool
• Shaper head collar
• Stop device
• Combination Allen wrench/testing tool
• Combination hex wrench/stop set screw wrench
• Depth plates
• Suction ring (fixed for LASIK)
• Suction ring handle
• Applanation lenses (used mainly for ALK)
• Barraquer tonometer
• Antidesiccation chamber (for free cap)
• Other accessories for LASIK
Corneal marker
Corneal spatula
Ultrasound pachymeter
Micrometer

Table 5-3
ACS CHECKLIST
1. Check that the suction ring is free from debris or BSS crystals.
2. Check that the suction ring hole is clean.
3. Connect the suction tubing and test for good suction.
4. Check the gears of the head.
• Visual inspection
• Manually turn gears; they must be smooth and without friction or resistance
5. Check the blade under a high magnification microscope.
6. Check blade oscillation with the testing tool.
7. Check that the correct depth plate is present and correctly inserted in the shaper head.
8. Check that the stop device is present, correctly attached to the shaper head and, if adjustable, correctly set.
9. Check that all the components have been properly connected.
• The shaper head to the motor
• The motor cable
• The suction tube
• The suction ring handle
10. Check the electric connections to the console and wall outlet.
11. Check the correct position of the pedals.
12. Insert the microkeratome on the suction ring and check that it is completely free to move (forward and reverse) along the track of the ring.

- The suction ring and its handle
- The microkeratome head, blade holder, and collar
- The plates
- The stop device (if it can be removed)
- Other surgical instruments required for the procedure

The following components must not be sterilized in the autoclave (do not use alcohol on acrylic components):

- The motor
- The electric cables
- The tonometer and antidesiccation chamber
- The applanation lenses

B. Surgical Technique

PREOPERATIVE MEDICATION

Thirty minutes prior to surgery, two to three drops of topical antibiotic are instilled as prophylaxis to infection, along with an NSAID to reduce inflammation and postoperative pain. Our preference is a combination of ofloxacin (Ocuflox) with sodium diclofenac (Voltaren).

Five minutes prior to surgery, one or two drops of topical anesthetic (4% lidocaine or 0.5% proparacaine) are instilled to anesthetize the cornea and conjunctiva. Anesthetic drops are repeated prior to application of the suction ring. Two or three applications are more than sufficient for inducing adequate anesthesia. Excessive use of anesthetic (in frequency and/or dosage) may cause edema of the epithelium and alter the thickness of the lamellar cut; it may also weaken adhesion of the epithelium to Bowman's membrane, causing sloughing during the microkeratome pass.

The conjunctiva is more difficult to anesthetize than the cornea, and in the majority of patients, anesthesia of the cornea is sufficient. However, in anxious patients, it may be useful to pursue deeper conjunctival anesthesia than that obtained with topical application of anesthetic drops. This decreases the patient's sensation of manipulation, pressure and discomfort during the procedure, enhancing their ability to cooperate. A good technique to do this is to have the assistant hold an anesthetic-soaked sponge in the inferior, then superior, cul-de-sac without contacting the cornea for about 30 to 45 seconds in each area.

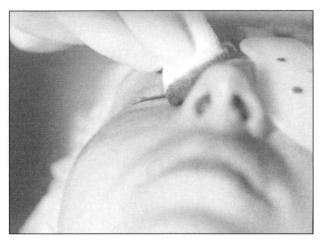

Figure 5-36. Betadine is used in preparation and disinfection of the operating field. The fellow eye is protected with a shield.

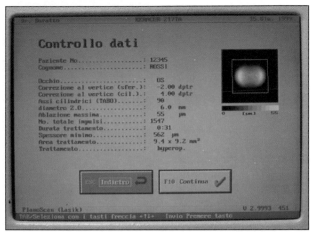

Figure 5-37. The patient's data is checked on the laser's computer.

Instruments

For LASIK with a nasal hinge, Buratto uses the ACS with the fixed diameter LASIK ring and the Keraor 217 laser (Bausch & Lomb Surgical, Claremont, Calif, USA) with a ceramic chamber. Brint uses either the ACS or Summit SKBM microkeratome with either the VISX Star or the Summit Apex Plus lasers.

Preoperative Check of Beam Quality and Data Entry

Prior to each LASIK procedure, the laser technician should check proper functioning of the laser. This includes:

Fluence tests to check the energy emitted by the laser and evaluate uniformity of energy distribution, or homogeneity of the laser beam. Also, the eye tracker must be centered with respect to the central ablation.

The surgeon should check that:

- The refractive correction is correctly entered into the laser's computer.
- Refractive data has been correctly transcribed from the medical record.
- The axis of astigmatism is correct and corresponds with that found topographically and by refraction.
- The minimum diameter of the ablation is appropriate to the patient's scotopic pupil diameter.
- The anticipated ablation depth will leave adequate residual stromal tissue.

Footpedals

The surgeon has three footpedals. They are:
1. The laser delivery pedal.
2. The microkeratome suction pedal which, once pressed, maintains negative pressure until it is pressed again.
3. The microkeratome motor pedal, which activates movement of the microkeratome and has three positions: forward, reverse, and off. Pressing the forward pedal advances the microkeratome, releasing stops the instrument. Pressing the reverse pedal reverses the microkeratome.

SURGEON PREPARATION

Clothing

LASIK is a surgical procedure and should be performed in a sterile environment suitable for surgery. Buratto personally wears a cap, mask, sterile gown, and gloves (powder-free). Brint prefers the no-glove technique with a thorough Betadine hand scrub between cases, drying with a lint-free cloth.

Prior to scrubbing for each case, the eyepieces of the microscope are set at the correct interpillary distance and optical correction. The chair should be positioned at the correct height and the arm rests correctly positioned. Finally, I ensure that the laser and microkeratome pedals are correctly positioned.

PATIENT POSITIONING AND PREPARATION

The patient is asked to lie on the bed. His or her head is positioned so that the forehead and chin are on the same level; a straight imaginary line passes through the feet, umbilicus, and nose (ie, the head must not be rotated). The operative eye is positioned under the operating

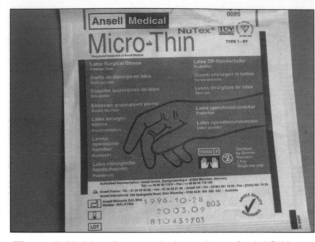

Figure 5-38. Very fine powderless gloves for LASIK.

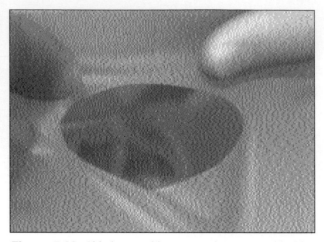

Figure 5-39. 3M drape with an opening surrounded by adhesive film.

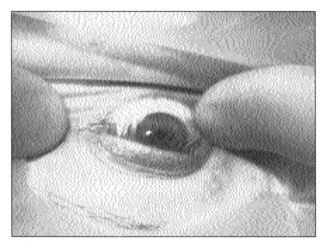

Figure 5-40. The drape is applied to the lower eyelid to exclude the eyelashes from the operating field.

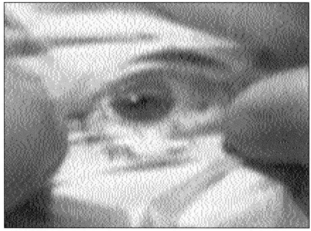

Figure 5-41. The same maneuver is performed on the upper eyelid.

microscope and the patient is instructed to look constantly at the fixation target.

The periocular area is prepared with a solution of povidone iodine and carefully dried.

Steridrape

A disposable self-adhesive aperture drape with a lateral pocket is applied to the lids and lashes.

The drape serves to:

- Isolate the surgical area and guard against contact between instruments or the surgeon's hands and nonsterile areas
- Prevent eyelashes from interfering with the advancement of the microkeratome
- The lateral pocket collects irrigating fluids
- The patient is asked to keep his or her eyes open, and the drape is applied to the margin of the lower eyelid first, then the upper lid, retracting the lids and isolating the lashes.

Lid Speculum

The Buratto speculum is gently inserted. Special care should be used to ensure that the speculum blades retract the drape completely over the lid margins; the end result is eyelashes that are completely excluded from the operating field. The speculum should be opened gently and gradually, but sufficiently to allow for placement of the suction ring and allow the microkeratome pass. Any obstruction in the pass must be removed (drape, eyelids, or lashes) or retracted prior to proceeding.

Correct speculum selection and placement is important to the success of the procedure and avoiding intraoperative complications. The speculum must retract the eyelids and allow advancement of the microkeratome without interference.

With the ACS microkeratome, surgeons tend to encounter impediments to advancement of the microkeratome more often when operating on the right eye. This

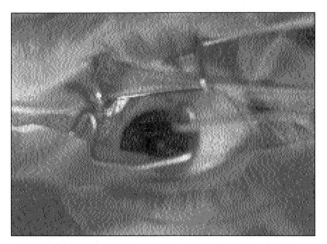

Figure 5-42. The first arm of the speculum is inserted so that the plastic catches the eyelashes.

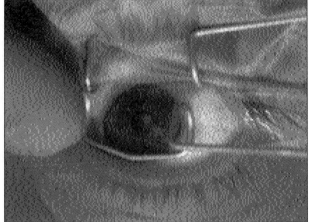

Figure 5-43. The same maneuver is performed for the other eyelid.

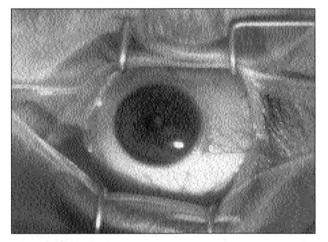

Figure 5-44. Once the speculum has been positioned, the eyelashes must be completely excluded from the operating field.

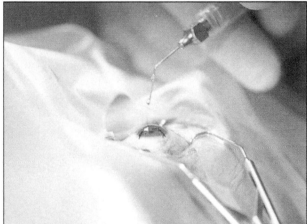

Figure 5-45. Three-radius marking of the epithelium with an Asico marker.

is because the stop mechanism is located superiorly and is more likely to hit the upper eyelid, speculum, or drape.

The speculum must be lightweight, thin, not bulky, and yet strong enough to withstand a forceful blink, while allowing reasonable comfort during insertion. A screw-type locking speculum is preferable. The cornea and the conjunctival sac are irrigated with BSS, and the conjunctival sac is then carefully swabbed with Merocel sponges to remove any secretions, eyelashes, or debris. This maneuver prevents any fluid in the conjunctival sac from being aspirated by the suction ring, thus preventing adequate elevation of IOP. An aspirating speculum can prove useful in removing any fluid present in the conjunctival sac.

Corneal Marking

The marker should enable alignment over the visual axis, at the same time marking the peripheral cornea across the flap margin to assist in the exact repositioning of the lamellar flap. Buratto uses a Buratto marker for this purpose.

Originally, the instrument had four radii. The radial line opposite the handle was removed so that when the instrument is placed on the cornea from the temporal side, no mark is made over the hinge. One of the three remaining radial marks has been bent in a pararadial direction. The optic zone has been elevated so that it does not touch the cornea (the dye or instrument itself may induce epithelial damage). The three radii have been shortened so the cornea is marked only across the peripheral flap margin near the limbus.

The radii are stained with methylene blue or gentian violet. The instrument is then applied to a dry cornea accurately and firmly so that three radii can be seen on the cornea (inferior, superior, and temporal). The three radial marks aid in correct flap repositioning. The parara-

119

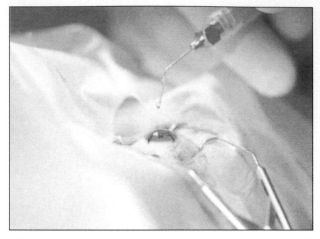

Figure 5-46. The cornea is washed to remove any residual dye.

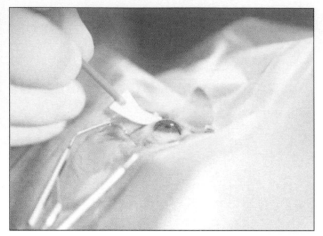

Figure 5-47. Excess liquid and impurities are removed with a Merocel sponge.

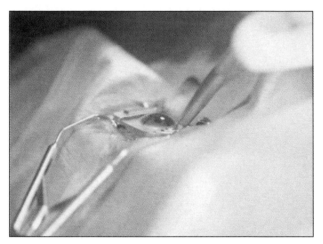

Figure 5-48. Positioning the suction ring.

dial mark is important for the flap replacement stromal side down in the event of a free cap.

Operating Room Ergonomics

The microkeratome, console, and instrument trays are located on a table to the left of the surgeon. The assistant also stands to the surgeon's left to hand off all instruments. As in all surgical procedures, it is important that instruments be handed to the surgeon oriented as they will be used—in particular, the microkeratome and suction ring. For right eyes, the suction ring is placed in the surgeon's left hand with the handle oriented inferiorly (the tubing will pass in front of the surgeon), and the microkeratome is placed in the surgeon's right hand. For left eyes, the ring is placed in the right hand with the handle oriented superiorly (the tubing passing behind the surgeon and over the right shoulder). The microkeratome is held in the left hand.

Reassuring the Patient

During a preliminary visit, the surgeon will have already explained to the patient that the operation is not painful, but may be slightly uncomfortable. The surgeon will also have explained the steps involved in the procedure. During preoperative preparation, the staff should reassure the patient and explain each step. More importantly, the surgeon should talk to the patient during the procedure, explaining step-by-step what is happening.

Suction Ring Application

Prior to placing the ring on the eye, check that the drape will not interfere with the microkeratome pass, that no eyelashes are exposed, and that the speculum provides adequate space for correct ring positioning. Widen the blades of the speculum by turning the adjustment screw, if necessary. Also check that the cornea is well centered in the intrapalpebral space. If there is greater exposure of sclera inferiorly, ask the patient to slightly raise the chin, this will induce a slight downward rotation of the eye to better center the cornea and allow easier placement of the suction ring.

The handle of the suction ring is oriented inferiorly for surgery of the right eye and superiorly for the left eye. The toothed track of the suction ring will thus align with the microkeratome gears to produce a nasally hinged flap. Remember that the serial number marked on the suction ring must always be on the temporal side of the eye.

Place the suction ring gently on the globe. Check that it is well centered on the cornea and that the corneal markings are visible. When certain that it is in correct position, firmly stabilize the globe and ask the assistant to engage suction, then wait a few seconds until the vacuum is adequate to firmly grasp the globe.

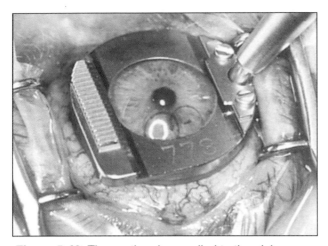

Figure 5-49. The suction ring applied to the globe.

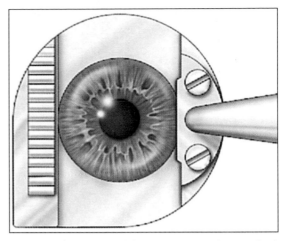

Figure 5-50. The ACS suction ring: the toothed track that allows movement of the microkeratome can be seen; the short track is on the right side to facilitate insertion of the microkeratome.

When the vacuum is activated, you will notice a slight increase in the diameter of the pupil. This is a good sign, indicating that the IOP has increased. You will also feel that the handle of the suction ring is no longer "free," and requires less support. At this point, release slight downward pressure on the globe, allowing it to return to its natural position inside the orbit. The suction ring's grasp on the globe can also be checked by slightly elevating the ring.

When treating simple cases of low myopia, it is better if the ring is well-centered on the cornea; if dealing with astigmatic or hyperopic patients, the ring should be decentered nasally 0.5 to 1.0 mm. This allows a hinge that is positioned slightly more nasal and out of the way of a large ablation, especially if the flap is smaller than planned. This amount of nasal decentration should also be considered in patients with steep corneas over about 46 D. As with the fixed LASIK ring, a large flap and hinge will be made, which may not be displaced enough even for a routine ablation.

If there is slight unintentional decentration of the ring after applying suction, the surgeon can proceed with the cut. If the decentration is marked, release the suction and attempt to reapply the ring. If there has been only a few seconds of suction applied this can be successful. If there has been 10 to 20 seconds of suction, apply a few drops of a steroid and vasoconstrictor and wait for the conjunctival edema and scleral groove formed by the suction ring to disappear. This will usually facilitate correct repositioning of the ring (if the ring is reapplied before the groove disappears, it will return to its previous placement, making the entire maneuver useless).

If it is difficult to correctly position the ring on the globe, place the index finger on the cornea to stabilize it in the correct position, then activate suction.

With the exception of a few seconds immediately prior to applying suction, avoid downward pressure on the ring. This causes unnecessary increase in IOP and allows bulbar conjunctiva to come around the ring, interfering with advancement of the microkeratome.

The surgeon should also avoid lifting the ring, as this may cause suction to be lost. If this occurs during the cut, it can cause serious damage. If the ring causes any subconjunctival hemorrhage, the surgeon should tell the patient that this is only a temporary cosmetic problem and will resolve spontaneously.

Tonometry

Prior to proceeding with the cut, it is mandatory to check that IOP is sufficiently elevated. Using the Barraquer tonometer, a meniscus inside the inscribed circle on the instrument indicates that pressure is above 65 mm Hg.

Accurate measurement is obtained when the cornea is almost completely dry. If it is too wet, the excess fluid will provide a pseudomeniscus that is falsely large. If too dry, the measurement will indicate falsely high IOP.

Indicators that IOP is elevated:
- Change in the sound of the suction pump when aspiration is blocked by the adhesion of the ring to the globe.
- The sensation when the tonometer is positioned that it is coming into contact with a rigid surface.
- The suction ring stays in position even when lightly supported by the hand.
- The pupil slightly dilates and the patient reports that he or she can no longer see the fixation light.

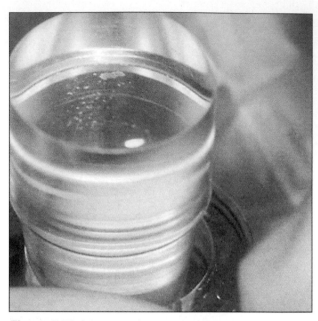

Figure 5-51. Intraoperative tonometry.

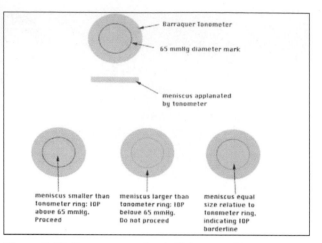

Figure 5-52. Barraquer method of intraoperative tonometry.

- Touching the cornea with the index finger gives the surgeon an idea of how firm the globe is.

It is important that pressure is adequate, otherwise the cut will not produce a flap of uniform thickness and diameter. If the tonometric reading indicates IOP is inadequate, it is better not to continue—release suction, reposition the ring, and try again.

Occasionally, despite repeated attempts, the surgeon is unable to achieve adequate elevation of IOP. Try other lid speculums such as the Barraquer wire, which allows the suction ring to be placed directly over it and then pushed downward in an attempt to proptose the globe, allow the ring to engage sclera, and obtain suction. With this technique, the patient must be warned not to squeeze during the microkeratome pass. Frequently, the conjunctiva will be aspirated into the orifice of the suction ring; in a tight orbit, the surgeon may not be able to stretch it to prevent this from reoccurring. In this situation, ask the patient to rest about an hour, then try the Hansatome, which has a nasal orifice, rather than one in the previously deformed spot. Rather than risk a serious complication, it is better to abort the LASIK procedure and give the patient the option of surface PRK, if appropriate.

Lubricating the Cornea and Suction Ring

Following tonometry, use a syringe-mounted cannula to apply a drop of ophthaine to the suction ring grooves that guide the microkeratome, then wet the cornea with two to three additional drops. This will aid in smooth movement of the microkeratome over the cornea,

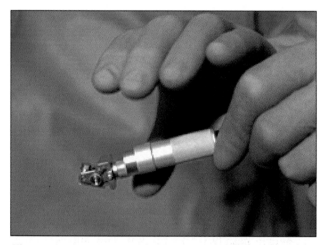

Figure 5-53. Holding the microkeratome, the assistant hands it to the surgeon who is ready to grasp it in the correct manner.

allowing a uniform cut to be performed. Too much liquid can be thrown from the microkeratome gears up onto the laser optics or mirror and damage them. An alternative technique is to paint the corneal surface and track with a very moist sponge soaked with proparacaine.

If the cornea is too dry during the cut, the cut surface may be uneven and epithelial damage is more likely to occur. If there is excess fluid, it may slow progression of the microkeratome and can be thrown, as mentioned, by the microkeratome gears up into the optics of the laser and microscope.

Engaging the Microkeratome Into the Suction Ring

When operating on the right eye, the microkeratome is held with the right hand; for left eyes, with the left hand. The microkeratome motor is grasped between the thumb and fingers with the palm facing downward.

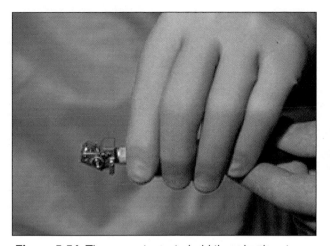

Figure 5-54. The correct way to hold the microkeratome.

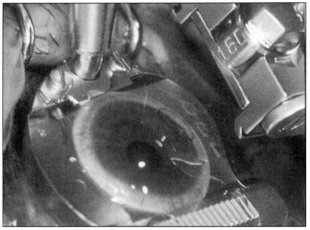

Figure 5-55. The microkeratome is ready to be inserted on the ring tracks.

The hand, arm, and elbow should be relaxed and aligned along the axis of the microkeratome. Insert the microkeratome into the suction ring. The microkeratome head is introduced into the suction ring by first sliding 3.0 to 4.0 mm of the wing on the bottom edge of the head into the dovetailed groove on the toothed track side of the suction ring. The other wing is then depressed onto the suction ring. Advance the microkeratome forward until it is stopped by the gears engaging the toothed track of the ring. Gently move the microkeratome up, down, and side to side, ensuring it is correctly secured in the suction ring (wobble test).

The hand is then moved from the motor to support the instrument by the connection cord. A neutral position should be maintained. Any pressure, torque, pushing, or lifting of the microkeratome can have a detrimental effect on smooth advancement of the instrument, which will compromise the quality of the cut.

The patient should be warned that pressure on the eye might increase slightly with engagement and advancement of the microkeratome, but discomfort will be minimal.

Engaging the Gears Into the Ring Teeth

Using the footpedal, advance the microkeratome until the gear catches the first or second tooth of the suction ring track. A final check is then performed to ensure that:

- The depth plate is correctly positioned
- The stop is correctly positioned
- The microkeratome path is free from obstructions

Performing the Lamellar Cut

This is the most critical phase of the entire operation. Carefully watching the advancing path of the microkeratome, the surgeon continuously depresses the forward portion of the footpedal. Alternately, this task may be delegated to the assistant who advances the microkeratome with the footpedal until it is prevented from continuing by the stop device. It is then reversed until it returns to its original position. At this point, the lamellar cut has been completed.

If the instrument has been well maintained, assembled, and used correctly, the microkeratome will normally advance and reverse at a constant speed. When the microkeratome reverses, it will return the cut flap to its original position on the stromal bed. Only upon lifting the flap can the surgeon verify that the cut has been made and judge its quality.

At this point, the most difficult and dangerous part of the operation has been completed and one can breathe a sigh of relief.

Microkeratome and Suction Ring Removal

When the microkeratome has returned to its starting position, the assistant releases suction by once again pressing on the pedal. The ring with the microkeratome still engaged is handed off as a unit to the assistant. After the procedure, the assistant will disassemble, clean, and sterilize them for the next patient.

We try to keep suction engaged for no more than 1 minute. This decreases the chance of vascular occlusion or damage from elevated IOP. When the procedure is uneventful, the lamellar cut can be completed in less than 30 seconds.

Additional Tips for Using the Microkeratome

The microkeratome gear teeth must insert accurately into those of the suction ring. If not, the microkeratome will not advance, in which case the surgeon must reverse

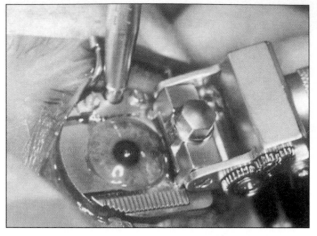

Figure 5-56. Insertion of the microkeratome on the tracks of the suction ring. The wing that enters the long track situated beside the toothed track is inserted first.

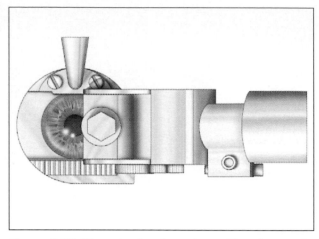

Figure 5-59. The microkeratome is positioned correctly on the tracks and the gears of the head are brought into contact with the toothed track of the suction ring.

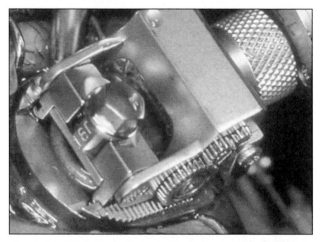

Figure 5-57. Intermediate cutting phase: the gears are about halfway along the toothed track.

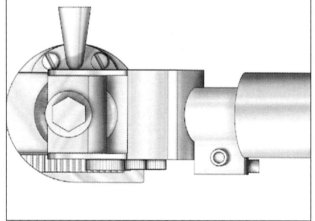

Figure 5-60. The intermediate cutting phase: the pedal that advances the microkeratome is depressed.

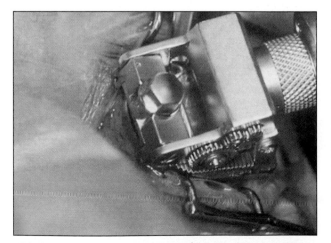

Figure 5-58. Final stage of the cut: when the microkeratome reaches the end of the pass, it will stop. Then, the reverse pedal is depressed and the instrument returns.

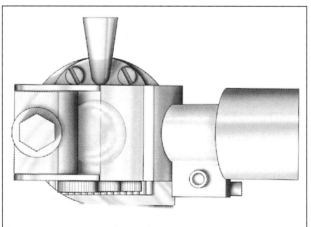

Figure 5-61. The cut has been completed. The stop device has come into contact with the suction ring and the microkeratome stops.

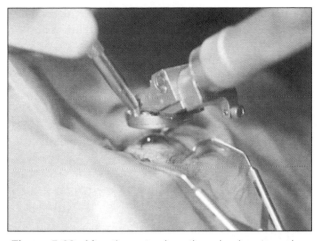

Figure 5-62. After the cut: when the microkeratome has returned, it, along with the ring, is lifted from the corneal plane.

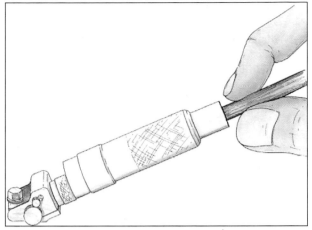

Figure 5-63. The ACS. Note how to support the power supply cable—it must not interfere with movement of the microkeratome in any way.

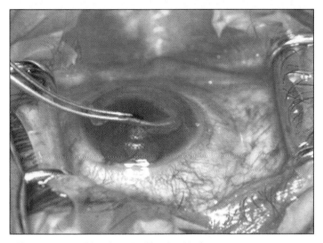

Figure 5-64. The flap is lifted with forceps.

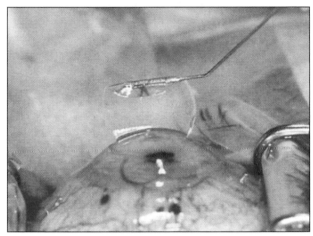

Figure 5-65. The flap is raised with a spatula.

the direction of the instrument, re-engage the head into the suction ring, and repeat advancement until the teeth mesh and the pass is completed.

The two wings on the microkeratome head must insert into the grooves of the ring so that the instrument will properly advance. Prior to beginning the cut, the microkeratome is gently rocked side to side (wobble test), first in one direction and then in the other to check that it is correctly seated in the suction ring.

Downward, upward, or forward pressure should not be exerted on the microkeratome because this may prevent smooth movement of the instrument, even binding the gears and stopping advancement prior to completing the pass.

Suction must be maintained during the pass; if interrupted, the resection will be incomplete and irregular. The procedure should be aborted, the flap perfectly repositioned, and a new cut attempted again after 3 to 4 months.

The microkeratome must traverse the entire track, stopped only by the stopping device. If stopped earlier by the speculum, drape, or eyelid, the cut will be incomplete and the surgeon will need to determine if the flap is large enough to allow for complete refractive ablation prior to proceeding.

If it is felt that the stromal bed is irregular, the flap has an irregular shape, the cut is incomplete, the flap is not of a uniform thickness, or there is a hole in the flap. The refractive ablation should not be performed. Instead, reposition the flap with sutures, if necessary, and wait a few months. Repeat the procedure using a depth plate that will provide a slightly deeper cut.

360° Cut (Free Cap)

In a free cap situation, the cap usually remains inside the microkeratome head. Ensure that the nasal epithelial side mark is still present. If not, make a short line with the marking pen on the protruding cap for future nasal and epithelial orientation. With a toothless or blunt-toothed forceps (Hoskin's forceps), gently remove the cap without stretching or pulling. A drop of BSS can help prevent it from sticking to the microkeratome and tearing. Carefully remove and place it in an antidesiccation chamber, preferably with the epithelial side down, on a single drop of BSS. Dry the stromal surface and examine the cap for shape and smoothness of the cut surface.

Examine the stromal bed, if it appears uniform and the diameter of the resection is sufficient to allow for the planned ablation, delivery of the refractive laser ablation can proceed. Then replace the cap, ensuring that stroma is against stroma and that the flap is exactly in its original position (this is easily done if the preoperative marking has been done correctly). If markings have faded, examine the cut surfaces very carefully, looking for landmarks that can aid in correct repositioning and orient the flap as accurately as possible on the underlying bed. Hopefully the surgeon has remembered to mark the cap while still in the microkeratome head as described above. If adhesion is good, sutures are not required; if there is any doubt, an external suture should be placed to prevent displacement and loss.

The main rule in managing free caps and incomplete or inadequate flaps is to avoid all but strictly necessary manipulations. Excessive manipulation can cause fold formation, alterations in Bowman's layer, epithelial disruption, and the introduction of foreign material into the interface.

Repositioning the Patient and Centering the Laser

Frequently during the microkeratome pass, the patient's head and eye move from their original position and must be realigned for delivery of the refractive ablation. The chin should be level with the forehead and an imaginary line should pass through the nose and between the feet. The eye must be directly beneath the fixation target and the two alignment targets must be focused on the cornea above the center of the pupil, or the reticule must be centered over the pupil, depending on the laser. The patient is instructed to fixate on the target light and continue to do so throughout laser delivery, even if the target appears out of focus.

The room lights and microscope light should be dimmed as much as possible, improving the patient's ability to maintain good fixation. Reassure the patient that the operation is proceeding smoothly and correctly. Recheck that the laser is perfectly focused and centered, then activate the eye tracker if appropriate.

A Buratto metal half-moon device (Asico) is placed on the nasal bulbar conjunctiva. The corneal flap is reflected onto this, preventing contact with the conjunctiva and potential contamination by secretions, fluids, or debris.

The flap is lifted using special toothless forceps designed by Buratto specifically for this purpose. Grasp the flap at its temporal edge, taking care not to damage the epithelium, and reflect it evenly onto the surface of the half-moon, avoiding folds as much as possible. If the flap folds over onto itself, it is straightened and immediately smoothed. Another technique to lift the flap (used by Brint) is to gently slide the open jaws of smooth tying forceps from the temporal margin of the wet cornea under the edge of the flap and lift it, nasally reflecting it.

THE REFRACTIVE ABLATION

The Refractive Ablation for Myopic Correction

It is interesting to occasionally take a pachymetry measurement of the stromal bed and determine flap thickness by subtracting this from the preoperative measurement to evaluate the flap thickness actually being obtained.

During delivery of the refractive ablation, it is mandatory to monitor centration and focus. The first optic zone or ablative phase is completed using the Technolas 217 laser.

At this point, a dry spatula is gently passed over the stromal surface to remove any fluid formed during the ablation. Alternatively, fluid can be dried using a Merocel sponge.

Subsequent ablation phases are then performed. During the last two phases, which have the greatest diameter, protect the hinge with a spatula or retract the flap to avoid it from being ablated, even briefly. This is especially important if the flap is small or decentered temporally.

The Refractive Ablation for Astigmatic or Hyperopic Correction

When with-the-rule astigmatism is treated, the flap must be protected at the hinge as the ablation will be performed along the 0° to 180° axis. This can be done with a spatula that is wide enough to completely cover the area.

If the myopic astigmatism is against-the-rule, the ablation is performed vertically, making hinge protection unnecessary.

In hyperopia, the ablation has an optic zone that is larger than in myopic or astigmatic corrections. The flap should be decentered nasally to remove the hinge from

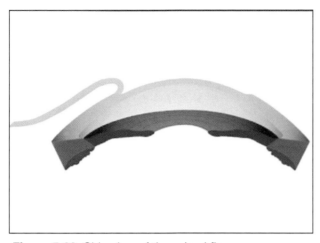

Figure 5-66. Side view of the raised flap.

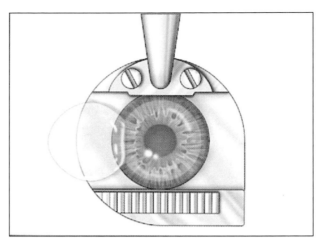

Figure 5-67. Some surgeons prefer to rest the flap on the suction ring where it is held in position without suction.

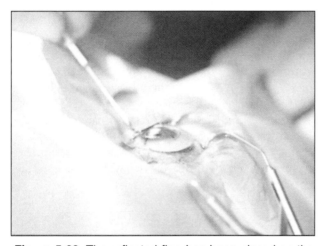

Figure 5-68. The reflected flap has been placed on the surface of the positioner during photoablation.

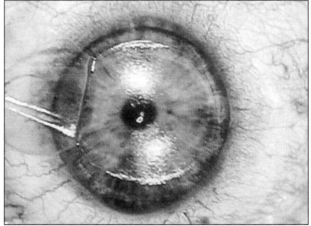

Figure 5-69. Ablation phase: in this case the flap is placed directly on the conjunctiva.

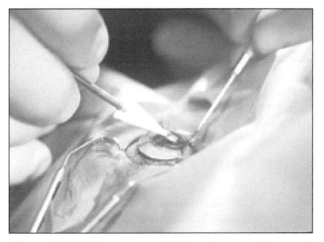

Figure 5-70. Between one ablative phase and the next, the excess fluid gravitating to the base of the hinge is continuously dried with a Merocel sponge.

the ablation zone. The hinge should always be retracted to increase the space available for the ablation while protecting the hinge and stromal surface from laser ablation. Using the ACS for hyperopic ablations is tricky, as generally the flap/bed is fine for myopia but borderline for the larger hyperopic ablation. With a steep cornea, a large bed can usually be obtained, with careful nasal decentration, there is adequate room for the ablation, even out to 8.5 mm. With flat corneas, which are more common in hyperopic eyes, the bed is smaller and there may be significant overflow of the ablation onto the hinge and epithelium outside the bed, stimulating epithelial ingrowth and hinge disruption. One should plan ahead and have alternative keratomes available for these situations.

During the Ablation

Continually monitor the focus and centration of the alignment targets. If the patient's eye has moved or the

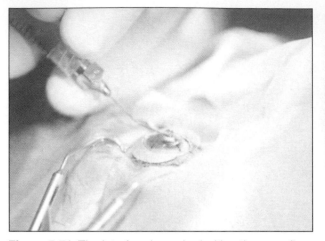

Figure 5-71. The interface is washed with a three- or five-channel cannula.

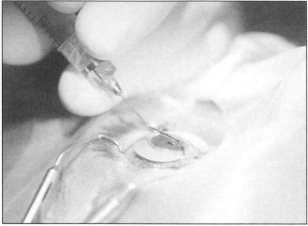

Figure 5-72. The edges of the flap are dried with a slightly damp Merocel sponge tip.

alignment targets defocus, stop the procedure. Proceed after recentering and focusing the targets. Perfect focus is of great importance when the eye tracker is being used. The infrared television camera of the eye tracker "sees" the eye obliquely; any upward or downward movement of the eye provokes a lateral displacement of the image, which will result in a decentered ablation.

If fluid forms on the stromal bed or along the flap hinge, interrupt treatment and dry the fluid with a Merocel sponge.

Try to proceed quickly, minimizing the exposure of stromal surfaces to air. If the stroma becomes dehydrated, the ablation will remove too much tissue, resulting in overcorrection.

Repositioning the Flap

To facilitate uniform distension of the flap, apply two or three drops of BSS to the in-situ stroma; the fluid is applied evenly onto the tissue using the curved back of a long, blunt 27-gauge cannula. Look for a symmetrical gutter to determine correct positioning as well as alignment of the marks (epithelium with the marks may slide; the symmetrical width of the gutter will not). The epithelium along the flap margins should be intact and a clean interface should be present.

If everything is perfect, the cornea is allowed to dry without further manipulation for about 1 minute. Then, using a blunt olive-tipped spatula or tip of a dry Merocel sponge, apply gentle pressure about 1.0 mm outside the incision to check flap adhesion to the underlying stroma. The surgeon should observe fine lines that extend toward the center of the flap (striae test). Warn the patient prior to performing the striae test to decrease the chance of sudden eye movement causing flap displacement.

Intraoperative Management of the Flap

Handle the flap with great care. Avoid excessive use of topical anesthetic drops. Avoid touching the flap with instruments or dry sponges; keep the flap well hydrated. Avoid allowing the flap to fold (decreasing postoperative striae and irregular astigmatism).

Treat the epithelium with extreme care. Avoid rubbing the flap with instruments, even if they are blunt.

Try to reposition the flap without exerting traction and pressure. We do not dry the flap with compressed air.

SPECULUM REMOVAL AND THE FINAL EXAM

To gently remove the speculum, first remove the inferior blade and then the superior, being careful not to touch the cornea and particularly not to displace the flap. Having the assistant retract the lids while the surgeon lifts the speculum up and away from the cornea facilitates this. Then remove the drape. The patient is asked to blink three or four times to check that the flap remains in position. Antibiotic (Ocuflox) and NSAID (Voltaren) drops are instilled. The patient is then asked to wait in the recovery area for about 30 minutes with his or her eyes closed and covered with protective shields.

Final Slit Lamp Exam

After 30 minutes, the patient is examined at the slit lamp. At the slit lamp, check:
- That the flap is well-adhered and smooth
- The gutter is symmetrical
- There is no significant debris in the interface

If at the slit lamp examination, the flap is not well-

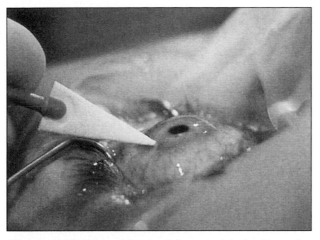

Figure 5-73. The striae test is completed with a dry sponge, or better still, with a button-tipped spatula.

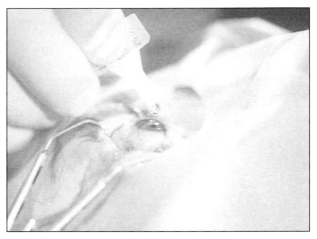

Figure 5-74. Medication with antibiotic eyedrops.

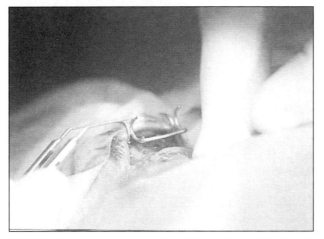

Figure 5-75. The speculum is gently removed.

aligned, has folds or striae, or does not adhere perfectly to the underlying bed, the patient is returned to a surgical microscope (not the laser microscope), the flap is lifted, the stromal bed is once again wetted, and the flap is repositioned correctly. If there is any debris, try to remove it. This may require stroking the underside of the flap and bed with a wet Merocel sponge, as irrigation alone sometimes will not wash out adhering particles. If the flap does not adhere to the underlying bed as quickly as usual, additional time is needed to allow the cornea to dry appropriately.

If all is in order, the patient is discharged with a prescription for the necessary medications and instructed not to rub the eye. On arrival home, the patient should go to bed and sleep for a few hours. Upon awakening, the superficial incision will have re-epithelialized, the cornea will be transparent, and he or she should begin to see clearly.

IOP Measurement During LASIK

Arturo Chayet, MD

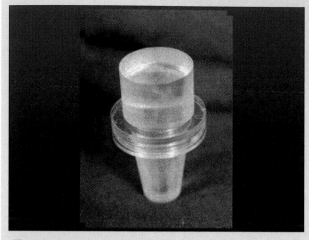

Figure 5A-1. A tonometer.

There are two major surgical components in LASIK: the creation of a corneal flap and the use of a laser to perform stromal ablation for optical correction. Several conditions are needed in order to achieve the desired dimensions of the flap, including:

1. Appropriate function of the microkeratome
2. Appropriate intraocular pressure (IOP) during the microkeratome pass
3. Appropriate attention to detail by the LASIK surgeon

Several studies have shown that the minimum IOP needed to create a good flap must exceed 90 mm Hg. During normal conditions, IOP exceeding this amount is achieved by most microkeratome suction ring devices. Poor IOP may arise from the following conditions:

1. Improper suction ring/vacuum unit function
2. Loose conjunctiva and/or chemotic conjunctiva
3. Eyes with very flat anterior segments (including flat corneas)
4. Improper suction ring alignment by the surgeon
5. Iatrogenic loss of suction during microkeratome use

The LASIK surgeon is capable of avoiding problems with the pass of the microkeratome due to low IOP in these conditions by measuring the IOP before passing the microkeratome head. The only way to prevent the pass of the microkeratome during iatrogenic loss of suction is by having an IOP sensor in the microkeratome unit that will disable the possibility of passing the microkeratome over the suction ring if the IOP is lower than 90 mm Hg.

In our clinic, at the time of this writing, I have performed more than 7000 lamellar procedures since 1994. In a retrospective analysis of all the procedures, we found eight eyes in which a small/thin improper flap was created; seven of those cases occurred during the first 200 cases and the last case occurred around case number 500. Until then, we used the Barraquer hand-held tonometer to measure IOP before passing the microkeratome. It was on the last case (feeling that I had already overcome my learning curve) when I realized that despite the fact that the applanation area was less than 65 mm Hg on the Barraquer tonometer, I had a bad flap; in order to have a precise number rather than a "ballpark" figure, IOP needed to be measured with an objective device that could provide an actual number. That is how we became interested in using the Pneumotonometer (Mentor, Santa Barbara, Calif, USA) to measure the IOP after the suction ring has been applied and prior to the microkeratome pass. Since that date, we have not had a poor flap again (in more than 6500 procedures). One may argue that one of the reasons for this may be the gaining of experience, a factor that, although partially true, is not completely correct. We have found a rate of 1:500 eyes in which the IOP is improper before the microkeratome pass. From those cases, in all but two eyes, we were able to re-apply the suction ring and achieve IOP over 100 mm Hg. In the other two eyes, we were unable to achieve good IOP (even in different sessions); therefore, we converted the cases to PRK with excellent results.

In summary, the ideal IOP necessary to create a proper flap during LASIK appears to be higher than 90 mm Hg. The Barraquer hand-held tonometer, although very useful, may lead to a false positive measurement. Therefore, we strongly recommend the use of the Pneumotonometer as the standard way of measuring IOP during LASIK, as this device has been proven to be the most accurate, reliable, and objective way of measuring high degrees of IOP.

DOWN-UP LASIK WITH THE HANSATOME: PERSONAL TECHNIQUE

6

Lucio Buratto, MD

INTRODUCTION

Following a decade of progressive improvements since its introduction, laser-assisted in situ keratomileusis (LASIK) has become the preferred surgical technique for myopia, astigmatism, and hyperopia. I established the foundation for the technique in 1989 when I used the excimer laser to perform intrastromal ablation on the lamellar cap first, then performed the first case in situ on an ametropic patient.

Between 1991 and 1996, LASIK was performed using an established, though evolving, technique. A microkeratome with automated advancement was used to cut a superficial corneal flap with a diameter 7.5 to 8.5 mm and a thickness of 130 to 180 microns. The cut began from the temporal side and was stopped nasally without completing the full pass, which left a nasal hinge of about 1.0 mm.

The flap was then raised to allow an excimer laser single or multizone in-situ ablation centered on the prepupillary area. The flap was then replaced without sutures. The entire procedure was performed under topical anesthesia in a laser center, office-based, or day hospital (outpatient) setting. Most frequently, the microkeratome used to create the flap was the Automatic Corneal Shaper (ACS), and the laser most frequently used internationally was the Technolas Keracor 117 (Bausch & Lomb Surgical, Claremont, Calif, USA), while in the United States the Summit Apex Plus and the VISX Star were used within the US Food Drug Administration (FDA)-approved limits. In 1996, I introduced a modification to the technique that involved performing the cut from below (inferior) upward (down-up). This created a hinge in the superior position, which is more "natural" than the nasal position. The advantages of such a hinge will be examined in detail later in this chapter. Techniques and instruments for refractive ablation have also evolved since this time. Presently, flying spot lasers using an eye tracker are producing significant improvements in the refractive and functional results.

THE COMPONENTS OF THE HANSATOME

This section examines what we consider the most suitable microkeratome for the superior hinge cut—the Hansatome microkeratome. Although the Hansatome, like other microkeratomes, consists of three parts a motor, a head fitted with a blade, and a suction ring—it is actually quite different from the others. Visually, the instrument differs because the motor and head are oriented vertically (ie, the motor is inserted above the suction ring and consequently above the eye). The cutting action is different; while all the other microkeratomes cut from temporal to nasal except for the Moria C-B unit, the Hansatome cuts from below upward (inferior to superior) with a fan-like movement through rotation of the head around a temporally situated pin. This produces a corneal hinge in the superior position, which is this machine's truly innovative feature. However, this microkeratome can also perform cuts with nasal, temporal, inferior, or angled hinges.

In cases of astigmatism, I advanced the idea of positioning the hinge along the axis of the astigmatism. However, in the cases studied, this actually did not seem to impact the final outcome. This is because the large flap created with this microkeratome did not cause interference with the ablation, regardless of the axis and amount of astigmatism. The down-up technique was thus used even in cases of high astigmatism, regardless of axis. The Hansatome can produce large-diameter high-quality cuts with a thickness that matches surgical need. This instrument has proved to be easier, safer, and more accurate. The various parts of the instrument as well as assembly and disassembly will now be examined.

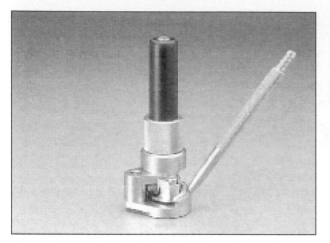

Figure 6-1. The Bausch & Lomb Hansatome microkeratome complete with suction ring, motor, and head.

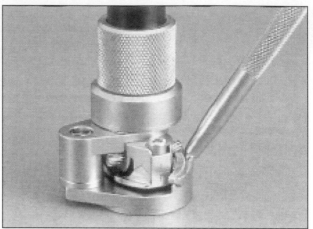

Figure 6-2. Close-up of the Hansatome: suction ring, head, and motor.

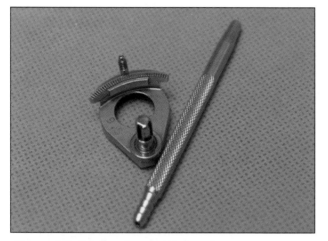

Figure 6-3. Suction ring and its handle.

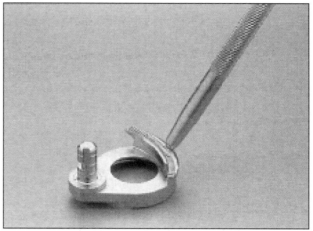

Figure 6-4. The assembled suction ring: on the right, the pin can be seen. The microkeratome head is inserted here and rotates around it during the cut. The handle can be seen on the left, below the curved toothed run. The stop mechanism lies below this. The surface of the suction ring has no tracks.

The Suction Ring

The suction ring consists of two components: the handle, which is connected by tubing to the vacuum pump in the console, and the suction ring itself. The handle is shorter to allow easy positioning under the excimer laser microscope. Inferiorly, the ring has a concave portion that comes into contact with the conjunctiva and sclera. There is just one suction orifice, but it is sufficient to allow the ring to firmly adhere to the globe. The ring is designed to provide excellent contact with the tissues and create excellent adhesion when suction is activated, which is mandatory for achieving good quality cuts and for reducing the risk of complications associated with inadequate suction. Suction has never been lost in more than 2000 LASIK procedures personally performed with this instrument.

The superior part of the ring is completely different from others in that the toothed track is circular and elevated to assist in avoiding obstruction. This aids in making the procedure simple and repeatable. Lamellar surgeons are well aware of problems related to the track and gear mechanism, such as debris along the pass that can interrupt the action of the microkeratome. Because the surface of the Hansatome ring is smooth, movement along the ring occurs easily, with no interference or obstruction.

Near the suction handle, the ring has an arch-shaped elevated toothed track, which engages with complementary gears on the instrument head and creates the automated cut. The elevated position of the toothed track with respect to the blade's cutting plane prevents the

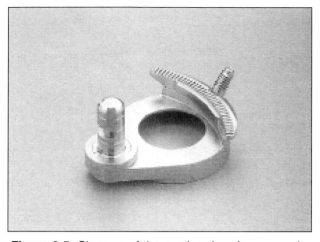

Figure 6-5. Close-up of the suction ring. An arc can be observed below and left of the toothed run: this is the stop mechanism. The toothed run is raised with respect to the cut plane.

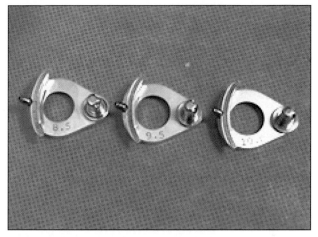

Figure 6-6. Three rings for cuts of different diameter.

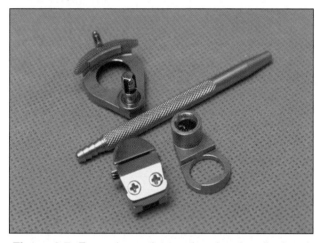

Figure 6-7. From above, the suction ring, handle, head, and the right/left separator (right).

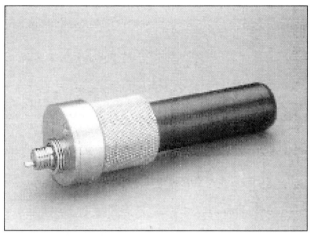

Figure 6-8. The microkeratome motor. This is screwed vertically onto the head of the microkeratome. The eccentric is similar to those of other microkeratomes. It is used to induce blade oscillation.

gear mechanism from coming into contact with the speculum, eyelids, or eyelashes. These features make the machine easier to use, as well as safer.

Anterior to the toothed track and on a slightly lower elevation, the ring has an arch-shaped protrusion that stops progression of the microkeratome at the appropriate completion of the pass. This stop mechanism is fixed and prevents many of the problems associated with incorrect stop assembly or calibration.

Opposite the suction handle is a pin for the vertical insertion of the head. The head rotates around this pin in a fan-like fashion. This pin has two grooves to ensure correct head position. By rotating the head on the pin at a predetermined point of rotation, the microkeratome drops in the grooves and rests on the suction ring plane.

The automated mechanism of the head can only then come into contact with the toothed track of the ring and successfully perform the cut. Because of this mechanism on the suction ring, the head maintains a precise fixed relationship with the suction ring and ensures a constant and uniform cut surface (and therefore thickness of the flap). This ensures that the cut will only be performed when the head and its blade are in tight apposition with the suction ring and a constant cutting planc is maintained.

In summary, the Hansatome microkeratome creates correctly sized hinges and lamellar cuts of uniform thickness. The suction ring adheres easily to the globe, and the instrument has proven to be reliable, comfortable, and safe to use.

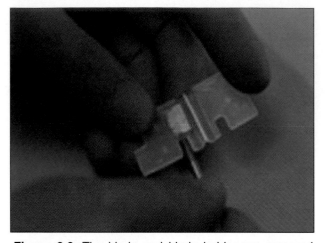

Figure 6-9. The blade and blade holder are removed from the sterile container.

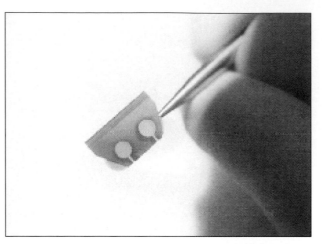

Figure 6-10. The blade with the plastic blade holder mounted on the instrument for insertion on the head.

The Motor

The Hansatome motor is fitted with an eccentric that rotates at a speed of 9600 revolution per minute (RPM) to activate blade oscillation. The motor also activates the advancement of the microkeratome along the toothed track of the suction ring. This high-speed rotation has a positive effect on the quality of the cut, particularly on the quality of the stromal bed surface.

The Hansatome motor differs from others because it is positioned vertically during the operation. Having the motor above the ring and globe confers stability and uniformity of traction during the cut. A microkeratome that cuts from temporal to nasal, on the other hand, creates traction force tangential to the ring as it is being inserted into the suction ring. If this traction force becomes significant, it may detach the suction ring from the globe or, alternatively, dislodge the ring with consequent decentration of the cut. The same may occur during advancement of the instrument on the suction ring. The position of the Hansatome motor vertically above the ring, as well as its weight, makes it adhere more firmly to the globe.

The Blade

The Hansatome blade is a traditional steel blade that comes mounted on a self-lubricating Teflon blade holder. The blade holder is inserted in the microkeratome head through a lateral slit—it may be inserted in only one way. Having the blade supplied on a ready-to-use plastic blade-holder greatly simplifies the insertion procedure and avoids useless manipulation of the blade itself. Since it cannot be resterilized in the autoclave (because the plastic will melt), single use of the blade is ensured. In the upper part of the blade holder is a preformed groove that engages the motor eccentric. This is another feature that adds safety and precision to the operation. The

groove receives the eccentric of the motor, and the motor activates the blade's oscillatory movement. During the cut, the blade is at a 25° angle. The oscillation rate is 9600 RPM.

MICROKERATOME ASSEMBLY

Initial Connections

Connect the 110 or 220 volts (V) electrical supply, which must be grounded. Next, connect the suction and motor activation pedals to the power unit; connect the cable between the microkeratome motor to the power unit and the aspiration tubing to the power unit.

SUCTION RING AND VACUUM CHECK ASSEMBLY

Screw the handle securely onto the suction ring but do not overtighten. Inspect the suction ring under the microscope to ensure that it is smooth, undented, and free of debris. Carefully connect the suction tubing at the free end of the handle. The suction is activated with the suction ring unoccluded (ie, the orifice open) and the level of induced vacuum is checked on the manometer of the power supply. Unlike the ACS power console, the vacuum level is internally checked and should read approximately 26.0 mm Hg. Then, cover the lower part of the suction ring with your thumb and allow it to firmly adhere. Check the vacuum level once again to be sure that it reads between 25.2 to 26.2 mm Hg.

Test the vacuum level by raising your hand; if the suction ring continues to adhere to the thumb with the handle pointing down, you can assume that the induced vacuum is sufficient for a satisfactory cut.

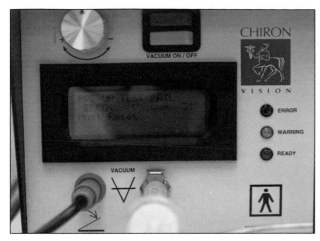

Figure 6-11. The power supply with the connectors for the electric cables of the microkeratome. Below and to the right are the connectors for the tube to the suction ring.

The Hansatome power unit is equipped with automatic electronic pressure control. (Note: pressure does not refer to intraocular pressure [IOP] but to the vacuum induced in the aspiration tube). This allows the surgeon to perform the cut only when the vacuum has reached an appropriate level and makes the lamellar cut significantly safer. Additionally, the cut will be interrupted during the operation if the level of vacuum inside the aspiration tube drops below the desired level for any reason.

If vacuum precalibration does not correspond to the "normal" operational level, an error message will appear on the display, and it will not be possible to use the machine.

The Hansatome unit is normally delivered to the patient with relative vacuum equal to about 26 mm Hg. This is the value used at sea level (4.0 mm Hg below the barometric pressure indicated by the display). The value is reduced by about 1.0 mm Hg for every 330-meter increase in altitude. If not already calibrated, vacuum can be calibrated as follows:

- Connect the electrical cable to the power supply
- Connect the vacuum pedal and pedal for advancement of the motor (do not connect the suction tubing).
- Completely rotate the knob for vacuum regulation counterclockwise toward the (-) sign.
- Turn on the power unit.
- Turn the knob three consecutive turns in a clockwise direction toward the (+) sign.
- Push the pedal that initiates vacuum (without the tube connected) and check that the "patient vacuum" value lies between a minimum of 25.2 mm Hg and a maximum of 26.2 mm Hg.

If the unit indicates error during the operation with the relative warning light turned on, push the vacuum footpedal once again, reset the unit by pushing the red button, and rotate the knob an additional three consecutive turns in a clockwise direction toward the (+) mark. Repeat this procedure until the above value has been reached. Once the desired vacuum value has been reached, the instrument will be permanently calibrated.

THE HEAD

The head is a single component, which makes assembly and disassembly of the unit simpler and faster, helps to lower surgical costs through added efficiency, and shortens the learning curve of the novice surgeon. The upper part of the head has a threaded opening for inserting the motor, and the central part has a groove where the blade is inserted. Anterior to this is a curved groove that receives the corneal flap during the microkeratome cut.

In the anterior lower part, the head has a fixed plate that determines the thickness of the cut. This plate is attached to the head and is removed only for periodic service by the manufacturer (in the newest models, it is no longer removable). A fixed plate is an important safety feature because it prevents the most serious complication of LASIK—corneal perforation. With earlier microkeratomes, it was possible to forget to insert the plate in the head during assembly or to insert the plate incorrectly or incompletely. The cornea could be perforated during the cut and, together with the high IOP induced by the suction ring, the consequences were disastrous. The fixed, nonremovable plate in the head is also an important safety feature for the surgeon because it removes the fear of forgetting to insert the plate, inserting it incorrectly, or using the wrong plate.

There are two gears on the two sides of the head, depending on whether the right or left eye is being operated on. One of these is to be inserted in the toothed track of the suction ring. For automatic advancement of the head, a specific right or left eye adapter device is inserted between the motor and the head. The adapter allows the head to rotate clockwise or counterclockwise depending on how it is installed. When performing surgery on the right eye, the adapter covers the letter "L" stamped on the head and indicates that the device is configured for right eye surgery. Conversely, when performing surgery on the left eye, the adapter covers the letter "R" stamped on the head and indicates that the device is configured for left eye surgery. The two gears of the head have been designed so that they come into easy contact with the toothed track of the suction ring, which simplifies the procedure. In addition, as a safety feature, the gear will come into contact only when the head is correctly inserted in the track.

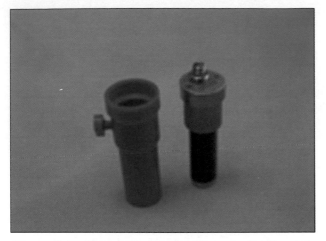

Figure 6-12. Motor with a sterilizable cover (by Buratto).

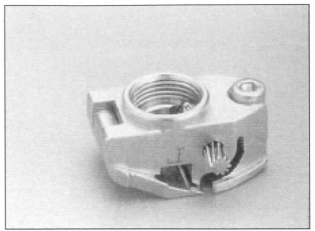

Figure 6-13. The microkeratome head. Top: screw channel for the motor. Center (to the left of the L): the gears that induce automated forward movement of the motor on the suction ring's toothed run. Below right: a slit for blade insertion; anterior to the slit is the fixed plate. Below to the left of the gears is a slit to house the cut flap.

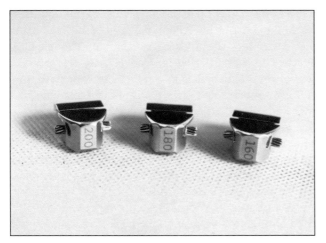

Figure 6-14. Three different heads of the Hansatome for cuts of different thickness.

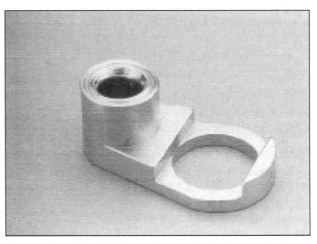

Figure 6-15. The device to be inserted between the head and motor to rotate the motor in a clockwise direction (left eye) or counterclockwise (right eye).

Assembly of the Head

Insert the metal pin in the opening of the blade holder with the sterile packaging of the blade sealed, and then peel open the package. Remove the blade from the package and examine it carefully under a high magnification microscope to ensure that it is perfect. Then, using the pin, insert the blade holder/blade into the groove of the head. Unscrew and remove the pin.

Holding the anterior and posterior part of the head between the thumb and index finger, insert the right or left eye adapter and position it so that the "R" (right) visible when performing surgery on a right eye (the opening for the pin would be on the right side of the instrument); and vice versa for operation on the left eye.

Insert the motor and screw it firmly, but without overtightening, into the threaded opening in the upper part of the head; this must be done so that the eccentric is positioned inside the groove of the blade holder. At the end of assembly, by rotating the motor in both directions through a half turn, the blade should oscillate uniformly if the eccentric has been inserted properly in the groove. Uniform oscillation confirms proper attachment of the blade to the motor.

Connect the cable to the power unit and turn on the power supply. When the reserve tank is completely full a green light turns is visible. Activate the motor to check for perfect function and regular blade oscillation. When the head is ready for surgery, the blade protrudes from the inferior plane of the microkeratome and is no longer protected. Be careful not to set the head down with the blade pointing downward, as this may damage the blade.

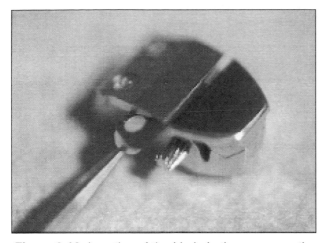

Figure 6-16. Insertion of the blade in the groove on the head.

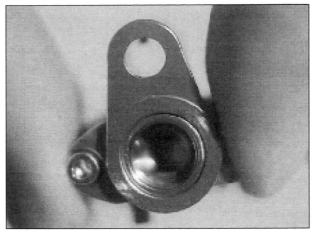

Figure 6-17. After having inserted the blade, a device is applied that determines the direction of the microkeratome's progression. Above is the hole that slides over the suction ring pin. At the center of the head there is a channel for screwing on the motor.

TESTING THE MOTOR AND GEARS WITH THE HEAD CONNECTED

As previously mentioned, the blade is inserted in the head during assembly. Wet the blade with a few drops of proparacaine (Ophthaine) or sterile double-distilled water, and insert it in the slot for lubrication prior to activation of the motor and to prevent the edge of the blade from being blunted during the test run. Now run the blade for a few seconds in both directions. The motor current must be between 50 and 60 mA (milliamps). A value higher than 100 mA indicates abnormal resistance. If the value exceeds 200 mA, the warning message "motor 40" will appear. This is associated with a flashing yellow light emitting diode (LED) and warning sound. Usually, high current is caused by compressed salt crystals lying between the blade track and bearings, or from difficulty of blade oscillation. Complete the test with the head connected to the suction ring. The motor current must be approximately equal to that of the previous test or the system is faulty.

BLADE TESTING

After inserting the blade into the microkeratome head, examine it very carefully under the operating microscope at maximum magnification to check the condition of the blade edge. All the parts of the blade and blade holder must be flawless before proceeding with the cut. Discard and replace a blade with notches or dings. Very small irregularities on the blade margin can also be detected by observing the reflection of the microscope's light on the edge of the blade.

With the blade tightly positioned on the insertion handle, slide it backward and forward in the slot. If even minimal friction is detected, the blade must be removed and replaced.

The blade should slide through the slot to the opposite side with gravity or a gentle tap. If not, replace the blade. Also do not activate a dry blade in the head of the microkeratome for more than a few seconds. Prolonged dry movement may damage the edge of the plate in the head.

It may be useful to keep some reserve blades that have functioned well with smooth oscillation and have demonstrated correct current draw within the 50 to 60 mA limits. If oscillation is smooth with these reserve blades, the problem may be due to dirt in the head or damage to the edge of the head itself.

Hot spots can develop due to friction from metal rubbing against metal (called galling) in the presence of specific conditions of temperature and pressure, lack of sufficient lubrication, or motor speed. Also, if the blade is too thick or the surface is irregular, the sharp edge may be blunted very easily when the motor is activated. In such situations, the current draw will be much greater than normal. If the blade is removed, a scrape or scratch on the surface may be visible. Also, a rough spot may be visible in relief on the inferior plate of the head, and the surface will not appear smooth and shiny as expected. The contact between this rough spot and a perfect blade produces scrapes on the new blade. Lubrication of the blade, even with sterile distilled water, will minimize the effect of heat friction that causes this damage. Once damage has been detected, the head must be serviced. Every blade must be checked to ensure that it does not damage the head.

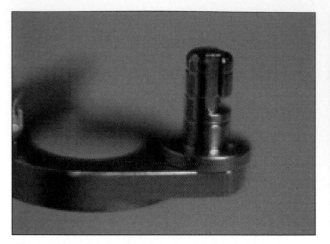

Figure 6-18. Close-up of the pin with the notches for correct head positioning.

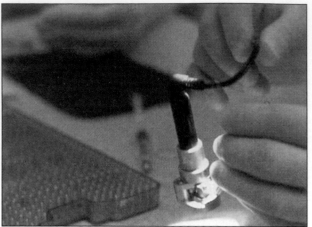

Figure 6-19. The microkeratome is mounted on the suction ring during the test run prior to use in surgery.

HEAD PERFORMANCE TEST

Position the opening of the head over the pin of the suction ring, located on the side opposite the handle. Using the index finger of the right hand, rotate the head so that it locks into one of the two vertical grooves on the pin. At this point—and only at this point—the head can descend spontaneously on the pin and seat itself on the suction ring at the appropriate level for the lamellar cut.

By depressing the footpedal, the head advances along the track for a test run on the suction ring. Although an alarm indicates when the microkeratome has reached the end of its pass, the surgeon should also visually memorize the end of the pass. If during advancement, the speculum obstructs the microkeratome and interrupts the run, the computer may interpret this interruption as the end of the pass. When the head reaches the end of the pass, push the footpedal once again to return the microkeratome to its starting point. At this point, rotating the head through half a turn in the opposite direction to insertion raises the head along the pin until it detaches from the suction ring. During advancement, the current on the display must not exceed 100 to 110 mA. The instrument is now ready for surgery.

Motor Test (Head Not Connected)

Prior to assembling the motor and head, the motor must be activated forward and backward. With the machine at room temperature, the motor current must read between 15 mA and 30 mA. If the value exceeds 50 mA, the internal mechanism must be serviced prior to using the instrument.

Hot Pump Message

This message indicates that the pump is beginning to overheat. The surgeon must complete the procedure and then stop to allow the pump (turned off) to cool down. If the surgeon continues, the pump will turn off automatically, even if the level of vacuum is maintained.

THE POWER SUPPLY

The new power supply features increase safety of the procedure for both patients and surgeons. The more important innovations include:

- Internal diagnostic test to check for correct performance of the system prior to beginning every operation.
- Visual and auditory indication of the suction level and microkeratome function.
- Cutting is possible only if the machine has reached the appropriate level of vacuum; the cut will be immediately interrupted if the vacuum drops below the safety threshold level.
- A back-up system that permits the surgical procedure to be completed in the event of power failure.
- Vacuum control that permits the surgeon to adjust the amount of suction.
- A reserve of vacuum that permits the surgeon to complete the operation in the event of intraoperative breakdown of the pump.
- An electronic sensing system that identifies the position of the stop, minimizing stress levels on the motor and gears.
- Maintenance of the advancement speed. If the microkeratome encounters any impediment during the cut, it is detected by the power supply and a greater amount of electrical energy is supplied to overcome the obstacle (however, this should not exceed certain limits).

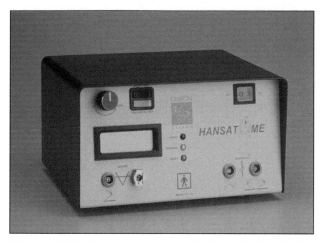

Figure 6-20. The power supply. Center left: the display indicates the operating values of the instrument.

- When the power supply is turned on, the surgeon must wait until the reserve tank is completely full (during this operation a yellow pilot light will be lit). When filling has been completed, the yellow light turns off, and a green light comes on automatically.

Power Failure

The Hansatome uses reserve nonrechargeable lithium batteries that are activated automatically to supply the microkeratome and electrical circuit in the event of a power failure. These batteries can work independently for more than 10 years if they are not discharged by improper use. Immediately after every normal operation, you must push the foot pedal for the vacuum to disconnect and protect the batteries. If this is not done, the electronic circuit will continue operating and the batteries will completely discharge in less than 30 minutes. The batteries will then have to be replaced.

DISASSEMBLY AND CLEANING

Unscrew the motor from the head. Detach the right-left lock from the head. Remove the blade from the head. Remove the suction tubing from the handle and detach the handle from the suction ring.

Cleaning the Head

The head, lock-in device, handle, and suction ring are immersed for 1 to 2 minutes in a cleaning solution consisting of 100 parts warm water and two parts Palmolive liquid soap (normal fragrance-free dishwashing liquid); alternatively, another neutral liquid soap can be used. The various components are carefully cleaned with the supplied brush. All the pieces are then washed and rinsed

in distilled water and dried under compressed air. Air from a cylinder (medical-standard air) is recommended, as it has already been filtered and is free from aqueous residues. If a cylinder is not available, a millipore filter must be applied to the exit channel of the air to trap any impurities. The components are then sterilized in an autoclave. Do not place the suction ring or connection tubes in any liquid if they are still connected to the supply.

Cleaning the Motor and Power Supply Unit

The exterior of the unit should be cleaned with a soft, damp cloth after detaching the electrical connections from the wall sockets. Do not use liquid cleaner. Always keep the protective plastic shield on the end of the microkeratome motor during cleaning in order to protect the eccentric. Do not use any type of lubricant or sterilizing gas for the motor.

Then, cut the plastic shield and immerse the terminal part of the motor (2.0 to 3.0 mm) in absolute or 99% isopropanol. At this point, activate the motor and turn it in both directions for 15 to 30 seconds. Then remove the instrument from the alcohol and dry it with a dry Merocel cloth. Squeeze the eccentric to facilitate removal of any liquid from the inside. If the sponge is at all discolored, repeat the process until no further discoloration is observed.

Continue to run the motor with the tip downward for at least 1 minute to dry it thoroughly on the inside. Finally, lay the motor to rest with the tip facing down to ensure that the residual alcohol drips out. The remainder will evaporate. This cleaning procedure with alcohol may also be used to dissolve or remove salt crystals or other debris from inside the rotary chassis, which often solves the problem of overloading the motor.

Dry the outside of the motor using a dry, gauze-free Merocel cloth or equivalent. It is important to keep the tip of the instrument pointing downward to prevent liquid from penetrating to the interior mechanism. To ensure the use of a sterile motor during the operation, drape the motor with a cover made of a sterilizable plastic material (Buratto motor cover).

Cleaning the Blade

A good blade can be easily inserted in the head. Cleaning and resterilization of the blade is mentioned only to discourage its use. The Hansatome blade is supplied with a plastic blade holder that prevents the blade from being sterilized in the autoclave (because the plastic will melt). This prevents the surgeon from using the blade more than once.

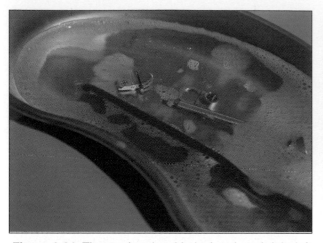

Figure 6-21. The suction ring, blade, head, and right-left separator are soaked in a water-Palmolive solution.

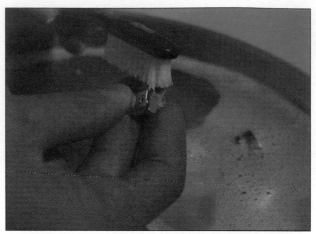

Figure 6-22. The head is carefully brushed with a toothbrush.

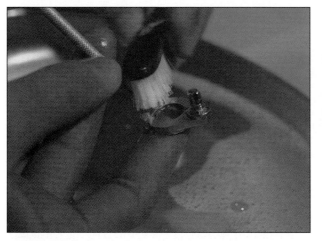

Figure 6-23. The suction ring is cleaned in the same way.

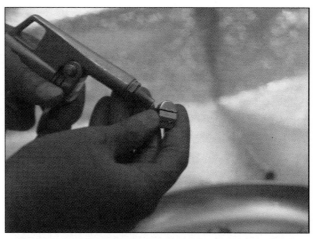

Figure 6-24. The head is dried under compressed air following washing with distilled water.

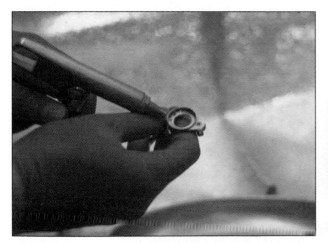

Figure 6-25. The suction ring is dried under compressed air following washing with distilled water.

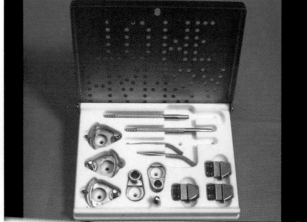

Figure 6-26. Personalized Hansatome set contains three different suction rings (8.5, 9.0, and 10) and three different heads (160, 180, and 200).

Cleaning the Instrument Between Surgeries

It goes without saying that the instrument should be cleaned and sterilized after every operation. Even when the operation is bilateral, some surgeons prefer to use a new blade and newly autoclaved microkeratome for each eye, while others prefer to use the same proven unit for the fellow eye. The easiest way to use a fresh unit for each eye is to have two suction rings, two motors, and two heads. Then, at the beginning of a bilateral operation, two instruments can be sterile and ready for use. Between one operation and the next, the ring, microkeratome, and electrical cable can be changed. A new blade ensures the best conditions for an optimal cut, while a blade that has been used once before has already demonstrated the ability to achieve a good cut, but may possibly be damaged between the two eyes. Sterilization of the instrument between operations avoids the remote possibility of infection transmission from one eye to the fellow eye. The frequency of infective complications with LASIK remains very low.

If the same instrument is to be used for a bilateral LASIK operation, it may be washed with sterile double-distilled water. A jet of sterile distilled water can be forced through a syringe into the entrance opening of the motor in the head. This will flush out any residual epithelial or stromal material from the first eye surgery. Any residual water must be dried, as it may damage the motor.

The following components can be placed in the autoclave for sterilization:
- The suction ring and its handle
- The microkeratome head

The following must not be sterilized in the autoclave:
- The motor
- The electrical cables
- The blade holder and blade, as the heat will damage the teflon of the blade holder and possibly dull the blade

Remember that the tonometer, which is made of acrylic material, must not be treated with alcohol and should not be sterilized in the autoclave.

ADVANTAGES & DISADVANTAGES OF THE HANSATOME

Advantages

Superior Hinge Advantages
This microkeratome can perform the cut from the bottom upward with the formation of a superior hinge.

Its inherent advantages include:
- Vertical continuous movement of the upper eyelid, along with the compression effect, keeps the flap in place and encourages distention and centration of the flap.
- The superior hinge reduces the incidence of superior epithelial defects.
- Patients have minimal foreign body sensation during blinking.
- Gravity tends to position the flap in the best way to promote healing.
- If the eye moves during surgery, the flap will have a greater tendency to return to its original position compared to a flap with a nasal hinge.
- The spatula that protects the hinge, if necessary, is placed superiorly and will not interfere with the normal function of the eye tracker, regardless of whether it is positioned to the side (as in the Technolas Keracor 217 excimer laser) or inferiorly (as in the Technolas Keracor 117 laser).
- The superior hinge helps keep the operating field dry.
- In the event of enhancement, repositioning is much simpler, healing is more rapid, and any induced foreign body sensation is decreased because the superior portion of the cornea remains intact.

Large Diameter Cuts
The Hansatome creates large diameter cuts, thus permitting broad ablations with wide transition zones. As a result:
- It is used for treating hyperopia, astigmatism, and any condition that requires a wide ablation area.
- It makes exact centration of the cut less critical.
- It is rarely necessary to retract the flap to prevent it from being even partially involved in the ablation.
- The distension-compressive effect of the superior eyelid inhibits the formation of microfolds in the flap.
- The resection line reepithelializes more rapidly because it is closer to the limbus, where cellular proliferation is faster.
- Any epithelial defects (usually along the resection line) are less disturbing to the patient because they are more peripheral.
- Greater contact surface (compared to a small diameter flap) allows better adhesion of the flap to the underlying stroma.
- Postoperatively, the healed wound line is "stronger" because it is closer to the limbus.

Fixed, Nonremovable Plate

As a result of the fixed, nonremovable plate, it is impossible for the surgeon to forget to insert the plate or position it incorrectly. This makes the operation safer and reduces assembly maneuvers and assembly time.

Single-Piece Head

The single-piece head makes assembly and disassembly simpler and faster. In addition, flap thickness is more reproducible and consistent. If necessary, the thickness may be modified by changing the head (eg, by replacing the 160-micron head with a 180- or 200-micron head).

Well-Designed Suction Ring

Because of the well-designed suction ring:

- There is good contact with the tissue and strong adhesion.
- There are no guide rails on the suction ring, which eliminate the difficulties associated with ring insertion. The procedure is simple because the microkeratome runs on the ring without impediment of the guides and runs on a flat surface.
- Because the toothed track of the suction ring is more elevated than the cutting surface, there is less possibility of obstruction by the speculum, eyelashes, or eyelids.

Fixed Stop Device

There is no need to set the correct position of the stop because the stop is fixed. Furthermore, the hinges created are always the same length.

Reduced Chance of Complications

The automated device is simple and safe, reducing the need for the highest level of surgeon dexterity for the keratectomy procedure. The likelihood of complications is therefore greatly diminished. The cut is made only when the vacuum has reached the appropriate value and when the microkeratome has been correctly inserted into the suction ring and the cutting phase is interrupted if, for any reason, the vacuum drops below the level required for a good quality cut during the operation.

Instrument Use is Comfortable

The surgeon is comfortable when using the instrument because it is easy to use for both right and left eyes. Also, the instrument is easy to use under the microscope of the excimer laser because the handle is short. The microscopes of the Technolas Keracor 117 and the Technolas Keracor 217 excimer lasers have a range of magnification for excellent observation during every surgical phase. The microkeratome cut should be performed under low magnification.

High Quality Lamellar Cut

The quality of the lamellar cut surface is very high due to the microkeratome technical features and the quality of the blades. This correlates to the high quality of postoperative vision and speed of visual recovery.

Batteries to Back-Up Power Supply

The reserve of nonrechargeable lithium batteries, if used correctly, will last for more than 10 years.

Internal Diagnostics

The instrument is fitted with internal diagnostics that check for correct function of the system prior to every operation, these include:

- Visual and audible indicators of the suction level and performance of the microkeratome.
- Vacuum control that allows the surgeon to regulate suction level.
- An electronic control for motor speed. If there is greater resistance by the speculum or eyelids, the motor will be supplied with more current to overcome resistance.
- An electronic stopping system that identifies the position of the stop to minimize stress on the motor and gears.
- The creation of vacuum and its release at the end of surgery occurs gradually, which reduces stress on the vascular structures of the globe.

Rapid Assembly

In general, the instrument can be assembled rapidly and easily, is easy and safe to use, and is easy to disassemble.

Disadvantages

- The blade is poorly protected and must be handled very carefully to avoid damage, particularly when the instrument is placed on the surgical table.
- The surgeon cannot observe the lamellar cut as it is being created.
- With very large diameter cuts, bleeding of the limbal corneal vessels may occur.

PERSONAL DOWN-UP LASIK TECHNIQUE

Preoperative Medication

Thirty minutes prior to surgery, instill one to two drops of topical antibiotic, such as ofloxacin (Ocuflox) as prophylaxis against infection and an NSAID (nonsteroidal anti-inflammatory drug) such as sodium

Table 6-1

HANSATOME PREPARATION PRIOR TO SURGERY

Checks to be performed

1. Check the blade under high magnification of a microscope.
2. Assemble the microkeratome head under the microscope and check that all components have been inserted correctly.
3. Check gears for any debris.
4. Check that the gears can be moved manually without friction.
5. Visually check blade movement.
6. Visually check that the suction ring is
   - free of debris
   - free of BSS crystals
7. Check that the suction ring orifice is clean.
8. Place the microkeratome on the suction ring and check its complete movement (backward and forward) prior to placing it on the eye.
9. Check that all components are in top working order.
10. Check the electrical and suction connections with the console.

Other preparations

1. Connect the supply unit to a grounded 110 or 220 V socket.
2. Connect the vacuum and microkeratome movement pedals to the power supply.
3. Connect the microkeratome motor cable to the supply unit.
4. Connect the suction tubing to the supply unit.
5. Connect the handle to the suction ring.
6. Select a 160 to 180 micron microkeratome head, depending on the requirements.
7. Use a sterile blade, remembering that the emblem on the container must face upward.

8. Slide the blade holder into the groove situated on the right of the container, checking that it is flat.
9. Open the container and, using the blade holder, lift the blade itself and examine it under the microscope under high magnification; then position it in the blade groove in the head.
10. Position the adapter for OD/OS so that the letter "L" is visible for the left eye (OS) and the letter "R" is visible for the right eye (OD).
11. Check that the adapter has been fully inserted into the groove.
12. Screw the motor into the head.
13. Turn the unit over and rotate the motor in both directions for one or two turns; check that the blade moves smoothly and is locked in place.
14. Connect the motor to the power cable.
15. Connect the suction ring to the suction tubing.
16. Turn on the control unit and wait until the reserve tank has completely filled (a yellow light will be on); once filling is complete, the yellow light will go off and the green light will come on.
17. Depress the pedal that controls microkeratome movement and check that the blade moves smoothly.
18. Lock the microkeratome on the vertical pin of the fixation ring and then depress the footpedal for movement. Continue pressure until advancement is stopped, accompanied by a warning sound. During advancement, the current in the machine must not exceed 100/110 mA (visible on the display).
19. The microkeratome is now ready; it may be placed on the surgical table, taking care not to damage the blade.

diclofenac (Voltaren) to reduce inflammation and postoperative pain. As soon as the patient is lying on the operating bed or chair, apply one to two drops of topical anesthetic (4% lidocaine or 0.5% proparacaine) to anesthetize the cornea and conjunctiva. Repeat application of anesthetic prior to insertion of the speculum and prior to applying the suction ring. Do not apply excessive anesthetic, which can be toxic to the cornea and induce epithelial edema.

Laser Calibration and Input

The Technolas Keracor 217 excimer laser is used. It is fitted with an eye tracker and ceramic cavity and operates at 50 Hz with PlanoScan 2000 software. Between surgeries, the laser technician must perform a fluence test to check the efficiency of the laser. Prior to surgery, I check the refractive correction setting, the axis of any astigmatism, and the minimum and maximum diameter

of the ablation. I also check the axis of the astigmatism against the topographic and/or refractive axis.

Finally, I verify these numbers against those recorded on the patient's clinical record sheet and the eye to be treated.

Footpedal Control

I operate the pedal for the laser and the pedal that activates the microkeratome. The pedal that controls the vacuum is located on the instrument cart and is manually controlled by the assistant (it is covered by a sterile drape). The Hansatome console is situated on the cart beside the laser.

Checking Microkeratome Function

Assemble the microkeratome separately under the operating microscope. Before starting the surgery, be sure to:

- Check that suction is working correctly by placing your thumb inside the suction ring to simulate suction on a globe; when vacuum has been achieved, adhesion between the suction ring and the thumb must be optimal.
- Check the console to ensure that the manometer needle for the vacuum reading has stabilized on 23 or the desired setting.
- Check for correct forward and reverse of the microkeratome movement on the ring.
- Check the reading on the voltmeter to ensure that the blade is moving correctly.
- Ensure that the blade is in perfect condition.
- Listen to the sound of the motor for the appropriate frequency (9600 RPM).
- Listen to the sound of the blade oscillation frequency after the motor has been inserted (8600 RPM).

Surgical Environment

LASIK necessitates a sterile environment that is suitable for surgery. I personally wear a sterile hat, face mask, gown, and powder-free surgical gloves.

Positioning and Preparing the Patient

Have the patient lie down on the bed, placing his or her head so that the chin and forehead are on the same plane. Position the eye to be operated on under the operating microscope and have the patient correctly fixate on the target light. Cover the fellow eye with a plastic shield to avoid cross fixation. Swab the skin of the eyelids with a solution of povidine iodine and carefully dry. Apply a disposable self-adhesive drape (fenestrated is easier to apply), complete with a lateral pouch. Ask the patient to open both eyes as wide as possible. To exclude the eyelashes from the operating field, apply the drape at the edge of the inferior eyelid. Do the same with the upper eyelid.

Speculum Insertion

Gently position a Buratto speculum or, alternately, the Buratto-Machat speculum, and open it gently and gradually. Check that the opening is sufficient for application of the suction ring and microkeratome pass. Remove any obstacles (pieces of plastic from the drape, eyelashes, etc) before continuing. Irrigate the cornea and conjunctival sac with BSS or proparacaine (Ophthaine), and then clean the conjunctival sac carefully with a couple of Merocel sponges to remove any secretions, eyelashes, and other debris, as well as any liquid from the conjunctival sac. If not removed, the liquid will be aspi-

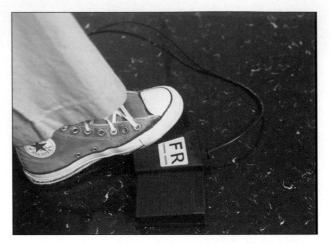

Figure 6-27. The foot switch: F for forward and R for reverse.

rated by the suction ring and may interfere with perfect adhesion of the ring to the globe. It may also damage the microkeratome. Remember to distend the conjunctiva smoothly over the underlying sclera in the area where the orifice of the suction ring will be positioned.

Corneal Marking

Recommended corneal markers are the Buratto markers, both of which mark the peripheral cornea well and allow exact repositioning of the flap at the end of the operation. The underside of the marker is stained with methylene blue and then applied to the dry cornea, precisely and firmly. Three radial marks will be seen on the cornea (nasal, inferior, and temporal). These radial markings are also important for flap replacement in the event of a free cap. Irrigate the cornea and conjunctiva carefully with BSS to remove any excess dye and then dry the conjunctiva carefully with a Merocel sponge.

Suction Ring Test Pass

In my clinic, the chairside assistant, who is positioned to the left of the laser where the other instruments are arranged, hands me the ring in the correct position for use. If the right eye is to be treated, the ring is placed in my left hand. The suction tubing passes in front of me and the handle of the ring is positioned nasally. Obviously, I hold the microkeratome in my right hand. If the left eye is to be treated, the suction tubing passes once again in front of me; it is caught by the right hand and is positioned with the handle nasally. The tube passes around my wrist so that any traction exerted on the suction tubing does not interfere with the cut, I hold the microkeratome with my left hand.

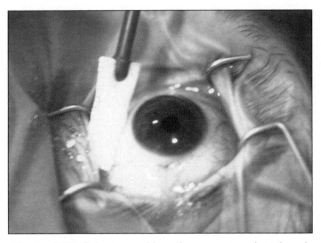

Figure 6-28. Prior to marking, the cornea and conjunctiva are dried with a slightly damp sponge, which also removes any secretions.

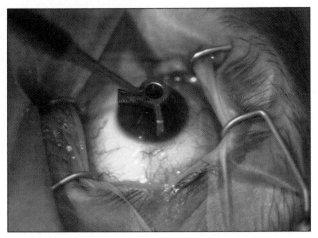

Figure 6-29. Marking with a three-radius marker.

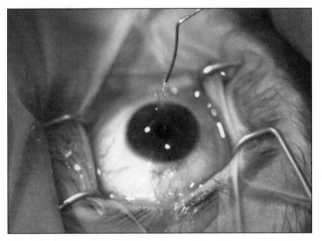

Figure 6-30. The cornea is washed to remove any excess dye.

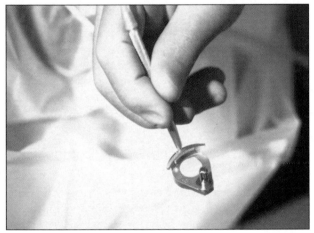

Figure 6-31. The surgeon receives the suction ring from his assistant.

Reassuring the Patient

Prior to applying the suction ring, I reassure patients and tell them what to anticipate. They are told:
- The procedure is short, painless, and produces only a slight feeling of discomfort and pressure.
- They will have to fixate constantly at the laser's target, which may disappear from view for a few seconds.
- They may smell burning, but must stay calm and keep both eyes wide open with the body relaxed and motionless. If necessary, a member of my staff holds the patient's hand for the few critical moments of the procedure.

Suction Ring Application

Prior to applying the suction ring, I ensure that the speculum has created enough space for insertion of the ring and its correct positioning; if this is not the case, I enlarge the opening by turning the adjustment screw on the speculum. With the handle positioned nasally, I gently place the ring on the globe and center it well on the cornea and pupil. When I am certain that it is in the correct position, I allow it to adhere by exerting a certain degree of pressure downward and carefully distend the conjunctiva under the orifice of the suction ring. I then ask my assistant to activate suction and wait a few seconds until the vacuum increases and there is good adhesion. Once vacuum has been achieved, the pupil diameter increases slightly. This is desirable, as it indicates that IOP has increased and the ring has adhered correctly to the sclera. When the vacuum in the aspiration line has reached the desired value, the power supply emits a signal. After this, the cut can be performed.

I then check the exact centration of the ring on the cornea and pupil. Because of the very large flaps (diam-

145

eter 8.5 to 10 mm) created with the Hansatome, exact centration of the cut is less important as compared with smaller diameter flaps in which centering is of major importance. Nevertheless, good centering is useful because it reduces the risk of bleeding from perilimbal corneal vessels. I then re-examine the operating field, making sure that the plastic drape is retracted from the globe and the microkeratome pass, that there are no eyelashes in the way.

Tonometry

Prior to initiating the cut, I apply the Barraquer tonometer to the cornea to check that the ocular pressure is sufficiently high. If applanation by the tonometer on the cornea lies inside the circle inscribed on the inferior surface of the tonometer, pressure is approximately 65 mm Hg. In using this tonometer, the cornea must be dry but not dehydrated. If the cornea is wet, the fluid meniscus will show an area of applanation wider than it actually is. If, on the other hand, the cornea is dehydrated, the area of applanation will appear smaller than it actually is, and the pressure will appear artificially high. If tonometry indicates a "soft" eye, the vacuum value can be increased by activating the "operate" mode and rotating the regulation knob through one complete turn in a clockwise direction.

Wetting the Cornea and Suction Ring Track

Following tonometry, I apply a few drops of liquid on the cornea to wet it. This facilitates gliding of the microkeratome's plate on the cornea, and thus helps create a good quality cut. The microkeratome manufacturer advises against use of BSS or other saline solutions prior to the lamellar cut because the salt is damaging to the motor/driver unit. It causes electrolytic corrosion and may cause the chassis to block if it precipitates into crystals. If these salt solutions are used, they must be completely eliminated prior to the keratectomy. Proparacaine can be used instead of BSS. It does not contain salt, has a balanced pH, and contains glycerin, a lubricant that facilitates the cut. In any case, excessive liquid should not be used, as it may be sucked into the inside of the motor under the effects of centrifugal forces, causing a deterioration in performance. One or two drops of liquid can be applied to the suction ring pin to facilitate insertion of the microkeratome and reduce friction during the cut.

The Microkeratome

The microkeratome is inserted on the suction ring pin and rotated gently until it locks into the grooves on the pin itself. The microkeratome first descends about halfway down the pin, and, by rotating it further, it

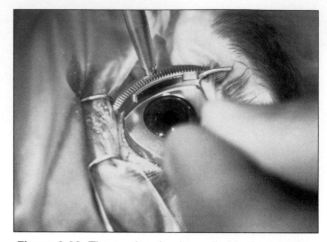

Figure 6-32. The suction ring is applied to the eye. One hand is on the handle and the other pushes on the pin to make the ring adhere firmly to the bulb.

descends to the end of the pin and comes into contact with the cutting surface of the ring. At the same time, the toothed gear of the head comes into contact with the toothed track of the suction ring. In the event of difficult insertion, I squeeze the microkeratome pin block of the suction ring between the thumb and index finger to facilitate insertion. The instrument is now ready for the cut. The patient will be aware of further pressure on the eye, but discomfort is minimal.

The Lamellar Cut

This is the most important and delicate phase of the entire procedure. I push the footpedal, causing the microkeratome to pass forward along the suction ring for about 6 to 7 seconds until it is interrupted by the stop device. At this point, I push on the other pedal and reverse the pass direction, returning the microkeratome to its original position (which takes an additional 6 to 7 seconds). The microkeratome progresses slowly and gently at a uniform speed for the forward and return pass. The cut is performed from the bottom upward with the hinge formed at 12 o'clock.

During the Cut

The teeth in the microkeratome's mechanism must mesh exactly with those of the suction ring or the microkeratome will not advance. If so, I return the instrument to its original position and attempt the pass again when I have managed to make the teeth mesh. I avoid exerting upward or downward pressure, as this will interfere with the pass and try only to support the connecting cable, allowing the instrument to move on its own accord. Since any debris on the toothed track of the ring will make microkeratome advancement difficult or impossible, I carefully inspect the intended path preoperatively to pre-

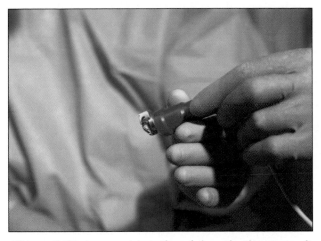

Figure 6-33. Incorrect transfer of the microkeratome. It should be handed to the surgeon in the correct position for the cut.

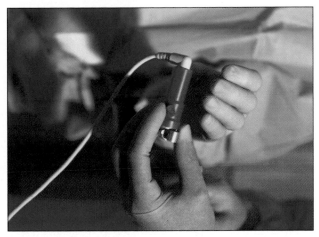

Figure 6-34. Another incorrect transfer of the microkeratome.

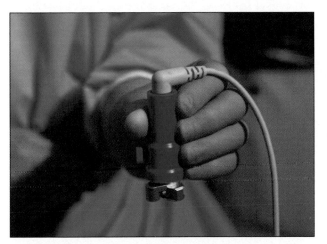

Figure 6-35. Correct hold of the microkeratome.

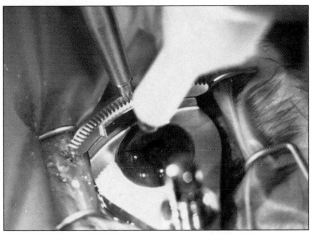

Figure 6-36. A drop of anesthetic on the cornea and pin to allow the microkeratome to slide more easily on both.

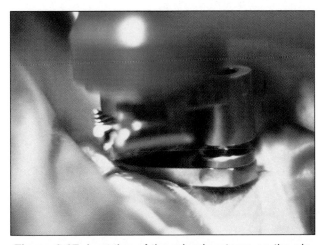

Figure 6-37. Insertion of the microkeratome on the pin. The instrument has still not reached the correct operating plane.

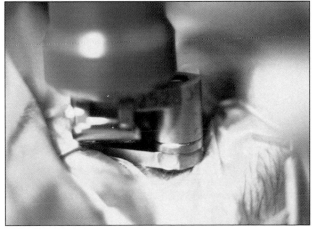

Figure 6-38. The microkeratome is correctly inserted on the suction ring.

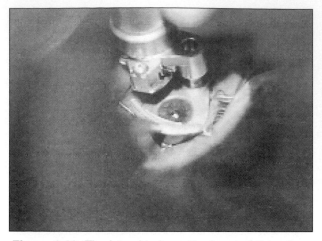

Figure 6-39. The lateral hole on the head of the micro-keratome is slipped over the ring's pin.

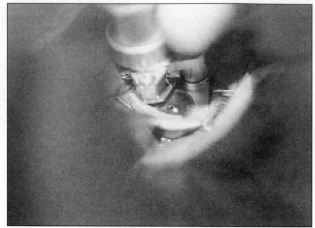

Figure 6-40. The microkeratome head is rotated in the direction of the denticulated route on the suction ring. In this way, the microkeratome can slide down the pin onto the cutting plane on the suction ring. At this point, the gears situated laterally on the head can come into contact with the toothed run of the suction ring.

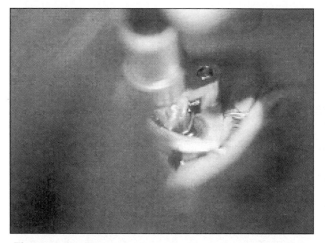

Figure 6-41. The pedal is pushed to activate blade function and automation of the microkeratome. The instrument starts to rotate around the suction ring's pin.

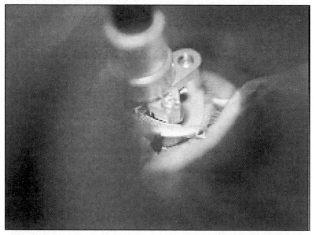

Figure 6-42. The microkeratome has almost completed the lamellar cut.

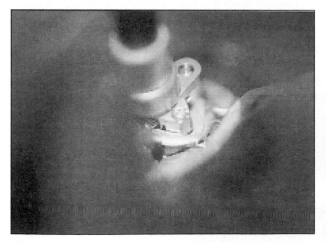

Figure 6-43. The cut has been completed.

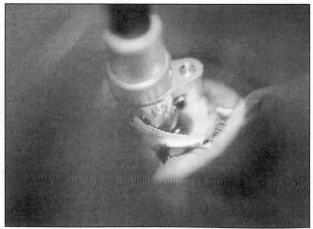

Figure 6-44. The return pedal is activated and the micro-keratome returns to its starting position.

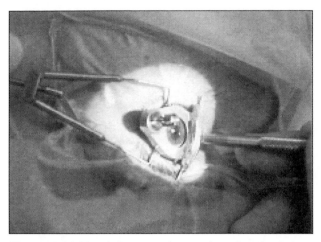

Figure 6-45. The Asico speculum and suction ring in correct position.

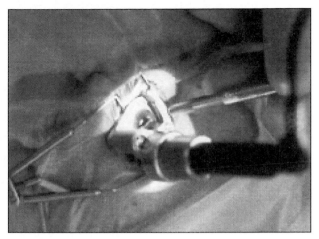

Figure 6-46. The microkeratome is inserted on the pin.

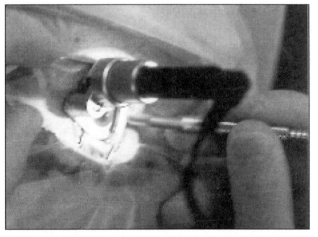

Figure 6-47. The cut is initiated.

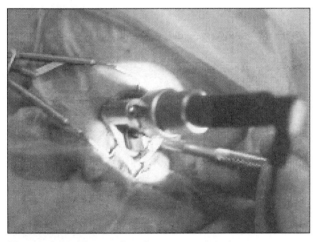

Figure 6-48. The cut has been completed.

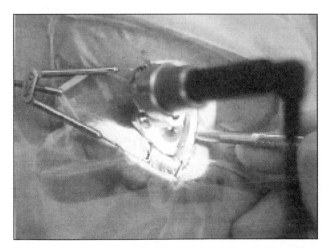

Figure 6-49. Return of the microkeratome.

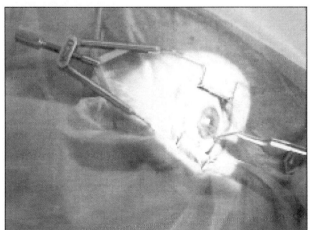

Figure 6-50. The flap with the superior hinge raised.

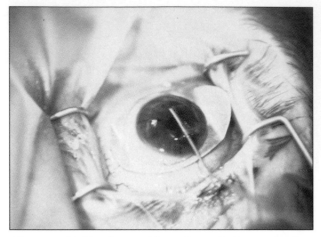

Figure 6-51. The flap positioner is applied, then the flap is raised using a spatula that has been carefully introduced at the interface.

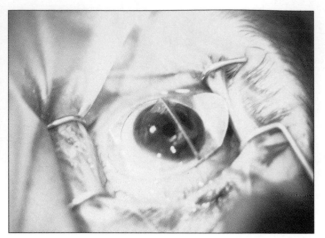

Figure 6-52. Initial phase of raising the flap.

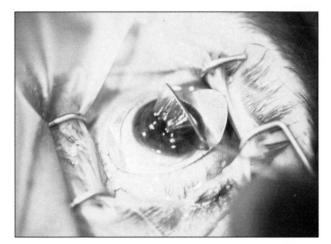

Figure 6-53. Intermediate phase of raising the flap.

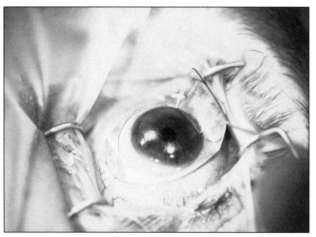

Figure 6-54. The flap rests on the positioner.

vent any obstruction of the pass. Such obstructions are rare.

Suction must remain active during the entire cut. If it is interrupted, the instrument will stop automatically and the cut will be incomplete. Although the operation will have to be aborted and postponed for a couple months, an incomplete cut normally does not damage the cornea. Also, if the microkeratome does not progress as far as the stop, the cut will be incomplete and the operation will have to be aborted. The microkeratome pass must be impediment-free (no speculum, drape, eyelashes, etc). The surgeon should not rely only on the acoustic signal but should also visually remember the end of the pass because any obstruction during advancement can cause the computer to interpret the interruption as the end of the pass.

Microkeratome Removal

When the microkeratome has returned to its starting position, my assistant releases the suction by pushing the

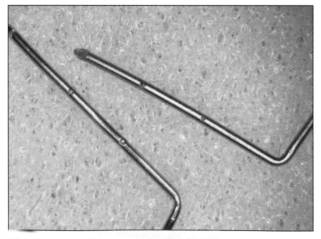

Figure 6-55. The cannula for washing the interface. Observe the spatulate tip and four orifices: two inferior and two superior.

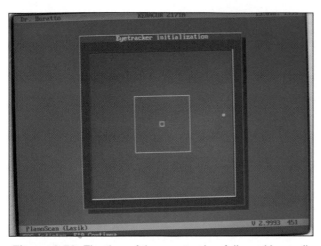

Figure 6-56. Fixation of the eye tracker followed immediately by the ablation.

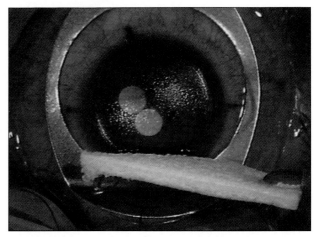

Figure 6-57. The ablation. To highlight the impact spots, the stroma has been stained with fluorescein (for demonstration purposes only).

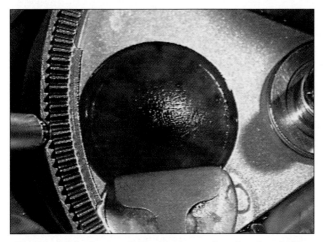

Figure 6-58. Some surgeons keep the ring in position during the ablation. If there is a wide ablation, the flap should be retracted and protected.

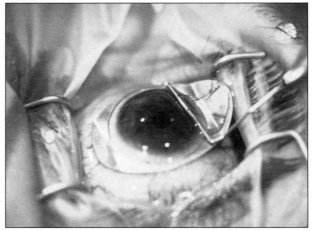

Figure 6-59. Following ablation, the in-situ stroma is wet using Buratto's five-orifice cannula.

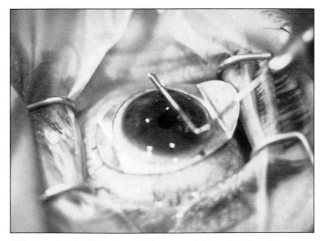

Figure 6-60. The flap is then positioned using the cannula. This is inserted under the flap near the hinge and the flap is positioned with a downward movement.

footpedal. Then, I remove the ring together with the microkeratome. I hand the two instruments to my assistant, who will disassemble, clean, and sterilize them. I try to have less than 1 minute between the start and finish of suction to avoid possible damage to the internal vascular structures from prolonged IOP elevation. When all goes as expected, the time lapse is about 30 seconds or less. With the Hansatome, the increase and release of suction is gradual.

Centering the Laser and Repositioning the Patient

Quite frequently, the head and eye move from their original position during the cut and must be repositioned for surgery. The patient's chin must be on the same plane as the forehead and parallel to the floor. The eye must be under the fixation target, and the two targets must be well focused on the corneal stromal above the pupil center.

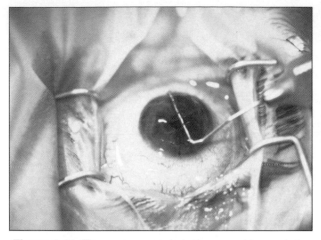

Figure 6-61. The same cannula is then used to wash the interface.

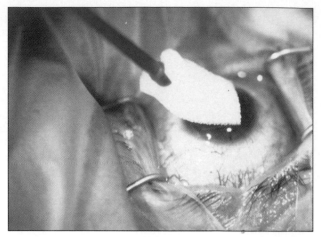

Figure 6-62. A damp sponge is used to gently dry the epithelium and distend the flap.

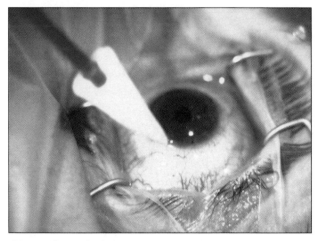

Figure 6-63. A damp sponge dries the gutter.

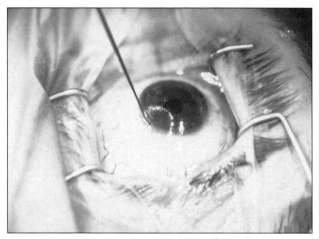

Figure 6-64. The Slade striae test.

The patient is then asked to fixate on the target light and continue to hold that position even though it may go out of focus after a few minutes. I use a special type of toothless forceps that I designed to raise the flap or a special spatula that I also designed. I use it to grasp the lower edge of the flap, taking care to avoid damaging the epithelium. I reflect the flap superiorly and rest it on an accessory specifically designed for that purpose. Occasionally during the refractive treatment, I retract the flap with a flap retractor. I decrease the intensity of the ambient room light and the light on the laser to reduce the amount of glare for the patient. This also permits the eye tracker to perform better. I then tell the patient that everything is proceeding according to plan, check focus and centration of the laser, then engage the eye tracker.

The eye tracker is a system of high-speed image sequencing that tracks the center of the pupil to ensure a well-centered laser ablation. Once the corneal center has been identified, the eye tracker follows eye movements and targets the laser beam on the most appropriate corneal zone. The laser automatically stops when the eye tracker is no longer in a position to identify the preset center, and will also stop if the eye moves more than about 1.5 mm from the preset center. The eye tracker may be turned off and surgery continued with the patient fixating on the target light.

The Refractive Ablation

The refractive ablation can now begin. I push the laser footpedal, check that the cornea is centered and in focus, and perform the first ablation phase. I pass a dry spatula over the stromal surface to remove any liquid that has formed during the ablation and proceed to the other ablation phases. Between one phase and the next, I pass the spatula over the in-situ stroma. Alternately, a dry Merocel sponge can be used. During the ablation phases, I rarely retract the flap to protect it because the Hansatome creates very large flaps that are not affected by the ablation. When treating with-the-rule astigmatism, the ablation occurs along the 0° to 180° axis and the flap does not need to be protected near the hinge. If the astigmatism is against-the-rule, however, the ablation will be vertical and the hinge will need to be protected. The large flaps created with the Hansatome make hyperopic ablations as easy as other ablations because wide-diameter optic zones (up to 6.0 mm) can be used.

During the Ablation

I continuously monitor centration of the reference target and the patient's focus. If the patient has shifted fixation or the targets are not focused, I stop the procedure and adjust the situation. Perfect focus is particularly important when the eye tracker is used because its infrared television camera "sees" the eye obliquely, and any upward or downward movement of the eye (ie, every displacement from perfect focus) shifts the image laterally and induces decentered treatment. In the event of refocusing, the surgeon should proceed using the F4 function. If any liquid forms near the hinge, it must be dried.

Flap Replacement

To encourage uniform distention of the flap, I apply two to three drops of BSS to the stroma in situ and spread the liquid evenly using the curved back of a long blunt cannula (27-gauge). The liquid forms a "water bed" that allows the flap to distend easily and evenly on the underlying corneal bed and return to its original position. I reposition the flap by inserting the cannula, on the epithelial face at the limit of the hinge, and pull the flap toward the center of the cornea. I pass the curved cannula, which adapts well to the shape of the cornea, two or three times over the cornea, starting from the hinge and moving in the opposite direction. This facilitates removal of any liquid at the interface. I then pass a damp Merocel sponge over the cornea, gently and delicately three to four times from the superior to inferior margins to further distend the flap, dry any liquid remaining at the edge of the incision, and encourage flap adhesion to the underlying stromal bed.

Checking Flap Position

I increase magnification and brightness of the microscope and carefully check that the preoperative marks of the flap align with those of the peripheral cornea (marking test). Then I check the circumference of the flap to see that the margins are symmetrical to those of the bed (the gutter test) and check for intact epithelium along the entire circumference of the cut. I also check for debris in the interface. If everything is in order, I rest for about 1 minute and wait until the cornea dries. Then, with a blunt olive-tipped spatula, I gently push about 1.0 mm outside the incision to check adhesion of the flap to the underlying cornea. Fine lines radiating toward the center of the flap should be seen (Slade striae test). I warn the patient that I am about to place the spatula on the eye to avoid sudden movement (from discomfort or pain), which may dislocate the flap or damage the epithelium.

Speculum Removal and Final Check

I gently remove the speculum, first the superior arm, then the inferior one, taking care to avoid contact with the cornea or displacing the flap. Finally, I ask the patient to blink three to four times and check that the flap has remained in position. I instill one drop of ofloxacin antibiotic (Ocuflox) and NSAID (Voltaren), and remove the adhesive drape. The patient then returns to the recovery room to rest quietly with the eyes closed for about 30 minutes. The eye is not bandaged or patched. After 30 minutes, I examine the patient's eye at the slit lamp. If everything is in order, the patient is instructed to not rub the eye that has been operated on and is discharged with a prescription for postoperative medication. The patient leaves the laser center protected by a pair of dark glasses and is also given a protective eye shield to be used at night. On arrival home, the patient should go to bed and sleep for a couple hours. Upon awakening, the cut line will have epithelialized, the cornea will be transparent, and he or she will begin to see.

INTRAOPERATIVE TECHNICAL PROBLEMS WITH THE HANSATOME

Difficulty Inserting the Suction Ring

The ring of the Hansatome has a diameter slightly greater than the rings of other instruments and this may occasionally create difficulty with insertion between the open arms of the speculum. Insertion is performed by opening the arms of the speculum (using the screw) or by inserting the ring obliquely, first the superior portion and then, with the help of the other hand, positioning the inferior portion. The ring must be pushed downward and centered, then suction is activated. When the appropriate level of suction has been achieved, the surgeon can slowly raise the ring with the globe to position it more suitably for the cut.

Difficulty Inserting the Microkeratome onto the Pin

It stands to reason that the surgeon must be familiar with the instrument and understand how it is inserted to obtain a good result. The ring is positioned horizontally

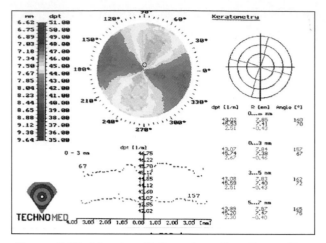

Figure 6-65. Myopic with-the-rule astigmatism with a 160° axis.

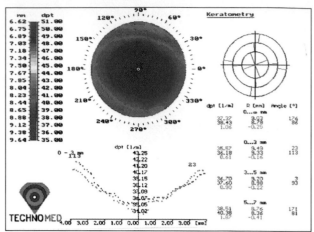

Figure 6-66. Postoperative map that highlights excellent correction.

with the pin positioned vertically. Insert the microkeratome vertically and allow it to slide down the pin. If this proves difficult, remove and reinsert it. Application of one to two drops of Ophthaine or distilled water to the pin may help. If after two to three attempts the microkeratome does not slide properly, the pin and microkeratome opening are either contaminated by debris or have been mechanically damaged (careless cleaning, etc). Rotate the microkeratome gently until it reaches the right point for spontaneously descending. When it has reached the lower plane of the ring, rotate it until the teeth in the head come into contact with the toothed track of the ring.

Instrument Blockage During the Cut

This occurs very rarely and the cut is usually completed because the instrument continues its pass. Possible explanations include:

- Breakdown in the power supply to the motor, in which case all the contact points must be checked to restore power.
- A faulty footpedal. You must move it with your foot, remove your foot, and repeat the forward pressure.
- The motor itself is faulty (optimal function of the motor should always be checked prior to surgery). Activate the advance footpedal a number of times, check whether there are any mechanical impediments to advancement (speculum, etc), or electronic faults in the power supply. Send the instrument to the manufacturer for service. Think back over the entire operation, focusing on any hints of poor function or indication of error or faults. In the event of blockage, if the suction levels have been maintained, push the footpedal several times to activate forward movement and com-

plete the cut. Never perform a forward-backward movement followed by another forward movement, as there is a high risk of cutting the flap.

Microkeratome Blockage at the End of the Pass

If the head does not return to its original position when the return pedal is pushed (a rare occurrence), repeatedly push the pedal up to 10 times. If this has no effect, release the suction and allow the whole unit to slide gently downward at a slight inclination, thus allowing the flap to detach from the microkeratome. At this point, move the patient away and treat the head of the instrument as follows. Rotate the motor of the head through a few degrees to supply reverse power, which should immediately retract the head. If not, place the assembled motor and head in a basin containing isopropyl alcohol no deeper than 3.0 mm above the inferior part of the head of the microkeratome and apply the reverse current. If this has no effect, repeat the procedure using a basin of alcohol and an ultrasound cleaning device. If this still has no effect, send the instrument to the manufacturer for service.

Alternately, detach the power supply cable to the microkeratome, unscrew the head, detach the right-left adapter, and remove the entire unit, taking care not to damage the cornea.

PROS AND CONS OF DOWN-UP LASIK

Below is a comparison of the pros and cons of the classic LASIK nasal hinge technique to the down-up LASIK technique (also known as the superior-hinge or top-hinge technique).

Flap Position Following Creation of a Nasal and Superior Hinge

In the classic LASIK technique, the flap is nasally attached to the underlying cornea, so that the tissue that remains attached cannot prevent the flap from moving under the pressure of vertical blinking movements of the eyelids. The flap remains attached to the underlying tissue secondary to the endothelial pump and other factors as opposed to mechanical effects. Therefore, the flap with a nasal hinge can potentially move, and this displacement is the most common postoperative complication during the learning curve of this procedure. It happens largely because of incorrect positioning of the flap at the end of the operation, through inadequate adhesion of the flap to the underlying bed in the immediate postoperative period, and occasionally, because of epithelial defects or excessive tearing.

In the down-up technique, the continual up-down movement of the upper eyelid helps keep the flap in position and actually contributes to its smoothing. Moreover, gravitational forces tend to position the flap in the best position for healing.

During the Surgery

The superior hinge helps keep the operating field (stromal bed) dry. Normally, most of the liquid is found at the superior conjunctival fornix. The patient's attempt at blinking, obstructed by the speculum, creates a sort of "pump" that makes the liquid flow to the operating field, particularly when the flap is in a nasal position. With a superior hinge at 12 o'clock, it is easier to keep the operating field dry.

Spherical and Astigmatic Ablation with Nasal or Superior Hinges

In the classic LASIK technique, the cut flap is positioned nasally during laser ablation. If the flap diameter is small or the ablation is done with a large optical zone, the superficial stroma of the reflected flap could also be ablated. Thus, the hinge needs to be protected with a flat spatula. The nasal hinge actually reduces the amount of ablation in the nasal area, which may affect final visual function (an untreated nasal area remains). This is particularly important in with-the-rule astigmatism because the ablation occurs along the horizontal axis and the treatment involves wider ablation zones.

Astigmatic treatment is greatly facilitated by the absence of the nasal hinge in the down-up technique. An astigmatic ablation (and even more so a spherical one) can be performed with a wide optical zone. With-the-rule astigmatic treatment is especially facilitated because the surgeon can make full use of available laser software.

This is particularly true for lasers with scanning technology. In any case, any ablation limits with the down-up technique lie superiorly (ie, in the area of the cornea covered by the upper eyelid).

Centering and Smoothing the Flap

In the classic LASIK technique, the flap may be repositioned incorrectly (ie, it may be decentered slightly upward, downward, or nasally). It may also be incorrectly distended and intralamellar microfolds (striae) may persist, which will cause marked functional disturbances postoperatively. In the best case scenario, eyelid movement will not worsen the situation, but in the worst case scenario, movement may increase the amount of displacement, the number of folds, or both. In the down-up technique, the up and down movement of the upper eyelid, together with its compression effect, encourages distention and centration of the flap, even if it is slightly decentered temporally or nasally.

Flap Diameter

With currently available microkeratomes used for the classic LASIK technique, flap diameters less than 8.5 mm are obtained. This partially limits the possibility of performing ablations with wide zones or creating appropriate transition zones because of the presence of the nasal hinge. On the other hand, flaps obtained with the latest microkeratomes are typically large (9.0 to 10 mm) and permit the use of larger ablation zones. In most cases, protection of the hinge is not necessary. These very large flaps also make astigmatic and hyperopic ablation very simple.

Intrastromal Microfold Formation

Laser ablation removes tissue. The central depth of the ablation is proportional to the degree of myopia, the chosen optical zones, and whether treatment is single or multizonal. If, for example, the surgeon is treating 10 D with a single 5.5 mm zone, the ablation at the center will be 110 microns, and there will be a difference in thickness of 110 microns between the center of the ablation and the untreated area. The intrastromal space left by the laser ablation will be filled by the superficial flap, which will adapt to the underlying bed. However, there is a price to pay since flap microfolds will form in relation to the depth of the ablation. Postoperatively, these may also have a negative effect on visual performance.

Because of the nasal hinge in the classic LASIK technique, flap position cannot be uniform and regular over 360°, and microdisplacement of the flap, which will encourage formation of these microfolds, may develop. In the down-up technique, on the other hand, the distention-compression effect of the superior eyelid tends to limit formation of these microfolds and distribute them more evenly over the surface. Since the surgeon can perform large ablations with suitable transition zones, the folds tend to be less obvious and fewer in number.

Temporal or Inferior Cut

In the classic LASIK technique, microkeratome insertion from the temporal side is relatively easy and advancement is straightforward. However, the microkeratome does not always run smoothly on the tracks, the globe is not always sufficiently exposed, and the eyelids may not be opened wide enough. In the down-up technique with the Hansatome, the procedure is easier, safer, and more precise because the instrument is positioned above the suction ring and, as a result, enters more easily in the intercanthal space. Once the surgeon has carefully assembled the microkeratome, all he or she has to left to do is apply the suction ring correctly. The microkeratome will then do its job with ease because of its precise automation, thus the risk of complications is greatly reduced.

Working Under the Laser or Surgical Microscope

The classic LASIK technique is usually performed under the laser's microscope. This can be difficult because not all lasers are equipped with microscopes suitable for surgery. They may lack zoom function, a focusing device, coaxial illumination, etc. The Hansatome, however, is easy to use even under the excimer laser. It is compact, the suction ring handle is short, and it is in general very easy to use.

The Surgeon's Comfort

In the classic LASIK technique, the surgeon is usually in a reasonably comfortable position when performing the cut, particularly if he or she is operating on the right eye. Comfort is reduced for left eye surgeries because the cut has to be made with the left hand. Generally, temporal access is comfortable and simple. In the down-up technique using the Hansatome, the surgeon is seated much more comfortably compared to surgery with a traditional microkeratome, largely because the surgeon has a predominantly passive role during the cut.

OTHER ADVANTAGES OF DOWN-UP LASIK

Postoperative Topography

The treated area of patients who underwent down-up LASIK appears more homogeneous and uniform on topography in a shorter time than compared to the clas-

sic LASIK procedure. Best visual acuity is reached more rapidly, to the satisfaction of both patient and surgeon.

Postoperative Foreign Body Sensation

Epithelial microlesions producing irritation or foreign body sensation along the cut line may appear during blinking following the classic LASIK technique. This may induce tearing (with the flap tending to float in the lacrimal fluid) or the patient may rub the eye in an attempt to relieve the foreign body sensation. The flap may be displaced in either of these situations. The superior position of the hinge with the down-up technique reduces the possibility of superior epithelial defects. Moreover, foreign body sensation during blinking is reduced to a minimum and is considerably less than after the classic LASIK technique.

No Interference with an Eye Tracker

If a laser with an eye tracker is being used, an instrument placed nasally to protect the reflected flap will block the action of the eye tracker, and the advantages of this important precision device will be lost. In down-up LASIK, the instrument, which protects the hinge, is at the top and will not interfere with the normal activity of the eye tracker.

Safer in the Event of Eye Movement

During the operation, the patient's eye may move. With the flap positioned nasally, the stromal bed can easily be contaminated by lacrimal fluid, or the flap may wander uncontrollably over the corneal bed, which may introduce cells and/or debris to the interface. If the eye moves during the down-up technique, the flap tends to return to its original position on the corneal bed, with less chance of contamination.

Enhancement

Enhancement with the classic LASIK technique involves raising the flap at the temporal side, folding it back nasally, and performing in-situ treatment to correct the residual defect. As a result, partly because the flap is stretched as it is raised and partly because the epithelial defect occurs superiorly, foreign body sensation may follow, particularly during blinking. In addition, flap distention may not be optimal. With the down-up technique, repositioning is simpler and healing is more rapid but, above all, there is less discomfort because the superior portion of the cornea is intact.

In conclusion, down-up LASIK (superior-hinge LASIK or top-hinge LASIK) procedures are a true step forward in the keratomileusis procedure, particularly when the techniques are performed with the Hansatome microkeratome.

SURGICAL ATLAS: CASE 1

Down-Up LASIK With the ACS

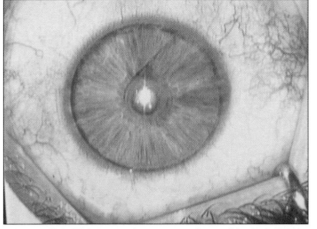

Figure A-1. This operation was performed in June 1996. It was the first down-up operation, which begins with corneal marking.

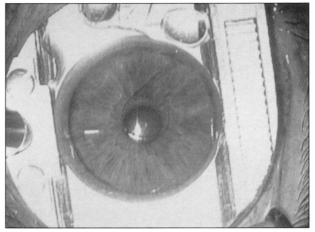

Figure A-2. The suction ring is applied with the tracks vertically.

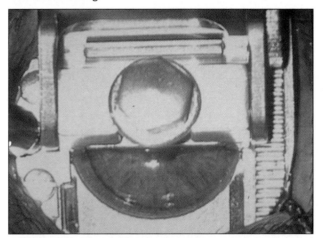

Figure A-3. The ACS microkeratome cut is performed from down upward; the globe must be well-exposed.

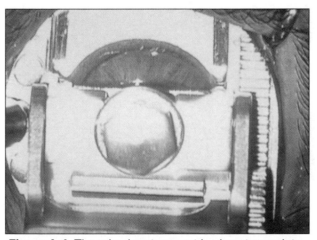

Figure A-4. The microkeratome cut is almost complete.

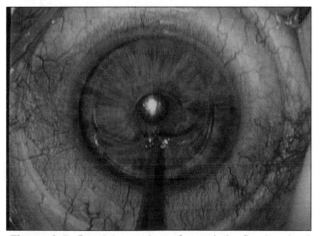

Figure A-5. Once the cut is performed, the flap is raised from down upward and it is positioned superiorly. The ablation is performed as usual.

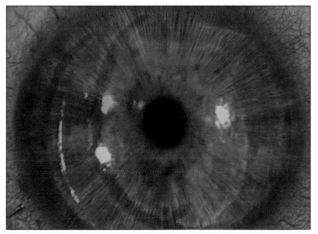

Figure A-6. The flap is repositioned at the end of surgery.

SURGICAL ATLAS: CASE 2

Down-Up LASIK With the Hansatome

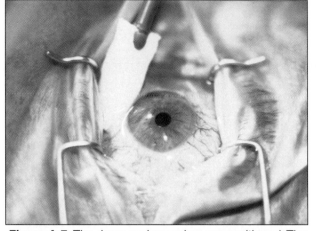

Figure A-7. The drape and speculum are positioned. The operation starts by drying the cornea and conjunctiva.

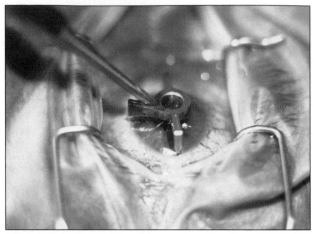

Figure A-8. Corneal marking.

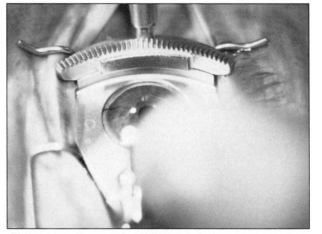

Figure A-9. The suction ring is applied and held in position with both hands until the ring has firmly adhered to the globe under the effect of the vacuum.

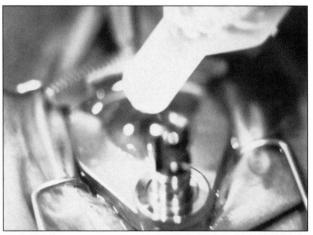

Figure A-10. The cornea and pin are wet with anesthetic to facilitate the pass of the microkeratome on the cornea and ring.

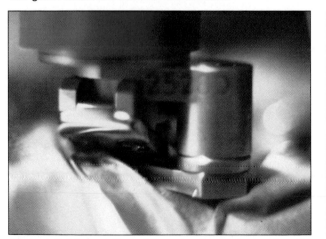

Figure A-11. Insertion of the microkeratome on the pin and the cut.

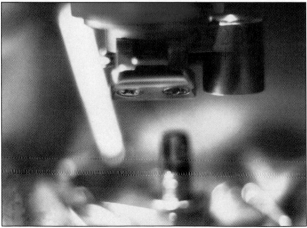

Figure A-12. At the end of the cut, remove the microkeratome first and the ring second.

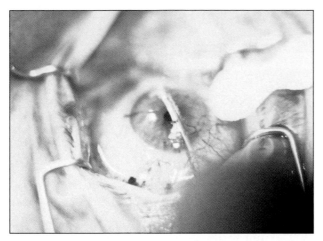

Figure A-13. The flap is raised with the spatula.

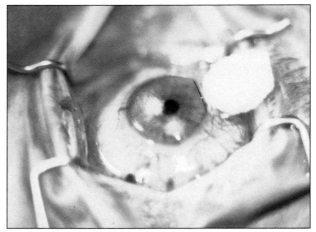

Figure A-14. The flap is positioned on a sponge and the sponge is closed.

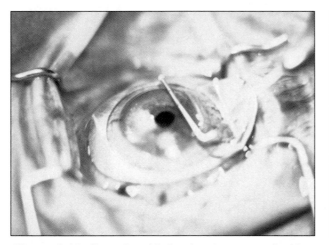

Figure A-15. Once the ablation has been completed, a drop of BSS is applied to the stroma and evenly spread.

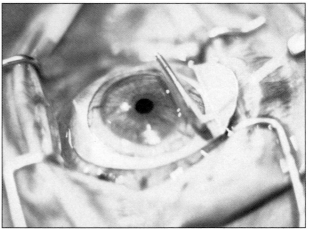

Figure A-16. The flap is repositioned using a cannula inserted below the hinge.

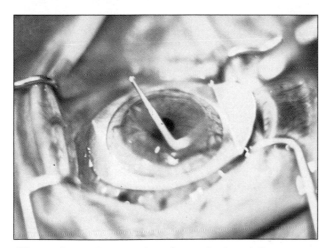

Figure A-17. The interface is washed and the cornea dried with a slightly damp sponge.

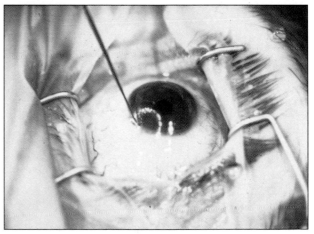

Figure A-18. The operation ends with the striae test followed by careful removal of the speculum and drape.

SURGICAL ATLAS: CASE 3

Down-Up LASIK With the Hansatome

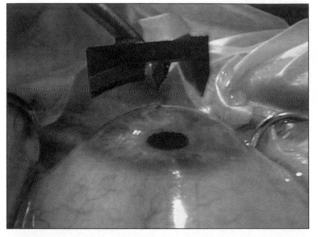

Figure A-19. Three-radius marker approaching the cornea.

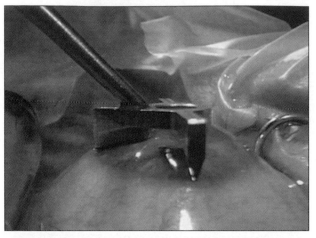

Figure A-20. The marker makes a slight indentation in the cornea.

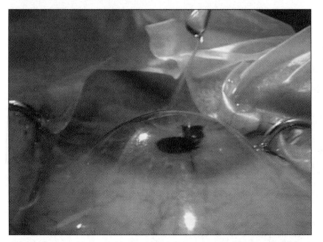

Figure A-21. Washing the cornea to remove any excess dye.

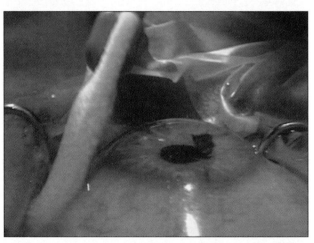

Figure A-22. The conjunctiva is dried to remove the dye and any secretions.

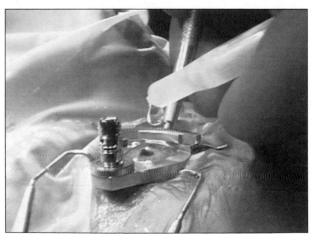

Figure A-23. Application of the microkeratome and wetting the cornea.

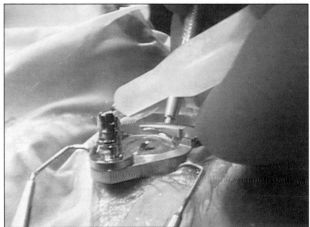

Figure A-24. The pin is wet.

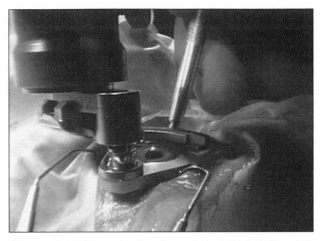

Figure A-25. The microkeratome is inserted on the pin.

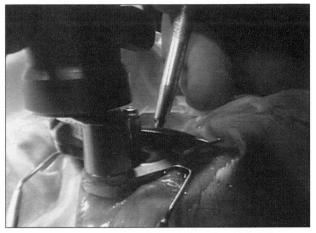

Figure A-26. The microkeratome has descended well on the pin and is ready to perform the cut.

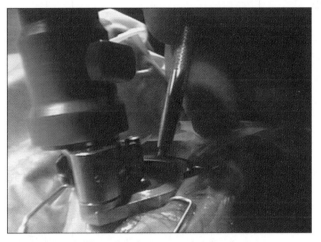

Figure A-27. The microkeratome cut begins.

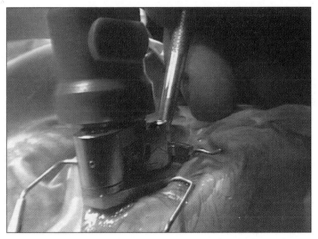

Figure A-28. The microkeratome has almost completed the cut.

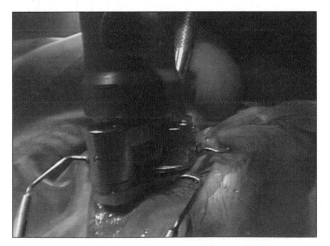

Figure A-29. The microkeratome at the end of the run. It is then returned to the starting position.

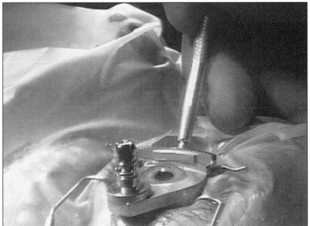

Figure A-30. Removal of the microkeratome.

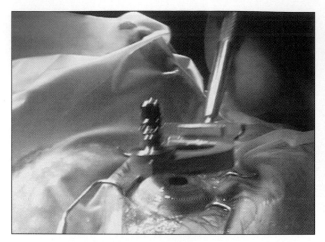

Figure A-31. Removal of the ring.

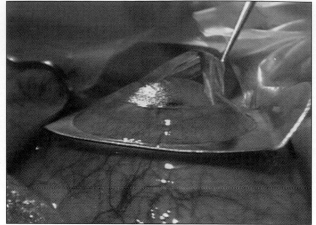

Figure A-32. The flap is raised with a spatula following positioning of the positioner.

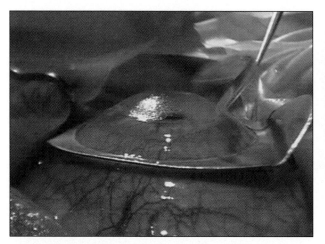

Figure A-33. The flap is partially raised.

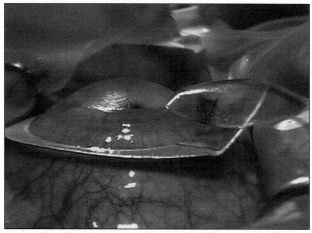

Figure A-34. The flap is positioned superiorly on the positioner.

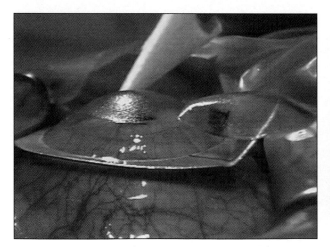

Figure A-35. Drying the stroma prior to the ablation.

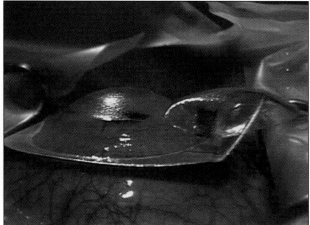

Figure A-36. The ablation.

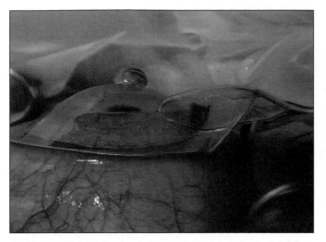

Figure A-37. At the end of the ablation, a drop of BSS is placed on the stroma.

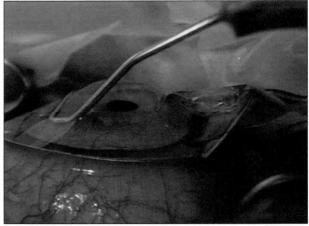

Figure A-38. A cannula is used to spread the fluid over the stroma.

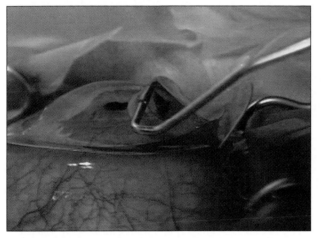

Figure A-39. The cannula is inserted under the flap and the flap is repositioned.

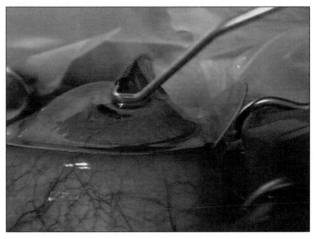

Figure A-40. Intermediate phase of flap repositioning.

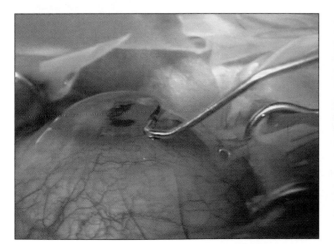

Figure A-41. Washing the interface: initial phase.

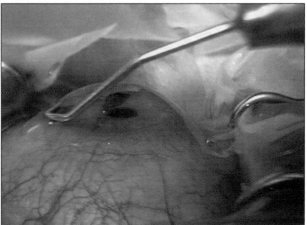

Figure A-42. Washing the interface: final phase.

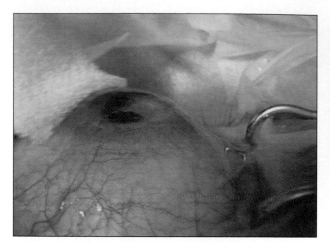

Figure A-43. Drying the flap and cornea.

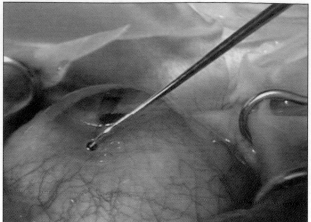

Figure A-44. Slade striae test completes the operation.

LASIK: Large Flap or Small Flap?

Lucio Buratto, MD

Keratomileusis is a surgical technique that was created and developed by Jose Barraquer in 1949.

Through the years, the operation has significantly evolved, resulting in the current technique of LASIK with a superior hinge as originally proposed by Lucio Buratto.

There are two basic steps in the operation: the lamellar cut using the microkeratome and the refractive cut (now a laser ablation rather than a mechanical cut). The lamellar cut is the focus of this discussion.

It is desirable to obtain a cut that has the following characteristics:
- Smooth and uniform cut surfaces
- Uniform depth cut
- Well-centered cut over the pupil
- Regular and suitable diameter for the refractive ablation
- A hinge that is sufficiently large as well as displaced from the ablation

Traditionally, the cut has had a diameter of between 7.0 and 8.0 mm. In my opinion, the diameter should be greater. A resection between 9.0 and 10 mm affords numerous advantages.

INTRAOPERATIVE ADVANTAGES OF A LARGER FLAP

- A larger stromal area is available for myopic, astigmatic, and hyperopic ablations.
- It is easier to perform ablations with large transition zones.
- The corneal hinge is protected from laser ablation.
- The hinge is more displaced from the center of the ablation, thus any collection of fluid at the hinge is less likely to interfere with the ablation.
- Comfort during surgery is greater.
- There is less need to protect the hinge.
- A reduction in surgical time is obtained, as there is less need for retracting, drying, and protecting the hinge.
- The flap is more easily repositioned at the end of the operation.
- There is no interference with the use of the eye

tracking system (retracting instruments are avoided).
- LASIK is easier to perform in special cases (LASIK following PKP, EPI, RK, AK, LTK, etc).

POSTOPERATIVE ADVANTAGES OF A LARGER FLAP

- There is a larger area of adherence to the underlying tissue (the area of a 7.0 mm flap is 38.5 mm^2; the area of a 9.5 mm flap is 70.7 mm^2).
- The cornea has more stability because of the greater area of adhesion of the flap.
- The flap is less likely to be displaced either spontaneously or if the patient rubs his or her eye.
- Larger scar circumference (scarring occurs along the periphery of the cut, from Bowman's to Bowman's).
- Re-epithelialization is rapid, as the new epithelium forms peripherally.
- The minimal foreign body sensation (superior hinge, peripheral epithelial damage).

DISADVANTAGES

- There is a possibility of bleeding because the cut will encroach on the limbal blood vessels.
- The cut must be automated to ensure that the large cut surface is uniform and regular.
- It is more difficult to lift the flap if enhancement is required.

CONCLUSION

Technically, it is difficult to obtain a cut of a large diameter. A state-of-the-art microkeratome is required using a suitable ring and very sharp blade; the microkeratome must also have automated movement to provide constant uniform speed, resulting in a smooth cut with no chatter.

At the present time, the only instrument that has all these characteristics is the Hansatome. The larger, smoother cut provided by this instrument is giving excellent clinical results.

LASIK WITH THE SKBM AND SUMMIT LASER: PERSONAL TECHNIQUE

Stephen Brint, MD

7

INTRODUCTION

My laser in situ keratomileusis (LASIK) technique has evolved with the procedure—through the work and collaboration with dedicated surgeons from all over the world. I use the Summit Apex Plus (Waltham, Mass, USA) and the VISX Star excimer lasers routinely in my LASIK procedures. My early experience with the Steinway microkeratome for myopic keratomileusis (MKM) procedures, through its evolution and subsequent manufacture and distribution by Chiron Vision, led me to continue using the ACS (Automated Corneal Shaper) microkeratome as I began performing LASIK. Currently, I continue to use the ACS as well as the Hansatome and the new SKBM (Summit Krumeich-Barraquer Microkeratome). Although it does not approach the cost of an excimer laser, the microkeratome is not only expensive but also the most important tool in LASIK. It enables us to create a corneal flap and thus preserve the outer layers of the cornea.

The description of the assembly, disassembly, and maintenance of each of these microkeratomes is carefully detailed in other chapters of this book. Strict adherence to the respective protocol for each microkeratome is mandatory.

When possible, allowing for adequate residual stromal bed thickness (225 to 250 microns), I prefer a 160-micron flap. I have found that this is what I normally obtain when I use a 180-micron depth plate with the ACS and the 160-micron fixed heads of the Hansatome and the SKBM. This thickness leads to smoother, more manageable flaps.

Why is a thickness of 160 to 180 microns used? In general, the thinner the flap, the less stable it is and the easier it is to wrinkle and form striae, which lead to irregular astigmatism and poor vision. In contrast, the thicker the flap, the more stable it is. However, less tissue is available for ablation in high myopia with a thicker flap. Considering this, a thickness of 160 microns is probably the best compromise in higher amounts of myopia. In a very thin cornea, a thickness of 130 microns may alternatively be used, but thicker or thinner flaps should be avoided.

With regard to possible complications, the depth plate is the single most important part of the ACS. Should the surgeon forget to insert it or should the depth plate be improperly seated, the eye will be penetrated during the cut. This results in iris damage, damage to the lens, and possible vitreous loss. Amazingly, these complications have actually occurred in a small number of cases. It should be our foremost duty to prevent a complication as disastrous and as easy to avoid. However, the only way to do this every time with utmost security is by using a checklist. The newer microkeratomes, such as the Hansatome and SKBM, have fixed plates to avoid this problem. Only a standardized procedure that involves routine use of a checklist will guarantee maximum results. We use several checklists depending on the microkeratome, which summarize all key items and contain the absolute minimal requirements to successfully complete the LASIK procedure. These include materials set-up, microkeratome assembly and testing, patient preparation, and a final surgeon's checklist.

Microkeratome assembly and performing laser testing is completed by our assistants, but the surgeon is responsible for performing a final test immediately prior to LASIK. I designed a very simple checklist that is attached to my laser within easy view of both my assistant and myself. My standard procedure is to review the laser settings and fluence performance, beam homogeneity, helium-neon (He-Ne) alignment, laser disc cassette, and Axicon alignment tests. Prior to patient entry into the laser suite, I carefully go through this final checklist. With the Summit Apex Plus, the morning start-up consists of checking He-Ne alignment, beam homogeneity,

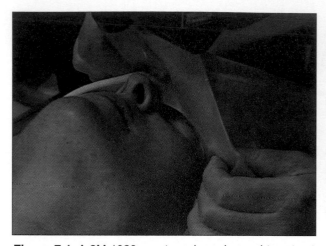

Figure 7-1. A 3M 1020 aperture drape is used to retract the eyelashes and eyelids.

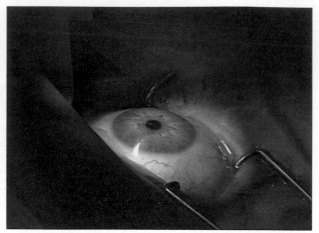

Figure 7-2. A Liebermann locking-style lid speculum is used for maximum exposure.

fluence, laser disc cassette alignment, and Axicon lens alignment. We also cut a polymethylmethacrylate (PMMA) disc.

PATIENT PREPARATION

Careful patient preparation cannot be overemphasized. During preparation for LASIK in the preoperative area, the patient receives instruction and information regarding the procedure. The eye(s) are irrigated to remove tear film debris. Initial topical drops of the antibiotic ofloxacin (Ocuflox), as well as a nonsteroidal anti-inflammatory drug (NSAID) such as sodium diclofenac (Voltaren) are instilled approximately 30 minutes prior to surgery. The operative eye(s) are marked with a color-coded sticker. Patients wear surgical caps and shoe covers, and a blanket is provided in the preoperative area and laser suite (the required ambient temperature makes the area uncomfortably cold for most patients).

When the patient is comfortably situated in the reclined laser chair, the first drops of 0.5% proparacaine (Alcaine, Alcon, Fort Worth, Tex, USA) are instilled bilaterally to initiate anesthesia and decrease the blink reflex in the fellow eye. I then begin a routine Betadine surgical hand scrub. The patient's lids and lashes are prepared with Betadine swabs and an additional proparacaine drop is used in the first eye to be operated.

PROCEDURE

I isolate the lashes and retract the lids very carefully using a modified 3M 1020 drape (Figure 7-1). A locking Liebermann-style lid speculum, which gives maximum exposure and slightly proptoses the globe, is then inserted and slowly opened (Figure 7-2). The disadvantage is discomfort to the patients, especially in small lid apertures and deep-set eyes. In any case, the speculum must be strong enough to withstand forced closure of the lids. Otherwise, the patient may forcefully squeeze his or her eyes during the cut, which would dislodge the suction ring and keratome, resulting in dissection of an irregular cap.

Alternately, if good exposure cannot be obtained with this or another locking-style lid speculums, a Barraquer wire speculum may be used. The technique here is to place the suction ring on top of the speculum, push down, the eye is proptosed, and exposure and suction can usually be obtained. The risk is that the patient is able to squeeze and may dislodge the suction ring during the microkeratome pass, creating an irregular flap.

The position of the patient's head is rechecked and adjusted once he or she has been prepared for the procedure. The head must be in a horizontal plane to avoid decentration of the ablation, which can occur when the head is tilted up, down, or to the side.

To ensure proper flap repositioning, it is mandatory to mark the cornea prior to the cut. Both radial and pararadial marks are used (Figure 7-3). The pararadial marks are important in case a free cap is dissected, as they will ensure that the flap is replaced properly with the stromal side down. Marking or not marking can mean the difference between minor nuisance (free cap, replaced properly as marked) and a major complication (free cap replaced epithelial side down and lost during the first night) (Figure 7-4).

Many high-volume surgeons have abandoned the marking step, as they feel it is unnecessary and have confidence in dealing with the rare free cap. I did not mark for approximately 1000 cases without encounter-

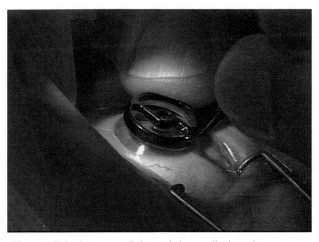

Figure 7-3. A pararadial mark is applied to the cornea, taking care to use a minimum amount of gentian violet.

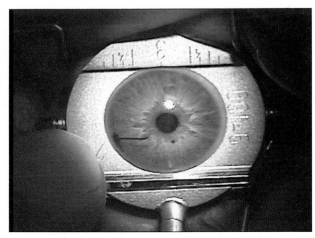

Figure 7-4. The suction ring of the SKBM is applied to the eye and decentered slightly nasally.

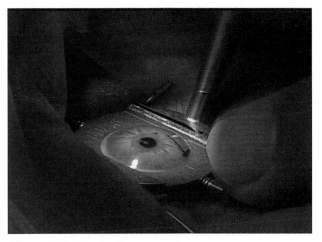

Figure 7-5. Suction is engaged.

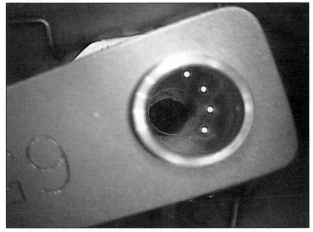

Figure 7-6. The SKBM Barraquer tonometer is used to verify that the applanated area is well within the circular mire on the tip of the tonometer.

ing a free cap. I felt, however, that I was returning to the laser suite too often to reposition a slightly displaced flap detected at the routine postoperative flap check. Reinstating the pararadial mark into my routine has significantly decreased this occasionally unnecessary effort.

The suction ring is now placed on the eye with slight nasal or superior decentration depending on the microkeratome, to allow for a more peripheral placement of the hinge out of the way of the ablation. In eyes with average keratometry of less than 41.5, a smaller flap, bed, and hinge are produced. In these cases, the suction ring needs to be well centered (Figure 7-5). Anticipating the possibility of later retreatment with recutting a new flap, slight nasal decentration is recommended for the initial procedure; this ensures a fresh entrance cut when the suction ring is later placed centrally for the enhance-

ment cut. It also allows room for hyperopic ablation if needed later with either a lift of the original flap or a new cut.

Adequate suction is verified using an applanation tonometer on a dry cornea to check the pressure. The applanated area must be smaller than the reference circle engraved in the tonometer (Figure 7-6). After tonometry indicates that the intraocular pressure (IOP) is appropriately high and after moistening the corneal surface with proparacaine (avoiding salt crystals) (Figure 7-7), the microkeratome is inserted into the suction ring (Figure 7-8). Prior to making the cut, verification that the advancing path of the microkeratome across the eye is unobstructed is mandatory (Figure 7-9). With the SKBM microkeratome, the diameter of the applanated cornea is visualized and this data is entered on the console to assure correct hinge size.

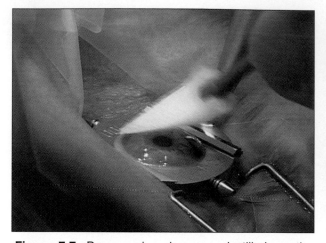

Figure 7-7. Proparacaine drops are instilled on the cornea; the excess is carefully removed from the suction ring surface.

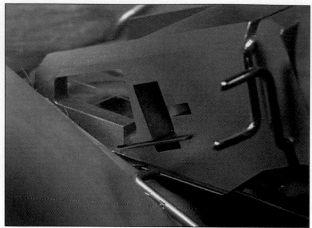

Figure 7-8. The SKBM, checked and seated in suction ring, is ready to advance.

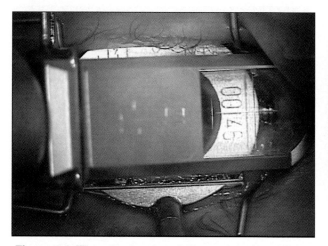

Figure 7-9. The microkeratome's forward motion stops at the end of the pass.

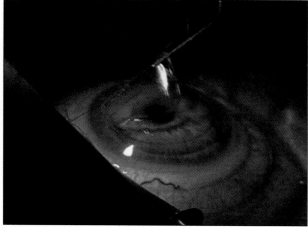

Figure 7-10. The flap is lifted and rotated nasally using the open blades of a tying forceps, taking care not to actually grasp the flap.

In summary, there are four essential steps that guarantee a perfect cut:

1. A perfectly functioning and checked microkeratome
2. Tonometry to verify sufficient pressure
3. A moist cornea (not wet)
4. The path of the microkeratome must be unobstructed

These essential steps are again verified using our checklist.

Once the cut is completed, I carefully remove the suction ring, turn down the direct illumination, and immediately loosen the lid speculum for patient comfort. I use blunt, smooth, open tying forceps to slide in under the flap margin opposite the hinge, lift the flap, and lay it smoothly toward the hinge side (Figure 7-10). During a 15-second period the stromal bed is gently wiped with a Merocel sponge, and then I briefly wait to obtain consistent corneal hydration. I focus and center the red aiming beams of the Summit Apex Plus at the central pupil margins or use the reticule of the VISX Star. During the ablation, I constantly monitor centration and fixation. The flap hinge is protected from inadvertent ablation using a blunt metal instrument (I use a Tooke knife) or a moist Merocel sponge. The metal protector is easier to control. A Merocel sponge is used to remove any visible fluid that frequently collects at the hinge of the flap or collects centrally during a prolonged ablation.

The 3.4.1 software presently being using with the Summit Apex Plus in the CRS study allows single-zone treatment (surgeon adjusts from 1.0 to 6.5 mm) from 1.0 to 9.9 diopters (D) of myopic ablation (Figure 7-11). We generally use a 6.0 mm zone up to -7 D at the spectacle plane per US Food and Drug Administration (FDA)

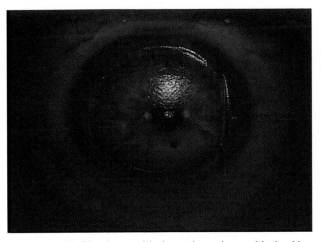

Figure 7-11. The laser ablation takes place with the He-Ne beams diverging and centered at the 3 and 9 o'clock positions.

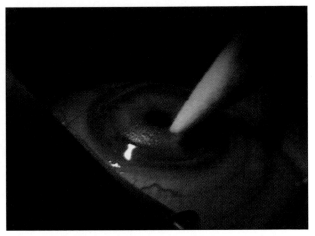

Figure 7-12. During long myopic ablations, the bed may be periodically dried to avoid central island formation.

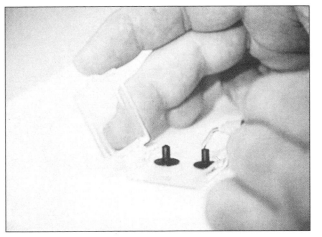

Figure 7-13. A dust-free, single-use suction cup is applied to the pneumatic forceps for transferring the laser disc to the Emphasis cassette (photos used with permission from Machat JJ, Slade SG, Probst LE. *The Art of LASIK. 2nd Edition.* Thorofare, NJ: SLACK Incorporated; 1999).

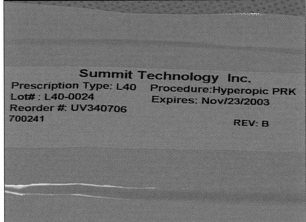

Figure 7-14. A hyperopic laser disc is supplied in a foil-type wrapper.

approval for this amount of myopia. From 7 to 15 D (the software actually allows 22 D) of myopia, I use the aspheric program, which creates a 5.0 mm ablation that smoothly blends out to 6.5 mm, removing less tissue in these higher myopes. Central island prevention treatment is used with all ablations and is generally preprogrammed to deliver an additional 10% of the total anticipated ablation pulses to the central 2.5 mm treatment area (Figure 7-12). With the VISX Star, the FDA-approved internal software used in the United States predetermines the pretreatment amount and zone (single or multi) size.

Toric correction is provided by the toric laser disc (Figures 7-13 through 7-19), which is placed and aligned to the minus cylinder axis in the Emphasis cassette. The

laser displays the appropriate disc to use once the desired refractive correction is entered. Laser discs are supplied in a consignment similar to intraocular lenses. Up to 5 D of astigmatism may be corrected simultaneously with the myopia, creating a very smooth ablation surface of 5 x 6.5 mm size (soon to be enlarged to 6 x 6.5 mm, as is being used internationally) (Figures 7-20 and 7-21).

Likewise, spherical hyperopia to 6 D (L disc) (Figures 7-22 through 7-24) and mixed and compound hyperopic astigmatism (P disc) can be corrected with a 6.5 mm ablation zone. Blending out to 9.5 mm with the Axicon lens (Figures 7-25 through 7-27) creates predictable and stable hyperopic correction. As the Bausch & Lomb/Chiron ACS microkeratome generally creates an 8.5 mm flap (depending on the steepness of the cornea), the newer Hansatome and SKBM unit, which create larger flaps, are preferred for these larger hyperopic ablations.

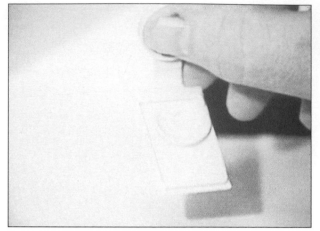

Figure 7-15. The laser disc is removed from the foil wrapper and stored in a contact lens case.

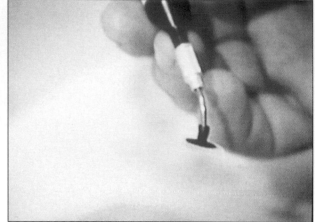

Figure 7-16. The disc is grasped by the suction cup from the contact lens case.

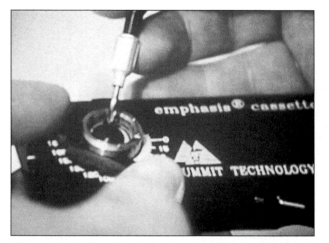

Figure 7-17. The disc is firmly seated in the Emphasis cassette and locked into place.

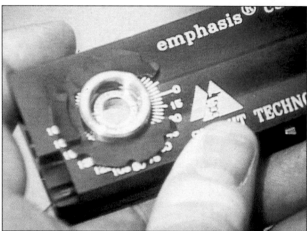

Figure 7-18. The toric disc is aligned with the minus cylinder axis, taking care to avoid error of parallax.

With the VISX Star, the amount and axis of the cylinder to be corrected is programmed into the laser computer and is delivered by the opening iris diaphragm and closing slit blade technique.

Once the ablation is complete, I place a drop of BSS on the bed, then gently sweep the flap temporally or inferiorly with closed tying forceps (Figure 7-28). I follow with irrigation of the interface with balanced salt solution (BSS) using the Slade cannula—the primary purpose of which is to allow the flap to float back to its original position as guided by the hinge, as well as to remove any potential debris (Figure 7-29). The flap is then painted into place with a moistened Merocel sponge (Figure 7-30) and the position checked primarily by making sure the gutter is symmetrical all the way around, as well as by verifying alignment of the corneal marks. Once the flap is perfectly centered, a 2- to 3-minute drying period allows the flap to adhere while the central epithelium is

kept moist with a drop of methylcellulose (Celluvisc). Even though Celluvisc has been said to increase drying time and possibly decrease adherence, I have found the opposite. I feel it provides good flap distension and adherence with a decreased incidence of immediate slight flap displacement when the speculum is removed and the patient blinks. After flap adhesion is verified, the lid speculum is carefully removed (Figure 7-31). The patient is then asked to blink while looking up and down, which again verifies flap adhesion. Ocuflox and Voltaren eye drops are instilled prior to the patient sitting up and leaving the laser suite.

POSTOPERATIVE

After surgery, patients are escorted into an exam lane for a slit lamp flap check, followed by postoperative instructions. Tobradex eyedrops and nonpreserved artifi-

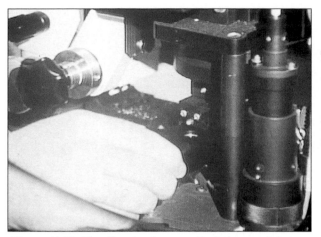

Figure 7-19. The Emphasis cassette is inverted, inserted into its slot, and locked into place in the laser down tube.

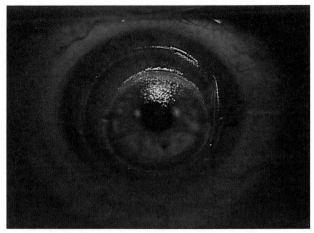

Figure 7-20. A hyperopic ablation is demonstrated.

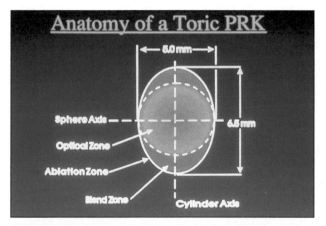

Figure 7-21. The currently available toric ablation pattern of 5 x 6.5 mm, soon to be enlarged to 6 x 6.5 mm.

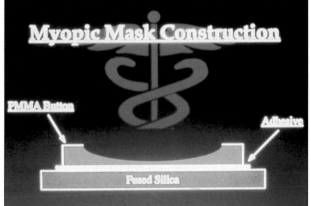

Figure 7-22. The PMMA laser disc, mounted on a silica plate, is typical of the myopic and toric disc.

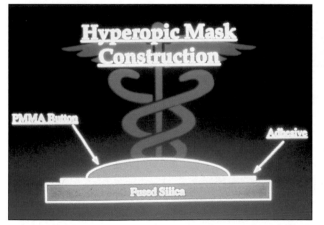

Figure 7-23. Hyperopic disc construction.

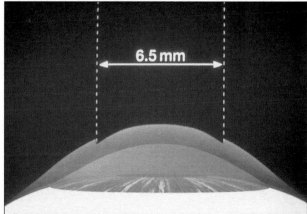

Figure 7-24. An illustration of the hyperopic correction obtainable using the L-mask.

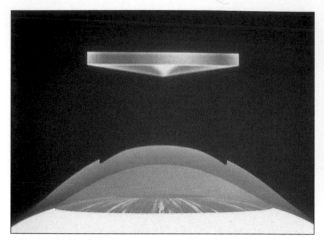

Figure 7-25. An illustration of the Axicon lens in place, which diverges the laser light.

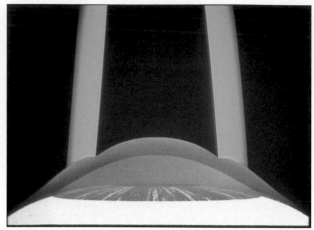

Figure 7-26. The divergent laser light blends the edges off the hyperopic ablation, extending the transition zone out to 9.5 mm.

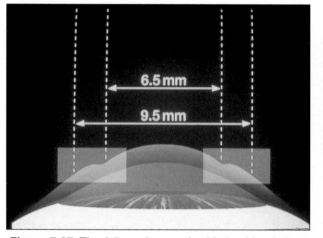

Figure 7-27. The 6.5 mm hyperopic ablation blended out to 9.5 mm with the aid of the Axicon lens.

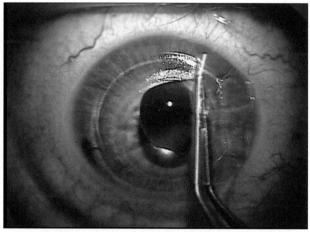

Figure 7-28. The flap is stroked back into place by placing closed typing forceps underneath the hinge and flipping the flap back onto a moistened bed.

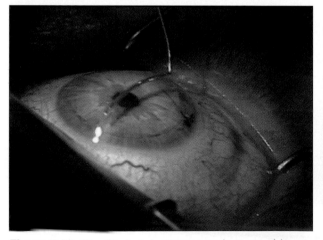

Figure 7-29. The Slade irrigating cannula is used to irrigate the interface, removing any potential debris and creating a lake of fluid, which allows the flap to float back into perfect position.

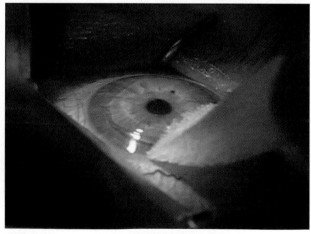

Figure 7-30. The flap is very gently painted, nasally to temporally, into position with a moistened Merocel sponge and then allowed to dry in place for 3 minutes.

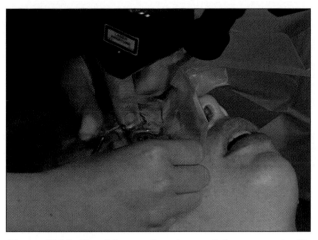

Figure 7-31. The lid speculum is carefully removed with the aid of an assistant to prevent dislodging the flap while removing it and the drape.

cial tears (Genteal, CIBA, Atlanta, Ga, USA) are instilled and written postoperative instructions are reviewed. At the slit lamp, I verify proper adhesion, centration, and smoothness of the flap, and that the interface is clean. The flap is rechecked approximately 20 minutes later by another doctor prior to leaving the center.

Patients are instructed to use an eye shield(s) (in the postoperative pack) during the night for 4 nights. In addition, Tobradex (qid for 4 days) is prescribed and the patient is instructed to immediately begin using the non-

preserved artificial tears every 30 minutes while awake for the first 2 weeks and tapered as needed thereafter. We are increasingly finding that one of the most frequent problems post-LASIK is dry-eye syndrome. This is being seen as an older population is interested in LASIK, especially hyperopic LASIK in the presbyopic age group. Many of these patients are female, having undergone cosmetic lid procedures and already experiencing dry-eye symptoms prior to the procedure. We are even using collagen punctum plugs prior to surgery in many of these patients, as well as recommending copious amounts of the tear substitutes. We check the patients the first day after surgery and return them to the care of their comanaging doctor for the 1 week (5 to 10 days after surgery) postoperative exam. Other routine exams are scheduled after 4 to 8 weeks, 4 to 6 months, 12 to 14 months, and 24 to 26 months.

Frequent evaluation of our clinical results is facilitated by an up-to-date outcomes database. Uncorrected visual acuity, as well as desired versus achieved correction, is the main criteria used to assess the effectiveness of a refractive procedure. This data is collected and entered into our outcomes program for every postoperative visit. Current statistics of this type allow us to not only make informed decisions about nomogram adjustments, but also give our patients a very real picture of the success of the LASIK procedure.

COMPLICATIONS OF LASIK

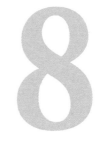

Lucio Buratto, MD and Stephen Brint, MD

INTRODUCTION

Surgical complications of any refractive procedure may be divided into the categories of preoperative, intraoperative, and postoperative. Either the anatomy or the visual quality of the eye may be altered.

Regardless of when the complication occurs (pre-, intra-, or postoperative), what really matters is the final result obtained from understanding and managing the problem correctly. Postoperatively, we may see complications analogous to those seen with other corneal surgery procedures, such as glare, halos, and reduced contrast sensitivity. Complications that are common to eye surgery in general may also occur, such as infections, loss of visual acuity in general or, decreased best-corrected visual acuity. Finally complications related to corneal lamellar surgery, such as irregular astigmatism, epithelial ingrowth and stromal melting can occur. It is naïve to believe that complications can be completely avoided as they are an inevitable part of any surgical procedure. What is important is to reduce them to a minimum in terms of frequency and severity. The patient should also be fully aware of the risks prior to the surgical operation, as part of obtaining the informed consent.

Increasingly, we are recognizing that the most common complications of refractive surgery are those associated with quality of the postoperative cornea. Even though the cornea may be perfectly transparent, there may still be functional problems derived from its altered structure. These functional problems cannot always be measured using standard Snellen charts, which measure vision only under conditions of high contrast. Low and medium contrast sensitivity testing is required. Refractive surgery frequently creates a reduction in contrast sensitivity, typically associated with glare.

Contrast is a fundamental part of the visual process, given that it is defined as the ability to differentiate a pale object from a dark one. As reduction in contrast and glare are dependent on light being improperly focused on the retina, the corneal contributions to this defocused light constitute just one of the complications of refractive surgery. These problems are not usually caused by a diffuse opacities of the cornea, but by several small areas of dense opacity and epithelial irregularity. The corneal refractive surface, despite being modified by the refractive procedure, maintains its nonspherical properties (the cornea does not focus light to a point as a lens would normally do), thus physiologic dilation of the pupil in darkness may induce poor night vision. Therefore, the pupil plays a key role in reducing the number of improperly focused light rays.

The most frustrating complication of refractive surgery, in terms of visual quality, is irregular astigmatism, because this increases the diffraction of the light rays, reduces contrast sensitivity and may create diplopia. Readers should remember that very minimal astigmatism may not be detected by computerized corneal topographies (CCT) but can sometimes be observed with routine keratometry performed by an expert.

At the present time, experienced LASIK surgeons typically have an incidence of minor complications such as epithelial ingrowth in the region of 1% to 2%, and an incidence of major complications (loss of the flap, corneal flap melting, etc) in the region of 0.2% to 0.3%. Understanding the etiology of complications is the first step toward their prevention.

Complication avoidance is multifactorial and includes:

- Correct preoperative preparation and testing of the instruments
- Correct patient preparation
- Accurate preoperative examination and evaluation of the patient
- The majority of complications involve the lamellar cut (ie, correct microkeratome management)

Theoretically, LASIK complications can be avoided or minimized if the surgeon pays maximum attention to the finer details of the surgical procedure. It is essential that an accurate preoperative evaluation of the patient so that patients with clear contraindications to surgery, such as unstable refraction, keratoconus, active corneal or intraocular inflammation, will be excluded. It is of the utmost importance for the surgeon to:

- Have an accurate stable refraction
- Have accurate pachymetry measurements
- Be thoroughly familiar with the instruments
- Ensure that the microkeratome is cleaned and assembled correctly, followed by preoperative testing
- Ensure that all parameters of the laser are checked
- Ensure that the patient's fixation and ablation centration is correct

PREOPERATIVE COMPLICATIONS

Anesthesia Complications

We prefer topical anesthesia because it is simple, efficacious, appreciated by the patient, and avoids complications that may result from retrobulbar and para/peribulbar anesthesia. As soon as the surgeon is comfortable with the microkeratome and use of the laser, he or she should use topical anesthesia. The patient prefers topical anesthesia because it eliminates the need for a patch, (a clear shield may be used immediately or only at night for the first 4 to 7 days) and the improvement in vision is usually obvious immediately, while continuing to improve over the next few hours. General anesthesia should be used in LASIK only in cases of patients who are extremely anxious, uncooperative, mentally unstable, or handicapped.

Retrobulbar anesthesia may rarely be used for inducing good exposure of sunken eyes or eyes with very narrow interpalpebral spaces. This facilitates placement of the suction ring and completion of the cut, however, it also induces dilation of the pupil, decreased ability to fixate, which increase the risk of decentration. Other risks include perforation of the globe and retrobulbar hemorrhage in these highly myopic eyes. If retrobulbar anesthesia is used, it must be performed correctly and with great care and attention. There are better ways to deal with sunken globes and narrow fissures, which will be described later. A drop of topical anesthesia should also be applied to the fellow eye to reduce the patient's blink reflex.

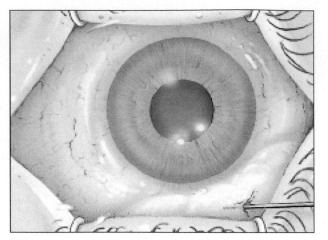

Figure 8-1. Conjunctival chemosis: complications of injection anesthesia. It may prevent adhesion of the suction ring.

Chemosis

Chemosis of the conjunctiva may occur following para/peribulbar anesthesia secondary to diffusion. This may interfere with placement and grasp of the suction ring and the inability to maintain high intraocular pressure. Repeated placement of the suction ring also induces chemosis and should be avoided if at all possible. If there is a large amount of chemosis, it is better for the surgeon to stop and postpone the procedure. If the chemosis seems to be a minor problem, rather than postponing the procedure the surgeon can attempt to correct the problem by using the blunt side of a curved cyclodialysis spatula or forceps to "milk" the edema (or blood in the event of a subconjunctival hemorrhage) into the fornices.

Epithelial Toxicity

Topical anesthesia should be carefully dosed. Usually one to two applications are sufficient (one drop per application) during the 5 to 10 minute period prior to surgery. Excessive applications can have a toxic effect on the corneal epithelium, creating edema manifested as a reduction in the adhesion of the epithelium to Bowman's layer. If a corneal abrasion or sloughing occurs during the microkeratome pass, visual recovery is significantly delayed and may even create a thin or buttonhole flap. Dry corneas, poor adhesion of the epithelium, as observed in diabetic patients, or basement membrane disease may aggravate this situation. The ideal anesthetic agent appears to be 0.5% proparacaine, as it seems to cause the lowest degree of epithelial toxicity. A 0.5% concentration of tetracaine is also available as a sterile single-dose dropper, but this has proved to be the most toxic of the agents available. Nonpreserved xylo-

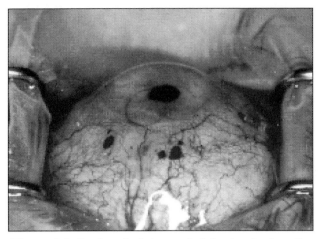

Figure 8-2. Conjunctival chemosis following the lamellar cut.

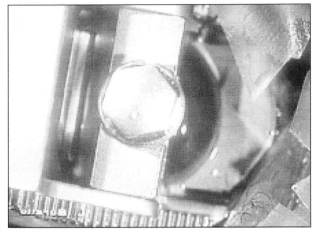

Figure 8-3. Fragments of the drape may interfere with the microkeratome pass. Excessive magnification will restrict the overall vision of the surgical procedure and make surgery more difficult.

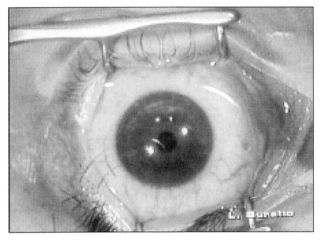

Figure 8-4. Eye exposure prior to surgery. The speculum has been positioned correctly. Some eyelashes are lying on the conjunctiva. These may interfere with adhesion of the ring and lodge into the interface during the lamella cut.

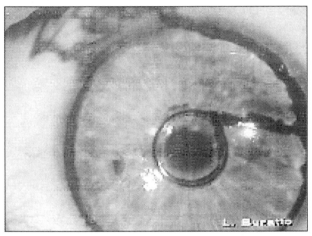

Figure 8-5. An excessive amount of dye will be toxic to the epithelium.

caine in a concentration of 2% or 4% is less toxic than tetracaine, but its action may be excessively prolonged. Another alternative is 0.4% oxybuprocaine. The cornea should be moistened with a glycerine-based topical anesthetic (proparacaine) just prior to the microkeratome pass in order to minimize trauma to the corneal epithelium and prevent salt build-up in the microkeratome mechanism. One should minimize contact between the anesthetic agent and the cornea: a single application of anesthetic is sufficient to anesthetize the cornea. The surgeon should also attempt to anesthetize the fornices and conjunctiva using a Merocel sponge soaked with the anesthetic agent, rather than applying with anesthetic agent directly to the cornea. Using this technique, the lamellar cut and vacuum created by the suction ring are generally well-tolerated. Following instillation of anesthetic drops, the patient should keep his or her eyes closed to avoid corneal drying because the blink reflex has been reduced. Tobramycin or a fluorquinolone is preferred as the preoperative antibiotic drop rather than gentamycin, which is epithelial toxic.

Tip for prevention: topical anesthesia should be used sparingly. A minimum of a nontoxic or low toxicity anesthetic agent should be used in limited contact with the cornea.

Drape and Speculum Complications

The drape should simultaneously cover and retract the eyelid margins, removing the eyelashes from the operating field. This helps to improve sterility of the operating field and prevents the lashes from being engaged during the microkeratome pass, which may pre-

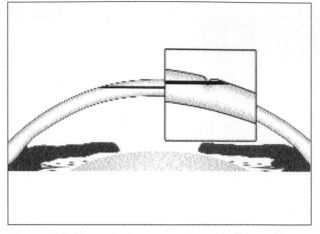

Figure 8-6. Excessively aggressive epithelial marking or marking made with a cutting instrument.

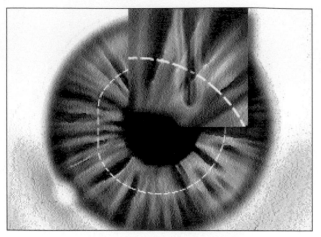

Figure 8-7. Close-up of Figure 8-6.

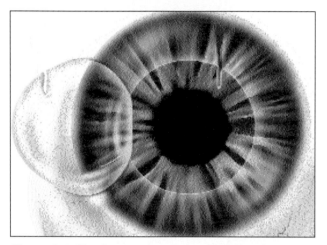

Figure 8-8. The flap may be damaged by overly aggressive marking.

maturely stop the pass. The drape, if not well retracted and carefully observed, may also interfere with the pass. Adhesive drapes are recommended, as they are easier to manage. The assistant on one side and the laser technician on the other may be of great help to the surgeon in providing further assurance that the lashes, drapes, and speculum are away from the microkeratome pass. The drape should be applied and retracted as carefully as possible to avoid corneal abrasion. The same considerations apply to the selection and placement of the lid speculum during its insertion and removal. Again, the assistant's retraction of the eyelids can aid in safe removal of the lid speculum.

Tips for prevention:
- The drapes and speculum should be handled with great care
- Adhesive drapes should be used
- The arms of the speculum should be checked for smoothness
- An appropriate speculum should be used
- One drop of balanced salt solution (BSS) should be applied prior to applying the speculum

Complications from Tear Film and Conjunctival Secretions

Prior to the patient entering the laser room or once the surgeon has placed the drape and speculum, but before applying the suction ring, the cul-de-sac should be irrigated to remove debris and oily tear film. This also provides a more aseptic operating field. Any excess liquid should be removed from the conjunctival sac using a dry Merocel sponge, taking care to remove any secretions and debris, leaving the cul-de-sac dry to avoid fluid aspiration by the suction ring, which may result in poor suction.

Tips for prevention: the surgeon should make sure the operating field is clear of obstructions and that the fornices are perfectly clean and dry. Another useful tip is to use one of the newer speculums equipped with an integrated aspiration system.

Corneal Marking Complications

The cornea should be marked with a pen or one of the various corneal markers that are available. The pen must be soft, moist, and fine. A dry, rough pen or one contaminated with dye deposits may cause epithelial abrasions. Gentian violet, commonly used, is toxic to the epithelium and should be used in minimal quantities only, with the excess irrigated away. Marking within the central 3.0 mm zone should be avoided. Dried fragments of gentian violet deposited on the corneal surface may create irregularities in the epithelium during the lamellar cut or may be deposited in the interface and should be irrigated or gently stroked away with a moist sponge. Methylene

Table 8-1

PREOPERATIVE COMPLICATIONS

Etiology

General anesthesia
- Patient unable to cooperate/fixate
- Risks associated with the anesthesia itself

Para/peribulbar
- Retrobulbar hemorrhage
- Globe perforation
- Mydriasis
- Conjunctival chemosis
- Subconjunctival hemorrhage

Topical anesthesia
- Epithelial toxicity, edema, fragility
- Epithelial defects and sloughing
- Drape

Epithelial trauma
- Inadequate lid/lash covering and retraction
- Speculum

Fluid/secretion in the fornix
- Malfunction of the vacuum pump
- contamination of the field

Corneal marking
- Pen (gentian violet)
- Epithelial toxicity
- Contamination of the interface with dye debris
- Epithelial irregularity during the cut

Metallic marker
- Epithelial defects
- Inadequate marking

Prevention
- Topical anesthesia preferred
- Reduced dose topical anesthesia
- Retrobulbar anesthesia must be performed correctly
- Use an adhesive drape positioned carefully with a moist cornea
- Carefully control/speculum positioning
- Irrigate the fornices prior to applying the suction ring; then dry the fornices
- Check integrity and smoothness of the marker/use only a small amount of gentian violet/sufficient but not excessive impressions

Treatment

In the event of problems (conjunctival chemosis, etc), delay for a few hours or postpone the operation

blue is toxic to the cornea and may contaminate the interface. Metallic markers may damage the epithelium if their surfaces are rough; moreover, the markings may be inadequate. Complications associated with incorrect marking, (eg, the axis of astigmatism) failure to mark, or the mark washing off may occur and will be discussed later. Aggressive marking that leaves deep impressions on the cornea induces an irregular surface that can be a

source of potential problems with the microkeratome resection.

Tips for prevention:
- Check the condition of the marker
- Make a light but clear mark
- Avoid methylene blue
- Use as little gentian violet as necessary and remove dye fragments

INTRAOPERATIVE COMPLICATIONS

Although some intraoperative complications may be associated with the suction ring, the majority are the result of surgeon inexperience or over-confidence with the microkeratome. The microkeratome is a precision instrument with which the surgeon should be intimately familiar, and which must be carefully checked prior to every operation.

Suction Ring-Related Complications

Inadequate suction, or the total loss of suction, is a potential source of serious problems during LASIK. The surgeon should be alert to situations, which may lead to poor suction. The suction ring frequently induces minor subconjunctival hemorrhage of minimal clinical significance. Conjunctival chemosis may be induced by repeated attempts to place the suction ring if the first attempt is not correct. Chemosis often prevents good suction and may not allow adequate fixation by the patient. If chemosis is induced from repeated suction ring placement, an incision in the conjunctiva may allow drainage of excess fluid; alternately, blunt instruments such as a Merocel sponge, the handle of a swab, or a forceps can be used in an attempt to "milk" the fluid away from the limbus. In

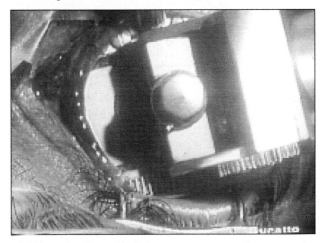

Figure 8-9. Excessive ring pressure on the eye may cause conjunctival chemosis, which will interfere with the advancement of the microkeratome.

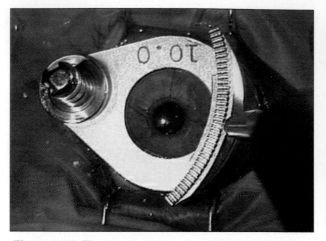

Figure 8-10. The ring has been correctly positioned prior to the cut.

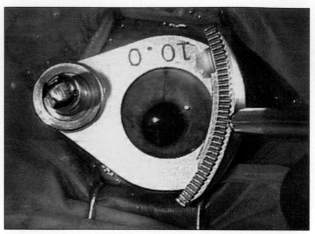

Figure 8-11. The ring has been decentered at the end of the cut.

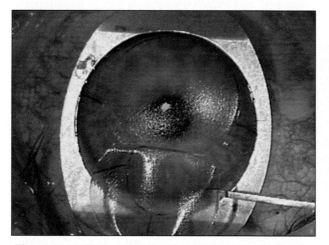

Figure 8-12. The cut has been decentered following the downward and nasal displacement of the ring during the lamellar cut.

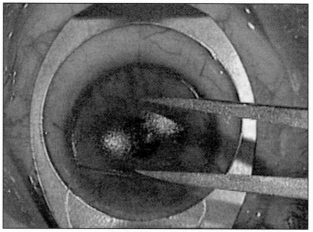

Figure 8-13. If the surgeon has doubt about the tissue available for ablation, he or she should measure it.

rare instances, a conjunctival peritomy may be performed to allow suction with the ring positioned directly onto the sclera. A better alternative is to wait 30 to 45 minutes and then try again. It is best, if possible, to simply postpone the procedure for 1 to 2 days and allow the subconjunctival edema to reabsorb. Loose conjunctiva will also create difficulty with suction ring grasp, and may need to be stretched by depressing the speculum posteriorly.

Inadequate Exposure

With poor exposure, the suction ring is difficult to position and good suction may not be obtained. Room for microkeratome passage may also be compromised. A lateral canthotomy may be indicated when placement of the suction ring is difficult. Alternately, it may be possible to operate without using a speculum or by changing the speculum. If a speculum is not used, one must ensure

that the eyelashes and eyelids do not overlap and cover the ring, especially the track. In small eyes, an axial length measurement performed preoperatively allows the surgeon to select the correct ring diameter for the operation (under the circumstances, the standard 11 mm suction ring may not be suitable). A retrobulbar injection to proptose the globe has been suggested. This is a valid technique but may induce chemosis-related problems described previously, as can repeated attempts to place the ring. Photorefractive keratectomy (PRK) should be considered if appropriate when suction cannot be obtained.

Poor draping may create a pseudo-eyelid slit smaller than a real opening. The drape should be kept taut until it adheres to the eyelid. The eyelids may be separated manually and the lid margins and lashes retracted as the drape is being applied.

With a prominent brow, the patient should be posi-

Table 8-2

INADEQUATE GLOBE EXPOSURE

Etiology
- Orbit anatomy: sunken eyes, small eyes
- Prominent brows
- Narrow palpebral fissures
- Tight eyelids
- Squeezing
- Previous surgery of the orbit or eyelids
- Previous trauma to the orbit or eyelids
- Poor drape application and retraction
- Poor choice of speculum

Results
- Difficult to position the suction ring
- Difficult to achieve suction
- Incomplete microkeratome pass
- Interference from the speculum
- Interference from the drape
- Interference with eyelashes

Prevention
- Accurate positioning of the drape to maximize exposure
- Use an appropriate speculum
- Have alternate speculums available
- Position the patient's head with the chin up or down as needed to obtain better exposure
- Have the assistant exert downward pressure on the speculum during the microkeratome pass

Treatment
- Lateral canthotomy if necessary
- Retrobulbar injection if necessary
- Perform the operation without a speculum

tioned with the chin raised slightly, as this will maximize exposure.

Tip for prevention: the assistant should push down gently on the speculum while the microkeratome is being inserted. This tightens the conjunctiva where the suction ring adheres in addition to proptosing the eye and avoids drape and lid problems during the microkeratome pass.

Dislodgement of the Suction Ring

Patient Induced

Uncontrolled forceful blinking can dislodge the suction ring. The surgeon should be alert to squeezing during the preoperative exam or during drape placement. When this occurs, it is important to talk with the patient and try to make him or her feel more relaxed. This can have a more powerful effect than drug-induced sedation. Excessive sedation may reduce patient cooperation, leading to poor fixation and decentration of the ablation.

Surgeon Induced

Loss of suction may be iatrogenic. Accidentally pressing the footpedal a second time following initial activation will induce immediate loss of suction. Some systems require constant pressure on the footpedal to control the suction level. Diligence by the surgeon or delegating control of the suction to the assistant is the best form of prevention. Irregular, thin, or incomplete flaps may be the result of inadequate or total loss of suction. These complications may also be caused by the microkeratome.

Induced by Inadequate IOP

It is mandatory that intraocular pressure (IOP) be at least 65 mm Hg following the application of the suction ring. Insufficient pressure will result in a multitude of complications, such as thin flap, perforated flap, or free cap. Redundant conjunctiva can simulate adequate IOP (pseudosuction), as it obstructs the orifice of the suction ring. Even though the pump may suggest good suction at the console, the IOP may not be adequate. It is thus mandatory that IOP be measured using either the Barraquer tonometer (part of the microkeratome set) or the pneumotonometer, as suggested by Chayet. Any further manipulation of the suction ring, speculum, eyelids, drape, etc, may cause a loss of suction and thus the pressure should be rechecked prior to the microkeratome pass. Alterations of the globe secondary to previous vitreo-retinal surgery may make application of the suction ring difficult. The following should be considered:
- The presence of a Lincoff sponge
- The scleral hourglass
- Low IOP from vitrectomy
- Conjunctival irregularities from a prior conjunctival peritomy

Microkeratome-Related Complications

Microkeratome-related complications usually result in a lamellar cut that is:
- Too short
- Too long
- Too superficial
- Too deep
- Of poor quality and irregular

Corneal Perforation

Although completely avoidable with good surgeon and staff training and by diligent following of a "preflight" checklist, this is without doubt the most serious complication encountered during LASIK. Perforation is due to the absence or incomplete seating of the depth plate of the microkeratome. If the plate is absent, the cut

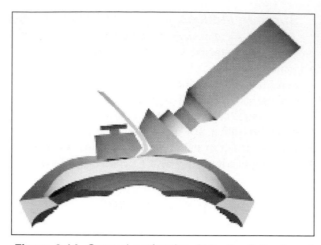

Figure 8-14. Corneal perforation. Note the flattening of the anterior chamber.

will be 900 microns deep, greater than the entire corneal thickness. This may also occur with a cut on a cornea that is thin in localized areas following an ulcer, wound, keratoconus, or previous refractive surgery. With corneal perforation, both the anterior and posterior segments will be damaged. Damage to the anterior segment will be magnified by the considerable difference created between increased IOP (65 mm Hg) and the sudden drop in IOP caused by the perforation, which may be accompanied by expulsion of the intraocular contents. Rarely, there may be only a simple perforation of the cornea if the surgeon is quick to respond to the appearance of the aqueous. Response time is usually inadequate because the pass is extremely rapid. Typically, a large opening of the anterior chamber is created with problems ranging from athalamia to total compromise of the eye with total or partial loss of the iris and crystalline lens, and damage to the posterior segment, including expulsive hemorrhage. If the plate has been inserted but is poorly positioned, the crystalline lens cannot become involved. Perforation can only occur through a total lack or inadequate insertion of the depth plate.

It is thus mandatory to check that the plate has been inserted correctly prior to every use. Improper seating of the depth plate increases the space between the terminal part of the plate and the blade edge, and the cut will be deeper than planned. Vibrations that result from blade oscillation may cause the partial disinsertion or complete detachment of the plate with sudden exposure of the corneal dome to the blade edge. If ocular damage is to be limited, the surgeon must promptly recognize initial leakage of aqueous during the microkeratome pass. The power and suction must be stopped immediately and the damage repaired. This is very difficult to achieve, as the microkeratome pass is very rapid.

Table 8-3

INADEQUATE SUCTION

Etiology
- Suction pump malfunction
- Small diameter cornea with redundant conjunctiva
- Conjunctival chemosis
- Relaxed conjunctiva
- Squeezing of lids
- Excessive elasticity in severely myopic eyes because of an excess in orbit fat
- Iatrogenic reasons: the suction pedal is accidentally depressed
- Intraoperative manipulations of the suction ring, drape, or speculum
- Previous vitreoretinal surgery

Results
- Thin or superficial flap
- Buttonhole or interrupted flap
- Irregular flap

Prevention
- Preoperative patient sedation
- Good globe exposure
- Keep the suction ring firmly against the globe until suction has been activated correctly
- Practice using the pedals
- Avoid manipulating the suction ring, drape, and speculum once good suction is achieved
- Treatment
- Always measure IOP
- Always remeasure IOP if there has been manipulation
- Treat any induced chemosis
- Conjunctival incision
- Conjunctival squeezing (milk the chemosis into the fornix)
- Conjunctival peritomy
- Wait 30 to 45 minutes
- Postpone the operation

If a perforation occurs, the eye must be protected with a plastic shield. The patient must be transferred to an operating room and general anesthesia administered. An anterior vitrectomy must be performed, followed by the reformation of the anterior changer with air or viscoelastic; the iris and cornea must then be carefully sutured. A vitreoretinal surgeon should be available. Corneal and lens surgery with the insertion of an intraocular lens (IOL) may be necessary. Following initial repair, the road to full rehabilitation is long. Initially, an aphakic contact lens, possibly with an artificial pupil, may be needed. A scleral-sutured IOL may be considered as a second procedure.

Most modern microkeratomes have an integrated plate, thus the risk of corneal perforation is completely

Table 8-4
GLOBE PERFORATION

Simple perforation
- Cornea is thinner than usual in just one spot
- Old corneal ulcer scar
- Old corneal wound
- Keratoconus
- Previous refractive surgery

Perforation with damage to the iris and crystalline lens with no vitreous loss
- Incomplete insertion of the plate

Perforation that may also jeopardize the posterior segment, vitreous loss, expulsive hemorrhage
- Absence of the plate

Table 8-5
PERFORATION OF THE EYE

Etiology
- Absence of the plate in the microkeratome
- Incorrect seating of the plate in the microkeratome

Prevention
- Precise assembly of the microkeratome
- Check the microkeratome prior to use
- Obligatory preoperative examinations:
  - Slit lamp
  - Corneal topography
  - Pachymetry

Treatment
- Varies from case to case on the basis of severity of the situation

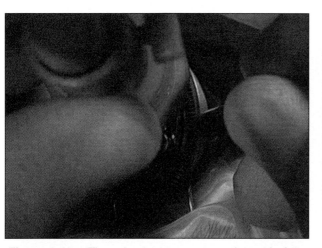

Figure 8-15a. The microkeratome stops the end of the pass. A first attempt is made to restart it manually if this fails.

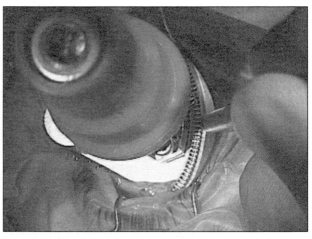

Figure 8-15b. The electric cable is disconnected. Then, holding the suction ring firmly, the motor is unscrewed and removed.

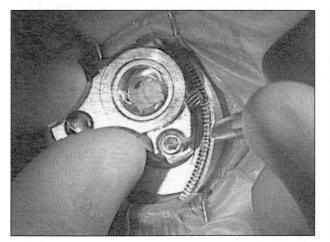

Figure 8-15c. At this point, the head is reversed manually to the starting point; the suction is deactivated and all the instruments are removed.

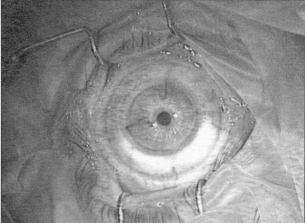

Figure 8-15d. With this technique, the flap is not damaged in any way and the cut surface is perfect.

avoided. One is the Hansatome, created specifically for the down-up technique. With these newer microkeratomes, perforation occurs only if the surgeon performs the lamellar cut on a very thin or irregular cornea, or a cornea with advanced keratoconus. It is therefore mandatory to perform accurate pachymetry at several points on the cornea.

In conclusion, if the preoperative evaluation and intraoperative technique are performed correctly, corneal perforation cannot and should not occur. Prevention is based on correct preoperative checks: topography, slit lamp examination, pachymetry, double-checking plate insertion (by the assistant and the surgeon), or better still, using modern microkeratomes with a fixed plate.

Incomplete Primary Cut (Short Flap)

Causes

- Incorrect setting of the stop device
- Electrical power failure
- Loss of power or motor breakdown
- Surgeon or assistant prematurely releasing the forward pedal
- Blockage of the microkeratome secondary to obstructions, such as the speculum, eyelids, drapes, cellular debris, salt crystals, or eyelashes caught in the gear/track mechanism
- Loss of suction
- Partial or total release of the microkeratome suction ring
- Inadequate slack in the microkeratome power cable
- Incorrect assembly of the microkeratome
- Poor cleaning of the microkeratome
- Salt crystal formation, which may impede the microkeratome pass can be avoided by using a salt-free solution to wet the cornea (topical anesthetic or distilled water instead of BSS) just prior to the pass. Excess fluid should not be used prior to the microkeratome pass and any sign of moisture in the motor should be immediately absorbed using a Merocel sponge at the end of each procedure when the microkeratome is disassembled.

Tips for prevention:

- Prior to beginning surgery, forward and reverse movement of the microkeratome should be tested.
- Exposure, speculum, draping, and path of advancement must be checked and clear.
- As an incomplete flap may be secondary to loss of suction, the surgeon should be alert to unusual movement of the globe or unfamiliar noises from the machine. The IOP should be rechecked prior to beginning the pass.

Management

If the microkeratome stops abruptly, the surgeon should reverse direction, release suction, and remove the suction ring. If the microkeratome has completely jammed, suction should be released and the microkeratome and suction ring, as a unit, should be gently removed with great care and attention. Even though the flap is incomplete, it is still partially inserted in the microkeratome and may be adhered to the blade. The ring-microkeratome should be slightly lifted and slowly moved away from the hinge. With the ACS, this would be a temporal movement. If this proves difficult, it may indicate that the flap is stuck to metal. The assistant should then irrigate the microkeratome cavity where the flap is located in an attempt to release it.

Two situations may result:

1. The cut allows sufficient space for a full ablation to be performed.
2. There is insufficient space for a full, well-centered ablation.

In the event of #1 above, the keratectomy may be extended slightly manually with a lamellar dissection blade, such as a Beaver 69, attempting to maintain the same dissection plane, which is not easy. Manual dissection should be avoided if at all possible. When in doubt, a 6.0 mm optical zone marker can be placed over the pupil to determine whether there is enough area suitable for ablation. Protection of the hinge using a spatula or moist sponge is required to prevent inducing irregular astigmatism and/or damage to the integrity of the flap and hinge.

In the event of #2 above, the flap must be replaced on the corneal bed with irrigation of the interface, and the procedure must be terminated. It may be repeated 4 to 6 months later assuming the postoperative course has been uneventful. With repeat surgery, a 180 micron plate should be used so that the cut is deeper than the previous one (160 microns), if the corneal thickness will permit it. The new cut should also be initiated temporal to the first one, if possible. Typically, the incomplete cut with replacement of the flap does not affect the refractive, topographic, or anatomic result. Induced astigmatism may rarely result with visual distortion regardless of whether the ablation was performed or not.

Irregular Cut

This cut is irregular in its shape, edges, or surface. A normal flap should be circular with regular clean-cut edges. A flap resulting from an irregular cut is unacceptable in terms of smoothness and uniformity.

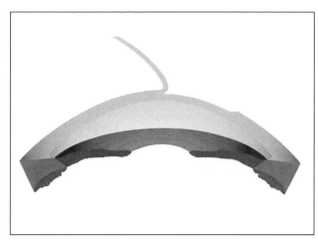

Figure 8-16. Side view of an incomplete lamellar cut.

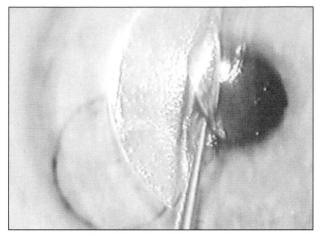

Figure 8-17. Incomplete lamellar cut due to premature release of the pedal.

Table 8-6

INCOMPLETE FLAP

Etiology
- Incorrect setting of the stop device
- Power failure
- Power loss or motor breakdown/malfunction
- Accidental blocking or stopping of the footpedal
- Microkeratome blockage due to obstacles along the pass
  - From the speculum
  - The drape
  - Cell debris
  - Salt granules from dehydrated saline solutions
  - Eyelashes
  - Eyelid margins of poorly exposed bulbs
  - Incorrect assembly of the microkeratome
  - Poor cleaning of the microkeratome
- Partial or total detachment of the suction ring/loss of suction

Results
- Unable to proceed with the ablation
- The ablation may be performed but with greater difficulty and decreased ablation size

Prevention
- Total surgeon and assistant comfort with the type of microkeratome used
- Adequate globe exposure using lateral canthotomy if necessary
- Perfect assembly—clean and check the microkeratome and suction ring prior to every procedure
- Make sure the microkeratome is advancing and returning smoothly in the track prior to each procedure
- Avoid excess fluid prior to using the microkeratome
- Avoid salt-containing solutions prior to the cut
- Pay attention to all clues that may suggest loss of suction

Treatment
- If the laser ablation is performed, protect the hinge with a sponge or metal protector
- If the ablation is not possible, reposition the flap and postpone the operation

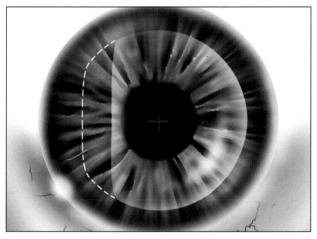

Figure 8-18. Incomplete cut: the cut surface is inadequate for a myopic ablation and even more so for a hyperopic one.

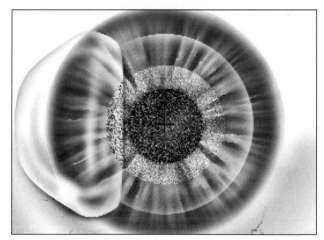

Figure 8-19. Incomplete cut: the theoretical ablation includes an uncut area.

Etiology

An irregular cut may be due to:

- Uneven movement of the microkeratome pass (plow-up phenomenon)
- Irregularity of the blade edge
- Surgeon-induced torquing or jamming of the microkeratome (hold in neutral position)
- Displacement of the ring on the globe because of globe asymmetry or clumsy movements by the surgeon
- Obstruction during the pass (speculum, eyelashes, drapes, redundant conjunctiva, etc)
- Loss of suction

Tips for prevention:

- The surgeon should perform the preoperative microkeratome testing pass both forward and backward
- The corneal surface and track should be moist
- The eyelid margins and speculum should be adequately retracted
- The blade edge should be carefully checked under the surgical microscope and replaced prior to every operation
- Correct plate thickness should be verified and as thick a flap as possible should be used to allow for adequate residual stroma
- The conjunctiva should be smooth, flat, and nonchemotic
- Avoid excess topical anesthetic

Pressure on the globe from the suction ring should be avoided. The suction ring should be held in a neutral, relaxed position. Excess pressure may induce chemosis as well as obstruct the pass of the microkeratome. A final check of relaxed surgical position, slack in both the power cord and noncrimped suction tubing, as well as correct readings on the microkeratome console should be performed.

Postoperative Symptoms

The surgeon should be aware that every tiny surface irregularity in the visual zone modifies transmission of light radiation, inducing annoying symptoms such as glare, monocular diplopia, and polyopia with poor or qualitatively insufficient functional recovery.

Management

With irregular cuts, the surgeon should not proceed with the ablation, but the flap or fragments there of should be carefully replaced and realigned to their original position using the gutter width as a landmark. The pieces should fit together like a jigsaw puzzle. Additional waiting/drying time is used and a bandage contact lens overnight may be considered if the epithelium is rough.

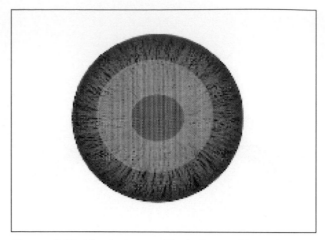

Figure 8-20. Keratectomy with chatter and irregular surface (plow-up phenomenon).

Table 8-7
IRREGULAR CUT

Etiology
- Irregular speed of microkeratome pass (plow-up)
- Uneven blade edge
- Microkeratome slips because of accidental movement by the surgeon
- Block during the cut phase from:
  - Speculum
  - Eyelashes
  - Drape
  - Redundant conjunctiva
- Loss of suction

Result
- Irregular cut surface in terms of smoothness and regularity of the stromal surface

Prevention
- Test the microkeratome pass prior to each procedure
- Check the blade edge and replace it before each patient or procedure
- Wet the track
- Make sure there are no obstacles in microkeratome advancement
- Check that the correct depth plate has been inserted
- Check that the orifice of the suction ring is open and free
- Check that the conjunctiva is smooth and flat
- Avoid excessive topical anesthesia that may cause detachment of the epithelium
- Assume a relaxed, comfortable operating position
- Make sure all cords, tubes, etc are unrestricted and will not bend
- Check the values of voltage and current (voltmeter and ampmeter)

Treatment
- Smooth the cut stromal surface using the excimer laser (PTK)
- Abort the ablation, reposition the flap, and repeat the operation 3 to 6 months later, or perform a homoplastic operation at least 6 months later

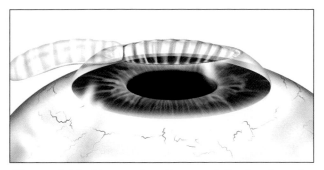

Figure 8-21. Uneven lamellar cut following irregular advancement of the microkeratome. It occurs more frequently with manual microkeratomes.

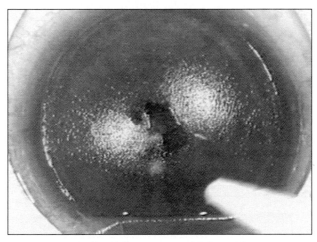

Figure 8-22b. Superficial cut: an island of Bowman can be observed at the center of the cut.

Four to 6 months later, the keratectomy can be repeated using a thicker plate and initiating the cut more peripherally. In more serious situations, it may be necessary to perform a lamellar keratoplasty at least 6 months after the initial operation.

Thin and Buttonhole Flaps

Thin and even buttonhole flaps are one of the more common complications during the learning curve. Fortunately, the incidence decreases dramatically to about 0.2% with increased surgeon experience.

Common Causes

Mechanical
- Poor suction resulting in inadequate IOP and firmness of the globe from:
  - Obstruction of/or poor tubing
  - Obstruction of suction ring
  - Suction pump malfunction
  - Altered conjunctival anatomy
- Lack of blade sharpness or damaged blade; a new blade should be used for each patient

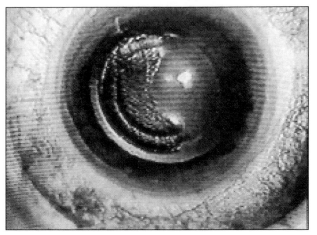

Figure 8-22a. Incomplete superficial cut due to loss of suction

- Incorrect choice of plate; excessively rapid microkeratome advancement
- Sloughing of epithelium due to excessive anesthesia or basement membrane dystrophy, inducing the microkeratome to pass over the clump of epithelium
- Epithelial edema
- Excessively dry cornea
- Malfunction of the microkeratome

Anatomical
- Very flat corneas (a rare occurrence)
- Very steep corneas (perforation of the flap)
- Severe irregular astigmatism

Typically, the procedure should be aborted and the recut scheduled 4 to 6 months later. However, if the thin flap is intact and the stromal bed is smooth, with no evidence of Bowman's membrane showing centrally, the procedure can continue but all manipulation must be much more delicately than usual.

Prevention

The creation and maintenance of good suction is the single most important factor in preventing perforated flaps. Redundant conjunctiva should be stretched by gentle depression of the speculum to avoid pseudosuction. Patients with extensive vitreous syneresis, prior retinal detachment, or vitrectomy are at risk because of difficulty achieving sufficient pressure. Excessive anesthesia, which creates epithelial edema and reduces adhesion, should be avoided, as sloughing will cause the epithelium to bunch up as the plate traverses over it, creating a thin central flap. The suction ring orifice should be clean and the correct and adequate depth plate should be selected. Finally, the blade should be inspected prior to each operation. Many surgeons use the same blade for

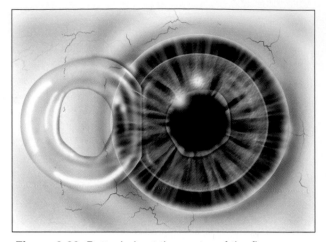

Figure 8-23. Buttonhole at the center of the flap.

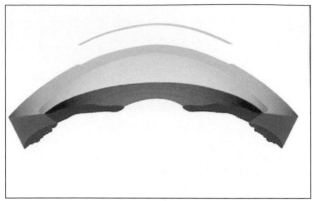

Figure 8-24. A 360° keratectomy (free cap) with reduced thickness of the entire cut surface.

both eyes (in bilateral simultaneous surgery), as the blade has already demonstrated a good cut on the first eye. Multiple reuse and autoclaving should be avoided, as each cut becomes progressively thinner.

Management

In the event of an excessively superficial cut, there is a significant risk of tearing or damage if it is raised or manipulated. Avoid the temptation to lift. If the flap is lifted, it should be repositioned very carefully and the operation repeated 3 to 4 months later. If, on the other hand, the flap has cleared Bowman's layer and has some stroma included, it can be lifted and photoablation can be performed, paying special attention to alignment and being careful not to induce wrinkles during repositioning. Visual recovery will be slow. The second eye should be postponed and etiology should be taken into account before operating on the second eye.

If the flap is centrally perforated or torn into several pieces, it should be replaced and allowed to heal for at least 3 months prior to further treatment. The flap alignment should be as accurate as possible. With multiple fragments, the surgeon should reconstruct it like a jigsaw puzzle. Excessive manipulation should be avoided and, if possible, the flap should not be raised at all. The surgeon should resist the temptation to raise the flap to examine what damage has been done underneath!) The surgeon should simply irrigate the interface to remove any infiltrated epithelial cells. In these complicated cases, it should be kept in mind that the thickness of the corneal flap is greater peripherally and the gutter may be the best reference for alignment. Irregularities of the stromal bed must match those of the flap. This will be impossible if ablation has occurred. Once the flap has been repositioned, additional time should be allowed to ensure that the flap fragments are well adhered prior to removing the

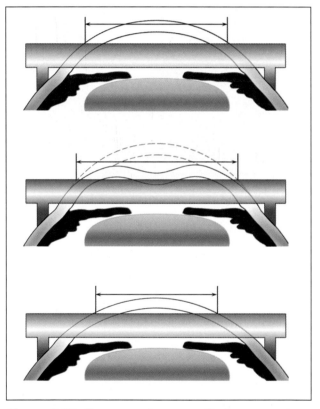

Figure 8-25. Top: normal cornea. Center: very steep cornea. Below: very flat cornea. The steep cornea lends itself to developing a buttonhole due to possible inferior bending during the cut. A very flat cornea lends itself to a superficial cut due to poor exposure of the tissue to the blade edge.

speculum. Most patients return to their original functional and refractive status following central perforation of a flap. In some less fortunate cases, there may be ingrowth centrally with associated melting, not only originating from the edge of the flap but also from other perforations and ruptures. It is almost impossible to clean the epithe-

Table 8-8

THIN OR PERFORATED BUTTONHOLE FLAP

Etiology
- Inadequate suction
- Corneal anatomy
- Very flat corneas
- Very steep corneas
- Irregular surface curvature
- Severe astigmatism
- Torsion induced by the weight of the microkeratome
- Poor blade quality

Results
- Impossible to perform the ablation
- Risk of epithelial growth
- Risk of irregular astigmatism

Prevention
- Do not begin the pass with less than perfect suction (IOP measurement)
- Caution patients with high or low keratometry readings of the increased risk
- Check that the plate is inserted correctly
- Consider using a thicker plate on steeper corneas
- Check the microkeratome each time before using
- Use a new blade for each patient
- Gently support the handle of the microkeratome during the run

Treatment
- Carefully replace the thin or perforated flap
- Carefully examine the flap and check adhesion
- Continue the operation if it is possible to lift the flap, despite it being difficult
- Recut the flap 2 to 3 months later with a thicker plate
- Use contact lenses
- Total removal of the flap in severe cases

lial cells from the interface. In this dire situation, the flap will have to be removed and the epithelium allowed to regenerate as in PRK, necessitating amputation and phototherapeutic keratoplasty (PTK) smoothing of the hinge.

The long-term approach to these eyes may be:
- Soft contact lenses
- Gas-permeable contact lenses
- Retreatment with LASIK 3 to 6 months later if adequate thickness remains
- Transepithelial PRK (high risk of haze and irregular astigmatism)
- Complete flap removal with PTK
- Decentered flap

Etiology

Decentration of the cut is caused by:
- Surgeon error in centering the suction ring to allow room for the desired ablation
- Spontaneous decentration of the ring following activation of the suction pump
- Lack of patient cooperation during surgery

Management

If the surgeon detects that the suction ring has spontaneously decentered and will not allow an adequate ablation following the cut, the case should be postponed a day or two to allow the scleral anatomy to return to normal. If the cut is performed and the area of ablation is adequate, the surgeon may proceed with a laser treatment, possibly with a slight reduction in the optic zone. If this is not possible, the flap is repositioned and the operation repeated 3 to 4 months later. This is particularly important in hyperopic or astigmatic treatments, and when a large ablation zone is planned.

Tips for prevention: The surgeon should monitor the corneal marks, centration of the optical axis, the astigmatic axis, and the keratometry values, which determine flap size. The cornea can be stabilized with the surgeon's index finger prior to initiation of suction to prevent torquing when suction is engaged. If the suction ring is decentered, stop immediately and try again. If the ring returns to its original decentered position, delaying the procedure is advisable, for at least 2 days.

Patient fixation should be confirmed. The surgeon should never attempt to operate if the pupil is dilated, as this will make centration and patient fixation more difficult.

Decentered Flap

Etiology

Decentration of the cut is caused by:
- Surgeon error in centering the suction ring to allow room for the desired ablation
- Spontaneous decentration of the ring following activation of the suction pump
- Lack of patient cooperation during surgery

Management

If the surgeon detects that the suction ring has spontaneously decentered and will not allow an adequate ablation following the cut, the case should be postponed a day or two to allow the scleral anatomy to return to normal. If the cut is performed and the area for ablation is adequate, the surgeon may proceed with laser treatment, possibly with a slight reduction in the optic zone. If this is not possible, the flap is repositioned and the operation repeated in 3 to 4 months. This is particularly important in hyperopic or astigmatic treatments and when a large ablation zone is planned.

Table 8-9
DECENTERED CUT

Etiology
- Surgeon error in centering the optic axis
- Error in paracentral marking
- Incorrect centration of the suction ring on the corneal surface
- Globe torque when suction is engaged
- Poor patient cooperation during surgery

Results
- Inadequate exposure of the central stroma for a well-centered complete ablation

Prevention
- Check centration of the optic axis
- A nonmydriatic pupil to center the optic axis
- Accurate marking
- Center the suction ring correctly and stabilize the cornea as suction is engaged
- Patient education and reassurance
- Postpone the procedure instead of re-attempting to reapply the suction ring

Treatment
- Perform the ablation if adequate bed is available
- Replace the flap and repeat the operation after 3 to 4 months

Table 8-10
CUT WITH IRREGULAR THICKNESS

Etiology
- Interference with the suction ring
- Scleroconjunctival cysts and irregularities
- Pterygium
- Dents, damage, or debris on the suction ring tracks
- Inadequate suction during the cut
- Poor blade quality
- Lateral displacement of the microkeratome during the cut

Results
- Not a serious problem if excimer laser ablation is planned, as opposed to ALK

Prevention
- Check and clean the suction ring tracks
- Check the microkeratome
- Change and inspect the blade after every procedure
- examine the blade edge under high magnification

Tips for prevention:
- The surgeon should monitor the corneal marks, centration of the optical axis, and the astigmatic axis and keratometry values, which determine flap size.
- The cornea can be stabilized with the surgeon's index finger prior to initiation of suction to prevent torquing when suction is engaged. If the suction ring is decentered, stop immediately and try again. If the ring returns to its original decentered position, at least a 2-day delay is advisable.
- Patient fixation should be confirmed.
- The surgeon should never attempt to operate if the pupil is dilated, as this will make centration and patient fixation more difficult.

Cut With Irregular Thickness

Definition
The flap does not have a homogenous thickness, but the thickness differs from zone to zone.

Cause
There are anatomical and mechanical causes. If there are superficial alterations on the scleroconjunctival plane, cysts, neoformations, pterygia, or blebs, they may interfere with the good resting position of the ring on the

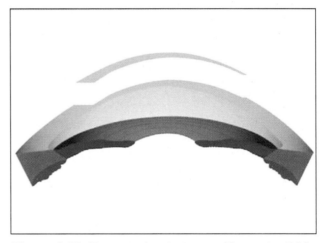

Figure 8-29. Free cap keratectomy with greater thickness in the final part of the cut.

tissue plane, creating a final cut with a nonhomogenous thickness.

Mechanical causes include:
- Irregularity, damage, or debris on the suction ring tracks
- Insufficient suction during the cut
- Insufficient blade cutting ability
- A blade with a good cutting edge in one section and a blunt cutting edge in another
- Lateral displacement of the microkeratome during the cut

Finally, it should be kept in mind that some instruments are fitted with suction rings with a single wing. This may create lateral displacement of the microkeratome and cause a parallel cut. This is not as serious a

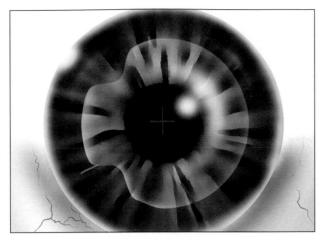

Figure 8-26. Irregular cut shape.

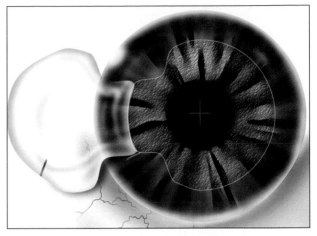

Figure 8-27. Exposure of the stroma is sufficient for a myopic ablation and fairly good for astigmatic treatment (depending on the axis). It is not suitable for hyperopic ablation.

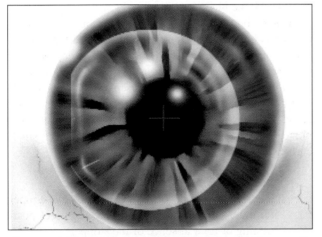

Figure 8-28a. Cut decentered nasally, which permits excellent ablation.

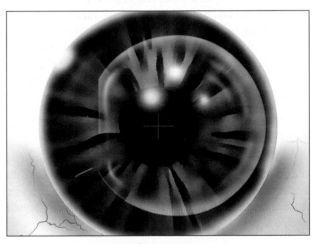

Figure 8-28b. A cut decentered temporally is not usually suitable for correct ablation.

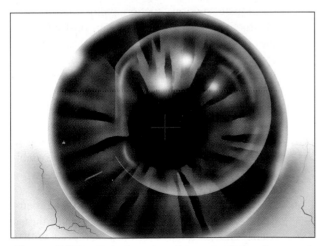

Figure 8-28c. Cut decentered temporally and upward, which is not suitable for correct ablation.

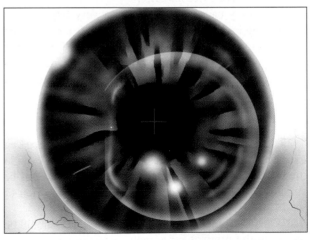

Figure 8-28d. Cut decentered temporally and downward, which is not suitable for a good ablation.

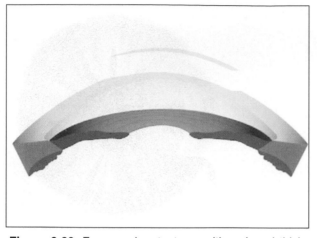

Figure 8-30. Free cap keratectomy with reduced thickness in the final part of the cut.

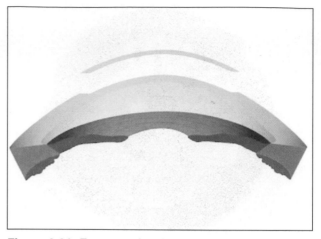

Figure 8-31. Free cap of uniform thickness.

problem if the refractive cut has been scheduled with the excimer laser and not with mechanical means.

Tips for prevention: exam and clean the ring tracks and microkeratome to avoid any conditions that may reduce the correct degree of suction. The blade should be changed after every cut and examined under the microscope prior to every procedure.

Free Cap—360° Flap Cut Without Hinge Formation

A complete cut without creation of a hinge rarely is the source of serious problems, as for many years in situ keratomileusis was normally performed in this manner. Today, however, a free cap is a nuisance that we would prefer to avoid.

Etiology

Anatomical Predisposition

A primary cause of free cap is a very large cornea (measuring in excess of 14.5 mm), which is also very flat (mean keratometry of less than 41 diopters [D]). A flat cornea protrudes slightly less than a steep cornea through the suction ring, thus the portion of the cornea presented to the microkeratome's blade has a smaller diameter and stops too late. A flat cornea makes the applanation lens meniscus appear smaller than normal.

There are suction rings designed to avoid a free cap even when used with corneas of 36 D; however, even in these cases, the corneal flap and hinge created will be smaller and therefore at a greater risk of dislocation or total loss.

When a repeat cut is planned, the new cut should be based on the original keratometry and not on the value resulting from the first operation, as the midperipheral

unaltered cornea is the first part that is presented to the microkeratome blade.

Ironically, flat corneas with a small corneal diameter are not as much at risk of a free cap. In this situation, the cornea protrudes to a greater extent inside the ring because the ring is situated on the surrounding limbus. The microkeratome blade is presented with a steeper, larger cornea, resulting in a larger flap compared to the corneal diameter. Peripheral neovascularization may induce bleeding following flap resection in these small corneas.

Mechanical Problems

- Incorrect assembly of the microkeratome stopper on older models of the ACS with incorrect positioning or total absence of the stopper
- Use of a ring that provides insufficient corneal exposure
- Inadequate suction, suction pump malfunction, obstruction of the suction tubing, obstruction of the ring orifice, poor positioning, or surgeon torquing of the suction ring
- Reduced intraoperative IOP, usually secondary to previous ocular surgery
- Removal of the suction ring to which the flap has adhered, secondary to dehydration in those cases in which the surgeon leaves the suction ring in place (without suction) to assist in globe stabilization (not recommended)

Tips for prevention:
- Always be aware of corneal size and keratometry
- Make sure the stopper is firmly seated and adjusted
- Make sure adequate suction is achieved with a tonometer (Barraquer or Pneumotonometer)
- Make sure the corneal mark remains visible

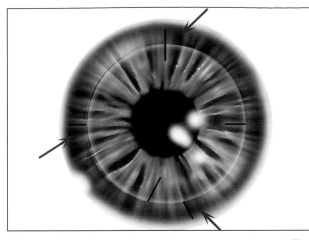

Figure 8-32. Pararadial markings are not aligned. The free cap is positioned upside down with the epithelium downward.

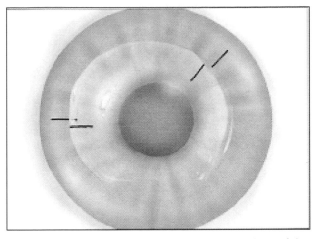

Figure 8-33. Partial rotation of a free cap and loss of the correct central position in relation to the corneal bed.

No matter how experienced the surgeon, corneal marking should always be performed with a special pararadial or other marker that identifies the epithelial surface and aids in correct alignment. One should take care that the mark crosses the resection, because if it is inside or outside the flap it is useless. Patients with very flat corneas should be warned of the increased risk of free cap as part of the informed consent.

Management

Anticipation is the key to successful management. With a free cap, the disc is placed epithelial surface down in the antidesiccation chamber over one or two drops of BSS. An in-situ ablation is then performed. A Barraquer fenestrated spatula atraumatic to the disc is used to transfer the disc back to the bed. Excessive swelling or drying of the free cap should be avoided. Do not place BSS on the stromal surface of the flap. Edema does not depend on the quantity of fluid but the time the tissue surface is exposed to it.

Once the ablation has been performed, place a drop of BSS directly in the middle of the corneal bed. The surface tension of the fluid will assist positioning and rotation of the cap on the stromal bed. The surgeon places the cap on the corneal bed, taking care to replace it exactly in its original position—always remember the preoperative pararadial epithelial marking; this will not be a straight line if the cap is placed upside down or is not properly aligned. The same principle applies to the four marking points for alignment in Machat's disparate double circle marker. A contribution to alignment is actually provided by an irregular resection. In this case, the irregularities facilitate alignment as they will have to "match" the corresponding irregularities on the stromal bed. In addition, the surgeon must also ensure that the gutter

margin is symmetrical 360°. The cap is rotated to correct position on a moist bed using moist Merocel sponges. If the bed dries, an additional drop or two of BSS may be placed under the cap. After the marks are aligned and the gutter symmetrical, waiting begins.

In the event of a free cap, instead of the normal 1- to 3-minute wait, the surgeon should wait 6 to 8 minutes before removing the speculum and allowing blinking. An adherence test is then performed, such as the striae test using a button-tipped spatula or dry Merocel sponge to exert slight pressure on the corneal limbus just outside the resection. Striae will form, which radiate toward the center of the cornea if there is good adhesion between the cap and stroma.

Sutures are almost never needed; however if the epithelium has been damaged, it is better to protect the eye with a bandage contact lens. If the epithelium is intact, a contact lens should be avoided as it may dislocate the cap.

The eye should be taped shut, but compressive bandages should be avoided, as they may dislocate the cap with eye movement. If the cap moves, it will remain in the fornix and will be lubricated. However, if it becomes edematous, subsequent replacement will probably require suturing. If there is any doubt as to adhesion, an eight-bite antitorque, an external compression ("bra"), or interrupted sutures should be used.

Because the marks may sometimes be difficult to see or be washed off, it may be useful to leave the free cap in the head of the microkeratome until the laser ablation has been completed. This may assist in the correct orientation of the free cap when it is repositioned on the stromal bed. Alternately, the epithelial surface of the free cap may be marked on the presenting edge of the blade with gentian violet, which indicates the nasal orientation of the pre-

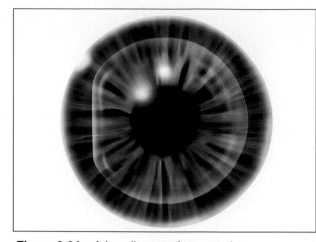

Figure 8-34a. A lamellar cut of correct size.

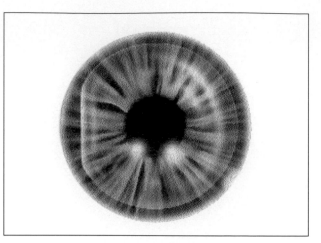

Figure 8-34b. Large diameter lamellar cut.

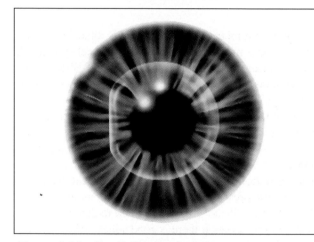

Figure 8-34c. Small diameter lamellar cut.

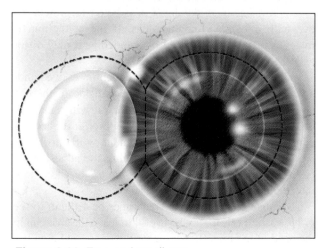

Figure 8-36. Free and small cap.

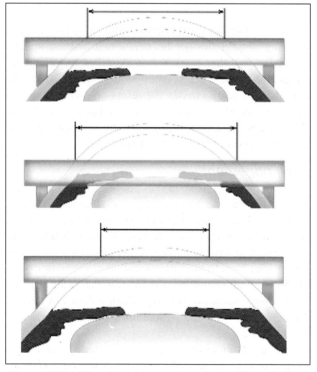

Figure 8-35. Top: the cornea protrudes sufficiently from the suction ring to provide a cut of correct size. Center: the cornea protrudes excessively and the cut produces a larger flap. Bottom: a globe that protrudes a small amount through the ring creates a small flap.

Table 8-11

FREE CAP

Etiology
- Corneal anatomy: large flat cornea (generally less than 41 D but also depends on the type of microkeratome)
- Inadequate suction
- Incorrect applanation of desired resection (when this is performed)
- A ring that does not allow sufficient exposure of the globe
- Low intraoperative IOP
- Removal of the suction ring with the flap adhered to it
- Incorrect positioning or setting of the stop mechanism
- Defective stop device

Results
- Free cap
- More difficult to reposition
- Easier to dislocate
- Easier to completely lose
- The ablation can be performed

Prevention
- Always mark correctly
- Check the microkeratome prior to every operation
- Check correct positioning and setting of the stop device
- Advise patients with flat corneas of the increased risk

Treatment
- Ensure that the mark is retained or remark prior to removing it from the microkeratome head
- Place the free cap in an antidesiccation chamber
- Replace the cap, right side up, on the stromal bed
- Correctly align the flap
- Ensure adhesion between the flap and stroma (wait 3 to 8 minutes before removing the speculum)
- Place sutures if necessary
- Use a bandage contact lens if the epithelium has been altered

senting edge as well as defining the epithelial side up.

Chatter marks from vibration along the edges of the bed due to blade oscillation can often be of assistance; in order to better highlight them, the surgeon should use the magnification and the high illumination of the microscope.

FLAP-RELATED COMPLICATIONS

Flap damage may occur at any time during the surgical procedure. Alterations and irregularities secondary to careless manipulation of the flap may alter the final refractive result. Any microtrauma, which may alter the characteristics of the flap, must be avoided. In addition, avoid:

- Prolonged operating time with excessive dehydration of the tissue.
- Manipulation with forceps, swabs, or other instruments unsuitable or not specific for LASIK.
- In rare cases, the damage may be irreversible; the flap must be discarded. Homoplastic tissue may be required to replace the flap; alternately, the stromal bed can be left to re-epithelialize as though PRK has been performed.

Other flap-related complications are:
- Dislocated flap
- Wrinkled flap
- Edematous flap (excessive irrigation)
- Contracted flap
- Stretched flap

Flap Dislocation During Surgery

Dislocation of the flap is typically seen postoperatively, but may also occur during the operation itself.

Causes

This occurs intraoperatively when:
- There is sudden eye movement when instruments are near the flap edge or during the striae test.
- Careless irrigation of the interface with the cannula displacing the flap.
- Excess fluid in the interface so that the flap has poor adherence.
- Patient blinking or squeezing as the speculum and/or drapes are being removed, related to Bell's phenomenon.

Tips for prevention: it helps to ask the patient to look temporally while the surgeon slides the speculum out nasally. The patient should try not to blink when the speculum and drapes are removed, which can be aided by the surgeon or assistant retracting the lids while the speculum is lifted up and away from the globe and removed.

Treatment

If the flap is displaced, it should immediately be refloated and smoothed. This is usually easy, as the patient relaxes and a typically less stressful speculum such as the Barraquer, is used. Folds or striae of the flap are rarely seen when the dislocation occurs during the surgical procedure and the flap is immediately repositioned.

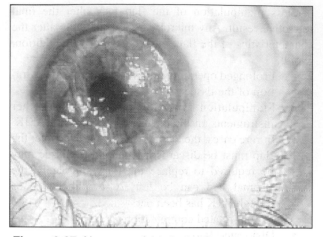

Figure 8-37. Numerous folds in the flap due to incorrect replacement.

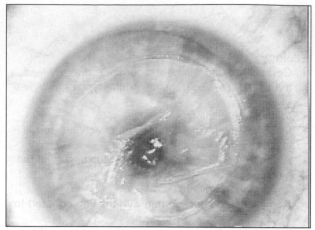

Figure 8-38. Dislocation of the flap at the end of surgery due to incorrect removal of the speculum.

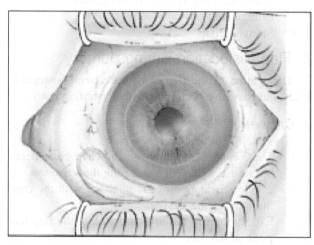

Figure 8-39. The flap has detached from the hinge and dislocated onto the conjunctiva.

Wrinkled Flap

Cause

Gentle repositioning of the flap and alignment are essential to avoid wrinkling. The flap should not be allowed to dry excessively during the ablation. Wrinkling occurs more frequently if the flap is thin, if it is not sufficiently wet prior to the cut, if air in the operating room is dry and drafty, and if the length of time the flap was raised is prolonged. During the ablation, it is helpful to position the flap on a damp Merocel sponge. A flap that rests on the conjunctiva of the fornix during ablation may become excessively dehydrated inducing wrinkles. On the other hand, excessive hydration will increase flap thickness and shrink its diameter. Once it is replaced and normal hydration is restored, wrinkles may develop.

Repositioning should be performed with the stromal bed damp or wet; this will facilitate immediate rehydra-

Table 8-12
FLAP THAT DISLOCATES DURING SURGERY

Etiology
- Sudden eye movement when an instrument is near the limbus
- Eye movement during the striae test
- Blinking or squeezing when the speculum and drapes are removed

Results
- Dislocation or wrinkling of the flap

Prevention
- Have the patient fixate at the light when the striae test is being done and warn the patient about pressure
- Ask the patient to not blink and stare straight ahead when the drapes and speculum are removed and have the assistant retract the lids during these maneuvers

Treatment
- Immediately refloat and reposition the flap

tion of the flap and allow the flap to float on the stromal bed with additional gentle irrigation performed underneath it, allowing the flap to float back to its original position. Excess irrigation, however, may overhydrate the flap, prolonging adhesion time as well as forcing debris from the tear film into the interface. The surgeon should then exert gentle pressure with a very moist Merocel sponge to express the fluid, starting from the hinge then smoothing from the center toward the edges, first seating the flap from the hinge to the opposite side, then smoothing in all directions. If the flap is touched roughly with a damp or excessively dry sponge, the flap may be distorted with the creation of wrinkles. The centrifugal motion of a blunt spatula may also express the fluid.

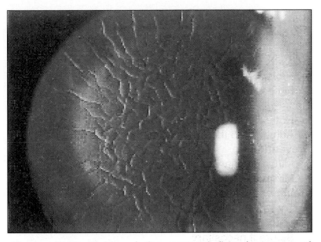

Figure 8-40. Folds of the corneal flap (courtesy of Enrique Suarez, MD).

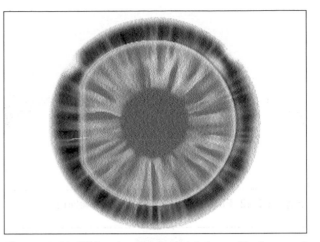

Figure 8-41. Widespread edema of the epithelium and flap.

Diagnosis

Some lasers have slit illumination that allows examination of the flap following repositioning. Wrinkles are more clearly visible with retroillumination, but this is not possible during surgery. The best guide under the laser microscope is an even gutter margin 360° and a smooth matte finish to the flap as it begins to dry before a drop of BSS or Celluvisc is applied during the waiting period.

Tips for prevention:

- The flap must be repositioned very gently and carefully
- The flap must not be allowed to dry out
- The flap should be adequately moistened prior to the cut
- Suitable humidity levels should be maintained in the operating room
- The time between lifting the flap and its replacement must be as short as possible
- During the ablation, the flap should be positioned on a damp sponge
- The flap should be repositioned on a moist stromal bed, or the surgeon should moisten the surface and irrigate under the flap
- Thin flaps should be avoided

Treatment

If there are wrinkles, the flap should be lifted and repositioned with additional brief irrigation of the interface. The flap should be repositioned and smoothed using a moist sponge or spatula, as previously described.

Flap Edema Secondary to Excess Irrigation

Cause

This may occur if the interface is excessively irrigat-

Table 8-13
WRINKLED FLAP

Etiology
- Incorrect positioning of the flap during ablation
- Excessive desiccation of the flap
- Rough manipulation of the flap

Result
- Wrinkling of the flap will cause irregular astigmatism and visual aberrations

Prevention
- During the ablation, gently place the flap in a cupped position on a damp sponge
- Use a moistened Merocel sponge to smooth from the hinge and then from the center to the edges
- Do not allow fluid to remain under the flap
- Using a spatula or sponge, smooth the flap with centrifugal motion

Treatment
- Gently replace the flap to its original position
- Epithelial wrinkling often disappears spontaneously within a few days; if it has not disappeared within 5 to 6 days, raise the flap and reposition correctly

ed. Good adhesion between the flap and stromal bed becomes more prolonged and difficult. If the fluid is not expressed completely after irrigation, it may form a meniscus of fluid in the interface; this may prevent the flap from attaching firmly, facilitating decentration or displacement (the "floating flap" phenomenon). Nonetheless, it is important to irrigate the interface following repositioning, not just to remove potential debris and epithelial cells from the interface, but also to reposition the flap with correct alignment. This meniscus is expressed as described above. If not, poor visual acuity and a pseudo central island appears, which may respond

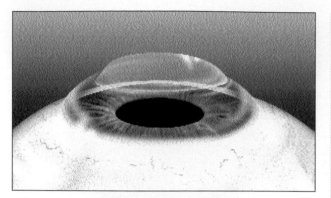

Figure 8-42. Flap edema with evident swelling.

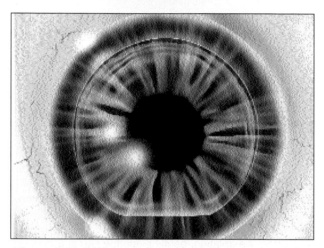

Figure 8-43. Shrinkage of the flap for more than 180°.

Table 8-14
FLAP EDEMA

Etiology
- Prolonged manipulation of the flap
- Excessive irrigation

Result
- Retraction of the flap edge
- Adhesion to the stromal bed is more difficult

Prevention
- Minimally manipulate the flap
- Minimally irrigate under the flap

Treatment
- Try to gently distend the flap with an almost dry sponge or blunt spatula
- Suture if necessary

Table 8-15
FLAP SHRINKAGE

Etiology
- Excessive dryness of the flap (due to delays during surgery)

Result
- The flap must be stretched
- Sutures may be required

Prevention
- Avoid delays during surgery
- Decrease time between flap reflection and ablation
- Decrease the time between ablation and flap re-positioning

Treatment
- Gently stretch and distend the flap
- Lift and rehydrate the flap a second time
- Suture if necessary

to the Caro island masher or resolve spontaneously as the excess fluid is absorbed.

Flap edema may create retraction, which may require stretching the flap using the tip of a dry sponge. The eye is immobilized using a Thornton ring. In extreme situations when edematous flaps are repositioned, as when there are large areas of epithelial loss, sutures may be required to avoid a deep groove forming around the flap with possible early dislocation of the flap.

Tips for prevention:
- Keep manipulation and irrigation of the flap to a minimum, enough to allow proper positioning of the flap, but no more.
- Carefully and methodically express the liquid from the interface after irrigation.

Flap Contraction

Cause

Flap contraction can be caused by both excessive dehydration or overhydration prior to repositioning.

Management

The contracted flap is managed as previously described for a wrinkled flap, with proper attention to hydration and smoothing. If there has been marked flap contraction, and it cannot be smoothed because of epithelial loss (eg, suturing may be required to align the flap and maintain its position in situ).

Stretching the Flap and Epithelium

There may be short-term stretching of the entire flap, with associated thinning. Sliding and folding secondary to the microkeratome or other instruments may stretch the epithelium itself.

Cause

The flap may be stretched through excessive manip-

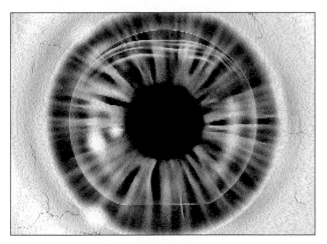

Figure 8-44. Incorrect flap position that is retracted inferiorly.

ulation. Rough manipulation or excessive smoothing of the flap with a damp sponge may stretch it. Sliding and bunching the epithelium may also be caused by excessive manipulation. Any maneuvers to smooth the flap must be done using a damp sponge and gentle touch.

If the epithelium has been detached or bunched by the microkeratome, further maneuvers used to smooth it may stretch the epithelium with fold formation, or it may stretch to overlap the edges of the flap. In this case, the epithelium should be carefully repositioned. When a large section of the epithelium has detached, a damp sponge should be used to manipulate the surface in localized spots rather than generalized smoothing.

Tip for prevention: manipulate the flap as little and as gently as possible.

Treatment

Delicately reposition the epithelium. It is rare that redundant epithelium needs to be removed. Once epithelium is considered satisfactory, a bandage contact lens may be used for a few hours or overnight. One should take great care in removing it by maintaining good hydration of the lens before sliding it over the flap.

Irreversible Damage or Destruction to the Flap

Cause

During the microkeratome pass, the flap may roll on itself, coming into contact with the blade, and be irreversibly damaged. Fortunately, this is rare and usually occurs on an excessively dry cornea.

Damage to the flap is caused more frequently by:
- Decentration of the photoablation, damaging the flap's stroma
- Lack of protection of the flap or hinge during the

| Table 8-16 |

STRETCHING THE FLAP AND DISPLACING THE EPITHELIUM

Etiology
- Prolonged manipulation
- Excessively aggressive smoothing and positioning

Results
- Difficulty in positioning the flap and/or epithelium
- Striae that affect vision

Prevention
- Minimize manipulation of the flap
- Delicately stroke with a damp sponge when smoothing or positioning the flap

Treatment
- Gently reposition the epithelium
- Eliminate redundant epithelium
- Use a bandage contact lens if necessary (there is a risk of flap dislocation when the contact lens is removed)

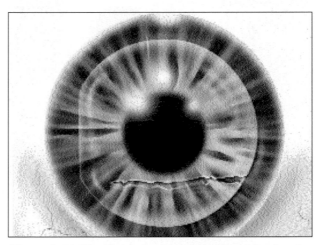

Figure 8-45. Significant damage to the flap following the microkeratome cut.

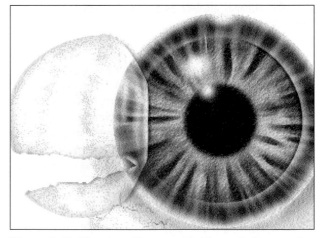

Figure 8-46. The case illustrated in Figure 8-45 once the flap has been lifted.

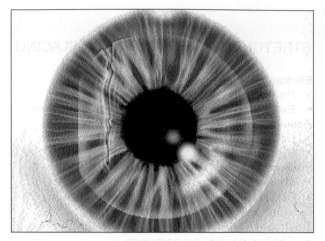

Figure 8-47. Flap cut close to the hinge. This is due to a lack of free movement inside the microkeratome head.

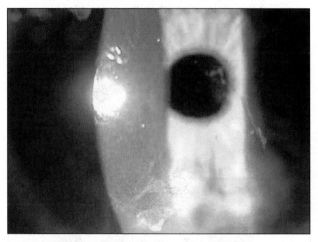

Figure 8-48. Corneal scar from a flap cut.

ablation, especially with large optic zones (correction of astigmatism and hyperopia)

Tips for prevention: prior to the lamellar cut, make sure the corneal surface is moist. Protect the flap and hinge during ablation.

Management

If the corneal flap is irreversibly damaged during photoablation, a homoplastic flap will be necessary to replace the damaged tissue. If no homoplastic tissue is available and the cut surface is sufficiently smooth, the surgeon may proceed with the ablation, using a contact lens to facilitate epithelialization. If the surface is moderately uneven prior to the refractive ablation, a standard PTK should be performed.

If the surface is extremely uneven, a number of options are available:

1. Extensive PTK can be performed, which will require a considerable amount of ablation.

Table 8-17

IRREVERSIBLE DAMAGE OR COMPLETE DESTRUCTION OF THE FLAP

Etiology
- Faulty blade
- Cut performed on an excessively dry cornea
- Significant ablation of the flap undersurface
- Lack of flap and/or hinge protection during the ablation

Prevention
- Prior to performing the lamellar cut, ensure that the corneal surfaces are not excessively dry
- Protect the flap and hinge during the ablation

Treatment
- Homoplastic tissue may be needed
- Proceed with the refractive ablation and apply a contact lens (PRK)
- Perform a PTK and then refractive ablation
- Perform a second very thin lamellar cut, followed by PTK, and then refractive ablation
- Abort the operation, use a bandage contact lens, allow re-epithelization, then perform a transepithelial PTK

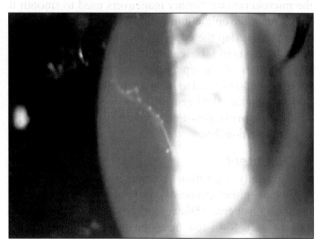

Figure 8-49. Corneal scar from a superficial cut.

2. A second very thin lamellar cut can be performed, using a plate of 70 to 80 microns (if available); this will allow the removal of the majority of irregularity. PTK is then performed, followed by the refractive ablation (the refractive calculation in such a case is very difficult). It is then necessary to use a lamella of homoplastic tissue because the corneal thickness has been considerably reduced.

3. The operation can be aborted, a contact lens applied, the epithelium allowed to regenerate, and then a transepithelial PTK performed, then the refractive ablation and homoplastic flap.

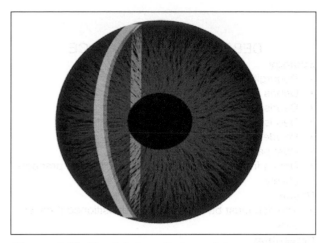

Figure 8-50. The interface is free of deposits or inclusions.

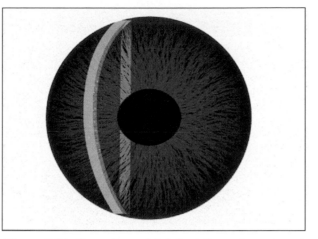

Figure 8-51. Deposits and debris at the surface viewed under the biomicroscope.

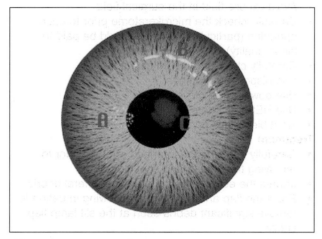

Figure 8-52. A. Deposits in the interface. B. Hypotransparent areas. C. Epithelial ingrowth.

Deposits in the Interface

Causes

Nonorganic material can be:
- Metal particles from the microkeratome or blade
- Metal particles from the cannula or spatula
- Particles from the sponge
- Talc from surgical gloves
- Lint from the drapes or gauze
- Dust in the air from the operating room

Organic material can be:
- Endothelial cells (from severed neovascularization)
- Epithelial cells
- Tear film debris

The presence of this debris may arise from:
- Reflux of tear film and debris from irrigation into the interface

- Poor microkeratome blade quality
- Cannulas and spatulas that are not clean from organic debris (cells, secretions, fat, etc) as well as lint
- Surgical gloves with talc
- Lack of HEPA air filters, which are helpful in removing airborne contaminants
- Use of incorrect lint-containing drapes
- Intraoperative corneal hemorrhage secondary to pannus or an eccentric cut

Diagnosis

It is advantageous if the laser incorporates slit illumination; otherwise, interface debris is usually not detected until the patient is examined at the slit lamp.

Tips for prevention:
- Clean cannulas and spatulas
- Use disposable syringes
- Use power-free surgical gloves or no gloves
- Use HEPA air filters to reduce airborne contamination in the operating room
- Adequately irrigate and dry the fornices
- Avoid excess fluid in the operating field
- Check the microkeratome carefully, paying particular attention to blade quality
- Use only lint-free drapes
- Treat blepharitis preoperatively
- Try to avoid the pannus if possible

Treatment

Typically, interface debris rarely interferes with functional recovery; however, if the optic quality of the cornea is compromised, the debris must be removed. Even small particles can interfere with visual acuity through one of the following mechanisms:
- Induction of astigmatism

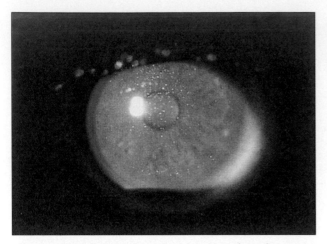

Figure 8-53. Central deposits in the interface (courtesy of Enrique Suarez, MD).

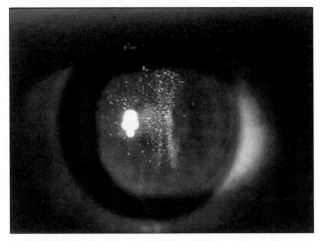

Figure 8-54. Central metallic deposits in the interface (courtesy of Enrique Suarez, MD).

- Induction of hyperopia
- Scar formation
- Epithelial ingrowth

If debris is observed during or immediately after surgery, it should be immediately removed. If debris is near the flap edge, a cannula can be passed under the flap to remove the particles. If debris is seen centrally, the entire flap must be raised and repositioned after irrigation, and perhaps both surfaces should be wiped with a moist Merocel sponge. The surgeon should avoid prolonged or repeated irrigation of the flap, because it may become swollen with the attendant problems mentioned earlier. If the debris is detected in the immediate postoperative period, it may be monitored and removed if inflammation is seen. It is usually of no consequence.

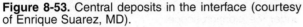

Table 8-18

DEBRIS IN THE INTERFACE

Etiology
- Regurgitation of fluid in the fornix
- Debris from sponge, drape, gauze
- Debris from the microkeratome blade
- Debris from the cannula, syringe, bottles
- Powder/talc from surgical gloves
- Dust particles in the operating room
- Debris from blepharitis that was not treated preoperatively

Result
- The flap must be irrigated and repositioned if necessary

Prevention
- Irrigate and dry the fornices preoperatively to remove any mucous/lipid debris
- Avoid excess fluid in the surgical field
- Carefully check the microkeratome prior to each operation (particular attention should be paid to blade quality)
- Carefully clean and dry all cannulas
- Use disposable syringes
- Use powder-free gloves
- Use HEPA air filters
- Treat blepharitis prior to surgery

Treatment
- Carefully examine the interface and flap prior to removing the drapes and speculum
- Irrigate the edges to remove any peripheral debris
- Raise the flap and reposition it following irrigation to remove significant debris seen at the slit lamp flap check

Epithelial Complications

Preoperative

Epithelial damage may occur preoperatively secondary, to excessive topical anesthetic, which makes the epithelium edematous and fragile. Damage may also be caused by abrasion from the drape and excessive marking.

Patients with anterior basement membrane dystrophy or recurrent erosions are at high risk for epithelial complications. It is a judgement call whether to cautiously proceed with LASIK or perform PRK on these patients.

Loose epithelium may roll and bunch, causing the microkeratome to ride over it creating a thin or buttonhole flap and increasing the risk of irregular astigmatism and both peripheral and central epithelial ingrowth.

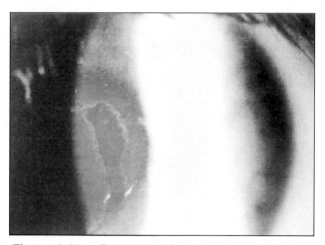

Figure 8-55a. Epithelial defect (courtesy of Enrique Suarez, MD).

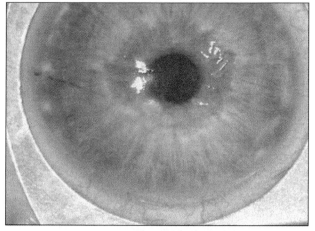

Figure 8-55b. Epithelial trauma secondary to the microkeratome pass.

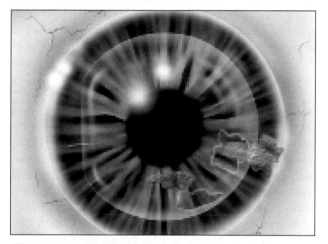

Figure 8-56. Multiple epithelial abrasions.

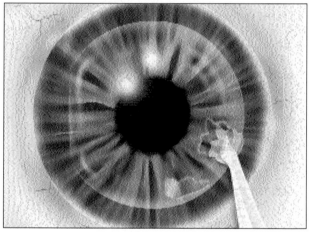

Figure 8-57. The epithelial fragments are carefully replaced.

Intraoperative

During surgery, damage to the epithelium may occur:

- When the cornea is dry, particularly if there is debris on the cornea or surface of the microkeratome.
- When the blade is not inserted properly and does not have unrestricted oscillation.
- From incorrect use of the forceps or spatula used to reflect the flap.
- When damage is observed more frequently along the incision edge—especially the superior edge— usually following passage of the microkeratome.
- From improper use of the sponge, particularly during the final phase when the flap is being smoothed or during striae testing.
- If the patient moves the eye as the speculum is being removed. The patient should be reminded that it is normal to feel speculum pressure even

though the cornea is completely anesthetized.

The detached epithelium, when possible, should be gently smoothed back into place after the flap has been repositioned and adhered. Care must be taken not to introduce epithelium into the interface during this maneuver. In those cases when repositioning the epithelium is not satisfactory, it should be removed. The surgeon should remember a single gentian violet mark may be lost if the epithelium is damaged in the marked area, thus multiple marks may be helpful.

Tips for Prevention: prevention is based on minimal manipulation of the flap, appropriate hydration of the flap, and minimal preoperative anesthesia. Operations on patients with advanced basement membrane dystrophy should be avoided. The patient should be instructed to avoid eye movement and blinking when the speculum is removed.

Table 8-19
EPITHELIAL COMPLICATIONS

Etiology
- Eye movement as the speculum is being removed
- Blinking as the speculum is being removed
- Incorrect insertion of the blade in the microkeratome
- The forceps or spatula used to reflect the flap
- Damage is encouraged by a dry flap
- Damage is increased in superficial corneal dystrophies

Results
- Discomfort for the patient
- Epithelial ingrowth
- Longer functional recovery
- Loss of the gentian violet mark

Prevention
- Avoid operating, or cautiously operate on patients with superficial corneal dystrophies
- Avoid excessive flap drying
- Reduce manipulation of the flap
- Reduce preoperative anesthesia
- Take care in applying and removing the speculum

Treatment
- In the event of displacement, reposition the epithelium
- Remove the epithelium if it cannot be replaced
- Apply a bandage contact lens
- Use antibiotic cover

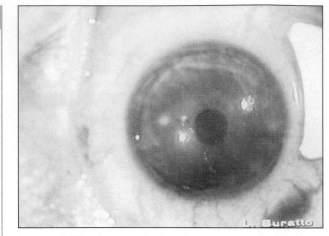

Figure 8-58. Blood in the interface at the end of surgery due to the cut passing through areas of neovascularization secondary to chronic contact lens wear.

Management

In the event of detachment, the epithelium is repositioned; if this is not possible, the epithelium must be removed. A loose-fitting bandage contact lens is used to protect the epithelium, with antibiotic coverage to avoid secondary infection. NSAID drops may be used minimally (twice daily for 2 days maximum), as these will slow re-epithelization.

This significantly slows visual rehabilitation and increases the risk of epithelial ingrowth. The bandage lens should be removed as soon as epithelization is nearly complete. It should be thoroughly hydrated with artificial tears and a drop of anesthetic, and floating on the corneal surface prior to gentle removal.

Intraoperative Hemorrhage

Corneal Neovascularization

Intraoperative corneal bleeding frequently occurs in patients that are long-term contact lens wearers and have superior, or more rarely inferior, neovascularization. If the microkeratome cuts through, these vessels will bleed, especially if pronounced.

Preoperatively, the surgeon should anticipate this potential situation and modify his surgical procedure if possible. A very steep cornea (keratometry in excess of 47 D) as well as a small cornea, may create a large flap that transects the pannus.

Bleeding not only reduces visibility and may create staining of the interface postoperatively, but also prevents proper laser ablation resulting in an asymmetric ablation. If blood enters the stromal bed, the ablation must be interrupted. The blood must be gently removed with a spatula or sponge and the surface of the bed dried with a Merocel sponge. Once ablation has been completed, the blood along the edges of the bed must be irrigated or gently removed prior to replacing the flap. A thin layer of residual blood can be removed by interface irrigation, with immediate sponging and smoothing of the flap to tamponade the vessels.

Prevention

A suction ring that provides a smaller cut may be used as long as it is compatible with the expected ablation diameter. This will avoid contact with blood vessels. The suction ring can also be positioned so as to avoid neovascularization, typically decentered slightly inferiorly, as the vessels are normally superior. Consider, however, that the inferior neovascularization may be involved, the flap position may be poor from excessive decentration, and it may be difficult to insert the Hansatome on the track. Alternately, an argon laser can be used to coagulate the vessels prior to surgery.

If the bleeding enters the fornix, it can be removed later; however, if it oozes toward the interface, the surgeon must ensure that there is no residual blood in the interface at the end of surgery. The flap should be allowed to dry for a longer period of time, but be sure bleeding has stopped prior to removing the speculum. If there is slight residual blood in the interface peripheral to the visual axis, it will not affect the patient and will spontaneously reabsorb.

Treatment

Bleeding can be minimized in the following ways:

- Apply a dry sponge to the bleeding area (if bleeding is localized) and exert slight pressure (sufficient to arrest it) or wick away the blood and simultaneously perform the ablation.
- A Gimbel-Chayet sponge may be used to prevent the blood from oozing into the bed, as well as elevating the flap and keeping fat and debris in the tear film from coming into contact with the interface.
- Leave the flap in position and wait until coagulation begins and bleeding diminishes.
- Drugs such as 2.5% phenylephrine, cortisone, or thromboplastin may be instilled, as eyedrops or better still, applied on a sponge at the bleeding area with slight pressure. With phenylephrine there is a risk of irregular mydriasis, which may create problems with the eye tracker or surgeon laser fixation on an irregular pupil.
- Pressurized air can be used as a vasoconstrictor and encourage coagulation.
- In uncontrolled bleeding, the suction ring may be reapplied and pressure reactivated for the duration of the ablation; this will arrest bleeding until the end of treatment, but should not be used longer than 30 seconds. A lower negative pressure would be better, which is available with some microkeratomes. A simple way of doing this is to perforate the suction tubing with a needle (the tubing will be discarded at the end of surgery). Pressure can be instantly activated as needed by occluding the perforation.
- Continual oozing at the end of the procedure is stopped by flap replacement, irrigation, and smoothing, which closes the interface and tamponades the vessels.

Retinal Hemorrhage

Literature reports cases of macular hemorrhage following LASIK in patients with high myopia. In reality, no cause and effect has been found between LASIK and macular hemorrhage.

It is always advisable to perform a preoperative examination of the retina, with photography and fluorescein angiography, to document the preoperative status of the macula. The possibility of macular hemorrhage as related to severe myopia should be part of the informed consent.

Table 8-20

INTRAOPERATIVE HEMORRHAGE

Etiology
- Corneal neovascularization
- Very large flaps
  - Very steep corneas
  - Very small corneas

Results
- Ablation delayed until bleeding is stopped
- Blood must be removed
- Reduced visibility of the surgeon
- Overhydration of the stroma
- Blockage of the incident laser ray (asymmetric ablation)
- Erroneous flap ablation

Prevention
Primary
- Inferior decentration of the suction ring and flap
- Preoperative argon laser photoablation
- Use a smaller diameter ring to have a smaller cut
Secondary
- Use a Chayet or Gimbel-Chayet sponge
- Use suction pressure briefly
- Use manual pressure on the ring
- Use 2.5% phenylephrine
- Use pressurized air flow

Treatment
- Interrupt the ablation
- Remove blood from the stromal bed
- Eliminate any blood in the interface by irrigating under the repositioned flap
- Leave the flap in position and wait for clotting; the operation can then be continued
- Apply a dry sponge to the bleeding, exert slight pressure and continue with ablation

Finally, it is possible that some peripheral hemorrhages are due to use of the suction ring, particularly in patients with diabetes and/or high blood pressure in which there is already anatomical alteration of the retinal blood vessels. Again, a preoperative examination of the peripheral retina is advisable.

LASER-RELATED COMPLICATIONS

Complications associated with the excimer laser may be serious. If the laser has been checked and programmed correctly, these can be almost completely avoided or at least reduced in terms of frequency and severity.

The laser beam must be centered, the energy level

must be appropriate, and the beam must be qualitatively homogeneous. The surgeon must never perform treatment without first having ensured that all laser calibration tests have been correctly performed.

Moreover, the laser company's service technicians (ongoing routine maintenance) must check the laser carefully and regularly.

The following complications may be laser related:
- Uneven ablation
- Decentered ablation
- Overcorrection
- Undercorrection
- Incorrect optic zone
- Incomplete treatment because of laser blockage

Uneven Ablation

Uneven ablation surfaces create loss of visual acuity, alterations in quality of vision, reduction in contrast sensitivity, and regression. It is therefore essential that the surgeon recognize the reasons underlying this complication, not only because they can be prevented by using the correct operating program but can also be avoided.

The ablation surface can be altered by:
A. Significant irregularities caused by:
- The patient suddenly moving his or her head or eyes
- Movements of the operating bed—a stable bed is therefore essential
- Poor cleaning of the stromal bed:
  - Debris, impurities
  - Uneven hydration of the bed
  - Bleeding that affects the laser ablation
- Inadequate evacuation of the plume from the laser
- Incorrect function of the excimer laser:
  - The mirrors may be dirty
  - The mirrors may be damaged
  - There may be defects in the laser optics
  - The gas may be inadequate (helium, fluorine, etc)
- There may be incomplete opening of the delivery system's diaphragm
- There may be problems with the mirror motor in flying spot lasers

Laser function is greatly influenced by temperature, humidity, altitude, barometric pressure, and air purity in the operating room. These parameters should be monitored constantly to avoid complications.
B. Micro-irregularities:
- These appear constantly during the ablation procedure through various types of movement:
  - Saccadic movements of the eye
  - Respiratory
  - Due to heart-beat

- Due to swallowing
  (The latter three are more common in athletes with obvious cardiac excess and who are slim)
- Due to the method of laser emission and its interaction with the cornea when the eye tracker is used
C. Small transition zone caused by:
- Inappropriate nomogram
- Interference with the hinge (this only applies to the area immediately adjacent to the hinge)
- Fluid near the hinge or in other areas
- Decentered and/or small hinge
- Lack of adequate examination of the topography in which the surgeon makes the mistake of treating all patients as though they were the same

Smoothing the ablated stromal bed with the excimer laser (PTK) can treat these three types of complications.

The real problem is whether the surgeon is really able to make an intraoperative diagnosis of a nonhomogeneous ablation. Actually, irregularities of the ablated surface can only be highlighted intraoperatively by using the Scheimpflug camera.

Smoothness of the ablated surface can be divided into three categories:

Grade 1: smooth, even surfaces or with fine granular irregularities. The edges of the ablation are not visible. The concentric steps around the ablation are visible under high magnification.

Grade 2: slight surface irregularities; the edges of the ablation are visible.

Grade 3: marked surface irregularities, significant decentration, and sharp ablation edge.

If these three groups are compared, the final postoperative visual outcome is better in the first group, worse in the second, and definitely poor in the third. Considering this, a smoothing treatment is advisable in LASIK in groups 2 and 3. This technique is comparable to therapeutic photoablation: a wide ablation is used (9.0 to 10 mm) as well as a masking fluid (the characteristics are described below). In order to obtain a better result with broadbeam lasers, the ablation should be performed with a low frequency beam (10 Hz) to prevent corneal overheating. This is not a problem with flying spot lasers.

Smoothing with a large diameter removes the same quantity of corneal tissue from the entire corneal surface. The induction of hyperopia is highly unlikely.

The masking fluid must have the following specific chemical physical characteristics:
- Low ablation frequency (as close to the stromal frequency as possible)
- Surface tension identical to that of the corneal epithelium

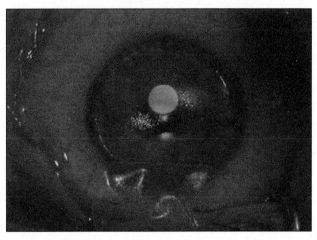

Figure 8-59. Stroma with a small amount of fluorescein so that the impact spots can be seen (under very low light intensity). If the surgeon suspects decentration, he or she may check centration to ablate.

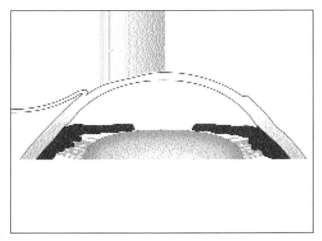

Figure 8-60. Decentered ablation with a broadbeam laser.

Table 8-21

DECENTERED ABLATION AND DECENTERED FLAP

Etiology
- Poor fixation by the patient
- Poor centration of the laser beam by the surgeon
- Poor eye stabilization if a ring is used

Results
- Irregular astigmatism
- Mixed astigmatism
- Problems with night-time vision
- Halos
- Ghost images
- Glare
- Reduced BCVA
- Diplopia

Prevention
- Calm, accurate instruction on patient fixation
- Use of a fixation ring if necessary

Treatment
- Proceed with the ablation if possible
- Reposition the flap and postpone the operation
- Enhancement in the event of undercorrection

- Low viscosity to ensure a thin, even distribution over the bed to be ablated
- Shear rate suitable for correct distribution with a spatula (such as VES); thus, slow movement of the spatula creates a thicker layer, whereas a more rapid movement creates a thinner layer

The product that provides the best results is hyaluronic acid, which is available in a number of forms (by varying the ratio between molecular weight and concentration the results are similar). The fluid must cover the entire corneal surface—no areas of dry cornea are allowed or the ablation will not be performed correctly. Careful intraoperative monitoring is therefore necessary.

The fluid will allow the stromal peaks to protrude, thus the irregularities can be ablated while the fluid protects the submerged structures from laser ablation.

Smoothing the peaks is much easier than trying to correct the troughs; some PTKs are therefore easier than others.

Instruments available for monitoring the ablated surface are:

- The Keeler Tearscope (IK). Used with the Placido disk inserted, it allows observation of the regularity of the surfaces and the distance between the rings. This gives the surgeon a good evaluation of the quality of the ablation. Given that the density of the rings is low, small central islands may not be clearly visible.
- Videokeratoscopy and corneal topography. This examination allows an accurate examination of the corneal surface. At the end of the smoothing procedure, the keratoscopic rings must be perfectly round, at a regular distance one from the other, clear, and continuous.
- Digital retroillumination with the analysis system of the anterior segment of the eye (Nidek EAS 1000). The image in retroillumination appears on the instrument's monitor. Through a series of transformations, an image is obtained that provides a representation of the optical quality of the cornea.

Another useful method: fluorescent under UV light to highlight the stromal areas that emerge from the masking fluid. The stroma has its own fluorescence, so strong illumination is required for this examination. In practice, it is easier to examine the areas where there is fluid break-up under high magnification.

Decentered Ablation

Decentration of the ablation may be caused by:
- Poor fixation by the patient:
  - Does not fix the laser target light correctly
  - Cannot see the target light correctly
- Incorrect head position
- Poor function of the eye tracker
- Loss of the eye tracker
- Incorrect test of laser beam alignment
- Carelessness by the surgeon
- Incorrect centration by the surgeon
- Malfunction of the laser
- Excess humidity, which may act as a mask and prevent the ablation of a specific area

Prior to initiation of treatment, the surgeon must check that the laser settings are correct and that the patient's head has been positioned so that the corneal surface is perpendicular to the ablation beam. The ablation is centered on the pupil and centration must be constantly monitored. If the patient moves his or her head or eye, the ablation should be stopped and the patient returned to the correct position; only then can the ablation be resumed.

During the ablation, fluid that may accumulate on the corneal surface must be dried with a sponge or removed with a blunt spatula. This is particularly important for ablations performed with broadbeam lasers, which tend to create a pool of liquid in the center. It is of little importance with flying spot lasers.

Generally, decentration will be inferior if the patient tends to close the fellow eye because of Bell's phenomenon; decentration will be superior if the patient tends to look downward.

With miotics, nasal decentration is likely, while mydriasis tends to produce superotemporal decentration.

Prevention

Ensure that the patient is always alert and continues to maintain fixation on the target point; for this reason sedation should be reduced to a minimum or avoided completely. The patient should be continually reminded to stare at the target light, explaining that the light will be blurry following the lamellar cut.

On the contrary, experience has demonstrated that general sedation (eg, with diazepam) may prove to be very useful. If it is not excessively strong, it will relax the patient and facilitate the ability to fixate the target light. Even the eye tracker appears to work better in these cases. If the patient is not sedated, his or her eye is likely to move abruptly.

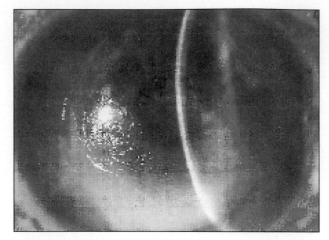

Figure 8-61a. Corneal abscess following LASIK (courtesy of Enrique Suarez, MD).

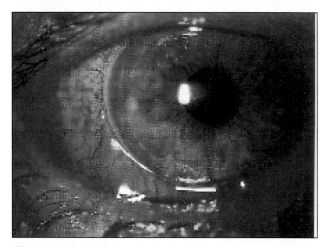

Figure 8-61b. Corneal abscess stained at 9 o'clock (courtesy of Enrique Suarez, MD).

Avoid a mydriatic pupil. In addition to making it more difficult to obtain good centration, blurring the patient's vision makes fixation more difficult even prior to the lamellar cut.

Reassure and relax the patient to help fixation. Detailed explanation of what is happening will improve cooperation. The patient should be reminded that the microkeratome and lasers will make a noise and unusual odors, but that he or she must not be alarmed.

Holding the patient's hand is a useful adjunct to calm; the surgeon should also give the patient clear, concise instructions. The surgeon should tell the patient to keep the fellow eye open instead of blinking under the drape.

If fixation proves difficult, it is better to interrupt the ablation and wait.

Unquestionably, lasers fitted with an active, sensitive eye tracker reduce or avoid problems related to decentration, even when the patient is uncooperative. Having said

Table 8-22
PAIN
Etiology
• Pressure from the speculum
• Pressure from the suction ring
• Poor apposition of the flap edge and bed
• Epithelium defects
• Dislocation of the flap
• Loss of the flap
Prevention
• Give accurate information to the patient
• Avoid any movements that may cause alteration to the flap or the epithelium
• Carefully reposition the flap
Treatment
• Check that the flap and epithelium are in place and intact
• Reassure the patient
• Use analgesics/sedation when appropriate
• Use NSAIDS
• Use bandage contact lenses when there is epithelial damage
• Artificial tears/ointment lubrication

Table 8-23
INFECTION
Etiology
• Bacterial
• Viral
Symptoms
• Pain
• Photophobia
• Blurring of vision
Prevention
• Cleaning, adequate sterilization of the instruments
• Cannulas
• Syringes
• Microkeratome
• Preoperative treatment of blepharitis
• Use a sterile surgical technique
• Avoid excessive intraoperative irrigation
• Postoperative antibiotic prophylaxis
• Avoid swimming and eye make-up for 2 weeks pre-operatively
• Avoid complications that will encourage infections
• Dislocated flap
• Lost flap
• Perforated flap
• Epithelial ingrowth
• Melting
• Debris in the interface
Treatment
• Diligent follow-up
• Antibiotic treatment
• Treatment with NSAIDs

that, it is preferable to have the patient fixate on the target light. The eye tracker has an angular speed of about 50° compared to 700° of the eye's angular speed. It can therefore not track the eye perfectly, so it should be considered a useful aid but not totally reliable.

The eye tracker must be checked preoperatively and an appropriate alignment test of the laser beam must be performed. If no eye tracker is available, in the case of nystagmus or immobility, the patient's eye can be stabilized using a Thornton or Fine-Thornton ring.

When this ring is positioned, the surgeon should avoid torsion of the eye, otherwise the treatment will be decentered.

Symptoms

A decentered ablation will create clinical-functional problems correlated to the degree and position of decentration.

Decentration of the ablation should not be confused with decentration of the lamellar cut. There will be few problems if the cut is moderately decentered (a situation that the surgeon will frequently create for a number of reasons) and the ablation is centered. If the cut is greatly decentered, the final refractive result may be impacted even if the ablation is centered. In this case, the ablated area is often incomplete; replacement of the decentered flap will induce a certain degree of astigmatism, which is likely to be irregular.

The eccentric ablation, as previously stated, creates functional and refractive problems: irregular astigmatism, mixed astigmatism (this should lead to suspicion of a decentered ablation), halos, glare, problems with night vision, ghost images and diplopia, and inclination or distortion of the images associated with the astigmatism.

Optically, there may be a reduction in best-corrected visual acuity through irregular astigmatism and uncorrected visual acuity through undercorrection because the area that has undergone a greater amount of treatment is not aligned on the visual axis.

Decentration greater than 1.0 mm may induce functional problems, and greater than 2.0 mm will create severe visual disturbances.

Diagnosis

In general, this is observed only during the postoperative follow-up period. The patient's functional recovery is not optimal, and he or she perceives the above-mentioned disturbances. Objectively, these problems can be highlighted with corneal topography.

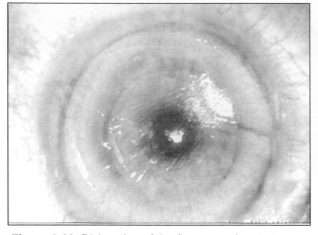

Figure 8-62. Dislocation of the flap secondary to trauma in the immediate postoperative period.

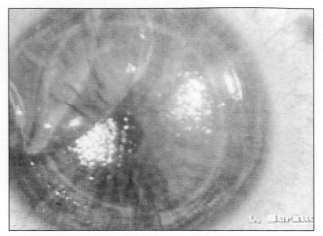

Figure 8-63. Dislocation of the flap due to aggressive eye rubbing.

The evaluation of a decentered ablation must not be performed using an axial examination, as this may produce a false diagnosis of decentration. It is essential that the examination be performed tangentially.

Management

Generally speaking, correction of a decentered ablation is relatively easy and possible with another procedure. The simplest and most effective method is an ablation correlated to the topography (topolink treatment). In this case, a CCT is performed and sent to a laboratory that processes the laser software; a personalized software package is developed to correct the error. In reality, it is not as simple as it would appear. Frequently, two ablations—one on top of the other—do not integrate well; there is often excessive removal of the tissue and residual astigmatism persists.

An alternative method for recentering an ablation without topolink treatment is to use a recentering system, such as the one devised by Vinciguerra. This method is based on the concept that with a decentered ablation, recentering requires the ablation of a larger, deeper area that will include the decentered area. In this way, the surgeon can obtain a correction equal to that originally expected.

A decentered ablation will cause asymmetry of the optic zone through excessive ablation in some areas and insufficient ablation in others.

This asymmetry is directly proportional to the amount of decentration. Moreover, the greater the decentration and the greater the visual defect to be corrected, the greater the visual reduction.

The visual problem is greater with the smaller the ablated area. In this type of situation, the corneal meridians modify their shape, transforming from spherical to parabolic. The corneal meridian that joins the pupil center to the treatment center will present the greater degree of error. At this meridian, there is a continual transition from the maximum to the minimum dioptric power.

The oblique meridians also present an oblique shape, but the dioptric slope decreases progressively with an increase in the distance from the meridian with greatest error.

The only round, arc-shaped meridian is found perpendicular to the axis of decentration. It stands to reason that only this meridian allows good focus.

In comparison to the conoid of Sturm, which presents meridians with infinite but regular radii of curvature, the Vinciguerra Nizzola conoid is irregular with different parabolic meridians due to the decentered treatment.

Correction

A secondary complementary ablation can be performed to produce an evenly ablated area.

Using algorithms, the depth of the new ablation is calculated. By evaluating a tangential corneal topography, the center of the decentered zone, the axis for retreatment, or the axis of decentration must be calculated.

In theory, a well-centered treatment is compared to a treatment that has been decentered by 1.0 mm, with point-by-point quantification of the ablative error. In order to do this, lines are marked that connect all the points of equal error.

From these profiles it is possible to design a series of metal diaphragms to be used in succession during retreatment, starting with the largest opening and ending with the smallest. These diaphragms must be well-centered and placed on the axis of decentration. It is preferable to insert the diaphragms in a specially designed suction mask.

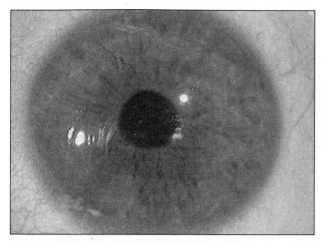

Figure 8-64a. Five days after surgery, the lower part of the flap has folded over, leaving a half-moon area uncovered.

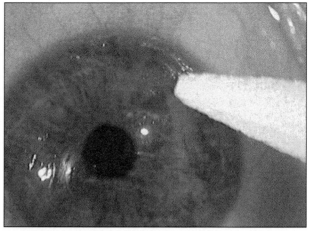

Figure 8-64b. Correction technique: the epithelium is removed from the area of stromal bed that remains uncovered.

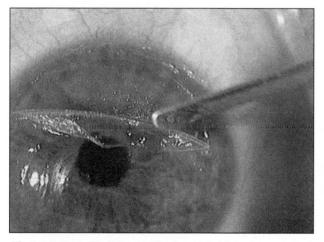

Figure 8-64c. The flap is lifted and the inferior part that has folded inward is peeled back.

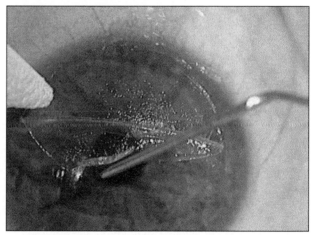

Figure 8-64d. Once the inferior part has been freed, the flap is repositioned.

The Vinciguerra system consists of:
- A suction mask with blocking positions of 45, 90, 135, 180, 225, and 270 degrees
- A cross-shaped reference point for centration
- 7 to 10 diaphragms

The procedure occurs in three steps:
1. The mask is centered on the visual axis by means of the centering reference cross. The arm of the cross is aligned on the axis of decentration (an imaginary line that joins the visual axis and center of the decentered area evaluated by corneal topography).

   At this point, the cross is removed and the first diaphragm is inserted in the same blocking position, where it is automatically centered.
2. Successive ablations are performed with each of the seven diaphragms.

3. PTK is performed under intraoperative topographic monitoring to smooth the newly ablated area with a topographic and refractive evaluation.

Generally speaking, it is advisable to use half of the total algorithm because experience has demonstrated that if 100% of the algorithm is used, decentration will occur again, now in the opposite direction. This may be due to the fact that the greater the degree of decentration, the less the validity of the topography. Therefore, it is more difficult to perform the calculations. In any case, it is easier to perform an additional treatment if 50% of the algorithm is insufficient, rather than fix an overcorrection. Once half of the algorithm has been used, topographic and refractive checks are performed to evaluate the result.

Result: the asymmetrical ablation obtained with this technique is complementary to the asymmetrical ablation resulting from the decentered treatment.

Table 8-24

POSTOPERATIVE FLAP DISLOCATION

Etiology
- Excessive lid squeezing
- Rubbing the operated eye
- Excessively dry eye
- Reduced blinking
- Anesthesia from lateral canthotomy
- Poor wetting of the eye
- From eyelid anomalies (lagophthalmus)
- From orbit anomalies (exophthalmus)
- Incorrect use of fluids during the operation
- Poor adhesion of the flap
- Due to disruption of the epithelium
- Due to poor intraoperative repositioning
- Due to excessive irrigation with edema of the flap and the stromal bed
- Postoperative trauma

Results
- Repositioning is required
- Risk of flap edema
- Risk of abrasion
- Risk of epithelial ingrowth
- Risk of striae
- Risk of infection
- Sutures may be required

Prevention
- Pay attention to anatomic abnormalities of the eyelids and orbit
- Check adhesion of the flap after repositioning
- Remind the patient:
  - To not rub the eye
  - To not squeeze
  - To wear a humidifying chamber for the first 24 hours and every night for the first week

Treatment
- Carefully reposition the flap
- Equally distend the flap in the event of folds and striae
- Use sutures in the event of persistent folds, prolonged epithelial defects, or if the flap had to be repositioned intraoperatively
- Keep the flap lubricated with nonpreserved artificial tears

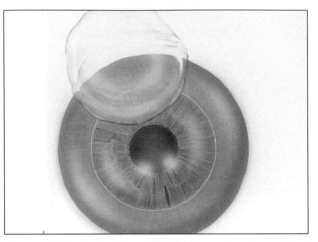

Figure 8-65. Dislocation of the free cap from its original position.

- Overcorrection: an excessively high energy level relative to normal levels or it may depend on an error in data input.
- Ablation on tissue that is excessively dry. Overcorrection may also be due to a poor refractive examination performed without cycloplegia, or alternately the laser was not calibrated for each individual patient.
- Undercorrection: an excessively low level of laser energy (ie, lower than normal levels). Undercorrection may also occur because the ablation was performed on excessively hydrated tissue or through an error in data input.
- Inappropriate optic zone: results from an error in setting the surgical program in the laser's computer. It may also be due to a lack of calculation regarding the bumps in the cornea, which will interfere with the bumps in the ablation.
- Stopping the laser during the ablation: may occur due to electrical power failure or for other technical reasons. If the computer has recorded the number of pulses emitted or they have been noted by the technician, the machine may be turned off, turned on again, the same treatment reset with the number of pulses fired prior to the power failure onto a test paper and the remainder on the patient's stroma.

While waiting, the flap should be replaced to avoid excessive dehydration of the stroma.

If the laser power cannot be restored for any reason, the procedure can be completed later.

Prevention of Complications with the Excimer Laser

- Accurate, continuous monitoring of the laser

The combined treatment and retreatment create a well-centered ablation, the optic zone is wider, the ablation is deeper, and the final refraction outcome corresponds to the value originally expected.

In order to do this, it is of the utmost importance to correlate the exact algorithm to the amount of decentration. All this produces a thinning of the cornea that is greater—the greater the decentration of the initial error to be corrected and the initial optic zone used.

Other complications related to the laser:

DECENTERED ABLATION

Etiology
- Poor fixation by the patient
- Carelessness by the surgeon
- Eye tracker malfunction

Result
- Irregular astigmatism
- Mixed astigmatism
- Halos
- Problems with night vision
- Ghost images
- Glare
- Reduced best-corrected visual acuity
- Diplopia

Prevention
- Careful patient education regarding fixation and what is about to happen during the procedure
- Optional use of a stabilizing ring

Treatment
- Proceed with the ablation
- Reposition the flap and postpone the operation
- Enhancement for the correction of undercorrection

- Hydration of the stromal bed must be carefully checked prior to starting the ablation and again while it is being performed
- The operating room environment should be controlled
- The electrical power supply should be controlled

Digital Retroillumination

During LASIK, retroillumination allows the surgeon to study the interface (ie, the surface cut by the microkeratome and ablated stromal surface). Irregularities on these surfaces may create disturbances of visual function.

Retroillumination is obtained by illuminating the fundus and using the light reflected from it toward the "bleached" cornea, naturally if the other refractive structures are transparent. This examination is very important because it also provides a picture of the optic quality of the cornea.

This may be altered by:
- Opacity in the tissues
- Surface irregularities
- Alteration of the refractive index

The latter in LASIK may be a consequence of non-uniform thickness or interstitial formation between the flap and the stroma; the latter occurs if the margin of the ablated surface is sharp (ie, with no transition zone) because the flap cannot completely mirror the stromal surface.

The most common reason for alterations of visual function is a surface that has been poorly cut by the microkeratome, poorly ablated by the laser, or without a transition zone.

Other reasons may be epithelial ingrowth or stromal hypertrophy. Digital retroillumination is obtained using an instrument produced by Nidek (the Nidek EAS 1000 system).

During the examination, it may prove useful to test different positions in order to obtain the best possible image of the area under examination.

The light tone of the instrument can be inverted so that the diffracted light provides a dark image. Where there is no diffraction, the image will be pale. Vinciguerra has drawn a scale of evaluation for the ablated surfaces; this is based on the nonuniformity observed according to the image obtained with retroillumination.

V0 = unobservable nonuniformity
V1 = slight nonuniformity
V2 = severe nonuniformity

Clinical Use

Digital retroillumination can be used preoperatively and both early and late postoperatively. It can also be used in PRK.

In LASIK, light diffraction is examined at the interface. As mentioned previously, there is no other means available for studying the interface.

The examination is very useful, for example, when a patient has visual disturbances even though the corneal map and slit lamp measurements are normal.

In this case, retroillumination that can highlight slight or important nonuniform surfaces may provide a feasible explanation for these phenomena.

At this point, it is possible to retreat the patient and achieve an interface surface that is smooth.

This examination can also be used intraoperatively; this will allow immediate correction of any irregularities of the ablated surfaces.

Scheimpflug Camera and LASIK

The Scheimpflug Camera (ESA 1000, Nidek Ltd) is an instrument based on Scheimpflug's principle. On the basis of this principle, the surgeon can obtain a clear image of a sloping plane on the condition that the plane of the eyepiece, the object, and the film cut the same point and the angles are the same.

The instrument and examination procedure were developed during the mid-1960s.

Initially (late 1970s to early 1980s), they were used to study the crystalline lens and its cataractous evolution. It provides a linear densitometry. The difference in the

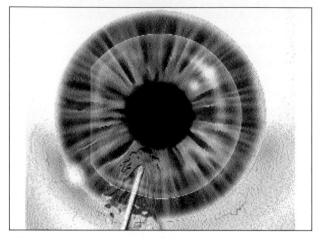

Figure 8-66. The interface is washed to remove foreign material.

darkening of photosensitive film corresponds to variations in the density of the opacity of the crystalline lens.

In refractive surgery, the Scheimpflug camera functions in a similar manner to computerized videokeratography; it serves to evaluate the extension and uniformity of the ablated corneal zones.

Two types of images are obtained: one in sagittal section, the other in retroillumination. By using the software available for the images in the sagittal section, it is possible to calculate:

- The radius of posterior and anterior corneal curvature
- The characteristics of any opacity: degree, depth, area, and volume

From the images in retroillumination, it is possible to obtain:

- Alterations of the stromal transparency
- Lines of tension or striae
- Uneven refractive

The software can calculate the area affected by treatment. With both types of images, it is possible to display the different images obtained with the various examinations (preoperatively and postoperatively).

POSTOPERATIVE COMPLICATIONS

Postoperative complications can be grouped most logically as anatomic or refractive.

Anatomic complications:
- Epithelial defects/epithelial displacement
- Infection
- Pain
- Foreign body/debris in the interface

Table 8-25
EPITHELIAL DEFECTS

Etiology
- Drying the flap surface, especially on the conjunctiva
- Manipulation of the flap
- Microkeratome pass
- Excessive topical anesthesia preoperatively
- Gentian violet markings
- A suction ring that has perilimbal support
- Suction transmitted through the suction ring
- Phototoxicity
- Microtrauma from forceps or instruments during the operation

Results
- Reduced oxygen pressure to the corneal surface, resulting in:
  - Reduced nourishment of the corneal stroma with
  - Reduction in corneal sensitivity
  - Reduction of cellular activity in the basal layer of the corneal epithelium
  - An accumulation of lactic acid with an intracellular osmotic effect and consequent epithelial edema
- Severe pain
- Photophobia
- Tearing
- Increased risk of infection
- Higher incidence of epithelial ingrowth
- Stromal melting

Prevention
- Adequate epithelium wetting
- Reduced manipulation of the flap
- Avoid or cautiously operate on patients with anterior corneal dystrophy
- Reduce topical anesthesia to a minimum

Treatment
- Daily exams of the patient to detect the appearance of any infection
- Antibiotic prophylaxis
- Pain therapy
- Use of a bandage contact lens
- Gently remove the contact lens
- In the event of epithelial slide or defect, treatment is the same as in the intraoperative period
- Artificial tears
- Autoserum

- Wrinkling of the flap/traction folds of the flap
- Flap striae
- Epithelial ingrowth in the interface
- Interface infiltrates
- Dislocation of the flap
- Loss of the flap/cap
- Interface haze
- Corneal ectasia and keratoconus

Table 8-26

DEBRIS AND FOREIGN BODIES IN THE INTERFACE

Etiology
- Metallic particles from the microkeratome, blade, spatulas, and cannulas
- Dust particles from air in the operating room and surgical gloves
- Fibrous particles from drapes, sponges, and gauze
- Impurities from vibrations of the microkeratome
- Blood or epithelial cell residues
- Inorganic debris in the operating room

Results
- Inflammation
- Surface irregularity
- Stromal melting
- Loss of BCVA

Prevention
- Carefully check the microkeratome blade
- Avoid excessive irrigation of the fornices
- Use lint/particle-free material (gloves, gowns, drapes)
- Reduce movement of personnel in the operating room
- Carefully check during and after surgery for the presence of any debris at the interface

Treatment
- See the *Intraoperative Complications* section of this chapter

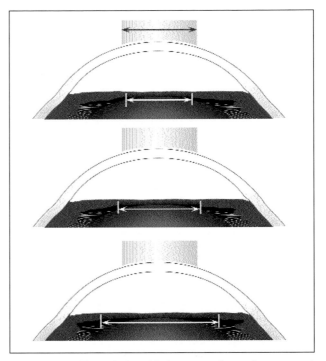

Figure 8-67. The relationship between the optic zone and pupil diameter in night lighting. Top: the optic zone is larger—excellent visual quality. Center: the diameters are the same—excellent visual quality. Bottom: the optic zone is smaller than the pupil—night symptoms.

- Stromal melting
- Central islands

Optical/refractive complications:
- Induced irregular astigmatism
- Undercorrection
- Overcorrection
- Regression
- Decentration

Pain

The majority of patients have minimal to no pain. Burning and tearing for the first 2 to 3 hours, slight foreign body sensation, slight photophobia, and slight discomfort are the most common symptoms. These symptoms are reported more frequently with enhancements that require flap lifting, as compared to primary treatments. Pressure exerted by the speculum and suction ring may be the source of an occasional complaint of orbital pain.

In general, narcotic analgesics are not necessary postoperatively, though sedatives or non-narcotic pain medication, such as ibuprofen, maybe helpful. If the patient reports pain associated with profuse tearing, the eye must be immediately examined at the slit lamp. One should suspect flap dislocation or significant epithelial disruption. Very severe pain may even indicate total loss of the flap.

Tips for prevention: the patient should be advised that it is normal to feel pressure from the speculum and suction ring. Follow all precautions to avoid epithelial trauma, and ensure good flap adherence.

Management

First, ensure that the flap and epithelium are intact. The surgeon should reassure the patient that there are no problems in terms of surgical wound healing. Additional analgesic and/or sedatives may be used once flap/epithelial problems are ruled out. It is useful to administer NSAIDs and use bandage contact lenses if there is epithelial damage, not only to keep pain levels under control, but also to avoid lid displacement of the flap with roughened epithelium. Lubrication is another important factor. As the flap is denervated for 1 to 2 months, tearing is reduced and nonpreserved artificial tears should be used as frequently every 30 minutes for the first 2 weeks, then tapering as needed. In more severe cases, punctum plugs and increased lubrication may be indicated, even prophylactically, in patients post blepharoplasty or with prior dry-eye history.

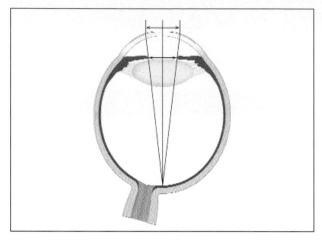

Figure 8-68. An optic zone with a diameter greater than the pupil allows good visual quality at night and during the day.

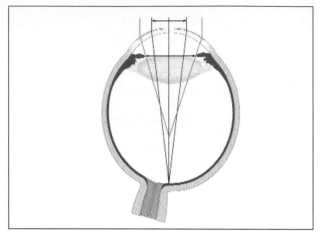

Figure 8-69. A pupil with a diameter greater than the minimal optic zone causes severe night glare symptoms.

Table 8-27

NIGHT GLARE AND HALOS

Etiology
- Optic zones that are smaller than the scotopic pupil diameter (spherical aberration)
- Subjects with unusually large scotopic pupil size
- Severe myopia
- Symptoms are aggravated by residual refractive errors

Results
- Disturbances of visual function
- Difficulty at night

Prevention
- New ablation algorithms with large transition zones
- Multizone technique or aspheric profile
- Central pretreatment

Treatment
- Symptomatic improvement with time and with bilateral treatment (cortex integration); the patient learns to disregard the problem

Table 8-28

STROMAL CLOUDING AND HAZE IN THE INTERFACE

Etiology
- Correction of high refractive errors
- Intrastromal edema from direct photoablation
- Intrastromal edema as a toxic reaction to substances used during the operation
- Intrastromal edema as a toxic reaction to debris in the interface

Results
- Reduced visual acuity
- Visual disturbances

Prevention
- Thoroughly clean instruments to remove any chemical residues

Treatment
- Transitory phenomenon
- Topical steroid treatment for 2 to 3 weeks

Infections

Infection following LASIK is a rare, potentially devastating complication. The reported rate of infective keratitis is about 1 in 5000.

With intact epithelium, introduction of bacteria is possible during the microkeratome pass and when the flap is elevated. Epithelial defects increase the risk of infection and should be carefully watched. Most corneal infiltrates are sterile but all need to be carefully monitored. Infective keratitis generally presents with infiltrates at the periphery of the flap.

Etiology
- Intraoperative infection due to bacterial contami-

nation of the operating instruments or field
- Poor patient compliance with the postoperative antibiotic regimen
- Predisposing factors, such as acne with blepharitis
- Patient's disregard for postoperative hygiene, such as avoiding eye make-up, swimming, etc, in the early postoperative period

Management

Late appearance (after days or weeks) of infective infiltrates on the surface or in the interface should be considered as a medical emergency to avoid corneal perforation and endophthalmitis with possible loss of the eye. Even though these late infections are extremely rare

(1:10,000), one should be prepared to recognize and institute emergency treatment.

The flap must be raised, cultures performed, and, if response to antibiotics is not rapid, may need to be removed. The patient should be hospitalized, and forti-fied topical and systemic antibiotic treatment should be administered with the patient examined frequently. It may be possible to save the flap, or penetrating kerato-plasty or lamellar keratoplasty may be necessary. The primary objective is to save the eye.

Tips for prevention: the operation should be per-formed under standard surgical conditions. Intraoperative irrigation should be minimized to avoid an influx of debris in the interface. The surgeon should use talc-free surgical gloves. Broad spectrum antibiotic cov-erage (fluoroquinolones) should be administered both 30 minutes prior to the procedure as well as postoperatively for 4 to 7 days. The risk is further reduced with appro-priate eyelid hygiene and Betadine lid preparation prior to proper draping to exclude the lashes from the opera-tive field.

Blepharitis should be treated prior to the operation. Eye make-up and swimming should be avoided for 2 weeks preoperatively.

Interface Infiltrates

As previously mentioned, most interface infiltrates are sterile. They may be secondary to a sterile inflamma-tory reaction or intraoperative contamination. The stro-mal interface is normally inert and does not react to trapped foreign bodies. This sterile inflammatory response in the interface, originally termed Sands of the Sahara, will be discussed in later in this chapter.

Flap Displacement

Intraoperative flap displacement has been previously discussed. Postoperative flap displacement results when a flap moves after is has been repositioned, and the patient checked and released.

Diagnosis

Diagnosis is typically apparent as soon as the patient enters the examination room. Instead of being white and comfortable, the eye is red, tearing profusely, photopho-bic, and very painful; vision is extremely blurred, usual-ly to counting fingers. Slit lamp examination using fluo-rescein shows the presence of a large stromal uptake of dye as well as the displaced or detached flap. In practice, it is very unusual for the flap to dislocate in the absence of trauma if the postoperative striae test and blink test are normal. Typically, the patient denies trauma or rubbing the eye, although later they may report hitting the eye with the protective shield during sleep. We have had two

Table 8-29
CORNEAL ECTASIA AND IATROGENIC KERATOCONUS

Etiology
- Excessively deep central ablation
- Thickness of residual stroma less than 200 to 250 microns
- Thickness of residual stroma less than 50% of the initial corneal thickness

Result
- Significant reduction of vision

Prevention
- Avoid ablations that are excessively deep
- Leave at least 200 to 250 microns of residual stroma under the flap
- Total thickness of residual stroma must be at least 50% of the initial corneal thickness

Treatment
- Contact lens
- Lamellar keratoplasty
- Penetrating keratoplasty

occasions where the flap was dislodged when the patient awoke from napping immediately following surgery, probably due to dry eyes when the lids opened. The dis-placement is usually about 1.0 mm, inducing peripheral or central corneal striae. It is rare for the flap to total-ly free and attached only by the hinge.

Cause

A complicated procedure or excessive stromal hydra-tion will facilitate dislocation. If refloating is necessary to reposition the flap during the procedure, additional drying time should be allowed for good flap adherence. Contrary to previous reports, I have found that placing a drop of Celluvisc on the surface of the flap after smooth-ing and initial adherence seems to distend the flap, diminish the gutter margin, and decrease the incidence of immediate flap displacement.

Predisposition to flap displacement:
- Flap hinge that is very short or thin
- Prolonged surgery time
- Excessive interface irrigation and subsequent insufficient intrastromal dehydration time, lead-ing to poor flap adhesion
- Incorrect final flap positioning
- Rubbing the eye by the patient usually in the first 24 hours
- Squeezing the eyelids in the immediate postoper-ative period
- Pressure patching of the eye, dislodging the flap with eye movement

Table 8-30

FLAP WRINKLING AND TRACTION FOLDS

Etiology
- Poor distention and repositioning of the flap/cap at the end of the operation
- Partial postoperative displacement of the flap
- Deep, highly myopic ablation with a relatively reduced optic zone
- Areas of greater traction (interrupted sutures)

Results
- Irritating glare
- Image distortion
- Poor quality vision

Prevention
- LASIK with superior hinge
- Examine the flap carefully at the end of the operation for symmetry and gutter alignment, and refloat immediately if necessary

Treatment
- Spontaneous resolution some weeks after suture removal

- Epithelial abrasion
- Accidental trauma

These may all induce dislocation or, more rarely, complete detachment and loss. Displacement of the flap is more unusual in myopic eyes as compared to hyperopic eyes because myopic flaps are typically thicker and have a larger diameter, equal to the diameter of the ring and plate used. Flaps in myopic eyes tend to seat in the bed better than hyperopic flaps, which have to drape over the increased steepness of the cornea.

Lateral canthotomy with its attendant orbital anesthesia and decreased reflex blinking predisposes it to flap displacement.

Tips for prevention:
- Avoid occlusive or pressure patching. Tape the lid shut if necessary and use a protective shield.
- Similarly, contact lenses should be avoided unless there are significant epithelial defects.
- Do not disregard the striae test, lid blink test, groove or gutter test, and iron test (this test applies stress to the flap instead of the peripheral cornea, also checking adhesion.

Treatment

Immediate intervention is necessary to avoid infection, to reduce pain, and to prevent permanent striae or damage to the flap. The patient is returned to the operating room, topical anesthesia is started, and the lids are prepared and draped. The flap must be elevated and reflected very carefully to avoid damaging the epithelium. It may be necessary to cut the epithelium along the flap edge. The surgeon should carefully remove any epithelium that has proliferated on the stromal bed or on the underside of the flap. If displacement is discovered late and there is significant ingrowth, a few pulses of PTK on the bed and underside of the flap may help eradicate residual epithelial cells. The flap must be repositioned correctly with irrigation of the interface to eliminate debris and epithelial cells.

Failure to act promptly increases the likelihood of permanent striae formation with decreased visual quality. Additional time should be allowed for smoothing and stretching the flap symmetrically into place. This can usually be achieved using moist Merocel sponges, allowing drying as smoothing proceeds to facilitate grasp on the flap, stretching of striae, and extending the flap so that it completely fills the bed. The gutter margins should be symmetrical and minimal. In cases where striae formation is more pronounced, the edges must be ironed out to fill the peripheral groove and eliminate striae. This is a laborious procedure, taking several minutes, but it works even after several months. The surgeon should be aware that striae will initially remain visible but will disappear over 24 to 48 hours if the flap has been fully distended. It is useful to remember to keep the eye well lubricated with sterile single-dose artificial tears if it is impossible to immediately reposition the flap, as a dry flap is more difficult to reposition and is more susceptible to trauma and striae formation. The lids should be taped and shielded if repositioning is delayed for any reason.

If epithelial ingrowth recurs, the flap must be lifted as described in *Management of Epithelial Ingrowth*.

Rarely, two or three interrupted sutures or an eight-bite antitorque suture may be necessary to maintain flap position until the situation has stabilized. The knots must be rotated to avoid symptoms or irritation that may provoke the patient to touch and rub the eye. A transparent plastic shield, which protects against accidental trauma and rubbing as well as increasing humidity around the eye, should be used.

Loss of the Flap/Cap

The reasons for flap loss are the same as those for flap dislocation. Free caps are more vulnerable, although we should remember that this was the normal technique for several years. A patient with a free cap should have the eye lightly taped shut overnight, following proper placement and adherence checks. Normally, patients with flap loss report sudden, severe pain with excessive tearing and reduced vision in the immediate postoperative period. The surgeon should always take these complaints seriously, since LASIK is normally such a pain-

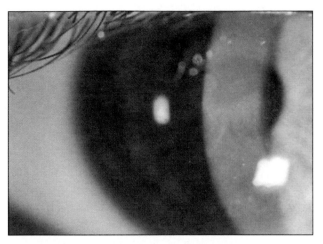

Figure 8-70. Moderate epithelial ingrowth.

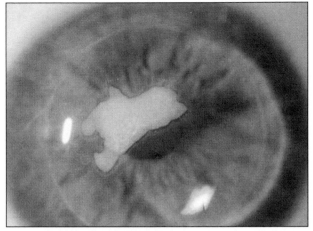

Figure 8-71. Significant epithelial ingrowth 6 months after surgery.

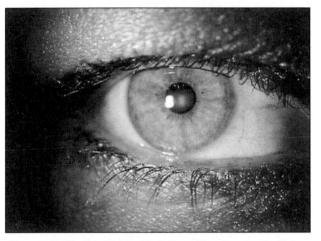

Figure 8-72. Central epithelial proliferation in the interface.

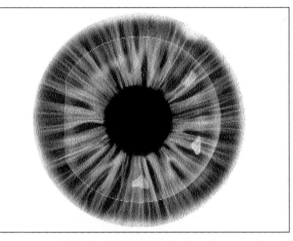

Figure 8-73. Multiple epithelial inclusions in a number of locations.

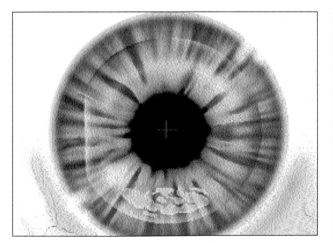

Figure 8-74. Inferior epithelial inclusions.

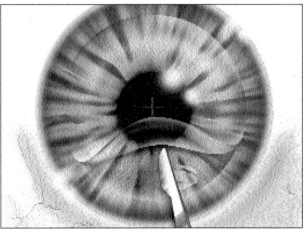

Figure 8-75. Peripheral or moderate extension removal technique: lift the flap in the specific area and mechanically remove with a blunt blade.

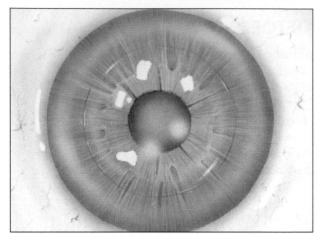

Figure 8-76. Islands of epithelium in the interface.

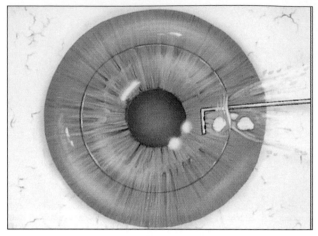

Figure 8-77. Small peripheral epithelial inclusions. Remove with a bent needle cannula, irrigate the epithelial material toward the elevated part of the flap that was used as the cannula's entrance route.

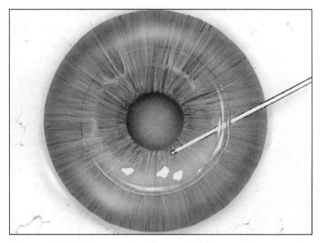

Figure 8-78. Removal with a straight needle cannula. The epithelial material is pushed by irrigation toward the area where the flap has been lifted.

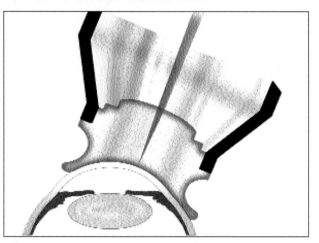

Figure 8-79. Removal of small localized epithelial inclusions using a YAG laser.

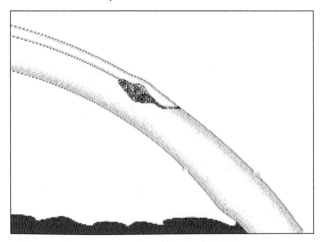

Figure 8-80. Cystic epithelial accumulation.

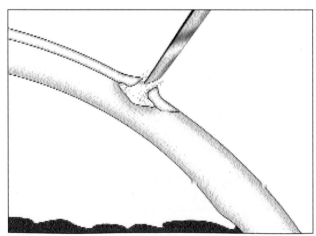

Figure 8-81. Removal technique: the flap is cut with a sharp blade tip and the material is then squeezed out.

less procedure. With total detachment of the flap, the flap may be completely lost. This may happen if the flap/hinge is too small and fragile and is torn secondary to trauma.

With a lost flap, if homoplastic material is available, the disc may be replaced using the adjustable ACS ring to remove a disc slightly smaller than the bed using either a whole globe or an artificial anterior chamber. If homoplastic material is not available, the cornea is allowed to re-epithelialize, as in PRK.

A soft contact lens should be used and the patient must be closely observed to monitor re-epithelialization. This normally takes 3 to 4 days. Some patients fully tolerate LASIK with cap loss and recover well with no significant visual problems. The eye is more likely to develop significant haze than with primary PRK. Generally speaking, haze is more common with deep ablations, in brown eyes and in younger patients. If the haze is marked after several months, the surgeon may perform PTK with the excimer following the complete removal of epithelium with the placement of a homoplastic corneal cap, as described above.

If the flap is found, we usually are faced with a flap that has been detached for a number of hours and has become very edematous, making it very difficult to distinguish the stromal face from the epithelial surface. The fine stromal granulation and occasionally the edges of the microkeratome cut can be used to identify the stromal side of the flap. Fluorescein may also be of assistance. If a bandage was used, the flap may actually be stuck to it, so on postoperative day 1 when the bandage is removed, the surgeon should closely examine it to see if the flap has stuck. In this situation, the flap will be severely dehydrated. If the flap is found, its stromal surface and stromal bed must be carefully cleaned to remove debris or epithelial growth; the flap may then be repositioned to its original location. This is not simple, as there are no marks and may be no landmarks.

Even when the flap has been found, cleaned, and oriented into position, it is highly unlikely that it will adhere without sutures. We prefer to use compression "bra" sutures anchored in the peripheral cornea over radial suturing of the edge of the cap, as this often produces scar tissue and irregular astigmatism. Single or double eight-bite antitorque sutures are also preferable to interrupted sutures. If the flap is irreparably damaged, it must be discarded.

Tips for prevention: prevention is based on anticipation and proper selection of rings, stops, diligent attention to operative detail, and thorough postoperative instructions to avoid rubbing and proper use of the protective shield.

Postoperative Epithelial Defects

Postoperative epithelial defects need to be managed aggressively and monitored frequently to avoid complications such as infection or corneal melting. Prevention is key.

Tips for prevention:
- Move methodically and quickly, avoiding epithelial drying
- Avoid excessive topical anesthesia, which loosens the epithelium
- Moisten the exposed corneal surface with a glycerin-based topical anesthetic (proparacaine) prior to the microkeratome pass to avoid trauma
- Use minimal gentian violet to mark, then irrigate the excess, also avoid the central 3.0 mm of the cornea
- Attempt to avoid placing the suction ring directly on the corneal surface
- Minimize phototoxicity
- Support the epithelial side of the flap on a moist Merocel sponge rather than the nasal conjunctiva
- Avoid microtrauma from the various instruments
- Avoid or be especially cautious of patients with basement membrane dystrophy

Physiology of Epithelial Trauma

Any trauma to the epithelium creates reduced oxygen pressure at the corneal surface, which persists for several weeks after the operation. Reduced oxygen supply leads to decreased nourishment of the corneal stroma. Persistent epithelial defects may have the following consequences:
- Reduction of corneal sensitivity secondary to reduction of acetylcholine at the corneal nerve endings (reflex mechanism)
- Reduction in cellular enzyme activity and mitosis of the basal layer of the corneal epithelium
- Reduction in the concentration of glycogen and glucose in the epithelial cells with secondary accumulation of lactic acid with intracellular osmosis and consequent epithelial edema

Sutures further destabilize the tear film; they alter even distribution of the superficial lipid layer in the paralimbal area. This encourages excessive evaporation of the water component with creation of so-called "dry spots," which are clearly visible under fluorescein examination.

Adjacent to sutures, filaments or nodules of mucopolysaccharides, due to excessive evaporation of the lachrymal film, develop. Moreover, subclinical irritation provoked by sutures increases the number of con-

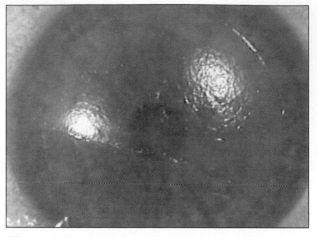

Figure 8-82. A clearly visible demarcation line can be seen under the flap. This is the advancing edge of epithelial proliferation (courtesy of Claudio Genisi, MD).

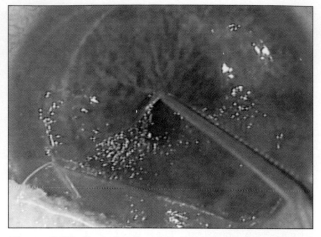

Figure 8-83. Once the flap has been lifted, the epithelial layer is separated from the stroma (courtesy of Claudio Genisi, MD).

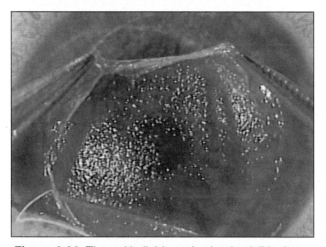

Figure 8-84. The epithelial layer is clearly visible (courtesy of Claudio Genisi, MD).

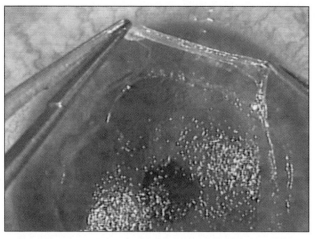

Figure 8-85. The epithelial layer is completely removed with two forceps (courtesy of Claudio Genisi, MD).

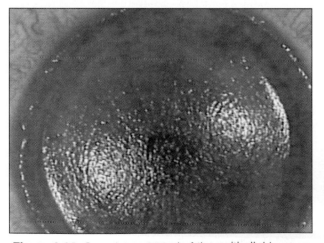

Figure 8-86. Complete removal of the epithelial layer on the stroma (courtesy of Claudio Genisi, MD).

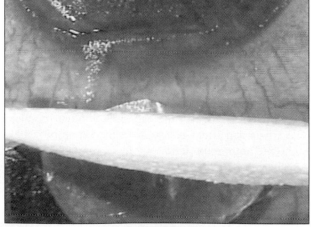

Figure 8-87. To remove any residual stromal cells on the flap, first the sponge is used, then PTK of about 15 microns is performed on both surfaces to destroy any residual cells (courtesy of Claudio Genisi, MD).

Table 8-31

EPITHELIAL INGROWTH

Etiology
- Poor adhesion of the flap edges
- Epithelial abrasions at the flap margins
- Poor flap alignment
- Perforated buttonholed flap
- Free cap
- Ablation at the edges of the stromal bed or beyond (especially hyperopic ablation)
- Epithelial irregularities at the edge of the flap (particularly with enhancement)
- Accidental introduction of epithelial cells during the cut with the microkeratome
- Manipulation of the intrastromal surfaces
- Introduction of cells following insertion of instruments in the interface (eg, cannulas, spatulas)
- The cap folds over on itself during the operation
- Inadequate irrigation and cleaning of the surfaces involved
- Previous radial keratotomy, especially with epithelial plugs and incisions

Results
- Reduced visual acuity
- Irregular astigmatism
- Discomfort (irregularity of the surface)
- Risk of stromal melting

Prevention
- Be kind to the epithelium
- Replace all torn epithelium to the edges of the flap
- Remove epithelial cells and debris from the stromal bed prior to repositioning the flap
- Avoid wide ablation zones on small beds and protect the area around the hinge if necessary

Treatment
- Small area (under 2.0 mm) that does not affect the visual area, monitor carefully
- Area that exceeds 2.0 mm even if it does not create visual disturbances, treat

junctival goblet cells leading to greater mucous production. This creates a veiling sensation and fluctuation in visual acuity. Extensive epithelial loss is associated with severe pain, photophobia, and tearing. This creates three potential complications: increased risk of infection, increased incidence of epithelial ingrowth, and increased likelihood of stromal thinning or melting.

Even minimal epithelial defects should not be ignored and should be closely monitored and treated if re-epithelialization is not rapid.

Management

The patient should be checked daily to detect the appearance of any infection. Antibiotic prophylaxis with double coverage (fluoroquinolone and aminoglycoside) should be initiated. Treatment of pain begins with patient reassurance, lubricants, bandage contact lenses, topical diclofenac, or ketorolac twice daily for no more than 48 to 72 hours (as they retard re-epithelization).

Another efficacious therapy for epithelial defects is the use of autoserum: 10 cc of autologous blood is centrifuged for 20 minutes; the obtained serum is administered as eyedrops 3 to 4 times a day.

A pressure patch is contraindicated, as eye movement beneath it may dislocate the flap.

Bandage contact lenses must be lubricated profusely, especially prior to removal, and then removed very gently. Proparacaine should be used, as it is the least toxic anesthetic agent for the cornea. With the patient looking upward at the slit lamp, the inferior edge of the contact lens is grasped with smooth forceps.

Debris/Foreign Body in the Interface

Particulate debris is frequently seen in the interface following LASIK, though this normally does not affect the final visual or functional outcome of surgery. Interface contamination may be organic or inorganic.

Inorganic debris includes talc from gloves, metallic fragments from blades and microkeratome vibration, lint, airborne contaminants, and rust from the autoclave. Organic debris includes blood, fat and oil from the tear film, and epithelial cells.

Result

Debris rarely induces inflammation or surface irregularities, but if this happens there may be loss of BCVA. There may also be inflammation-inducing melting. Management depends on location. If the debris is peripheral or paracentral, it typically does not create problems. However, if it is central in location and interferes with the visual axis, it may affect visual function in terms of quality, thus requiring surgical removal.

Management

If there are problems related to debris in the interface, the patient must be returned to the operating room and the debris removed.

Tips for prevention:
- Irrigate and remove debris prior to the microkeratome pass
- Avoid excessive irrigation, inducing reflux of fluid into the interface
- Consider a speculum with suction removal of excess fluid
- Careful intraoperative check during and following flap repositioning at the surgical microscope and at the slit lamp immediately postoperatively, with removal if present

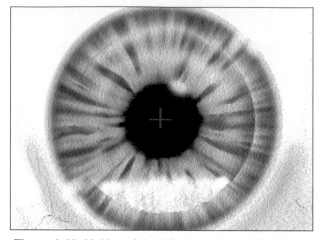

Figure 8-88. Melting of the inferior section of the flap.

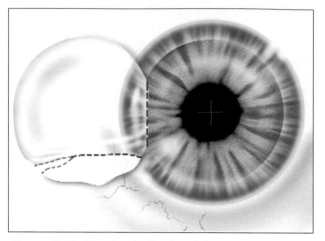

Figure 8-89. The flap is lifted and the damaged part is removed with scissors.

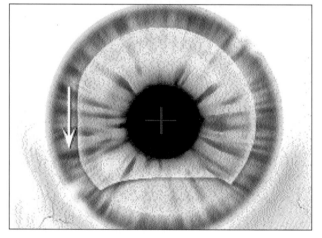

Figure 8-90. The flap is replaced and positioned in the usual manner.

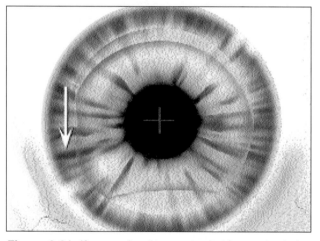

Figure 8-91. If excessive tissue removal is required, the hinge may be cut and the flap positioned over the center of the pupil.

Lamellar refractive surgery must be completely amoric (a word derived from the Greek language, meaning a = without, morion = particles). In amoric surgery, gloves, gowns, and drapes that release fibers, dust, or talc are avoided. HEPA filters should be used to attempt to remove airborne contaminants and movement in the room should be minimized.

Glare, Halos, and Night Glare

As was mentioned in the introduction to this chapter, now that the mechanics of LASIK are more understood and monitored, we are entering the era of attempting to achieve greater visual quality and minimizing visual complaints. Glare, especially at night, is one of the greatest problems, seen more frequently in patients with large pupils and high corrections. The abrupt edge slope created in high corrections defracts light, thus inducing halos.

Residual myopic refractive error aggravates these symptoms and should be treated if residual stroma is available.

This complication is more important in those patients with unusually large resting pupil diameters. The scotopic pupil diameter should be measured preoperatively and the patient counseled based on this and the amount of planned correction. This complication is due to an accentuated form of spherical aberration, with the diameter of the pupil under low luminance exceeding the effective optic zone created.

Increasing the optic zone is not always the answer as this means using an excessively deep ablation—a greater chance of inducing central islands—as in the case of a broadbeam laser. Patients with a disproportionately large pupil compared to the optic zone to be treated should be avoided. Phakic IOLs for higher correction should be considered, however large scotopic pupils may con-

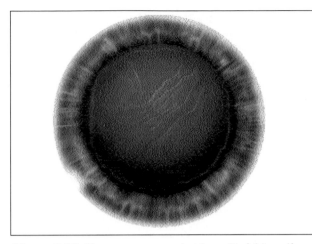

Figure 8-92. Numerous corneal striae with fairly uniform direction.

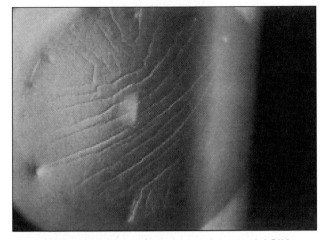

Figure 8-93. Wrinkling of the flap 1 day post-LASIK.

Table 8-32
STROMAL MELTING

Etiology
- Poor hydration by the lacrimal film with a consequent reduction in oxygen supply
- Epithelial ingrowth
- Reduced blinking
- Lacrimal film pathologies
- Thin flap

Results
- Patient discomfort
- Reduced visual acuity
- Loss of the flap

Prevention
- Copious lubrication
- Aggressive treatment of epithelial ingrowth

Treatment
- Lift the flap
- Clean the interface
- Use a bandage contact lens
- Use topical antibiotic and lubricant treatment
- Carefully monitor
- Perform a homoplastic lamellar transplant as a last resort

traindicate these as well. Luckily, the majority of patients improve with time. With bilateral treatment, the patient usually learns to ignore optical aberrations as a result of cortical integration.

Tips for prevention: multiple ablation algorithms have been attempted to achieve improved visual results in terms of quantity and quality, but all have to balance ablation diameter against ablation depth according to Munnerlyn's formula. A multizone or aspheric zone technique can be used with some broadbeam lasers to reduce ablation depth while attempting to maximize the effective optic zone, however the true effective optic zone remains small.

Flying spot lasers with newer software may be used to enlarge the effective optic zone, even with a residual refractive error near emmetropia if there is adequate residual corneal tissue for additional ablation.

Stromal Clouding and Haze in the Interface

Although rare, stromal haze following LASIK may appear even several months after the operation. Normally, it is associated with the correction of severe refractive errors and correlates with a certain amount of regression. The appearance is similar to that found in cases of PRK but it is less serious, as Bowman's membrane is not involved.

In some rare cases, slight haze can be observed as intrastromal edema due to direct photoablation or as a toxic cellular reaction to certain substances used in the operation (toxic residues from substances used to sterilize the materials) or the presence of debris in the interface.

This type of haze is transitory and normally disappears within a matter of weeks, following 2 to 3 weeks of treatment with an appropriate topical steroid.

Corneal Ectasia and Keratoconus

Preoperative pachymetry measurement is mandatory. This is essential so that the surgery can be planned to allow adequate residual corneal tissue following the creation of the flap and excimer ablation removal. Residual tissue resists the internal pressure of the eye so there will be corneal ectasia or true iatrogenic keratoconus. Actually, studies indicate that the important factor is not the final total postoperative thickness but the thickness of the residual stroma.

Preoperatively, the planned flap thickness results from taking into consideration the initial corneal thickness and the depth of the planned tissue ablation, so as to leave a bed with sufficient stromal depth. At least 200 microns, and preferably 250 microns, of stroma must be left in situ at the end of the ablation. A corneal flap of 160 microns is preferred when available, as it is easier to handle and less likely to develop striae, but a flap of 130 microns may be necessary with high corrections. At the end of the operation, total central thickness should be at least 350 to 400 microns. It has been shown that most flaps are thinner than actually predicted by the depth plate. The surgeon should perform intraoperative pachymetry to get a feel for the actual flap thickness he or she is achieving with a given depth plate. With my microkeratomes, Buratto typically achieves 140 microns with a 160 plate and 160 microns with a 180 plate.

Another school of thought is that the corneal flap added to the depth of the ablation should total less than 50% of the total corneal thickness. Munnerlyn's formula allows the calculation of stroma that must be removed for a given treatment diameter and amount. The formula is: ablation depth = optic zone^2 x diopters/3.

Generally, considered a contraindication, some surgeons have used LASIK to treat patients with keratoconus. To the present time, there has been no disease progression or additional postoperative corneal ectasia if a residual stroma of appropriate thickness is maintained. It is more difficult to calculate ablation depth considering the thickness of the cornea affected by keratoconus. We do not advocate performing LASIK on patients with keratoconus.

In summary, thickness of the residual corneal bed is the most important factor in avoiding ectasia and/or iatrogenic keratoconus. Cases of corneal ectasia and keratoconus that result from deep ablations combined with thick flaps have been reported, simply because with insufficient residual stroma even a thick flap is not able to prevent ectasia. If this serious complication occurs, penetrating keratoplasty will be required because of loss of transparency of the deep stroma and poor optics.

Flap Wrinkling and Traction Folds

Fine wrinkles of the flap due to shrinkage or traction may appear postoperatively.

Cause

Inadequate symmetric distension of the flap/cap at the end of the operation. The surgeon should inspect the cornea under high magnification at the end of surgery, especially ensuring that the gutter is small, and—more importantly—symmetrical around the resection margins. If there are folds or if the gutter is asymmetric, lift the flap, refloat it into place, and reposition it appropriately, taking care to smooth it with no displacement.

Postoperative partial displacement of the flap that must be immediately repositioned.

A deep ablation with a relatively small optic zone; the alignment of the two surfaces will not be uniform and the flap has a tendency to develop horizontal striae. In these cases, additional stroking and smoothing should be performed in all directions to attempt to minimize striae formation.

The folds are also the expression of areas of greater traction, such as when single interrupted sutures have been used. Fortunately, sutures are rarely needed.

Symptoms

If the folds are present in the visual axis, they can create irritating reflections and distortion, with decreased uncorrected and best-corrected vision. They seem to induce a small amount of hyperopia.

Tips for prevention: A superior hinge LASIK operation is performed because the natural blinking movement tends to maintain flap position and constantly smooth it.

The flap must be carefully inspected at the end of the operation, with immediate repositioning in the case of folds or an asymmetric gutter. Some surgeons recommend the use of a contact lens to reduce folds, but we feel the manipulations necessary for lens insertion and removal, and associated tearing, actually favor fold formation.

Management

There is usually spontaneous resolution of traction folds some weeks after suture removal. If folds are seen at the end of the operation, refloating and positioning should be done as described. Folds and striae that have been neglected by the surgeon, may be treated weeks or even months after the surgery, though the success rate declines with passing time. The technique is the same except that after the flap has been lifted and refloated, folds typically appear much more prominent than they previously did at the slit lamp. The principle of flap centration and peripheral smoothing is the same, except that much more vigorous "ironing" with the smooth side of a spatula or forceps (to distend the flap so that it fully fills the bed) is required. The epithelial surface should be allowed to dry so that adequate traction smoothing instrument is achieved. Similarly, dry Merocel sponges on a dry corneal surface may be used. After this 8 to 12-minute process, the epithelium is usually in poor condition and a bandage contact lens as well as careful follow-up is required, as described in the section on *Epithelial Defects* in this chapter.

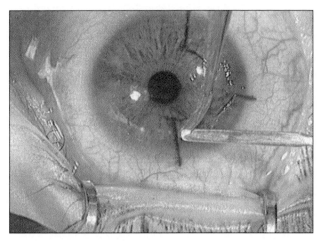

Figure 8-94. The flap is lifted with a spatula.

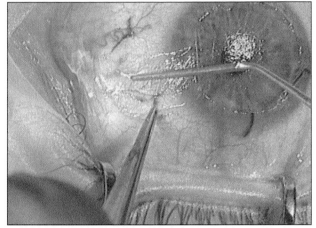

Figure 8-95. The flap is reflected nasally with a spatula and repeatedly smoothed.

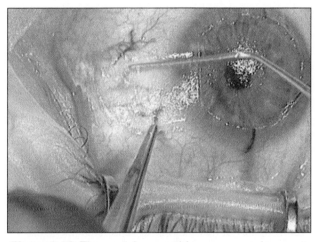

Figure 8-96. The spatula smoothing maneuver is repeated several times.

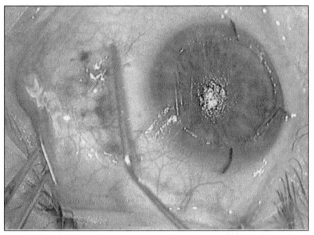

Figure 8-97. The spatula maneuvers are performed in a direction orthogonal to the previous one. Again in this direction, the spatula maneuver is repeated several times.

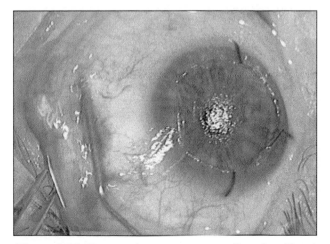

Figure 8-98. For spatula maneuvers, continue for at least 2 to 3 minutes in each direction.

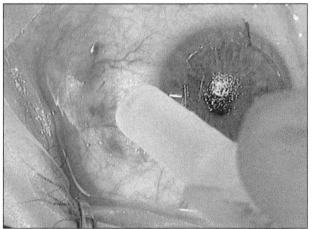

Figure 8-99. Finally, the flap is wet with a hypotonic solution to induce edema.

Epithelial Ingrowth

Definition

The proliferation of epithelial cells in the interface (ie, in the virtual space obtained with the lamellar cut). The incidence is about 2% and is usually observed in the first 2 to 3 weeks following surgery. With experience, incidence declines to 1% as the surgeon learns the maneuvers necessary to avoid introduction of epithelial cells into the interface. The incidence is higher with enhancement cases using flap lifting techniques and in hyperopic treatments.

Cause

- Poor adhesion of the flap to the stroma
- Introduction of epithelial cells during the micro-keratome cut
- Manipulation of the intrastromal surfaces
- The flap folding over on itself during surgery
- Incomplete irrigation and cleaning of the interface
- Previous radial keratotomy
- Epithelial abrasions at the edges of the flap
- Poor flap alignment
- Thin and buttonholed flaps
- Free caps
- Excessive ablation at the stromal bed margin (typically hyperopic treatments)
- Epithelial irregularities at the flap edges and bed with enhancement techniques

Risk Factors

- Anterior basement membrane dystrophy
- Recurrent corneal erosions
- Elderly patients
- History of epithelial ingrowth in the fellow eye

Symptoms

Clinically, the patient may be asymptomatic or he or she may have a foreign body sensation due to the irregularity of the epithelium. In general, the cells enter and proliferate at the peripheral margin and do not involve the visual axis, at least initially.

If epithelial ingrowth progresses centrally, visual acuity is affected. The topography and refraction are altered, inducing regular and irregular astigmatism and best corrected and uncorrected visual acuity. More importantly, these changes may be permanent due to melting of the adjacent stroma, thus immediate intervention is needed.

Diagnosis

Diagnosis of epithelial growth is performed by:

- Slit lamp examination
- Corneal topography
- Retroillumination with a dilated pupil

With direct tangential slit lamp illumination an area of epithelial growth that extends from the edge of the flap and has a spiral aspect can be seen. The edge of the flap may be gray, wrinkled, or necrotic. Fluorescein uptake may be seen at the edge or in the interface. Epithelial ingrowth can also be highlighted with retroillumination with the pupil dilated. Epithelial ingrowth is seen more frequently temporally when the hinge is nasal and inferiorly, or along the hinge, when the hinge is superior.

Evolution

Epithelial ingrowth and progression takes many forms. It may be central or peripheral, rapidly growing, stationary, or self-limiting. In the areas of previous epithelial ingrowth, haze may be observed that may also be present in areas with active growth. There may be surface irregularities corresponding to areas of epithelial ingrowth, which can be documented with corneal topography. In its most innocuous form, ingrowth appears as a fine white line at the edge of the flap, or as peripheral spots limited to the outer 2.0 mm of the flap edge. This form usually does not progress and may actually regress, but needs to be observed for at least 3 months. The more aggressive forms that tend to grow and, in general, require treatment are pearl-like, small islands, cysts (30 to 70 microns in size), sheaths, colonies, and strands. The final shape is usually a sheath. Regression is rarely seen and treatment should be initiated. Epithelial ingrowth may progress at the beginning and then be static or progress to stromal melting; the stroma found between the epithelium in the interface and the epithelium of the surface may become necrotic and melt secondary to collagenase release.

Care to preserve flap epithelium and closely approximate the peripheral gutter with good edge adherence is the key to prevention.

Management

Treatment is indicated when the epithelial ingrowth exceeds 2.0 mm from the flap edge, if progression is observed, if melting occurs, if it affects visual acuity, or if it induces astigmatism.

The specific treatment depends on the situation: if epithelial cells are present centrally, visual acuity is decreased due to the presence of cells, irregular astigmatism, and undercorrection. Cells must always be removed. Removal must be immediate to prevent extension of the cell mass and secondary stromal melting.

If areas of epithelialization are peripheral and do not affect the refraction or keratometry, they can be moni-

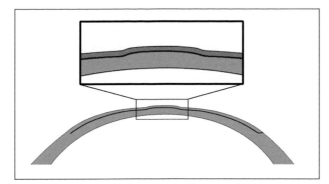

Figure 8-100. Central island with a magnified close-up.

tored regularly by biomicroscopy and photography during the postoperative checks to ensure that the situation is stable and not progressive.

In some cases, there may be spontaneous regression and disappearance of some moderately sized epithelial islands in the peripheral or paracentral zones. In order to evaluate whether there has been progression, the patient must simply be monitored 1 and 2 weeks, then 1, 2, and 3 months after surgery. If the epithelium does not disturb the patient's vision and is in the outer 2.0 mm with a demarcation line, it is probably safer to leave it alone, considering that removal may create folds or irregular astigmatism.

Machat has presented his classification regarding epithelial ingrowth on the basis of whether surgical intervention is required or not.

Machat Classification of Epithelial Ingrowth

Grade 1

Thin ingrowth, one or two cells in thickness, limited to 2.0 mm from the flap edge. Almost transparent and often difficult to identify. Often outlined by a white demarcation line along the front of the epithelial progression. Not associated with alterations to the flap and nonprogressive. No treatment is required, but the patient should be monitored at least monthly at first. This degree of ingrowth is more frequently seen at the margin of the bed when there has been enhancement with a poor flap lifting technique or at the time of enhancement in a previously unrecognized case.

Grade 2

The ingrowth is thicker and single cells can be seen inside the zone of epithelial growth. The area of ingrowth extents more than 2.0 mm from the flap edge. The cells are opalescent and easily identifiable at the slit lamp. There is no demarcation line. The edge of the corneal flap is normally thickened and may be rolled or gray.

Melting or erosion of the flap edges has not occurred. Normally, this condition is progressive. It does not require urgent treatment, but treatment should be planned within 2 to 3 weeks if there is any evidence of progression.

Grade 3

The ingrowth is marked and has a multicellular thickness. It exceeds the 2.0 mm distance from the flap margin. It is seen clearly at the slit lamp as an opacity. There are white areas of necrotic epithelial cells without the demarcation line; the edges of the corneal flap are usually wrinkled and appear eroded, thickened, white, or gray. Grade 3 progresses to areas of corneal melting secondary to the release of collagenase by the necrotic cells. Confluent haze develops peripherally at the edge of the flap as the flap detaches, leaving the stromal bed exposed to the epithelial surface. Urgent treatment is required with intensive follow-up. Frequent follow-up exams are necessary because the fact that the edges have been eroded means that recurrence is likely, which once again initiates the cycle.

Removal Techniques

If treatment is needed, one of several techniques may be used:

1. The flap may be lifted. The periphery of the flap nearest the epithelial island is lifted with the patient lying under the microscope (lifting is easier because of epithelial cells at the interface and lack of fibrosis). The surgeon looks for the demarcation line indicating the edge of the flap and incises the epithelium at the edge with a sharp Sinskey hook or one arm of a jeweler's forceps. Then, using two forceps, the peripheral portion of the flap is grasped and gently lifted without touching the central flap. Using a spatula (Suarez type) or chalazion curette, the epithelial island, which normally has a globular, cystic, almost encapsulated shape, is removed. (The stromal bed must also be cleaned even though the epithelium is normally adherent to the underside of the flap. The instrument used to clean (it must be cleaned after every stroke to avoid re-introducing epithelial cells. Alcohol, cocaine, and other toxic substances should not be used). Irrigation and brushing may be used if there is any doubt about total removal of the epithelium. Paying close attention, the surgeon should be able to remove all the material with a single stroke, reducing the chance of leaving cells and recurrence. If more than one pass of the spatula is needed, the two surfaces should be gently

scraped. Irrigation with abundant BSS to remove any residual cells and other debris from the interface should be done. It is advisable to direct the jet of irrigating BSS obliquely to the surface to be cleaned, using the flow to remove any occult cells or debris. Washing should always be in the same direction to allow the debris and cells to flow out of the interface. Once cleaning has been completed, the flap edges are reapproximated.

2. Incision and squeezing. A straight cut is made in the flap margin to reach the interface. The material is then squeezed out. If the growth is only in the periphery, squeezing is performed toward the edge. While this procedure is simple and quick, recurrence is frequent.

3. Removal using an Nd: YAG laser (for small peripheral epithelial islands only). The YAG laser, at a power level of 0.6 to 1.2 mJ, is slightly retrofocused to the epithelial plaque and 30 to 40 pulses are applied. The patient is re-examined 2 to 3 weeks later, and the procedure repeated, if necessary.

4. In severe ingrowth with melting and folds, it is better to remove the flap and allow healing, as with a PRK.

Stromal Melting

Definition

Stromal melting is the destruction of the normal stromal connective structure with thinning or abscess of portions of the flap.

Extremely rarely, days, weeks, or months after surgery there may be signs of epithelial and subepithelial tissue deterioration and thinning, caused by poor wetting by the tear film and subsequent lack of oxygen. Thus, all of the conditions associated with poor blinking or all tear film pathologies can easily lead to melting.

Predisposing Factors

Lacrimal pathologies such as ocular discomfort syndrome, filamentary keratoconjunctivitis, giant-cell keratoconjunctivitis, or decreased blinking (dehydration and exposure of the inferior segment of the flap) are predisposing factors. Moreover, patients with a thinner than normal flap or with epithelial ingrowth are at risk for stromal melting.

Symptoms

This alteration may be asymptomatic initially, may be perceived only as a foreign body sensation, or may be heralded by nonspecific symptoms, such as photophobia, mild pain, and blurry vision. It may also have a very rapid onset.

Diagnosis

The diagnosis is made with slit lamp examination. Objectively, the flap appears irregularly thin. It progressively loses transparency, and the anatomic integrity in the affected area appears to be precarious. There are erosions and areas of tissue loss initially appearing at the peripheral subepithelial portions of the flap. Compared to the normal postoperative edge scar, with melting there is an uneven white border with poorly defined edges, cysts, and epithelial inclusions. If these lesions are not treated aggressively, they may evolve into true melting of the stroma, ulceration, and infection of the flap. Loss of stromal tissue must be prevented if good anatomic and functional recovery is to be achieved. With delayed diagnosis, inadequate treatment, or poor tissue response to treatment, necrosis of the flap spreads with loss of flap integrity. This may require removal and replacement with a homoplastic flap.

Tip for prevention: the cornea must be kept well lubricated during and after the operation (using nonpreserved artificial tears and ointment, cyclosporin A, and punctum plugs as necessary). Treatment of epithelial ingrowth must be prompt.

Treatment

The flap should be lifted. It may not be possible to do this smoothly due to tissue alterations. The flap undersurface and stromal bed must be cleaned and gently debrided with a smooth spatula; all debris, impurities, or epithelial nests must be removed. The flap is then smoothed and repositioned following irrigation of the stromal surfaces with BSS. A bandage contact lens is recommended if significant epithelial defects are present. Treatment continues with topical antibiotic and tear substitutes under strict follow-up.

Despite aggressive management, melting may still occur. There may be necrosis of the flap with extension and loss of anatomic integrity of the flap itself. This situation requires rapid removal of the flap to avoid infection or necrosis spreading to deeper stromal layers. The damaged flap may require replacement with a homoplastic flap. (Remember the lamellar cut has no refractive power!) Homograph flap transplantation may induce a more intensive tissue repair response, with tissue haze requiring steroid treatment. It may also create peripheral epithelial hyperplasia of the flap, with induction of transient hyperopia.

Corneal Striae

Definition

The corneal flap has folds and wrinkles, which may

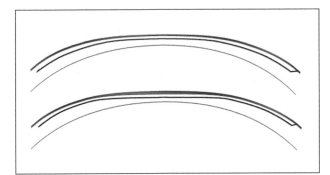

Figure 8-101. Top: normal epithelial thickness. Bottom: the epithelium has thickened—there is regression.

or may not reduce vision. Postoperative corneal striae result from:

- Prolonged folding on itself during the procedure
- Poor alignment of the flap during repositioning
- Slight flap displacement in the immediate postoperative period (ie, squeezing or excessive rubbing of the eyelids)
- Patients with high myopia; in these deep ablations, there may be poor conformance of the flap to the concavity
- A short hinge: the flap is unstable with increased risk of striae
- Asymmetrical or pear-shaped cut: forces across the bed are distributed unevenly making it easy for the flap to move with formation of striae
- Excessive and prolonged manipulation of the flap
- Flap striae test performed poorly, inducing striae

Symptoms

The striae induce irregular astigmatism and often induce hyperopia with reduction of best-corrected visual acuity.

Diagnosis

Striae are generally seen on postoperative day 1 at the slit lamp. They may be peripheral or central. Generally, striae are central if the flap is uneven in an area more than 1 mm from the margin. Normally the striae are oriented horizontally with a nasal hinge. The flap has a tendency to rotate in a counter-clockwise direction. Diagnosis may also be made during the operation itself if an oblique light source is available. Striae are usually identified the following day at the slit lamp after stromal edema has resolved. The index of suspicion begins with a reduction in best-corrected visual acuity, secondary to regular or irregular astigmatism. The diagnosis is confirmed at the slit lamp or with examination of the dilated pupil with retroillumination. If the striae are peripheral, indirect light of the slit lamp on the iris can highlight

them. Fluorescein dye may be used. Striae will be visible secondary to accumulation of the dye along the folds.

Treatment

If the striae cause a reduction in visual acuity or irritation to the eye, or if they are central, they must be treated. Otherwise, treatment is not necessary if visual acuity is as expected. Surgical treatment should take place as soon as possible. Normally, striae are visible even 1 hour postoperatively. Early management is easy, becoming more difficult the longer they are neglected. First, the surgeon must mark the location of the striae at the slit lamp. The patient is then transferred to the operating microscope. The flap is raised and reflected, using a cyclodialysis-type spatula. The flap is reflected nasally; the stromal surface of the flap is hydrated with filtered BSS, which swells the flap, making it easier to manipulate and replace, then smooth and stretch. The flap is repositioned and the edge is stretched toward the gutter. Depending on how long the striae have been present, stretching may be accompanied by anything from a slightly moist sponge, to a dry sponge, to the blunt edge of a forceps. The surgeon presses on the flap in a direction perpendicular to the striae, stretching and smoothing the flap. This takes several minutes, as the effect improves with time; and time must be allowed for the flap to adhere to its new position. Retroillumination serves to check whether the striae have disappeared. Improvement is not immediately visible. When good approximation is obtained, an antibiotic, steroid, and NSAID are instilled into the eye. The eye is then closed.

Twenty to 30 minutes later, the surgeon checks the eye; some striae usually persist but usually disappear after a few days. If they do not, the treatment may be repeated after 1 month. If for some reason the striae are neglected, there may be permanent loss in best-corrected visual acuity. The flap may require removal to reduce image distortion. Flap striae can be treated even after several months, but treatment becomes more difficult. The flap can be raised and detached from the stromal bed, even 1 year after surgery. At this point, the undersurface of the flap is treated with 10 microns of PTK; if there is residual myopia, the stromal bed is treated with a refractive ablation. If there is hyperopia, the surgeon should always remember that irregular astigmatism might be the cause and should not be treated, pending resolution of the striae. The use of PTK on the undersurface of the flap theoretically frees adhesions and allows the flap to be smoothed and stretched, reducing or eliminating the striae. The flap is then repositioned on the bed and stretched symmetrically for 8 to 10 minutes toward the peripheral gutter. The epithelial surface is allowed to dry and a spatula or the blunt edge of tying forceps is used to stretch the edges of the flap towards the edges of the stromal bed. An eight-bite antitorque suture to keep the flap stretched for several days has helped with resistant striae, but it may create regular or irregular astigmatism, or even new striae.

Abnormal Topography: Central Islands

Definition

A central or paracentral elevated area as measured with corneal topography, between 1 and 3 D in height with a diameter of between 1.0 to 3.0 mm due to localized central ablation deficiency.

Central islands are the most common topographic alteration following excimer laser treatment (PRK and LASIK). They are typically seen with excess hydration of the stromal bed during ablation or when optic zones 6.0 mm or greater in diameter are used with a broadbeam laser without incorporated anticentral island pretreatment. Lasers with an expanding diaphragm are more likely to create central islands than lasers with scanning beams, which have a lower-intensity acoustic shockwave.

Cause

Central islands are often multifactorial. Several suggestions have been made as to their cause:

1. Focal central epithelial hyperplasia. This applies only to PRK using laser epithelial removal and not to LASIK.
2. Vortex plume theory. The cloud created by debris from the ablation forms a central vortex, which shields the successive laser pulses. This has been demonstrated with high-speed photography.
3. Deterioration of laser optics. In reality, central islands can also be seen with carefully checked or new optics.
4. Theory of acoustic shockwave/differential hydration. Every pulse produces a shockwave, the shape of which is correlated to the energy profile and size of the laser beam. This shockwave has been demonstrated with special photographic techniques. The intraoperative stromal hydration is induced by the shockwave. Every pulse produces fluid. Shockwaves are formed secondary to the recoil from cloud formation. Lasers with a flat homogenous energy profile induce an accumulation of fluid centrally, which reduces the ablation. As a result, central islands appear. Nitrogen flow reduces this central accumulation of liquid, however induced haze with PRK and is no longer used. Scanning lasers produce very small shockwaves, thus central islands have not been seen

with them. At present the following reasoning seems valid: the occurrence of central islands is secondary to differential hydration of the corneal stroma (the central stroma is hydrated to a greater degree than the peripheral area and is therefore more resistant to photoablation because of the lower acoustic shockwave).

Predisposing Factors

- Older broadbeam lasers without anticentral island software
- Nonhomogenous beam that is "colder" in the center

Symptoms

Symptoms include blurred vision, fluctuation in vision, ghost images, and monocular diplopia that may be difficult to quantify with instruments. The patient's uncorrected vision is usually better than the postoperative refractive error would suggest.

Diagnosis

Biomicroscopy does not reveal central islands, but they may be seen with retinoscopy of the dilated pupil. At the time of this writing, only topography is capable of really documenting central islands, with elevation mapping being superior to placido disc mapping. Topographically, they appear as a central elevation (warm colors) 2.0 to 3.0 mm in diameter inside an outer flat area (cold color).

Tips for prevention: prevention is the best form of treatment. Broadbeam lasers now incorporate either automatic or surgeon adjustable anticentral island pretreatment software. Hydration of the corneal stroma during treatment should be closely watched. Some surgeons allow for slight central hydration, others remove excess fluid during the procedure. Blowing filtered compressed air over the surface or wiping with sponges or spatulas during the operation can reduce hydration. These are useful aids to avoid accumulation of liquid at the stroma. However, there is one advantage: stromal hydration improves the patient's fixation and reduces irregular astigmatism.

Central island pretreatment consists of an initial ablation of 30 to 40 pulses at a central corneal zone of 2.5 mm. Generally, pretreatment consists of a 1-micron ablation for every diopter; with multizone treatment, 0.6 microns is sufficient. This preoperative treatment has also been proved to produce a better final visual outcome.

Treatment

Central islands should be treated conservatively, as

they may tend to resolve spontaneously, though not as successfully as with PRK, which forces the epithelium to undergo more extensive remodeling. Patient reassurance is needed pending possible laser retreatment. Statistics demonstrate the incidence of central islands with broad-beam lasers is 80% in the first postoperative week, with a drop to 15% after 3 months and 5% after 6 months. When it persists for 6 months or more, one should consider treatment by laser ablation. Central islands are not seen with the flying spot laser. The amount of correction and diameter of the optic zone to be corrected depend on the corneal topography, according to Munnerlyn's formula. In order to avoid a hyperopic shift, the conservative approach is recommended. It is better to slightly undercorrect. Treatment involves raising the original flap and then using laser ablation, treat with PRK or PTK mode centrally where the islands are found.

Retinal Vascular Occlusion

For a perfect lamellar cut with the microkeratome, IOP must be raised. Bengerer's studies suggested that the ocular pressure should be at least 60 mm Hg and now many surgeons prefer 100 mm Hg. The question is often asked: can this pressure cause complications? Let us consider blood pressure. Arterial pressure is not a problem unless there is slight hypotension—in this case, the diastolic pressure could reach levels below that of the intra-operative IOP. Theoretically, there could be retinal vascular occlusion due to prolonged raised ocular pressure. This is more likely in patients with vasculopathies or diabetes. Venous blood pressure could possibly be lower than that measured inside the eye. Venous occlusion as opposed to arterial occlusion would therefore appear to be more likely. In actuality, literature does not report any case of venous or arterial retinal occlusion due to LASIK. It is possible that this is due to the short time in which IOP is raised. It is not known how long the eye pressure can remain elevated. However, no more than 2 to 3 minutes is advised. If the procedure becomes prolonged with the IOP elevated, it is better to abort the procedure. There are situations, such as vitreoretinal surgery or ophthalmodynamometry, during which raised IOP causes retinal vascular occlusion. Apparently even in these cases the risk would appear to be theoretical and not real.

REFRACTIVE COMPLICATIONS

As previously stated, postoperative complications are either anatomic or optical/refractive.

Optical/refractive complications:
- Irregular astigmatism
- Undercorrection
- Overcorrection
- Regression

Overcorrection is defined as achieving greater than the desired result. Undercorrection is achieving less than the desired result. Undercorrection must be distinguished from regression, in which the surgical result is not stable and the refractive effect decreases over time. Some studies have shown that the refractive result with LASIK is stable after about 3 months. Others show that 90% of the desired result is present 1 week after surgery. Variations from this statistical data outlines the regression pattern.

The surgeon should continuously input his or her postoperative results and monitor the achieved versus desired result. He or she can then modify the nomogram on the basis of these results, giving more precision using his or her own laser and operating environment.

Irregular Astigmatism

Definition

Irregular astigmatism is astigmatism with an irregular topographical pattern not correctable with spectacles and only with a rigid contact lens.

Improvements in LASIK technique have lead to a decrease in the induction of irregular astigmatism immediately postoperative. Low amounts of irregular astigmatism are quite common. For the most part, this disappears within the first few weeks or sometimes months. Less than 1 to 2% of patients develop irregular astigmatism that results in a permanent loss of two or more lines of BCVA. With less experienced surgeons, this percentage may reach 5% to 10%.

Causes
- Intraoperative problems (irregular or uneven cut), which translate into an uneven bed and uneven ablation
- Poor suture technique (this was the most frequent cause in the past when sutures were routinely used in this type of surgery), now a suture is rarely needed
- Decentration of the refractive ablation
- Incorrect flap repositioning at the end of surgery
- Folds in the flap
- Debris in the interface
- Epithelial ingrowth
- Incorrect marking of the axis of astigmatism to be treated
- Abnormal patient head position during the laser ablation
- Pre-existing irregular astigmatism (topography)
- Poor keratectomy (damaged or malfunctioning blade)

Table 8-33

DIFFERENTIAL DIAGNOSIS

Infective keratitis	**Sands of the Sahara syndrome**
Appears after 24 to 48 hours	Appears after 12 to 24 hours
Pain	Absence of or minimal pain*
Globe is soft to touch	Globe has normal consistency*
	Marked decrease in vision
	Slight decrease in vision
Objective findings related to symptoms and appearance	Objective findings not related to symptoms, even at stage 4
Treatment response to antibiotics	Treatment response to steroids

*At stages 1, 2, 3

- Incomplete, irregular, or decentered keratectomy

The most important of these factors is decentration of the ablation.

Tips for prevention: appropriate surgical technique must be used, particularly during the flap repositioning step. It must be replaced as accurately as possible. The size of the hinge is very important: a large hinge will better guide the flap to its natural alignment. Drying the flap with compressed air may cause the flap to unevenly shrink. If the surgeon recognizes a potential risk of irregular astigmatism, decentration of keratectomy, irregular keratectomy, etc, it is advisable to postpone the ablation, replace the flap and wait 3 to 4 months, then recut a new flap. Because the ablation has not been performed, repositioning the flap even after a bad keratectomy returns the patient to the preoperative situation. Performing the ablation on an uneven bed leads to irreversible irregular astigmatism.

Treatment

If the irregular astigmatism is secondary to an irregular keratectomy, an excimer laser PTK can be performed on the stroma prior to a successive refractive laser ablation. With irreversible irregular astigmatism, a rigid contact lens may be required.

Astigmatism Caused by Decentration of the Ablation

There are greater problems when the astigmatism is caused by decentration of the refractive treatment. Decentration of the laser ablation is a serious complication that is not easily remedied. It is due to poor fixation by the patient, poor fixation by the surgeon, or improper head position (head should be parallel to the floor). In cases of severe myopia and hyperopia, poor uncorrected visual acuity in addition to difficulty seeing through the cornea with the flap reflected may be the explanation for the patient not properly fixating. In these cases, passive fixation may be of assistance. A surgeon using the suction ring or a Thornton-type stabilizing device to center the eye will facilitate this. Eye-tracking systems have been incorporated into many excimer lasers and help avoid decentration. In these cases the patient sees across the sloping edge of the ablation, inducing irregular astigmatism, and resulting in loss of BCVA, diplopia, and ghost images.

With undercorrection, retreatment with the excimer laser may be attempted by slightly decentering treatment in the opposite direction using a large optic zone once the flap has been raised. The asymmetry is corrected by a complementary ablation. If a hyperopic correction is decentered, it will be aggravated by the fact that the thin part of the cornea may be located in the visual axis and additional ablation may be impossible, as there may be dangerous thinning of the cornea. In the event of a highly decentered ablation, penetrating keratoplasty is always an option.

Recently, Pallikaris described a method for moving the center of the ablation by creating arcuate incisions opposite to the decentered ablation. Decentrations greater than 1.0 mm have been corrected with considerable improvement in symptoms reported by the patient. With regular astigmatism, the surgical options are astigmatic keratectomy, LASIK with topolink, or LTK.

Undercorrection

Definition

Undercorrection means that even in the first postoperative month, there is residual, unexpected refractive error. Undercorrection is seen more frequently in high myopia above 10 to 12 D. In these cases, the surgeon may choose to err on the side of undercorrection rather than run the risk of overcorrection. It is easier to correct residual myopia than it is to correct hyperopia from overcorrection.

Cause

Undercorrection results from:

- Incorrect preoperative refraction (most common)
- Difficulty in performing a precise refractive evaluation (severe myopia with staphyloma, etc)
- Incorrect data entry in the laser computer
- Incomplete or decentered ablation
- Incorrect interpretation of the nomogram
- Unstable ametropia

Tips for prevention: correct evaluation of the refraction, avoid patients with unstable refraction, correct interpretation and setting the laser software, and correct postoperative management.

Treatment

Residual myopia will usually not please the patient. It may create anisometropia with the fellow eye and require temporary or permanent refractive aids. In all these cases, retreatment should be considered 2 or 3 months later, waiting longer in high myopia for stabilization.

There are several methods available for treating undercorrection:

1. Photoablative treatment in situ (lifting the flap and reablation). This is usually performed within 3 to 4 months of the first treatment and, generally speaking, no later than month 6. By this time, the patient's eye will have normally reached refractive stability and the wound will allow the flap to be delineated and lifted from the stromal bed without great difficulty. The surgeon looks for the faint scar between the flap and the uncut cornea. To do this, pressure on the center of the cornea is applied, allowing the surgeon identify the edge of the flap. A sharp Sinskey hook is used to demarcate the margin and incise the epithelium. At this point, the flap is held under tension with a fine-toothed forceps and lifted gently from the stromal bed using a blunt spatula to break any adhesions. This process exposes the underlying bed for successive ablation. It is preferable to use the largest optic zone allowed by the new corneal hinge. The flap is then gently redistended in its original position. The interface is hydrated to allow sutureless closure. Sutures are rarely needed.

This technique has a number of advantages:

- It is as fast as the original LASIK, but less complicated because there is no cut with the microkeratome
- Visual recovery is rapid
- Problems with haze, typical of PRK, are avoided
- Wound healing has a head start
- Very high errors of myopia and astigmatism can be corrected, as with the lamellar technique

This technique is preferable to a recut (ie, a LASIK with a new microkeratome cut) for a number of reasons:

- Risks inherent to the microkeratome cut are avoided
- It is very difficult to center the new flap on the previous one
- There is a high probability of cutting another layer, thus creating a double interface with dangling tissue

There are also some disadvantages:

- It is a surgical procedure complete with all the risks, the greatest being epithelial ingrowth at the interface
- Attention must be paid to the measurement of corneal thickness when evaluating the ablation depth to leave adequate residual bed

2. Lamellar technique or recutting a new flap (for myopias greater than 10 D). This should be performed at least 6 months after the initial surgical treatment. The in-situ operation is repeated with a slightly deeper cut than the primary cut (a 180-micron plate is normally used) and entering peripheral to the original cut, if possible.

3. Incisional techniques are an option but are not very predictable. They act on tissue that has already been flattened and where there is a different thickness between the centroparacentral and peripheral portions of the cornea.

4. Surface photoablation technique (PRK). Postoperative haze is significantly greater than in virgin eyes. This outcome and an unpredictable response rules this out as a real choice.

5. Homoplastic refractive keratomileusis. This is useful in extreme situations with significant flap opacity.

Overcorrection

If, 1 month after surgery, there is a refractive correction that exceeds the expected value, this is an overcorrection.

Causes

- Incorrect preoperative refraction
- Incorrect data entry into the laser computer
- Poor control of humidity levels in the laser room (too dry). This will create a certain degree of corneal dehydration, which is translated into refractive overcorrection. This is typically seen at high altitudes before satisfactory nomogram adjustment is achieved.

Tips for prevention:
- Precise evaluation of the refractive error
- Correct laser setting
- Appropriate humidity levels in the surgical room
- Careful attention to nomogram development
- Extra caution in the presbyopic age group

Symptoms

Compared to undercorrection, overcorrection will lead to greater discomfort and dissatisfaction of the patient. It is also more difficult to treat.

Treatment

The treatment possibilities are as follows:

1. LASIK (lifting the flap and re-ablating). Similar to myopic retreatment, it is possible to repeat the treatment for hyperopic values within 2 to 3 months. The surgeon raises the flap and performs a paraperipheral ablation of the anterior stromal bed, if the laser used has the capability of hyperopic ablation. It may be preferable to wait longer than with undercorrection to allow more time for regression. In addition, a larger flap may be necessary (recut) to allow the hyperopic correction and a recut should be done no sooner than 4 to 6 months.

2. Hyperopic surface photoablation (hyperopic PRK). This is not a central procedure, so it creates fewer functional problems correlated to the degree of haze generated, which will be greater than haze in virgin corneas. Hyperopia of 1 to 3 D can be corrected.

3. LTK with holmium laser (for hyperopia of 3 to 4 D). A fiber optic tip is used for contact (or noncontact technique) to produce localized corneal coagulation. The coagulated areas will create steepening of the central cornea with a subsequent decrease in the positive power. This can only be performed at least 3 months after surgery and should preferably be performed in an area external to the lamellar cut, as this will also limit any overcorrection that may occur due to the varied corneal consistency and shape. Treatment with the holmium laser should overcorrect, as there is a clear tendency to regress in time. It works better in older patients.

4. Incisional techniques with hexagonal keratotomy (for hyperopia of about 3 D). Hexagonal incisions are performed at about 90% of the depth with respect to the pachymetry readings in the incision zone and on the basis of topographic information using the nomogram presented by Mendez in 1986. The technique has been abandoned because of the unpredictable results.

5. Retreatment by hyperopic ALK. This technique is rarely used and may be useful with residual errors of 7 to 10 D. Following Casebeer's nomogram, the optic zone is considerably reduced with a resection thickness of 75% of the central pachymetry value. Correction is calculated as the relationship between the diameter and thickness of the cut. The technique involves a single cut with the microkeratome (the intrastromal refractive cut in this case is not performed). This technique has been almost completely abandoned.

6. Homoplastic keratomileusis for refractive error, as previously discussed.

7. Implantation of a positive refractive IOL.

Regression

Definition

Regression indicates that the refractive result of the LASIK procedure is not stable with continuing loss of effect over a few months.

Regression normally stops between 1 and 3 months after surgery. With slight to moderate myopia, refractive stability is reached at about 3 months postoperatively; with high myopia, stability is reached at about 6 months postoperatively.

Cause

No one has yet been able to give a good explanation for this phenomenon. Considering that the deep stroma is inert, regression should not occur. It may be due to a combination of epithelial hyperplasia and remodeling the stroma. The epithelium becomes thicker in response to flattening of the cornea. Large optic zones can reduce or limit the factors that cause central epithelial hyperplasia; these present a smooth and more progressive profile to the anterior corneal curvature. Moreover, central fibrosis is visible under corneal flaps of patients with severe myopia within the ablation area. This signals a certain degree of active stromal reshaping. In some patients, this fibrous reaction appears as reticular haze. These cases generally involve patients with myopia greater than 10 D and an excessively wet interface during ablation.

These patients have a marked wound-tissue reaction with myopic regression. Raising the flap for retreatment may prove difficult even early in the postoperative period. Rarely, there have been cases in which haze has developed at the interface several weeks after surgery (not to be confused with Sands of the Sahara syndrome), which may reduce acuity and quality of the patient's vision. Regression is more frequent in myopia greater than 10 D. It is also frequently seen in severe hyperopia and astigmatism. It appears to be more rapid than with PRK and has little to no response to steroids. If a single-zone technique is used to correct severe myopia and the optic zone is small to conserve stromal tissue, regression will be greater than with large optic zones or with the multizone treatments.

Treatment

The corrective options are the same as those described for undercorrection. Again, in this case the flap lifting and re-ablation technique is advisable. Topical steroids may be useful to control haze. However, prior to considering enhancement, the surgeon must be sure that regression has stabilized and is not due to progressive ectasia. Corneal ectasia or iatrogenic keratoconus occurs when the quantity of stromal tissue remaining after the laser procedure is insufficient. It is of utmost importance that the flap and ablation depth not exceed 50% of the initial preoperative thickness, or better still, the residual stroma should measure at least 250 microns.

Nonspecific Diffuse Intralamellar Keratitis

Nonspecific diffuse intralamellar keratitis is not infective, but is inflammatory. Its origins are still unclear. A sterile inflammation of the interface is present secondary to inflammation. Only polymorphonuclear granulocytic neutrophils are found in the interface.

Bobby Maddox, MD was the first person to describe this LASIK complication. Initially, he called it Shifting Sands of the Sahara (SOS) syndrome.

Other currently used names are:
- Nonspecific diffuse intralamellar keratitis (NSDIK)
- LASIK interface keratitis (LIK)
- Diffuse interface keratitis (DIK)
- Diffuse lamellar keratitis (DLK)
- Sterile interface syndrome (SIS)
- Nonspecific interface keratitis (NIK)

Causes

As previously mentioned, the etiology is still not completely known, though it is felt that a number of factors may be responsible. There is no universal theory as to causation.

Several hypothesis are considered:
- In acute polymorphonuclear inflammatory reaction (a nonspecific response to a corneal insult)
- An immune reaction to antigens or toxins in the interface
- Inflammation with a physical, not chemical, etiology, such as a reaction to thermal lesions on the stroma or toxicity from ultraviolet light

Table 8-34
NONSPECIFIC DIFFUSE INTRALAMELLAR KERATITIS **(Sands of the Sahara)**

Etiology
- Toxic reaction
- Immunological reaction
- Idiosyncratic reaction from:
  - Secretions from Meibomian glands
  - Exotoxins from gram-negative bacteria
  - Staphylococcal blepharitis
  - Material that has accumulated in the cannulas
  - Betadine
  - Ethylene oxide residue
  - Residue from cleaning solutions
  - Gentian violet
  - Residue of Merocel sponges
  - Red blood cells under the flap
  - Debris from the eyelid margin
  - Rust from the microkeratome or blade
  - Oil from the microkeratome gears or oil residue on the blade or from the motor
- Thermal lesions
- Toxicity from UV light
- Interaction between the laser and debris

Symptoms
- Reduction of visual acuity (including hyperopic shift)
- Discomfort
- Stromal melting with induced hyperopia
- Alterations in the corneal topography

Prevention
- Careful cleaning of the cannulas and syringes
- Careful cleaning of the microkeratome and suction ring
- Maintenance of the microkeratome by the manufacturer every 3 to 4 months
- Avoid cleaning the instruments with ultrasound
- Use topical steroids for 4 to 5 days after the LASIK operation
- Preoperative treatment of blepharitis
- Protection of the cornea from excess heat and UV damage:
  - Use cold BSS to cool the cornea
  - Check the laser's internal optics (UV filter)
  - Interrupt the ablation to allow the cornea to cool

Treatment
- Potent, frequent steroid drops
- Antibiotic prophylaxis
- Raising and cleaning the flaps for grades 3 and 4 (controversy in timing and steroid drop usage among various surgeons)

- An idiosyncratic reaction to substances present in the interface
- A possible interaction between the laser and sub-

stances present in the interface, but not a response to debris in the interface because it may develop even when the interface is clean. The substances that may be responsible for this reaction are various and diverse:

A. Originating from the eye or related structures:
- Sebaceous secretion from Meibomian glands
- Debris/bacteria from the eyelid margins
- Conjunctival debris
- Red blood cells under the flap secondary to corneal or conjunctival hemorrhage with neovascularization

B. Bacterial antigens:
- Antigens originating from gram-negative bacteria found in stagnant water of ultrasonic cleaners and autoclaves. These are exotoxins, lipopolysaccharides that are part of the external wall of bacteria. Sterilization destroys the bacteria but the exotoxins persist.
- Possible reaction from hypersensitivity with staphylococcal blepharitis.

C. Substances used to clean or sterilize the instruments or operative field:
- Betadine (following the first cases of sands, Maddox discontinued Betadine, but the sands persisted)
- Residual ethylene oxide
- Residue from cleaning solutions
- BSS or other material accumulated in irrigation cannulas (crystals of BSS have been observed in some cases). Filtered BSS did not decrease the incidence of sands. In any case, BSS seems to be the only common element in all reported cases of sands

D. Chemical substances used specifically for the LASIK procedure:
- Gentian violet
- Residue from Merocel sponges

E. Substances originating from the microkeratome:
- Rust or metal fragments from the microkeratome
- Rust or metal fragments from the blade
- Oil from the microkeratome gears

Initially, Maddox observed a rubbery substance on the blade, in the groove that houses the blade, and in the eccentric device of the motor. It was shown that this substance was a mixture of esters and hydrocarbons found in the microkeratome's motor. These substances are found in the lubricants, the pump's oil and the motor's oil. It is possible that the microkeratome blade comes into contact with these oils, particularly with the motor oil. Maddox removed the oil with acetone (it should be remembered

that acetone is toxic to the corneal epithelium, so every trace must be removed). This is one of many reasons why it is advisable to have the motor serviced by the manufacturer at least every 3 to 4 months. With acetone cleaning combined with the manufacturer's routine cleaning, Maddox has not reported further cases of sands. The syndrome, however, has been seen in cases of enhancement with flap lifting and no microkeratome use.

It has been suggested that there is a reaction to the latex of surgical gloves, which may come into contact with the instruments. The syndrome, however, has been seen even when the surgeon does not use gloves.

F. Others:
It has also been suggested that there is an interaction between the laser and substances found in the interface. The laser is thought to excite particles left behind following the microkeratome pass. The hypothesis that it is related to high corrections has been contradicted by the fact that it has been observed following ALK without the excimer laser.

G. Finally, another theory is that the syndrome has a physical etiology: a reaction to the thermal insult or to toxicity from the ultraviolet light. Several surgeons have measured corneal temperatures in excess of 50°C during ablation. Following hyperopic LASIK, Hatsis, having used three nonablatable shields (3.5 mm, 4.0 mm, and 4.5 mm) found the amount of "sand" was directly proportional to the amount of stromal exposure to the excimer laser ablation.

This syndrome has never been produced experimentally. In bilateral simultaneous LASIK, the syndrome may develop in only one eye—sometimes the first eye operated, sometimes the second, and rarely bilateral. The cases are usually sporadic but may be clustered in a group of eyes operated on in 1 day.

Risk Factors

Trauma and epithelial defects are occasionally associated with this syndrome and may be risk factors.

Clinical Signs

Typically, early signs are evident on the first postoperative day, but appear by days 5 to 7 at the latest. Normally, the reaction is denser centrally but may appear in specific sectors or only peripherally. On postoperative day 1, the patient usually has good uncorrected visual acuity. The eye is quiet but at the slit lamp, minimal widespread haze throughout the interface is seen. It is white or yellowish white with an undulating appearance, similar to waves of sand, especially along the ablation steps or chatter lines of the microkeratome. Extremely rarely, cells may be seen in the anterior chamber. At this early stage, the patient is asymptomatic. If untreated and progression occurs, by day 3 to 4, yellowish white opaque areas are apparent in the interface. Compared to the previous appearance, these are darker, granular, widespread, evanescent, fragmentary, and appear more like sand dunes. In some cases, the opacities are concentric, coinciding with the steps created by the laser diaphragm. In other cases they are joined to form a central disc that resolves slowly. A superficial punctate epitheliopathy may be seen. At this point, there is a reduction in visual acuity and contrast sensitivity. There may be photophobia, eyelid edema, epiphora, and discomfort. Without prompt intervention, this may result in stromal melting due to the release of proteolytic enzymes from the polymorphonuclear cells.

Topography is useful for following the evolution of the syndrome.

Differential Diagnosis

The primary differential diagnosis is infective keratitis. Infection appears 24 to 48 hours after surgery n o t usually after 12 to 24 hours. It is accompanied by moderate to severe pain, which is not present with Sands of the Sahara syndrome. Grade 4 SOS can present with photophobia, eyelid edema, anterior chamber reaction, and limbal injection, as in infective keratitis. In grades 1, 2, and 3, the globe is not painful or soft to touch. Even with grade 4, the objective examination is much worse than the symptoms. The symptoms are always less than one would expect upon examination of the eye.

Maddox and Hatsis have proposed a classification of the syndrome, which is useful in management.

Grade 1: Mild infiltration in the interface. At the slit lamp, there is a dusting in the interface that looks like grains of sand. It appears yellowish white in color and forms fine undulating lines alternating with transparent areas, similar to a target. It may be diffuse throughout the interface or in the peripheral area alone. Visual acuity and refraction are not affected. The patient is asymptomatic. Treatment: topical steroids every hour tapered over a period of 1 week.

The progression from grade 1 to grade 2 is often extremely rapid within 24 hours. In these cases, with topography the sand looks like a decentered ablation.

Grade 2: Total infiltration of the interface. The appearance is similar to grade 1, but widespread throughout the interface with greater density centrally. Grade 2 is the most frequent presentation. Treatment: topical steroids every 30 minutes with doses tapered after the infiltrate has disappeared over a 3 to 4 week period.

Grade 3: Dense total infiltration of the interface with aggregates or groups of cells. The release of proteolytic

enzymes may lead to stromal melting. Bowman s membrane may rupture and there may be scarring. Normally, BCVA is affected with the loss of one or two lines. Frequently there is a hyperopic shift. Stromal melting alters corneal topography, so the topographic picture is one of decentration or irregular astigmatism. Patients are symptomatic with decreased uncorrected or best-corrected acuity with or without discomfort. Treatment must be immediate and aggressive. Treatment: the flap should be lifted and cleaned and a topical steroid administered every 30 minutes beginning 2 to 3 hours after cleaning, with prolonged observation and tapering of the steroid.

Grade 4: Total infiltration of the interface with extra-corneal involvement (ie, cells in the anterior chamber, eyelid edema, edema of the flap, epiphora, extremely poor vision, photophobia, and perilimbal injection, discomfort). There is serious risk of flap melting. Treatment: similar to grade 3. Daily monitoring is necessary, as progression may be extremely rapid.

The Hatsis Classification

Grade 1: Partial infiltration of the interface

Grade 2: Complete infiltration of the interface

Grade 3: Dense total infiltration of the interface with aggregates or groups of cells

Grade 4: Total infiltration of the interface with extra-corneal involvement

Machat Classification

Machat has also used a classification that is used to determine treatment. He classifies three grades.

Grade 1 roughly corresponds to Hatsis grades 1 and 2.

Grade 2 corresponds to Hatsis grade 3

Grade 3 corresponds to the Hatsis grade 4

Grade 1: Very mild cases that resolve spontaneously within 1 month and may be widespread or peripheral. It is typically noted on routine postoperative day 1 or week 1 exams. At the slit lamp, it appears as a slight haze with no vision or refraction involvement. The patient is asymptomatic. Even though the case is mild, treatment with potent steroids every hour should be initiated, followed and tapered over a 2- to 3-week period to prevent progression.

Grade 2: This is the most common presentation, with more diffuse haze. Density is usually greater versus the periphery. Visual acuity is affected, with BCVA reduced by one to two lines. There may be a hyperopic shift in the refractive error. Patients are typically symptomatic with mild discomfort and perceive the deterioration in vision. Rapid progression may occur if massive treatment is not initiated. Potent topical steroids every hour the first day, then every 2 hours the second day are used, with the dose reduced gradually over 3 weeks.

Antibiotic cover with a fluoroquinolone is administered during the first week. If there is not a quick response, lifting and gentle cleaning is used, as previously described.

Grade 3: This is a very serious, but rare. It appears as a dense central infiltrate or plaque. The corneal flap may have striae overlying the infiltration. Though the infiltrate may resemble infective keratitis, the eye is usually quiet. There is no purulent secretion, hypopyon is absent, but rarely there may be a reaction in the anterior chamber. Generally, if there is breakdown of the flap epithelium, there will be a flare in the anterior chamber with endothelial precipitates. UCVA is usually 20/200 and BCVA is usually less than 20/60. Presentation is usually on days 5 to 7 after initially looking normal upon slit lamp examination on postoperative day 1, when steroid drops are no longer being used.

Treatment

Topical steroids are the mainstay of treatment. They should be potent drops (betamethasone, dexamethasone, and prednisolone) not the formulation that causes reduced mucous absorption (fluorometholone, clobetasone). They must initially be administered with high frequency in addition to a prophylactic antibiotic cover. Antibiotic prophylaxis is necessary, as infective keratitis cannot be ruled out even though the presentation is usually much more severe than nonspecific diffuse intralamellar keratitis (SOS). The fact that the response to steroids is extremely rapid suggests that this syndrome is of immune origin.

Milder forms of the syndrome resolve easily in 1 to 2 weeks with topical steroid drops alone. More severe forms of the syndrome have moderate to marked findings and are symptomatic with moderate to severely reduced vision. In these cases, the flap must be lifted, gently cleaned, and aggressive steroid treatment must be immediately started with the addition of topical antibiotics as prophylaxis. Topical steroids act specifically to prevent degranulation by the polymorphonuclar enzyme cells, limiting or preventing melting. In these cases, there may be a worsening of the clinical picture on day 2, stabilization by day 3, and the start of improvement by days 4 to 5.

Some surgeons have achieved good results by early cleaning of the flap alone. Healing may appear to have been more rapid than with steroids. The flap is lifted, the stromal surfaces are cleaned (both on the flap and bed), and the flap is repositioned. It is possible that on the next day the cells may reappear. There are arguments against early lifting and cleaning (there have been cases of melting after the flap had been raised). Flap melting and accompanying hyperopic shift occurs because of the immune response. It is felt by some that melting occurs independently of the flap being raised and is due to the severity of inflammation.

Follow-Up

Slit lamp examination on a more or less daily basis is necessary for at least the first week. Daily topography is also useful given that the migration of cells in the interface begins as occupied space and evolves into tissue melting. Topographic examination will highlight the current status.

Evolution

Generally speaking, if treatment is rapid and massive, there is improvement within 1 to 3 days after initiation, with complete resolution with 1 to 2 weeks—1 month at most. Improvement normally starts peripherally and progresses toward the center.

Treatment Protocol

Maddox – Hatsis (1999)

Hatsis Grades 1 and 2
- 1% prednisolone acetate eyedrops every hour for 1 to 2 weeks with gradual tapering.
- Antibiotic eyedrops: Ocuflox eyedrops and/or Polytrim eyedrops.

Hatsis Grades 3 and 4
Surgical intervention followed immediately (within 1 hour) by 1% prednisolone acetate eyedrops instilled every 30 minutes along with antibiotic (Ocuflox or Polytrim) eyedrops every hour. Taper with improvement.

Surgical Management

The flap must be lifted immediately and the interface irrigated. The flap surfaces and stromal bed are brushed delicately with a BSS-moistened Merocel sponge. The attempt is to eliminate the inflammatory cells along with the digestive enzymes. The most important factor is to remove the enzymes, not the cells. Potent steroid drops must be instilled every 30 minutes even through the night. At night, neutrophil granulocytes reform; the steroid prevents release of further digestive enzymes, thus preventing further tissue destruction.

Machat (1999)

Machat Grade 1
- Intensive topical steroid therapy

Machat Grade 2
- 0.1% dexamethasone phosphate eyedrops:
  - Every hour for the first day

- Every 2 hours for the second day
- Every 3 hours for the third day
- Four times a day for 3 weeks
- 0.3% ciprofloxacin eyedrops four times a day for the first 4 to 7 days

Machat Grade 3

- Surgical intervention immediately or at a later stage with close monitoring
- Topical steroid therapy for 3 weeks as for grade 2, beginning immediately

Surgical Treatment

1. The flap is raised—this is easy partly because fibrosis is absent from the interface.
2. Remove the inflammatory material. This has a grayish white milky appearance. It is easily removed; however, the surgeon must be careful to remove it gently, otherwise a hyperopic effect will be produced. Both of the interface surfaces must be carefully cleaned with a spatula, blunt blade, or Merocel sponge.
3. A 5-micron PTK is performed on both surfaces.
4. Finally, the flap is closed and the interface is irrigated.

Normally, steroids are started immediately after the operation.

Prevention

Preventive measures vary depending on the surgeon's opinion of the etiology.

Hypothesis: Injury from heat and ultraviolet radiation. Considering that the laser generates heat, the cornea must be protected from thermal and UV damage.

The excimer laser has internal optics with coatings that must be checked and maintained by regular servicing.

Use cold BSS as the irrigating solution to cool the cornea, placing a swab soaked in cold BSS on the corneal surface, irrigating and cooling the tissue for 1 to 2 minutes. The corneal temperature may be checked using a pediatric infrared optic thermometer. Treatment is recommended when the temperature is above 22°C (75°F)

Control the ablation time. Interrupt the ablation on a regular basis to allow the tissue to cool down. If broad-beam lasers are used, toward the end of the procedure when the spot reaches 6.0 to 6.5 mm, the surgeon should apply just five to 10 pulses, allow a short break, and then continue. The larger the diameter of the ablation, the greater the amount of heat generated with each pulse. If ablation time is increased, the surgeon may need to adjust his or her nomogram to prevent overcorrection because of exposure and drying. (It is felt that more "sands" are being reported with the 10 Hz rate with the VISX laser as opposed to the former 5 to 6 Hz rate.)

Once the ablation is complete, the eye should be irrigated with cold BSS. Steroids (1% prednisolone acetate eyedrops) should be started 3 to 4 hours after surgery.

Hypothesis: Damage from oil or other microkeratome residues.

Either the day before surgery or immediately after the operating session, the microkeratome should be cleaned carefully throughout, including the gears, suction ring, and blade housing cavity. The instrument is kept free from oil, grease, and metallic debris.

Acetone or 99% isopropyl alcohol is used for cleaning the microkeratome motor head. A dry toothbrush is used to remove the metallic debris, oil residue, and salt crystals.

The blades can be cleaned the day before surgery with acetone and with ether on a Merocel sponge.

The manufacturer should perform routine maintenance every 3 to 4 months. Once the operating session has finished, the microkeratome head must be stored downward so that residual BSS or cleaning solution does not enter the motor.

Hatsis pretreats the day before the operation with combination eyedrops, such as Tobradex. He also uses Endozime to first clean the instruments and blade. He then resterilizes the blades prior to surgery. He advises against ultrasonic cleaning of instruments. Water may stagnate in the ultrasound cleaning systems, which will become the source of bacterial exotoxins. Alternately, replace the cleaning fluid in the ultrasound between uses and at least daily with cleaning the ultrasound interior.

Bacterial cultures may be used to check the validity of this method. Pure, sterile, distilled water must be used to rinse the microkeratome and irrigating cannula prior to steam sterilization.

As a secondary prevention, the surgeon must:

- Routinely use topical steroid drops four to five times a day for 4 to 5 days following LASIK.
- Advise the patient to contact the surgeon immediately if there is even a minimal drop in visual acuity.

Night Glare and Halos

Fracesco Carones, MD

Night vision disturbances should be considered a very important side effect of laser surgery. The risk of this complication must be screened preoperatively through the measurement of pupil diameter, and adequate ablation strategies must be applied to minimize this side effect which, once occurred, is very difficult to deal with.

In addition to the accuracy and efficacy of a refractive surgical procedure, the quality of vision also plays an important role in assessing its success. When patients consider refractive surgery, they do not only aim at 20/20 unaided vision but also the same visual quality they had before surgery with their spectacles or contact lenses. Patients are certainly happy when they can see without glasses after surgery, but even in this situation they may be very dissatisfied if their vision significantly decreases at night or with dim illumination.

Night glare and halos are among the complaints most frequently reported by patients. I personally have some patients who had to change their profession because they were unable to drive at night after surgery. There is also a letter to the editor in the *Journal of Cataract and Refractive Surgery* (1997;23:1435) in which a patient treated by LASIK reported his night vision difficulties and solicited the ophthalmic community to consider this a major problem after refractive surgery. The problem of inducing halos and night vision problems must be taken into account and managed before treatment when planning surgery. Once induced, these disturbances are very difficult to solve.

Halos are determined by the scattering of light rays at the edge of the ablation. When the pupil is undilated, scattered rays cannot reach the retina because of the diaphragm provided by the pupil; when the pupil dilates, it can come through the eye and blur vision. In other words, the larger the pupil dilates, the worse the problem; and the larger the ablation diameter, the better.

Before surgery, the preoperative visit should include pupil measurements under different light conditions. There are several pupillometers available on the market and some of them are quite inexpensive. Alternatively, it is also possible to consider the pupil measurement provided by corneal topography systems, which is carried out at a fixed luminance level. This measurement does not provide information about pupillary diameter in low-light conditions, but at least it gives a standard pupil diameter in which to refer.

I personally use the following guidelines: once a patient is found to have very large pupils in dim illumination (> 7.0 mm), I discourage him or her from undergoing laser refractive surgery, or at least I inform him or her of the great risk of night vision problems, regardless of the correction. When the pupil does not dilate much (<7.0 mm), I consider the amount of correction as the greater predictive factor for night vision problems (the higher, the greater risk). Consequently, I advise patients with higher corrections of this problem and do not recommend LASIK to those patients who have significant night vision requirements, such as taxi or truck drivers. Using large ablation diameters and blend zones, my danger-zone dioptric corrections are -8.00 (myopia) and +3.00 (hyperopia).

Treatment should be planned by taking into account the pupil diameter. I always try to perform the ablation as large as possible to reduce risk of night vision problems, but sometimes this approach is limited by the relationship between the amount of correction to be made and residual ablation thickness. I never perform corrections smaller than 5.0 mm central spherical diameter for myopic corrections (this means plus transition zone for overall corrections of 6.5 to 8.0 mm) and smaller than 6.0 mm central spherical diameter for hyperopic corrections (overall corrections of 9.0 to 9.5 mm, depending on the laser used).

Once night halos occur, they are very difficult to manage. Usually they are more troublesome during the immediate postoperative period and tend to decrease with time. A mild miotic may help the patients in certain situations, for example if they plan to drive for long periods at night, but certainly it cannot solve the problem. I hope that topography or wavefront ablation-based ablations may, in the future, avoid this complication and allow retreatment of symptomatic eyes.

Corneal Melting in Lamellar Refractive Surgery

Juan Alvarez de Toledo, MD

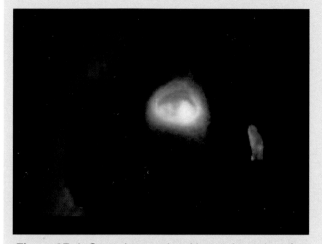

Figure 8B-1. Central corneal melting and scarring after epithelial ingrowth through Bowman's hole (central flap thickness 54 µm).

Corneal melting after lamellar refractive surgery is a potentially destructive condition that may end in a dense corneal opacity or perforation. Refractive surgeons must be able to identify this process in its early stages and start appropriate measures to correct it.

The best way to avoid this complication is its prevention. Careful medical history of the patient should be taken, ruling out active systemic immunological diseases than can affect the ocular surface (such as rheumatoid arthritis, relapsing polychondritis, Sjögren syndrome, Wegener granulomatosis, and other collagenopathies). If the systemic condition is actually quiescent, the patient should be informed of potential risks associated with his or her disease and surgery must be discouraged. Patients with a history of corneal herpetic disease must also be excluded. Several reports have shown serious recurrences of herpes with difficult management after PRK or LASIK.

Corneal melting can be caused by a misdiagnosed systemic condition, a reactivation of previous viral keratitis, an acute infection of the interface (bacterial, fungal, acanthamoeba), an epithelial ingrowth at the flap margins or through central holes, an acute inflammatory reaction to toxic substances left under the flap, and irregular or extremely thin cuts.

Epithelial ingrowth is the most frequent cause of corneal melts. It occurs when the flap is incorrectly positioned at the end of the procedure, after re-operations with keratorrhexis (relifting the previous flap), after peripheral intraoperative epithelial defects, or in central flap perforations. A sheet of epithelial cells grows from the cut margins, inducing a local elevation of the flap. If the distortion induces a "hole" in the tear film, flap stromal tissue melts without inflammatory signs. If the melted area is small it has no influence on final visual acuity. If epithelial ingrowth is progressing toward the center or there are clusters of epithelial cells in the optical area, the flap must be lifted and the interface cleaned on both sides. This should be performed as soon as possible, because epithelium stimulates keratocyte activation and haze formation at the interface level.

Severe immunological melting of the flap in systemic diseases can be triggered by the microkeratome cut or small epithelial defects produced during the surgery. In these cases, tear mediators can initiate an immunological cascade with a fast keratolysis. Aggressive management with intensive preservative-free topical lubricants, topical cyclosporine A 1% to 2%, and systemic immunosupression with high-dose steroids (1 to 1.5 mg/kg/day) and cyclophosphamide (1 to 3 mg/kg/day) has been proposed. If the corneal melting progresses, a soft bandage contact lens can be fitted. If the flap is considered lost, removal of the remaining tissue to obtain pathological studies can help in the diagnosis. As a last resort, lamellar or penetrating allograft can be performed to restore vision.

If a toxic reaction to foreign substances left in the interface is suspected, lifting up the flap and cleaning both interface sides is performed immediately. Thin, irregular cuts are often associated with focal melting. In these cases, careful observation is required until the process has healed. Then, optical measures like gas-permeable contact lenses or surgical repair can be considered if the amount of visual acuity lost is considered significant.

Infective Keratitis: Diagnosis and Treatment

Juan Alvarez de Toledo, MD

Corneal inflammation after lamellar refractive surgery may be due to two major causes: micro-organism infection of the surgical bed and sterile inflammatory response associated with systemic diseases, surgical maneuvers, or foreign material. It is very important to the refractive surgeon to know how to differentiate between entities in order to start the appropriate treatment.

Micro-organism infection of the interface is, fortunately, a very uncommon situation after modern LASIK surgery. Several cases have been described in literature from the last few years, typically due to rare corneal pathogens with a special antibiotic resistance.

In our clinical practice, we may experience two different presentations. First, the patient presents with acute onset of symptoms such as redness, tearing, photophobia, and blurred vision 1 to 4 days after an uncomplicated procedure. We observe a single or multifocal white or yellowish infiltrate at the interface level, surrounded by irregular flap edema, some descemet folds, and anterior chamber reaction. We must suspect aggressive bacteria such as streptococcus or pseudomonas. The second presentation is when the patient presents 2 to 4 weeks after surgery with slight pain, moderate ciliary injection, and slow decrease in his or her visual acuity. A small white or white-yellowish infiltrate, sometimes with small satellite lesions, is found at the interface level. The main lesion is surrounded by a halo. Its borders can be poorly defined and tend to spread outside, usually perforating the flap. Incipient stromal neovascularization can also be seen in delayed cases. This is a typical onset of fungal or slow-growth bacteria like mycobacteria or nocardia interface infiltration. Obviously, we can also have intermediate situations between these two particular cases.

A strict diagnostic protocol should be used when an interface infection is suspected. Samples of lid margins, tarsal and bulbar conjunctiva, and corneal lesions must be taken; and different aerobic, anaerobic, and fungal culture media must be inoculated. If the infiltrate is under the flap, we must lift it and obtain samples of both epithelial and stromal sides of the interface. If the flap

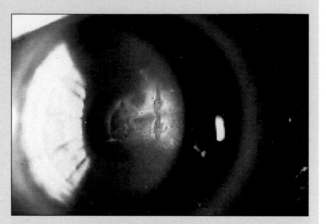

Figure 8C-1. Fungal infiltrate with flap perforation surrounded by an inflammatory halo.

status is considered lost, we can cut it at the hinge and send it for pathological and microbiological studies that can help in the diagnosis.

Initial empirical treatment will be based on clinical signs. In hyperacute and acute cases, a combination of topical fortified cephalosporin (ceftazidyme 50 mg/ml) and aminoglycoside (tobramycin 9 mg/ml) must be started. We can also combine fluoroquinolones (ciprofloxacin) with aminoglycosides. Each antibiotic is instilled one drop every minute for 5 minutes during each hour for 24 hours until culture results are known or a positive clinical response is observed. In subacute cases, the cephalosporin is combined with vancomycin 35 mg/ml using the same administration protocol. If a fungal infection is suspected, topical amphotericin B 2 mg/ml or natamycin 5% are combined with imidazolic agents (clotrimazole 2%) until drug sensibility is tested in vitro.

When the infection is under control, topical fluorometholone drops are started three to five drops a day to prevent interface scarring. If the flap has been surgically removed, we may treat the case like PRK, but normally a lamellar or perforating homograft keratoplasty is required to restore vision.

Progressive Induced Astigmatism in LASIK

Arturo Chayet, MD

As LASIK becomes more popular, a barrage of individuals with ametropia is invading the practices of refractive surgeons. Most of these patients have normal corneas, but very interestingly, I have found (compared to my general ophthalmology practice) an increased number of patients seeking refractive surgery, either with a case of keratoconus or with corneas showing a nonsymmetric nonorthogonal astigmatism. This latter group with topographical irregular astigmatism has been otherwise considered normal patients with ametropia by their former eye doctors who did not have the chance to evaluate their corneal topography.

At the time of this writing, I have performed more than 7000 lamellar procedures and found six highly myopic eyes (> -12 D) with evidence of post-LASIK keratectasia. In all cases, no evidence was found at the 1-year follow-up, and the first sign of keratectasia was diagnosed after 18 months. In addition, I found three eyes with progressive induced astigmatism, in which the corneal thickness was more than 500 microns and corneal ablation was less than 80 microns (always with a 160-micron thickness plate). In these three cases, patients experienced very good uncorrected visual acuity at the 6-month follow-up, and vision suddenly decreased around the ninth month. We have previously published information about regular regression due to epithelial hyperplasia following LASIK stabilized at 6 months, therefore, any change in vision along with a steepening of the cornea after this period should bring to mind the possibility of abnormal steepening, including the possibility of a case of iatrogenic keratectasia.

Currently, I do not perform LASIK in patients with one or more of the following preoperative findings:

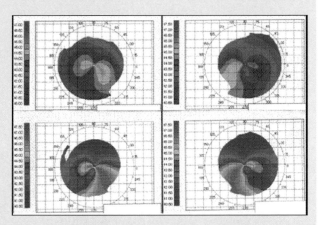

1. Myopia over 12 D
2. Corneas thinner than 490 to 500 microns (I suspect potential abnormality in thinner corneas)
3. Corneas with nonorthogonal astigmatism
4. Corneas with more than 1 D of topographic asymmetric astigmatism
5. When the untouched cornea may be less than 500 microns and/or the sum of flap/ablation exceeds 50% of the overall cornea thickness

We perform corneal pachymetry and two different cornea maps in every preoperative LASIK evaluation (no exceptions). In selected cases of low corrections in which one of the above parameters prevents us from doing LASIK, we perform PRK. It is my belief that by avoiding the lamellar cut and doing the ablation at a more superficial plane, the risk for ectasia or induced astigmatism is less than with LASIK. For higher corrections, phakic intraocular lenses have been found to be a better alternative.

Flap Displacement

Oscar D. Ghilino, MD

Flap displacement is directly related to patient habits, physiology of eyelid movements, and surgical technique.

To avoid flap displacement due to patient habits, patients must be instructed to not touch or rub their eyes for 2 weeks after surgery, no swimming for 2 weeks, and avoid activities that may cause trauma to the eyes.

It has been demonstrated by Carriazo in experimental work that with every blink, the eyelid paints the corneal surface, improves the position, and aligns the flap when the hinge is superior; but when the hinge is nasal, temporal, or inferior, every blink tries to dislocate the flap. Flap displacement is more common after irregular flaps, very thin or thick flaps, epithelial abrasions, free caps, or prolonged surgery. To prevent these complications, we must take into

account the particular characteristics, such as corneal curvature, globe size, and sunken eyes, prior to surgery.

To prevent equipment failure we must check our microkeratome and listen to the sound of the motor. Sometimes when there is debris inside, it moves slower and could even stop during the pass of the microkeratome. The blade quality should be checked—the cutting edge must be sharp and free of imperfections, and in the case of blades that have a plastic component, it should oscillate smoothly. The suction ring vacuum has to be checked and the microkeratome must run smoothly through the suction ring track to avoid displacement of the suction ring during surgery, promoting decentered flaps. Surgery must be smooth, clean, precise, and quick to achieve positive results and rapid rehabilitation.

Good exposure is necessary without eyelashes or skin that could make the microkeratome stop or jump producing abnormalities in the flap thickness, The surface of the cornea prior to the pass of the microkeratome should be moist with topical glycerin based anesthetic drops to have a proper and smooth pass and to prevent epithelial abrasions. The interface should be irrigated with BSS, but we must not leave too much water under the flap that could dislocate the flap. The use of compressed air to dry the cornea is unnecessary and can promote striae, just wipe the flap with a wet Merocel sponge from the hinge to the edge is sufficient to remove the liquid from the interface. The realignment of the flap, taking advantage of the paracentral marks to avoid dislocation and folds, should be perfect. One should move quickly to avoid dehydration of the flap and stroma, thus eliminating changes in the thickness that may lead to overcorrections and make flap repositioning difficult and facilitate epithelial erosions.

If dislocation of the flap appears, it must be treated immediately by lifting the flap, removing any epithelium from the bed and undersurface of the cap, hydration of the flap, and repositioning.

Free Caps

Jairo E. Hoyos, MD, PhD

When in situ keratomileusis became popular in the late 1980s, surgeons removed a complete corneal disc that was then sutured back onto the cornea. In 1991, the technique evolved to nonsutured discs, until the flap was developed in 1992. Today, whenever LASIK is performed, we try to create a corneal flap with the microkeratome in order to prevent disc displacement and loss.

In order to create the flap, we must stop the forward movement either before the microkeratome completes its full pass, or use a stopper on the microkeratome head. If the microkeratome does not stop at the right time or if the stopper is not well calibrated, the cut may result in a free cap. Probably the most frequent cause of this complication is a very flat cornea. Patients with flat corneas and a mean keratometry of less than 41 D are at a higher risk of having a free cap. A flat cornea will protrude relatively less into the suction ring compared to a steep cornea, thereby presenting a smaller cap diameter to the microkeratome blade. If the stopper is set for a small hinge, a free cap may result. This happens only in primary flat corneas because a flat cornea secondary to refractive surgery will behave exactly as the original cornea.

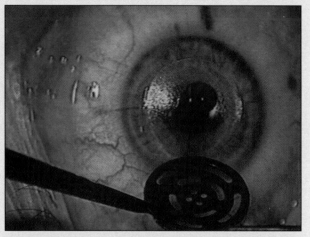

Figure 8F-1. Free cap disc replacement technique.

MANAGEMENT

Every LASIK surgeon must be alert to the possibility of a free cap and must prepare for it by always using epithelial reference markings. Surgeons must also know how to manage a free cap in order to be able to continue the operation without major complications.

We have found it very useful to place four radial marks and one pararadial mark on the cornea. We use a four-incision RK marker painted with gentian violet for the radial marks and add the pararadial mark with an astigmatic marker. We immediately wash the cornea with BBS in order to remove all traces of alcohol from the gentian violet, because of its toxic effect on the cornea. The pararadial mark helps identify the epithelial surface of the disc, and the four radial marks serve as reference points to replace the disc to its original position without inducing astigmatism.

While the ablation is performed, the disc should be kept in an antidesiccation chamber with the epithelial surface facing down. The disc should not be hydrated so as to avoid edema formation, although we do recommend the use of one drop of BSS on the epithelial surface for preservation.

Once the ablation is complete, the bed is flushed and dried with a Merocel sponge, and a drop of BSS is applied on the apex (Figure 8F-1). Using the Barraquer spatula, we retrieve the disc from the antidesiccation chamber and place it on the bed with the help of fine forceps. The BSS drop enables us to easily mobilize the disc with the help of two Merocel sponges until it is aligned with the radial markings. Finally, we thoroughly dry the edges and wait until the disc is attached to its bed.

We close the lids with two crossed adhesive strips for approximately 30 minutes. After that, we check the patient and if we find that the disc has moved, we reposition it and leave the lid closed until the next day. If the disc is found to be in the right position, the patient is sent home wearing only the ocular shield and is instructed to follow the instructions for normal flap cases.

Thin Flaps and Buttonholes

Melania Cigales, MD and Jairo E. Hoyos, MD, PhD

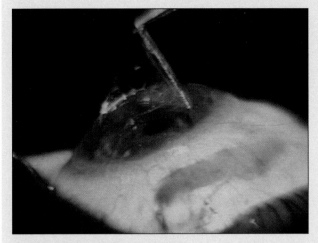

Figure 8G-1. A buttonhole flap.

The most common causes of thin flaps and buttonholes are inadequate suction, steep corneas, poor blade quality, and microkeratome malfunction.

Inadequate suction: The suction ring induces an ocular hypertension above 65 mm Hg, which is required to perform the keratectomy. We use the Barraquer tonometer to monitor this pressure. As the surgeon becomes more skilled and experienced, there is a tendency to discontinue use of the tonometer. However, it is important to remember that it is the sole reliable means to detect this complication and if the required pressure is not reached, the keratectomy must not be performed.

Lack of pressure may be due to a poor fit of the suction ring on the eye. This is usually the case in small sunken orbits and astigmatic eyes, in which it is difficult to place the ring.

There are other instances when the suction time is very long, creating conjunctival edema, or eyes with a very large axial length tend to go into hypotension. In the past, when in situ keratomileusis was performed using the microkeratome, we raised the pressure when it was not high enough with the help of a retrobulbar injection. However, now that we use topical anesthesia, we prefer to postpone the surgery (this is an infrequent situation).

Steep corneas: Corneal curvatures greater than 46 D cause thin, large diameter discs, which entail a risk of complication due to corneal buckling during the microkeratome pass. In the presence of a steep cornea, we recommend the use of a 180-micron plate or a blade with a larger gap (distance between the blade and the plate correlates to the thickness of the keratectomy).

Poor blade quality or sharpness: A dull blade creates a thin and perhaps irregular cut. Remnants of Bowman's membrane can sometimes be seen on the stromal bed. Blade quality varies considerably, and for this reason it is crucial to check and calibrate them under the microscope in order to reject those with an irregular edge or a small gap. Many surgeons reuse the same blade for four or five eyes. After each pass, the blade looses its sharpness, creating a thinner cut every time. We recommend using a new blade for each case.

Microkeratome malfunction: The microkeratome requires careful cleaning and assembly before each use in order to minimize any secondary complications due to malfunction. We also recommend sending the microkeratome to the manufacturer for periodic revisions and resetting. In 1993, we had three consecutive buttonhole cases (Figure 8G-1) resulting from keratome malfunction and the problem was corrected by simply changing the microkeratome head.

MANAGEMENT

We believe that whenever one of these complications occurs during creation of the flap, the best thing is to abort the procedure, replace the flap, and perform a new keratectomy 3 or 4 months later using a thicker plate.

It is not always easy to reposition these flaps because they tend to wrinkle and dislocate from lack of consistency. It is important to align the disc correctly and wait for as long as is necessary until it reattaches, and we recommend eye patching. When the resulting flap is practically epithelium only, we prefer to discard it and wait until new epithelium is formed.

The evolution is usually favorable. There is no leukoma or visual loss, although not in every case. In those cases where a central leukoma develops, we prefer to perform PTK prior to performing a new LASIK procedure.

Intraoperative and Postoperative Bleeding in LASIK

Thomas Kohnen, MD

Bleeding during refractive surgery is undesirable and should be avoided. The visual postoperative outcome after lamellar surgery can be reduced due to this problem.

There are three causes of intraoperative bleeding during LASIK:

1. Conjunctival bleeding due to the suction of the microkeratome ring
2. Bleeding of peripheral corneal vessels
3. Retinal bleeding due to the increased intraocular pressure during the suction process

Intraoperative conjunctival bleeding can occur during the suction process of the microkeratome, but this problem usually remains without consequences. Patients who are on anticoagulant medication will typically bleed. The best prophylaxis is to discontinue medication several days preoperatively and replace it with a systemic heparin treatment.

Bleeding of peripheral corneal vessels typically occurs in patients with a limbal pannus, usually due to long-term contact lens wear. The occurrence is higher in microkeratomes with larger diameter flaps (eg, 9.5 mm cut with the Hansatome. Prevention in these cases is either to use the same microkeratome but produce a smaller flap (eg, 8.5 mm for the Hansatome) or use a temporally cutting microkeratome with a smaller flap (Automated Corneal Shaper).

The surgeon should be prepared for this potential complication, because it may not be possible to stop intraoperative bleeding and blood remnants might persist under the flap. We have used adrenaline derivatives, but these drugs could interfere with the iris, causing intraoperative irregular dilation of the pupil. Therefore, our preferred drug is POR 8 Sandoz, a vasoconstrictor that does not affect pupil dilation. With a Merocel sponge soaked with POR 8, bleeding of peripheral vessels is generally stopped very quickly.

Retinal bleeding can occur because of the increased intraocular pressure during the microkeratome cut.

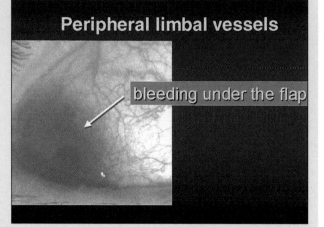

Figure 8H-1. Postoperative bleeding under a large corneal flap after LASIK using a 9.5 mm cut. The flap was relifted after 2 days, the interface was cleaned of erythrocytes, and this highly myopic Asian patient (preoperative spherical equivalent: 10.5 D) regained a quite useful uncorrected visual acuity of 20/30.

Peripheral retinal vessel bleeding might be undetected in most cases; however, if the bleeding interferes with the visual axis, visual acuity will be reduced after the LASIK procedure. In severe cases, vitreoretinal intervention may be necessary.

Postoperative bleeding after LASIK rarely occurs. Possible locations could be the conjunctiva, cornea, or retina (as described above). Conjunctival bleeding does not require treatment. Retinal bleeding requires treatment only occasionally. Because the flap is reattached quite strongly in a couple of hours, interface bleeding post LASIK is seen very rarely. However, if the blood remains under the flap, almost immediate cleaning is mandatory. In this case, the flap is lifted in the operating room and the stromal bed is cleaned with BSS. Prior to this intervention, the physician should search for potential systemic reasons for the bleeding and should treat the patient before the flap is lifted.

LASIK Interface Debris

Michiel S. Kritzinger, MD

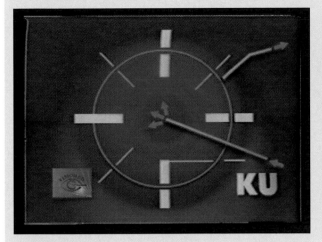

Figure 8I-1. One-way irrigation flow of BSS from underneath the flap to the fornix.

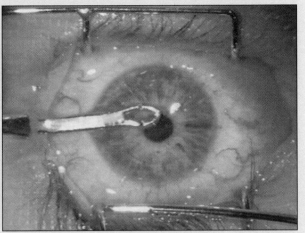

Figure 8I-2. K-U irrigation cannula in the surgical interface.

A postoperative LASIK cornea must have a pristine appearance. The ideal is to leave the cornea in a crystal clear finish, just as it was before surgery. Remember prevention is better than cure.

Interface debris is intimately related to flap complications, surgical technique, and instrumentation use. Debris increases the incidence of interface infections and inflammations, as well as halos and glare.

Types of foreign material in the interface:
- Pieces of lint from surgical clothes and dressings
- Dirt particles floating in operating room air
- Air bubbles with attached foreign material
- Conjunctival mucous
- Meibomian secretions
- Eyelashes cut by the microkeratome
- Spots of eyeliner, mascara, and eyeshadow
- Fluff from microsponges
- Metal dust from microkeratome blades, especially those that are turbo driven
- Oil and chemical lubricants from the microkeratome
- Chemical deposits of gentian violet marking ink
- Remnants of sterisolutions of Hibidal and or Endozyme cleaning material (diffuse lamellar keratitis [DLK])
- Wax oil on microkeratome blades (Sands of the Sahara [SOS])
- Red blood cells from peripheral corneal blood vessels
- Remaining residual water in the interface, producing interface haze patterns postoperatively

- Bacteria, fungus, or viruses introduced during the operation
- Glove powder
- Epithelial cells introduced with instruments, especially if too much local anaesthetic is used
- Entrapped tear film in the interface if no interface irrigation is performed
- Unknown agents causing DLK

How to prevent it:

Intraoperative technique:
1. Dry and clean the cornea and fornices before lifting the flap for laser ablation.
2. Do not wipe the corneal bed with a microsponge before or after the laser ablation.
3. Close the flap before performing any interface irrigation.
4. Create a one-way flow irrigation of the interface with a special irrigation needle and fornix suction needle.
5. Express excessive fluid from the stromal interface.
6. Use a damp microsponge to smooth the cap.
7. Use a dry microsponge to dry and seal the flap gutter area.

Postoperative approach:
1. Wash all foreign bodies out of the interface as soon as possible because they will not disappear by themselves.
2. There is always a grey halo inflammatory response around foreign bodies, which persists for a long time after removal of foreign bodies.

3. Rarely can all of the metal dust be rinsed out, but the remaining dust is fairly inert.
4. Red blood cells will disappear by themselves—no special irrigation has to be done.
5. Chemical deposits from blades and microkeratomes

must be washed out immediately to prevent DLK.
6. Remaining residual water haze patterns will eventually disappear.

Always be alert and meticulous with interface cleaning. There is no room for "slap-dash" surgery.

Corneal Ectasia Following LASIK

Francesco Molfino, MD

DEFINITION

Ectasia is a complication rarely observed following LASIK. It typically appears months after surgery, even though the initial outcome appears good. To date only a few rare cases have been reported. This text will attempt to answer three main questions concerning ectasia:

1. What causes corneal ectasia?
2. What is the mechanism behind corneal ectasia?
3. What steps can be taken to prevent iatrogenic corneal ectasia?

Our experience includes one case of corneal ectasia. The patient was 45 years old with a spherical equivalent of 14 D. Initial pachymetry was 535 microns and the corneal map showed symmetrical with-the-rule astigmatism. LASIK with a flap diameter of 8.5 mm and thickness of 220 microns was performed. The in situ ablation was 145 microns and the residual corneal thickness was 170 microns with an overall corneal thickness of 390 microns. In the 2 years following the operation, there was regression of myopia. At the patient's insistence, enhancement was performed; the original flap was raised and the residual error was treated. An optic zone of 6.0 mm and an ablation of 73 microns was performed. Three months later, the pachymetry value was 306 microns with signs of initial central ectasia, which required lamellar keratoplasty. During the postoperative exams, various biometry measurements demonstrated good stability.

In reference to the five cases reported in the literature, the residual posterior corneal thickness (ie, the thickness remaining after the lamellar cut and the refractive ablation) is not known; this makes the pathogenesis difficult to interpret.

WHAT CAUSES CORNEAL ECTASIA?

Thickness of the Flap

This may vary within a specific range for each type of microkeratome (it depends on how sharp the blade is, the speed of progression of the microkeratome during the cut, etc). The majority of surgeons use a plate that should create a cut of 160 microns. Actually, in more than 150 cases using the Chiron Automated Corneal Shaper, the mean pachymetry value of the flap was 134 microns ± 24 microns, with a range of between 87 and 227 microns.[1] It stands to reason that a thicker flap will reduce the thickness of the residual available stroma.

Ablation Depth

This value is based on the nomograms for refractive photorefractive keratectomy (PRK), which calculate the indices of ablation in reference to Bowman's membrane and the anterior stroma. Some authors report that ablation per pulse is greater in the middle of the stroma as compared to the superficial layer; the depth of the ablation in LASIK may be greater than the value calculated. This partially explains why many LASIK nomograms are based on reduction of the PRK nomograms. Moreover, the biomechanic qualities of the anterior stroma are different from those of the posterior stroma. This may bring about a greater ablation depth, particularly in high myopia.

Corneal Thickness in Thinner Areas

Standard clinical practice uses ultrasound pachymetry to obtain two or three measurements at the center of the cornea. This procedure is adequate; however, there are thinner areas that may not be analyzed on specific abnormal corneas. Does a cornea with an asymmetrical topography have thin irregular focal zones? If there is any doubt, ultrasound pachymetry should be supplemented by other technological means that measure the corneal thickness in a different manner (eg, using the scanning technology of the Orbscan unit).

WHAT IS THE MECHANISM BEHIND CORNEAL ECTASIA?

The exact etiology of iatrogenic corneal ectasia is not

known. The value of posterior corneal thickness following the ablation has not been established and the role of other concomitant factors is uncertain. These include the extension of the ablation (that may determine the shape of the thinned posterior corneal tissue), the nature of the postoperative scarring, and specific patient factors, including the structural rigidity of the cornea and the IOP.

In corneas affected by keratoconus, Andreassen[2] discovered a lower mechanical resistance as compared to normal corneas. Is it possible that there are variations in the mechanical characteristics of normal corneas? Is it possible that the safety value of the posterior corneal thickness may differ between healthy individuals?

Given our current state of knowledge, we can only evaluate the minimal corneal thickness necessary to prevent ectasia. Currently, the minimum acceptable posterior thickness would appear to lie between 200 and 350 microns. Barraquer[3] recommends a global corneal thickness of at least 300 microns. Seiler[4] recommends a minimum posterior thickness of 250 microns and a safety value of 325 microns.

Other surgeons calculate the acceptable minimum posterior thickness as a percentage of the total thickness. For example, a posterior stromal thickness of no less than 50% of the total corneal thickness could be left.

In reality, it seems advisable to make a percentage calculation of the posterior corneal thickness. If, for example, we have 200 microns as the thickness of the posterior corneal layer in a cornea of 450 microns, this represents 44.44% of the total thickness. However, this represents just 33.33% of the entire thickness of a 600-micron cornea. This may also have important clinical implications.

WHAT STEPS CAN BE TAKEN TO PREVENT IATROGENIC CORNEAL ECTASIA?

Until such time as the pathogenesis of this complication is understood, we can only suggest general guidelines to minimize its risk. Preoperatively:

1. Calculate the total final corneal thickness for every LASIK case on the basis of the refraction and optic zone.

2. Determine the minimum acceptable posterior corneal thickness. If the calculation shows that the treatment will remove an excessive amount of stromal tissue, the alternatives include either an adjustment of the operating parameters, reducing the refractive error to be corrected or the diameter of the ablation zone, or the choice of a different surgical technique.

3. Be very cautious when performing LASIK on eyes with dubious topography, excluding these patients from treatment, if necessary.

Intraoperatively:

4. Measure intraoperative flap thickness and posterior stroma (before and after ablation) in all patients so that in the event of ectasia, calculations can be made on known values.

Postoperatively:

5. Perform careful evaluation of topography and pachymetry prior to every enhancement operation and avoid performing it in eyes with reduced pachymetry values or with dubious topography.

6. Report cases of corneal ectasia in literature to increase understanding of its pathogenesis; examine excised tissue histologically, preferably in a center that specializes in corneal histology.

Until the pathogenesis of iatrogenic corneal ectasia is fully understood, we must handle our patients with extreme care and provide our colleagues with all information possible to increase our overall knowledge of this problem.

REFERENCES

1. Binder PS. Factors Affecting the Predictability of Current LASIK Procedures. In: Buratto L, Brint S, eds. *LASIK: Principles and Techniques.* Thorofare, NJ: SLACK Incorporated; 1998.
2. Andreassen TT, Simonsen H, Oxlund H. Biomechanical properties of keratoconus and normal corneas. *Exp Eye Res.* 1980;31:435-441.
3. Barraquer JI. *Queratomileusis y Queratofaquia.* Bogota: Instituto Barraquer de America; 1980:342.
4. Seiler T, Koufala K, Richter G. Iatrogenic keratectasia after laser in situ keratomileusis. *Journal of Refractive Surgery.* 1998;14:312-317.

Epithelial Defects

Marc Mullie, MD

Epithelial defects are the most common intraoperative complications in LASIK with the ACS. These occur most often as small abrasions superiorly along the edge of the flap between 10 and 2 o'clock. Sometimes the epithelium is not truly abraded but only wrinkled. The other type of abrasion is an unexpected large area erosion that covers the central one-third or more of the flap. In a retrospective review of our first 4000 LASIK cases with the ACS, the incidence of small abrasions was 1% (n = 40). There were six large area abrasions.

Epithelial defects are created as the keratome head passes over the epithelium under high pressure. There is usually an underlying congenital weakness in the attachment of epithelium to the basement membrane. For small superior abrasions, this weakness is well-known from PRK in which manual debridement shows us how easy it is to strip epithelium superiorly. For large area abrasions, there is not always an obvious basement membrane dystrophy, but when a PRK is done on the fellow eye, the epithelium is typically very loose and easy to debride. This underlying weakness, when combined with a rough footplate or dull blade, is enough to create a defect.

There are four basic ways to prevent epithelial defects:

1. Obtaining a thorough preoperative history to rule out recurrent erosions and a detailed slit lamp exam to screen for basement membrane dystrophies.

2. Anesthetic drops should not be instilled too far in advance of surgery to prevent toxicity and dryness. Patients should keep their eyes closed in the preoperative holding area.
3. Footplates and blades should be carefully inspected under the microscope to detect any rough surfaces or edges.
4. A small amount of lubrication (such as Celluvisc) can be applied to the leading edge of the footplate to assist the footplate in sliding over the eye. Also, the epithelium should be wetted with distilled water immediately before the keratome pass.

When small epithelial defects occur, it is best to fit the eye with a large soft contact lens that can act as a shield to protect the flap against lid movement. This lens can be removed the next day. These abrasions usually heal without problems. With large area abrasions, a decision must be made at surgery whether to proceed or not with the laser ablation. If the flap is of normal thickness, it is usually safe to proceed. A soft contact lens is then applied for 24 to 48 hours. In my experience, it is usually best not to perform LASIK on the fellow eye in such cases, but rather PRK or another procedure.

In LASIK, epithelial integrity is sacred. When this integrity is broken, cap edema and poor adherence can occur, leading to either cap displacement with macrostriae or epithelial ingrowth. It is therefore imperative to avoid epithelial defects at all costs.

Managing Partially Resected Flaps

Mihai Pop, MD

Partially resected flaps are small, thin and/or arcuate in one area, with excised or damaged epithelium in another area. The length of the partial flap usually extends to the expected hinge but, due to loss of suction, a defective microkeratome, or poor blade quality, the stroma and epithelium are resected in separate regions horizontal to the microkeratome's movement.

There are two main types of partial flaps: bisected and trisected. The bisected flap consists of one large or arcuate stromal region and excised epithelium on the opposite side. The trisected flap consists of two stromal regions on either side and excised epithelium in the middle. In the case of a bisected flap with removed epithelium outside the optical zone of treatment (6.5 mm

and larger), the LASIK ablation can still be performed since the defective flap will not affect the treatment.

It is mandatory to follow a strict protocol to ensure that stromal tissue is not discarded when cleaning and removing damaged epithelium: do not lift the flap before removing the damaged epithelium and debris. To identify the epithelium from the stroma, use a wet Merocel sponge irrigated with BSS to flatten and massage the flap from the hinge to the periphery. The epithelium over the flap will usually remain firmly attached to the stroma, even on a thin flap, while the damaged epithelium is stretched and loose.

Tape the eyelids closed and prepare the patient for slit lamp examination. Use a LASIK spatula (Katena K3-

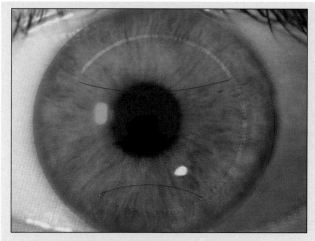

Figure 8L-1. Bisected flap before interaction.

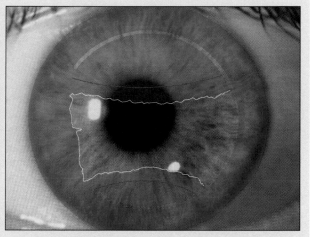

Figure 8L-2. Bisected flap after intervention.

2532) to remove remaining debris and loose epithelium. Never remove the epithelium that is adhered to the flap above the cut edge unless it is extremely long. Once the debris and epithelium are removed, go back under the laser microscope. Flip over the partial flap and remove debris. Using the spatula, massage the flap, then reposition and irrigate it using the flood technique.

The epithelium should extend over the stroma by at least 0.5 mm to decrease the risk of epithelial ingrowth.

Gently massage from the hinge to the periphery, making sure that the epithelium does not curl under the stroma. For trisected flaps, verify that epithelium from one flap is not under the stroma of the adjacent flap. Apply a soft contact lens.

Examine the patient daily until the epithelium is completely healed. Follow-up exams are scheduled in the same manner as for complete LASIK. Retreatment can be scheduled in 12 months.

Kit for Infection Emergencies

Paolo Rama, MD

MATERIALS REQUIRED

- Kimura disposable or reusable spatula with alcohol lamp or electric autoclave
- Sharp spatula (as used for corneal lamellar dissection)
- Glass slides with slide holders for smears
- Cytofix spray
- Sterile dacron or cotton-tipped applicator for swabs
- Transport media for bacteria
- Transport media for chlymydia
- Transport media for virus or vials with distilled solution for PCR

Preparation of Fortified Antibiotics

Cefazolin (50 mg/ml): General cefazolin is usually commercially available as powder (1 gram). The powder is diluted with 10 ml of BSS (equal to 100 mg/ml). Then, 5 ml of BSS are added to 5 ml of the diluted cefazolin (equal to 50 mg/ml). The preparation is stable up to 4 days.

Tobramycin (20 mg/ml): Fortified eyedrops can be prepared by concentrating the commercial eyedrops or making an extemporaneous preservative-free preparation. Both preparations are stable up to 30 days.

- Concentration of the commercial eyedrops: commercially available preparation is 5 ml of 3% solution (3 mg/ml). Remove 2 ml from the commercial eyedrops and add 2 ml of tobramycin for general use (100 mg/2 ml, creating a final concentration of 21.8 mg/ml).
- Extemporaneous fortified preparation: commercially available tobramycin for general use as a solution (100 mg in 2 ml) g/ml). Two ml of tobramycin are added to 3 ml of BSS to reach a final concentration of 20 mg/ml.

Vancomycin (50 mg/ml): Vancomycin for general administration is formulated as a powder (500 mg) that can be diluted with 10 ml of BSS to reach a final concentration of 50 mg/ml. It is stable up to 4 days.

Infections After LASIK

Paolo Rama, MD

Infection is a rare complication of penetrating ocular surgery. Nonpenetrating procedures, such as LASIK, present even lower risks but because refractive surgery is usually performed to correct optical defects in normal eyes, any complication affecting the quality and quantity of vision must be considered serious.

Fast and proper management of infection can influence the prognosis and outcome. For this reason it is important to always have the necessary tools available to carry out corneal scraping or biopsy. Specimen collection and preservation must follow strict protocols discussed with the microbiology center where the specimen will be referred.

PREDISPOSING FACTORS

Blepharitis must always be considered as one of the major risk factors for postoperative infective and noninfective complications. Blepharitis is often accompanied by a positive culture of gram-positive bacteria, or more often staphylococcus, which can become virulent after surgical procedures. Prior to planning any kind of refractive procedure, it is advisable to treat underlying blepharitis until it is under control.

Chalazion and hordeolum, often associated with blepharitis, can increase the risk of postoperative infections. All surgical procedures should be postponed until they disappear.

Conjunctivitis is an absolute contraindication to any ocular surgery.

History of herpes virus keratitis, or conjunctivitis, must be considered a high risk predisposing factor for herpes simplex virus reactivation. It has been clearly demonstrated that any trauma to the cornea, including keratectomy and excimer laser procedures, can reactivate the herpes from a latent state, causing serious recurrent keratitis.

CLINICAL SUSPECT

The type of onset, grade of inflammation, evolution of the infection, and clinical signs can lead to the suspicion of the possible infective agent (bacteria, fungi, viruses, etc). For example, some bacteria can have a very rapid and acute onset (also the night after the LASIK procedure), while fungi take longer to appear. Chlymidia more often causes a chronic infection, while recurrence of herpes virus can be acute.

Clinical suspicion is important for choosing the appropriate culture media and for starting the correct antibiotic therapy before receiving test results from the microbiologist.

DIAGNOSTIC PROCEDURES

When an infective complication is suspected, corneal scraping for smears and a culture should be performed before starting any treatment.

If the ulcer or the infiltrate is on the surface or at the border of the flap, scraping with a Kimura spatula is performed without raising the flap. On the contrary, when the infiltrate is within the interface, raising the flap is mandatory. After having scraped the material for smears and a culture, the interface must be copiously washed with antibiotic.

Smear: a gram stain makes it possible to distinguish the type of infective micro-organisms (bacteria, fungi, and acanthamoeba). Giemsa stain indicates the type of inflammation and shows intracellular inclusions, fungi, and acanthamoeba. The third smear is kept unstained for eventual further specific staining.

Culture: When possible, transport media must be avoided and specimens must be plated directly on the culture media; this enhances the chance of successful recovery of the infective agents.

Chocolate agar is an enriched medium that allows the recovery of most of the bacteria and fungi. It cannot recover anaerobic micro-organisms. It is the first choice if there is only enough material for one inoculation. Sabouraud's agar is a selective medium for fungi. Anaerobic blood agar is indicated for anaerobic bacteria.

Thioglycolate is an enriched medium used to cultivate any type of microorganism. It can be used when the material is scant or to rinse the spatula after having inoculated into the chocolate agar plate to increase the chances of recovering the infective agents.

Note: All media must be at room temperature before inoculation.

When a chlymidial infection is suspected, a specific transport media should be used.

When herpes virus is thought to be responsible of the infection, there are two options: using the specific transport media and then inoculating the material in the appropriate cell culture to detect the characteristic cytopathic effect, or analyzing the specimen with the polymerase chain reaction technique.

MANAGING INFECTIONS AFTER NORMAL HOURS

Smears can be fixed in air or with appropriate spray solution and submitted the following working day. Transport media can be used and kept at 4°C.

Treatment

Topical antibiotics must be started before having the sensitivity profile from the laboratory; for this reason, the drug has to be chosen according to the clinical suspicion and with a broad spectrum. The initial treatment must be aggressive (eg, eyedrops every hour during waking hours and ointment during the night for 5 days, then tapered to every 2 hours, and adjusted according to the clinical course).

Presently, fluoroquinolones seem to be the antibiotics with the best spectrum of activity and lowest toxicity. If the infection does not subside during the first 2 days, or if it gets worse, resistance to the antibiotic should be suspected and the drug changed. If the corneal scraping showed gram-positive bacteria, topical fortified cefazolin (50 mg/ml) or vancomycin (50 mg/ml) can be used. If gram-negative bacteria are detected, fortified tobramycin (20 mg/ml) can be used.

General antibiotics are usually not needed for corneal infection with no risk of perforation.

Topical steroids reduce the cicatricial reaction of the cornea, but they also reduce the host immunologic response and raise the risk of spreading the infection if the antibiotic is not sensitive. Steroids can be added to the antibiotic therapy as soon as the infection shows response to the treatment (not before 2 days) and the patient must be carefully checked.

Cycloplegics should be used only in case of congestion, fibrin formation in the anterior chamber and pain.

Pain can accompany corneal infections. Topical treatment with specific anti-inflammatory drugs can add toxic effects to the antibiotic therapy. It is preferable to use systemic treatment. If topical treatment is used, choose preparations without preservatives.

Severe infections within the interface may not respond to treatment because the drug cannot work as effectively as when it is in direct contact with the microorganisms. In these cases, one can choose to raise the flap every day for washing the infiltrate with antibiotic, remove the flap and keep it preserved in a short storage media (Optisol or similar at 4°C) or dehydrated in the air and then kept in a petri dish. Once the infection is successfully treated, the flap can be sutured back in place.

SUGGESTED READING

Tabbara KF, Hyndiuk RA, eds. *Infections of the Eye.* Boston, Mass: Little, Brown & Company; 1996.

Byrne KA, Burd EM, Tabbara KF, Hyndiuk RA, eds. *Diagnostic Microbiology and Cytology of the Eye.* Boston, Mass: Butterworth-Heinemann; 1995.

Avoiding Complications in LASIK

Olivia Serdarevic, MD

The flap should be meticulously created and handled with proper instrumentation and adequate, but not excessive, hydration to achieve optimal results and avoid flap complications in LASIK.

MICROKERATOME CONSIDERATIONS

Recent modifications in microkeratome design to simplify use by eliminating the surgeon's need to insert a plate, disassemble the head of the microkeratome for blade insertion, and place the blade in the blade holder, have decreased severe complications such as anterior chamber perforations from absent or faulty footplate insertion and very irregular flaps from damaged blades. However, many microkeratomes that were designed to simplify use precluded the surgeon's ability to modify flap parameters to prevent potential problems related to very flat or steep corneas, very large or small corneas, and thin corneas. Although surgeons can usually complete a procedure without considering these variables, meticulous attention to these details improves safety.

Variable Suction Rings and Stop Rings

Surgeons should remember that a microkeratome with the same thickness suction ring base creates wider flaps in steep and small corneas. A suction ring base with a thickness that cuts approximately a 9.0 to 9.5 mm flap in corneas with keratometry readings of 43 D to 44 D results in flaps smaller than 8.5 mm in very flat corneas with curvatures of less than 40 D, and results in flaps larger than 10 mm in very steep corneas over 46 D. Maintaining good suction can be difficult in very flat or steep corneas if only one suction ring with only one base thickness is used for all cases and, therefore, buttonhole formation is a risk in these extreme cases. Moreover, depending on stop ring location, free caps can occur in very flat corneas, particularly in large diameter corneas; and decentration of the microkeratome temporally when using a nasal hinge does not reliably prevent this complication. It is therefore important to choose the appropriate suction ring that, either on the basis of thickness or the internal diameter of the suction ring or both, allows adequate corneal protrusion to avoid complications even in extreme corneas.

Varying Flap Diameter

A very large diameter flap is not ideal in myopic patients with pannus because of intraoperative bleeding as well as more extensive and earlier wound healing at the flap edge, rendering enhancements with flap lifting more difficult. It is known that flaps too small in diameter in hyperopic and astigmatic eyes (with-the-rule astigmatism with nasal hinges) can preclude the surgeon's ability to obtain large optical zones and to prevent laser ablation of the hinge. Decentering the microkeratome (eg, decentering the microkeratome nasally when performing a nasal hinge) can partially obviate the problem of hitting the hinge while performing hyperopic ablations, but this measure is not reliable and can produce free caps.

Varying Flap Location and Width

Although I feel in many cases with narrow hinges that a superior hinge decreases the risk of displacement and folds (particularly when compared to oblique narrow hinges, which can be more difficult to handle), I do not use superior hinges in all cases. If a wider hinge is obtained and the flap is not too thin, can be equally stable no matter where the hinge is placed.

I prefer varying the location of my hinge depending on orbital configuration, the degree of meibomian secretions, corneal vessels, and the axis in which I am treating astigmatism. If a case involves an eye with little space superiorly or with a great deal of pooling in the superior cul-de-sac, I prefer to not use a superior hinge. If a patient has an oblique or against-the-rule astigmatism, I prefer to position the hinge obliquely or horizontally, particularly if the patient also has pannus; this keeps the flap as small as possible while still maintaining adequate space for laser ablation.

Varying Flap Depth

I prefer varying the depth of my flap depending on the amount of corneal tissue that needs to be ablated. I prefer cutting a flap about 180 microns thick to obtain extra flap stability if I have enough posterior corneal tissue remaining to perform an enhancement and still have more than 250 microns left. If the patient's cornea is thin or if I am correcting higher amounts of myopia in a cornea of normal thickness, I prefer cutting a flap of about 150 microns.

FLAP HANDLING CONSIDERATIONS

Marking the Cornea

Marking of the cornea is necessary to prevent folds and to ensure proper repositioning of the flap in case of a free cap. I find a single pararadial mark, which does not disturb the epithelium in the optical zone to be adequate.

For primary LASIK treatments without excessive or improper handling of the flap, repositioning of the flap using the mark makes the need for additional manipulation and alignment by the gutter unnecessary. However, for retreatments, I find that it is important to align the flap using both the epithelial mark and gutter repositioning.

Lifting the Flap

Careful lifting of the flap avoids tearing, folds, and epithelial ingrowth. For primary procedures, I use either forceps with blunt, polished tips, or a cannula.

For retreatments, after pressing on the flap with a moistened Merocel sponge to delineate the flap borders, I use my flap lifter with a tapered edge to facilitate sliding under and through the epithelium and opening adhesions at the flap edge (Figure 8O-1). This instrument allows me to lift the flap, even in the presence of more extensive wound healing responses in patients with wide flaps and pannus, without tearing the flap and without introducing cellular or other particulate debris.

I open 180° of the flap circumferentially with the angled lifter, gently lift and fold over the flap with the same device, then complete flap lifting with a capsulorhexis-like procedure using a moistened merocel sponge (Figure 8O-2).

I prefer to lift the flap for retreatments whenever possible, since recutting the flap can be problematic and can occur in different planes.

Hydration

Before laser ablation, any excessive pooling, occurring most often at the hinge border, should be lightly dried. Consistent hydration of the corneal bed, which should be neither too hydrated nor too dehydrated during each procedure is crucial for preventing undercorrec-

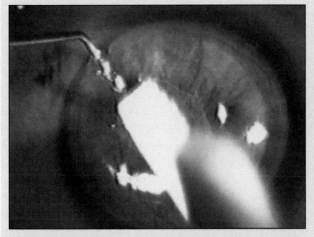

Figure 8O-1. After gently pressing on the flap to delineate the edge, the Serdarevic lifter (Storz) is used to open the flap 180°.

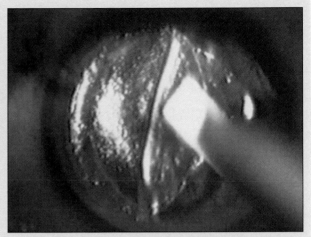

Figure 8O-2. After folding over the flap, flap lifting is completed with a capsulorhexis-like procedure using a sponge.

tions, overcorrections, or irregular astigmatism. On the other hand, excessive hydration of the flap can cause stromal swelling with slow visual rehabilitation and poor adherence.

Flap Repositioning

I reposition the flap after light irrigation of the stromal bed and posterior aspect of the flap.

In cases with a nasal hinge and without meibomian or other particulate debris, a moistened Merocel sponge can be used to reposition the flap. However, in cases with a superior or oblique hinge or with some particulate debris, I always use a double cannula with simultaneous irrigation of the stromal bed, posterior flap surface, and anterior flap surface. The cannula should be inserted on either side of the hinge and should be held parallel to the

hinge during repositioning. If done correctly, this maneuver precludes the need to reintroduce a cannula under the flap for cleaning, which can introduce epithelial cells under the flap and cause folds.

Flap Adherence

Gentle stroking of the flap from just in front of the hinge to just beyond the peripheral edge with a moistened Merocel sponge is my preferred method of ensuring proper flap adherence. Only about 20 strokes are required, but all the strokes must be in the same direction—perpendicular to the hinge—to avoid creating folds.

For retreatments, a little more manipulation consisting of drying the edges in the gutter and repositioning of epithelium outside the flap borders, may be necessary.

Treating Corneal Opacities with PTK and Lamellar Surgery

M. Farooq Ashraf, MD and Walter J. Stark, MD

INTRODUCTION

The excimer laser ablates corneal tissue with submicron precision without significant injury to the surrounding tissues. PTK is indicated for corneal scars and opacities in the anterior third of the cornea that interfere with visual acuity.

PREOPERATIVE EVALUATION

Preoperative evaluation includes visual acuity, visual

potential with pinhole, contact lens fitting, or potential acuity meter, pupil size, slit lamp biomicroscopy, and dilated fundus exam. A strong emphasis is placed on evaluating prospective candidates with a hard contact lens fitting. Many patients with scars or irregular corneas have reduced visual acuity from irregular astigmatism. A rigid or gas-permeable contact lens will correct the astigmatism, resulting in good visual acuity. The majority of patients who are referred to us for PTK leave without laser therapy, since these patients have good functional vision with just a contact lens fitting. Every attempt should be made to fit the patient with a contact lens, since a contact lens may be required after PTK because of induced flattening of the cornea and hyperopia. Preoperative evaluation should include an assessment of the depth of the corneal scar, as well as the overall thickness, with pachymetry or high frequency ultrasound.

SURGICAL TECHNIQUE

Under topical anesthesia, the epithelium may be removed manually or with the laser. If the epithelium is smooth, we remove the epithelium using the laser. The laser is set to the PTK mode with the desired depth, usually between 40 to 50 microns. An irregular epithelial surface is smoothed using masking agents such as 1% hydroxymethylcellulose prior to laser ablation.

The depth of stromal ablation is determined preoperatively and corresponds to the depth of the stromal scar or opacity. Any treatment should leave a minimum of 250 μm of stromal tissue to prevent corneal ectasia and/or haze. The total depth of tissue to be removed is calculated preoperatively with the optical pachymeter. As a rule, always remove less rather than more tissue because the procedure can be repeated. Therefore, caution should be placed on cutting any depth more than what had been planned preoperatively. We caution excessive smoothing or blending to remove a small area of irregularity. Postoperatively, resurfacing of the corneal epithelium will provide a smoothing of the anterior surface, and a contact lens can be used, if necessary, in the postoperative period for irregular astigmatism. Our preference is to remove the most dense area of the opacity. If irregular astigmatism is a problem postoperatively, this can be managed with a contact lens.

PTK will induce flattening of the cornea and result in 2 D to 6 D of hyperopia depending on the depth of the cut. We have modified the PTK treatment to reduce hyperopia. Initially, we induced approximately 4 D of hyperopia with this procedure. We have decreased this by half by creating a transition zone around the edge of the ablation. The epithelium is removed 2.0 mm peripheral to the PTK ablation. A 2.0-mm diameter spot size with a depth of 200 μm is used. The eye is grasped using two toothed forceps on the conjuctiva and episclera 180° apart. The eye is moved in a circular fashion so that the beam straddles around the peripheral edge. We have found that this technique reduces the amount of hyperopia by approximately 2 D to 4 D. In the future, hyperopic photorefractive treatment may be combined with PTK to reduce induced hyperopia.

Postoperative medications include antibiotics and anti-inflammatory agents. The eye is patched after antibiotic ointment (erythromycin or bacitracin) and a cycloplegic (homatropine) is applied to the eye. A therapeutic soft contact lens may be used for pain control. Patients are examined daily or until the epithelium completely covers the stromal bed.

RESULTS

Results of PTK treatment for corneal opacities vary with the etiology of the opacity. The success rate for corneal dystrophies such as lattice, granular, Reis-Buckler, and recurrent dystrophies in the graft is quite high (80% to 100%). Corneal scars, however, have a decreased success rate of approximately 50% to 60%. Deep corneal scars and those from herpes simplex virus do not do as well. Future techniques may involve using a microkeratome to access deep corneal scars or opacities.

Intraoperative Epithelial Complications

Jerry Tan, MBBS, FRCS Ed, FRCOpth, FAMS

Intraoperative epithelial complications are a common complication of LASIK surgery. As a surgeon gains experience, the incidence of this complication falls. The most frequent intraepithelial complication is a corneal abrasion.

Predisposition to a corneal abrasion during LASIK surgery can be caused by:

1. Pre-existing corneal pathology
   a. Recurrent erosion syndrome

   b. Diabetic corneal problems
2. Intraoperative conditions
   a. Epithelial drying
   b. Epithelial edema
   c. Epithelial toxicity from dyes and drugs applied to the cornea
   d. Foreign bodies on the cornea
   e. Blunt microkeratome blades and nonoscillating blades

PRE-EXISTING CORNEAL PATHOLOGY

Recurrent erosion syndrome is an uncommon corneal problem. However, some patients with subclinical recurrent erosion syndrome may unintentionally seek corrective refractive surgery, as they may be having problems with contact lens wear. They may also be looking for a cure for poor spectacle vision from irregular astigmatism caused by epithelial folds and reduplication of their basement membranes. A careful history and thorough examination with retroillumination are most helpful in determining this diagnosis. Their best spectacle-corrected vision is usually much poorer than their contact lens visual acuity. A photokeratoscopic (placido disc) picture in these cases is superior to a corneal topography, as most of the corneal topographers smooth over small irregularities with their algorithms. Fortunately, all topographers can create the placido ring picture; this is invaluable in revealing small corneal irregularities. Finally, many patients with recurrent erosion syndrome will rarely volunteer a typical history of recurrent pain and tearing upon awakening at night. They usually attribute their symptoms to their contact lens wear or dry eye.

Diabetic patients, especially the those with juvenile onset, have two problems that result in poor epithelial adhesion. First, corneal epithelial hemidesmosome and anchoring fibril formation is defective as a consequence of epithelial basement membrane thickening. Second, the loss of corneal sensation from diabetic neuropathy results in poor epithelial regeneration.

Diabetes, especially if there is loss of corneal sensation, is a relative contraindication for LASIK surgery and more so for PRK. Epithelial healing is usually slower and if a large abrasion occurs, flap adhesion is poor, resulting in a higher risk of epithelial ingrowth. Abrasions also increase the risk of infection, especially in patients with diabetes. The approach to diabetics should be individualized and they have to be warned of a slightly higher risk of epithelial complications before surgery.

The older the patient, the higher the risk of epithelial abrasions. Older patients also have poorer hemidesmosome formation due to a thickened epithelial basement membrane. There is a linear increase in the epithelial basement membrane thickness with age. Patients over 45 years old need to be warned about this increased risk and may need to wear a contact lens postoperatively. Warning patients at risk about this minor complication preoperatively will reassure even anxious patients. Since patients are awake during surgery, they tend to notice something different immediately during the LASIK procedure, especially if their second eye is being operated on.

INTRAOPERATIVE CONDITIONS

Epithelial Drying

The beginning LASIK surgeon always takes excessive time in the placement of drapes, lid speculum, eye position, and application of the suction ring. This results in excessive drying and dehydration of the cornea. In some cases, an excited novice surgeon may forget to thoroughly wet the cornea before making the microkeratome pass. This will result in a large and severe corneal abrasion. The microkeratome must flatten the cornea anterior to the advancing blade and the friction of a dry microkeratome will abrade the corneal epithelium.

As the LASIK surgeon becomes more experienced, he or she learns how to move efficiently and quickly; placement of drapes, lid speculum, assessment of adequate exposure, marking the cornea, and application of the suction ring can be done in less than 20 seconds. This short period of time will reduce the risk of epithelial erosion. Before the microkeratome pass, an abundant amount of BSS or topical glycerin-based anesthetic is flushed across the cornea to thoroughly wet it. The use of artificial tears, such as Celluvisc and Refresh Plus, has been advocated by some surgeons. However, the effects of long-term use on the microkeratome mechanism is unknown. Also, the effect of these drugs trapped between the corneal flap and corneal stromal bed is not well-documented. This may be a contributing factor in the incidence of the Sands of the Sahara syndrome, which I believe is multifactorial.

Epithelial Edema

Unfortunately, the surgeon that wets and lubricates the cornea too long and excessively runs the risk of causing epithelial swelling and edema. This edema increases the risk of epithelial abrasions during the microkeratome pass. Liberal use of local anesthetics increases cell membrane permeability and epithelial edema. While this is an advantage in PRK for epithelial removal, it is a disadvantage in LASIK.

It appears to be a "between the devil and the deep blue sea" situation. Too much lubrication causes abrasions as does too little lubrication. The longer the cornea is exposed to lubricants, the higher the chance of edema. The faster the surgeon performs the keratectomy after lubricating the eye the better. Some surgeons have their assistants wet the cornea immediately after suction is applied, minimizing the exposure time of the corneal epithelium to the lubricants.

Pharmacological Toxicity

Many experienced LASIK surgeons do not check intraocular pressure by applanation or mark the cornea for orientation. They have enough experience to feel the increase in intraocular pressure. They also use the signs of pupil dilatation and loss of vision as indicators of adequate suction. I have always done applanation tonometry and marked the cornea for orientation. This has, in many cases, saved me from making a thin flap or free cap.

One should never mark the cornea extensively. The ink and even the impressions made on the cornea by the various marking devices may cause epithelial breaks and irregularities from which an abrasion can originate. A single short pararadial ink mark from a thin round-bodied instrument is more than adequate to assist in orientation. Multiple radial, circular, or pararadial marks so commonly found on many elaborate markers, are unnecessary. By applying so many marks on the cornea, the time taken for corneal marking is longer and this predisposes the cornea to dehydration and epithelial abrasions. There is also an increased possibility of epithelial staining and toxicity caused by the marking ink.

Exposure to various drugs like ophthalmic povidone for sterilizing the operative field and anesthetic drugs with and without preservatives will contribute to epithelial toxicity. These should be minimized both in strength and exposure time. If possible all topical medications should be preservative-free.

Foreign Bodies on the Cornea

Lint, pieces of drape, and lashes can get dragged across the corneal epithelial surface during the keratectomy. The operative field must be flushed quickly and thoroughly, and the fluid in the operative field must quickly be drained away to wash away any debris. The use of lint-free drapes, positive air pressure operating rooms, and HEPA-filtered air can decrease the incidence of lint contaminating the operative field. Careful placement of the drapes, making sure that all lashes are covered and away from the operating field, is also essential.

Blunt Microkeratome Blades and Non-oscillating Blades

In many third-world countries, microkeratome blades are reused (some surgeons reuse the blades anywhere from four to 14 times!), and in other countries "copy" blades from independent manufacturers are used. Unfortunately, these blades have been known to be inferior to the original manufacturers blades. Any bluntness in these blades will result in a shallow cut, smaller flap, and ragged epithelial edges. These ragged edges will increase the risk of epithelial ingrowth and poor flap edge-bed apposition.

A nick in the edge of a blade due to manufacturing defect or poor handling will result in a shredded flap or epithelium. Unfortunately, if one does not inspect the blade preoperatively, the patient's cornea may be permanently scarred. All surgeons should assemble the microkeratome themselves, check the blade edge under the microscope, and check blade oscillations. In many cases, if a microkeratome is driven across the cornea and the blade is not oscillating, a flap will not be created, but an epithelial abrasion resulting in a postponement of surgery and an upset patient. Fortunately, most patients with epithelial abrasions have no permanent damage to their corneas.

MANAGEMENT OF INTRAOPERATIVE EPITHELIAL COMPLICATIONS

The main thrust of management is the prevention of an epithelial complication. However, even in ideal situations and the best of hands, a patient with occult recurrent erosion syndrome may undergo LASIK and after the keratectomy pass, a large flap of epithelium has shifted or torn off.

Management of this problem is divided into:
- Intraoperative management
- Postoperative management

Intraoperative Management

1. Preserve as much epithelium as possible; rearrange it back into the original position before reflecting the flap. This will prevent the epithelium from flipping wrong side up. Do not tear away or throw away any loose pieces of epithelium. Do not wet the epithelium, as it will start to swell and fail to adhere to the Bowman's layer.
2. Reflect the flap from the internal stromal surface. Do not hold the flap with a forceps, as this may tear away more loose epithelium.
3. Proceed with the laser ablation. The bed must be free of epithelium, as this will lead to uneven ablations and irregular astigmatism. Irregular astigmatism is very difficult to treat and almost impossible to resolve spontaneously in LASIK. PRK is much more forgiving in that aspect.
4. After the ablation, use a very wet Merocel sponge to brush the stromal bed thoroughly, but gently, to prevent any possibility of epithelial nest inclusion. Use the sponge and gently roll back the flap from the stromal side. Do not brush the epithelial side. This will tear away the epithelium and contaminate the sponge with loose epithelium.

5. Insert the irrigating cannula and flush vigorously and thoroughly, especially at the hinge and the edges. Next, float the flap back into position. Do not brush the flap down.

6. Use a nontouch technique to allow the flap to sink down into its bed. Dry the groove of the cut only and allow more time for flap dehydration and adherence.

7. Make sure there is no epithelial flaps or edges rolling under the flap. Try to rearrange the surface epithelium to cover most of the Bowman's layer. This must be done with the epithelium wet. A deft touch is essential. Once the epithelium starts to dry and adhere, it is difficult to move, so speed is essential.

8. Always test for striae and, if necessary, wait about 5 minutes for epithelial and flap adherence. Reducing the intensity of the microscope light increases patient cooperation and prevents rapid and excessive dehydration of the epithelium and flap. Working at the highest magnification allows exact placement of the epithelial pieces. Epithelium that does not stick to the Bowman's layer may be wrong side up.

9. Large epithelial defects can cause poor flap adherence. Always use a bandage contact lens to splint the flap and loose epithelium at the end of surgery. The contact lens should have a relatively low water content, large diameter, and flat base curve.

Postoperative Management

Early

1. The contact lens fit should be checked immediately postoperatively at the slit lamp. It should have slight movement upon blinking with no more than 0.5 mm vertical movement. If the contact lens is too tight, it should be changed to a flatter base curve, while a loose lens should be replaced with a steeper base curve. A good starting base curve is 9.0 or 9.2 mm.

2. The eye should be well-lubricated with preservative-free artificial tears, and a repeat check of the contact lens fit should be made at least 1 hour later.

3. Pain with the contact lens wear is a sign of problems. Most patients will have no pain, making use of topical NSAIDs like Voltaren unnecessary except in large corneal abrasions. These NSAIDs may slow re-epithelialization and should be discontinued after 4 days, if used.

4. Standard topical steroids and antibiotics are used over the contact lens.

Late

1. The following day, the patient is examined for flap position, re-epithelialization, and infection. The contact lens is removed as soon as the epithelium has healed.

2. If removal is done too soon, the patient will experience pain and discomfort with tearing and blepharospasm.

3. The epithelium will still be slightly irregular and visual recovery will be slower.

Patients who develop intraoperative epithelial complications range from minor tears of the epithelium, shifts in the epithelium, to large abrasions. They can be treated successfully without any risk of epithelial ingrowth. The standard LASIK technique need not be changed in cases of small abrasions, while it is essential to preserve as much epithelium and use a contact lens in large abrasions. With such techniques successful LASIK can be performed in cases of recurrent erosion syndrome, and enhancements can even be performed without difficulty. In fact, the fine-curved scar of the LASIK flap may help epithelial adherence and prevent further attacks of epithelial erosions.

Infections and Keratitis

Michiel S. Kritzinger, MD

Infections can be the most serious and visually threatening complication after LASIK surgery. Fortunately, the incidence is rare, about 1:1000 cases. It usually manifests between 1 to 4 days postoperatively and happens more frequently during the surgeon's learning curve. In bilateral LASIK surgery, infection rarely occurs bilaterally but can affect either eye in bilateral surgery.

Infecting agents can be:
1. Bacteria (eg, staphylococcus aureus, epidermis, seratia marcescens, pneumococcus, or pseudomonas aeruginosa)
2. Fungi (eg, aspergillus)
3. Virus (eg, herpes)
4. Acanthamoeba

Clinical symptoms:
1. Red, tearing, photophobic eye
2. Blurred vision
3. Swelling of the corneal flap and eyelids
4. Foreign body sensation
5. Painful eye

HOW DOES THE INFECTION PRESENT?

1. Flap edge infection and melting, more frequently the superior and inferior flap edge.
2. Mild stromal interface dot infiltration.
3. Severe stromal infiltrate interface infection.

How to prevent it:
1. Autoclave and chemical sterilization (with Endozyme).
2. Preserve epithelium as much as possible during surgery.
3. Perfect gutter-flap edge sealing.
4. Intact proper flap.
5. Eyelid care and hygiene.
6. Sterile environment and surgical technique.
7. Irrigation of the stromal interface after closing the flap to reduce foreign bodies and infective agents.
8. Prophylactic postoperative antibiotics.

Treatment:
1. Flap edge infection
   a. Amikacin 25 mg/ml one drop hourly

b. Vancomycin 50 mg/ml one drop hourly
   c. Pred Forte one drop every 2 hours
   Do not lift the flap because you will spread the infection. Use fortified eyedrops.
2. Mild dot interface infection
   a. Use fortified eyedrops as with flap edge infection.
3. Severe infiltrate infections
   a. Lift the flap and scrape both surfaces for laboratory MCS.
   b. Irrigate the interface with BSS and fortified antibiotic eyedrops.
   c. Do not perform an anterior chamber tap with an interface infection. It is unnecessary and you will spread the infection.

DIFFUSE LAMELLAR KERATITIS

DLK (diffuse lamellar keratitis) is also referred to as nonspecific diffuse intralamellar keratitis or Sands of the Sahara (SOS) syndrome. The incidence of this condition is rising for unknown reasons.

Etiology

Currently, etiology is unclear, but it is suspected that wax and oils from the blades of microkeratomes induce this condition. With bilateral LASIK surgery, it usually happens to the first eye but rarely to the second eye. At present, it manifests clinically, usually within the first week postoperatively.

Treatment

Although this condition responds dramatically to high dosages of topical steroid eyedrops, I still prefer to lift the flap and scrape out this grayish gel infiltrate from the interface bed as well. By having this aggressive surgical approach, the treatment healing time is short with steroid eyedrops.

Complications like basement membrane haze and fibrosis are also negligible. Visual recovery is usually faster and the incidence of postinflammation refractive errors is minimal. Usually with the steroid-surgical approach, antibiotics (Exocin) are added as well.

Early diagnosis and an aggressive treatment regime will give good visual results.

POSTOPERATIVE FOLLOW-UP

Lucio Buratto, MD and Stephen Brint, MD

INTRODUCTION

Follow-Up: Examination Schedule

1. **Immediate postoperative period** (ie, within the first hour after surgery). Some surgeons check the patient immediately after leaving the operating room to ensure that the flap is well positioned and there is no debris in the interface. They allow the patient to then rest for 20 to 30 minutes and recheck to ensure that the flap has not moved from blinking or rubbing and that there are no visible striae, with perfect gutter alignment. Some surgeons forgo the initial check and just perform the second check. The disadvantage of this is if flap dislocation is seen it perhaps could have been fixed 20 minutes earlier.

2. **Postoperative day 1.** Perfect flap position and absence of striae is checked again. Corneal topography may be performed to check centration of the ablation. Uncorrected visual acuity is checked and refraction may be done if indicated. If there are problems, it is much easier and safer to intervene by lifting the flap at this time as opposed to later.

3. **Subsequent exams** are typically done at 1 week, 1 month, 3 months, 6 months, and 1 year after surgery.

Visits at 3, 6, and 12 months allow the surgeon to check refractive stability. If necessary, at about 3 to 4 months postoperatively, the surgeon can plan to perform an enhancement operation.

Patients with regression or undercorrection while they are waiting for the second operation must be offered spectacles or contact lenses.

The patient should not use contact lenses for at least 2 weeks after surgery; after this time, we can be reason-ably sure that the flap has firmly adhered to the stromal bed.

Disposable contact lenses are essential given the need for frequent changing until the refraction has stabilized. Disposable lenses are very thin, highly flexible, and adapt well to the new corneal surface, in addition to being well-tolerated. A semirigid contact lens should not be used; these will often form a liquid meniscus between the contact lens and cornea, as well as producing blurry vision and altered refraction. Semirigid contact lenses must also be avoided, as they will modify corneal topography while the patient is waiting for the enhancement. Contact lenses must be used with artificial tears.

Additional Exams

Visual acuity is checked at each postoperative visit. At the initial check, visual acuity will usually be quite good but will improve even over the first week. In the majority of cases, the maximum final uncorrected visual acuity is present at 1 month after surgery.

By the third month, visual acuity should have stabilized; stabilization may occur later only in those cases in which there were intra- or postoperative problems or when the treated myopia was extremely high.

Stabilization of the refraction can also be confirmed with cycloplegia and corneal topography. These should remain more or less unchanged after the first month. If there is glare or irregular astigmatism at 6 months after surgery, these phenomena are likely to be permanent. Treatment should be considered if possible at this time.

The cornea, refraction, topography, subjective evaluation, and treatment are summarized at the various time intervals following LASIK:

1. **Immediately postoperative** (within 1 hour after surgery):
- Refraction: reduced visual acuity.
- Subjective report: irritation and discomfort. The

patient can feel the flap edge that has not yet re-epithelialized and there is slight burning and tearing.

- Conjunctival injection and edema.
- **Cornea**
  - The resection line of the flap edge is visible.
  - Mild corneal flap edema. This edema may give the ablated area an irregular eccentric appearance
  - Possible epithelial defects. If small, the defects will heal spontaneously with no further consequences; if they are larger, frequent follow-up will be necessary to monitor possible epithelial ingrowth.
  - Possible debris and/or blood residue in the interface.
  - Possible conjunctival and/or corneal hemorrhage.
  - Rarely, an air bubble may be seen under the flap. It will spontaneously reabsorb but the flap may not be perfectly distended.

2. **Day 1**
- Refraction: visual acuity is usually 75% or 80% of the maximum potential value (BCVA). There may be overcorrection of 1 to 2 diopters (D).
- **Subjective**
  - The patient reports good quality vision, but not perfect (he or she may complain of glare and ghosting). Generally, the patient is quite satisfied with the obtained result.
  - If there is undercorrection in a hyperopic patient, the patient may complain of poor near vision. The opposite applies to myopic patients.
  - There may be moderate photophobia but without excessive tearing.
  - If the tear production is excessive, the surgeon should carefully check the flap and its edges; there may epithelial defects or flap displacement.
- **Cornea**
  - The flap resection line is no longer visible; however, a very fine peripheral line can be seen.
  - Usually the flap is well-distended. On close examination, some microstriae may be seen, particularly with a nasal-hinged flap.
  - The corneal flap edema will have almost disappeared. Thus, the area of ablation will be more centered and regular. If the edema persists, particularly if significant, it usually indicates problems during surgery. Steroid eyedrops may be used to reduce it. The surgeon must carefully look for flap striae. If the flap has been aligned correctly and just a few fine folds are observed, it is likely that the folds were actually caused by

the edema and will disappear once the edema disappears. More frequent checks are necessary in this situation because edema can also encourage the dislocation of the flap. An apparent dislocation can be observed if the flap is edematous and the edema is not uniform. In this case, absence of folds and correct alignment of the markings (that are still visible) will indicate that the dislocation is only apparent. If there has been true dislocation of the flap, the patient must be returned to the operating room for refloating and repositioning. Persistent edema unrelated to epithelial defects is not normal. It may indicate infection, epithelial ingrowth, Sands of the Sahara syndrome, and debris in the interface.

- Possible epithelial defects. These can be seen with fluorescein staining. These must be monitored daily until they are resolved. These defects may indicate localized edema, poor flap adhesion, which creates a risk of epithelial ingrowth. If the epithelial defects are small, current therapy can be continued. However, if marked, steroids should be suspended for 2 to 3 days. A contact lens can be applied if necessary.
- Possible conjunctival incision with inclusion of blood or blood residues at the interface.
- Possible low-grade haze interface.
- Debris in the interface.
- Corneal topography: even at this early stage, this examination is useful; it serves to check whether the ablation is centered and whether the ablated area is sufficiently uniform and extensive.

Postoperative Therapy

Combination antibiotic steroid drops four to five times per day for 7 days, artificial tears five times a day for at least 2 weeks, and even more frequently the first few days.

3. **After 6 to 8 days**
- **Refraction**
  - In the majority of cases, uncorrected visual acuity will be near its potential.
  - Corrected visual acuity may have returned to its preoperative level, except in severe myopia or hyperopia in which a greater amount of time is required; in the majority of cases, in the absence of complications, the visual acuity should exceed 75% of the preoperative value. Initial overcorrection should have decreased. This may disturb near vision in presbyopic myopic patients; the surgeon should reassure the patient that this was intentional in order to achieve a good final outcome. Temporary spectacles may

be prescribed to correct near vision in presbyopic patients. During this examination, the surgeon gets a feel whether the correction is adequate or if there is a tendency for undercorrection. In the latter case, this will increase over the next few weeks.

- **Subjective**
  - Quality of vision has improved considerably. Glare, ghost images, etc, will have almost disappeared. Some patients complain of difficulty with night driving, particularly severely myopic patients and those with large pupils; this complaint will tend to diminish with time. Residual myopia compounds this problem and should be corrected with temporary spectacles.
  - Some patients notice vision fluctuation throughout the day; it is a frequent phenomenon but decreases with time.
  - The flap should be checked for dislocation if there is any sudden appearance of excess tearing postoperatively. If so, prompt repair as previously described should be performed.
- **Objective corneal findings**
  - The white peripheral demarcation line of the flap (ie, the surface cut at Bowman's layer) is easily visible.
  - The flap is generally well-positioned.
  - Under retroillumination, flap microfolds may be seen, which do not cause the patient any disturbance.
  - Sometimes, isolated groups of cells can be observed that may give rise to areas of epithelial ingrowth.
  - Corneal topography: This may highlight central islands, decentration, and astigmatism.
  - Therapy: Combination antibiotic steroid drops five times a day until day 7, and monodose artificial tears four times a day.
  - Prevention: The patient should be instructed to refrain from contact sports for at least 1 month (as this carries the risk of flap displacement) and to avoid swimming for 2 to 4 weeks (as this carries the risk of infection). Eye rubbing should be strictly avoided.
4. **One month**
- **Refraction:**
  - Uncorrected visual acuity will have reached its maximum value.
  - Corrected visual acuity will normally have returned to its preoperative levels (but may be further delayed in severe myopes). At this time, the surgeon can usually tell how effectively the refractive error has been corrected (with severe

astigmatism, there will be an improvement in vision as compared to preoperative values). If visual acuity is not as good as expected, the surgeon should try to identify the reason. He or she should check for decentration of the ablation or central islands. Microstriae do not normally interfere with visual acuity unless they are through the visual axis. Small residual errors should be corrected. If the error is more than 1 D and the patient was not a high myope, further enhancement can be considered. Pachymetry must be performed to check the residual corneal thickness. As previously mentioned, further surgery at 3 to 4 months postoperatively allows lifting the flap mechanically without having to cut a new flap; this involves minimal risks for the patient and excellent functional results. Steroids are temporarily useful; but do not affect regression. The patient may use contact lenses (one-a-day disposables are preferable).

- **Subjective**
  - The quality of vision has improved. Glare, ghost images, etc, have almost disappeared in uncomplicated cases. In some cases (severely myopic patients in particular), there may be complaints of disturbances at dusk or at night.
  - A residual refractive error will aggravate these vision disturbances. They may be corrected with spectacles or contact lenses to improve the quality of vision.
  - A check of ablation centration and pupil diameter may also prove useful under conditions of mesopic light. In some cases, administration of 0.5% pilocarpine at dusk for 1 to 2 months may improve symptoms.
  - Undercorrected patients will normally be disappointed with the partial correction. Prior to suggesting an enhancement treatment, the psychological profile of this patient should be carefully evaluated.
- **Objective corneal findings**
  - There are no problems in the majority of cases. The edges of the flap are difficult to see.
  - There may be areas of epithelial ingrowth.
  - There may be central islands—these will require monthly checks. When refraction and topography have stabilized, the islands can be treated.
  - Intrastromal haze is almost absent.
- **Topography**
  - This examination should be repeated to document centration.
  - In the event of reduced visual acuity, this test also serves to define any central islands or astig-

matism; it helps the surgeon to understand any refractive variations.

- **Therapy**
  - Monodose artificial tears can be used when needed.

5. **Three months**
- **Refraction**
  - Uncorrected and best-corrected visual acuity will be almost completely stabilized (with the exception of some cases of high myopia and some complicated cases). Any residual astigmatism (more than 1 D) can be corrected.
  - If necessary at this point, an enhancement treatment can be planned.
  - Subjective: Evening discomfort is reduced. Some patients complain of dry-eye sensation.
  - Objective corneal findings: Microstriae may sometimes be seen.
  - Corneal topography: This test generally shows little to no change from the first month.

Table 9-1
FOLLOW-UP
Immediately postoperatively: Check the flap and interface
Day 1: Check the flap and interface, measure refraction (optional), visual acuity, and topography
Week 1: Measure refraction and visual acuity, check the flap and interface
Month 1: Measure refraction and visual acuity

6. **8 to 12 months**
- The situation should be unchanged from the 3-month exam. If the refractive error has increased, corneal topographies and biometry must be compared to evaluate whether it is a question of regression or increase in the axial myopia.
  - If the patient still complains of night glare and irregular astigmatism, these phenomena can be considered permanent.
  - If necessary at this stage, enhancement can be scheduled. However, in this case, a new microkeratome cut should be performed.

ENHANCEMENT AND LASIK IN SPECIAL CASES

10

Lucio Buratto, MD and Stephen Brint, MD

INTRODUCTION

An enhancement procedure should be considered when residual refractive error requires correction (myopia, hyperopia, or astigmatism). Laser-assisted in-situ keratomileusis (LASIK) can be used to enhance not only those patients who had LASIK as a primary procedure, but also patients treated with other refractive techniques, or patients with surgically induced refractive error.

LASIK ENHANCEMENT

Enhancement is more commonly needed with higher refractive errors. The surgeon should advise these patients prior to their primary procedure that enhancement may be necessary in order to obtain an acceptable refractive result.

The decision to enhance is normally based on the 1- to 3-month postoperative refraction. At this point, refraction is stable and the LASIK flap can still be easily lifted. The majority of myopic regression occurs within 1 month and stability is normally reached within 3 months. Enhancement procedures can be planned between 1 to 3 months following the primary procedure.

In theory, the lower the amount of pre-LASIK myopia, the earlier the enhancement can be done. Preoperative myopia of -3.0 diopters (D) can safely be enhanced at 1 month postoperatively; however preoperative myopia of –12.00 D should not be enhanced for a full 3 to 4 months after the primary procedure. Enhancement of overcorrections should be delayed even longer, even up to 1 year, especially if the preoperative refractive error was high. There is a tendency toward myopic regression that may eliminate the need for enhancement.

Astigmatic refractive errors stabilize quite rapidly allowing for early enhancement.

Because hyperopic LASIK requires a longer period of time to stabilize enhancement should be delayed until a stable refraction is demonstrated.

Preoperative Evaluation

A complete pre-enhancement evaluation should include a through review of the original procedure in order to identify any unusual elements. The patient's refractive history should be re-evaluated.

With a new patient (the surgeon did not perform the original procedure), the surgeon should attempt to obtain the following data:
- The original refractive error
- History of previous refractive procedures
- Healing process
- Initial quality of vision and subsequent
- Changes in visual acuity
- Progression of the ametropia (this will aid in determining the cause of the postoperative refractive error)

When planning an enhancement procedure, the ocular and refractive evaluation must be accurate. The exam should include both subjective and cycloplegic refraction. Keratometry and topography are useful in evaluating corneal curvature and determining corneal stability or ectasia. Pachymetry determines whether the corneal thickness is sufficient to allow for enhancement without risking postoperative ectasia. Pre-enhancement pachymetry is mandatory and should be verified by repetition.

When planning hyperopic enhancement of undercorrected hyperopic LASIK, pachymetry should be performed centrally and also 3.0 mm from the central cornea. Ideally, residual thickness at 3.0 mm following hyperopic LASIK should be 350 microns or more.

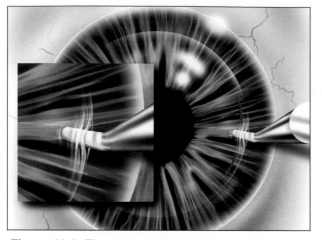

Figure 10-1. The enhancement spatula separates the scar between Bowman's membrane.

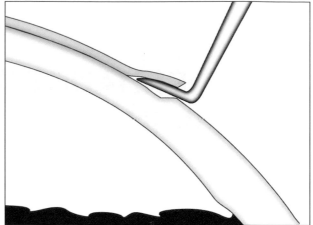

Figure 10-2. Close-up of Figure 10-1: the spatula that separates the flap from the underlying cornea.

Corneal transparency should be examined with the slit lamp. Any opacity or haze should be stable before enhancement is considered. Refractive lamellar keratoplasty may be preferable when dense opacities interfere with vision. If epithelial ingrowth or striae are noted, the surgeon should plan to correct this during the enhancement procedure.

Corneal topography or corneal videokeratography are essential for centering the ablation and ruling out a central island or decentered ablation. If there are any doubts, computerized retroillumination and topography with an Orbscan elevation type instrument may be useful. This provides posterior corneal curvature and pachymetry over the entire cornea.

Enhancement can be performed in two ways:
1. By cutting a new flap with the microkeratome
2. By lifting the LASIK flap

Whether the first or second technique is preferable is the subject of much controversy. Following is a closer look at both.

Lifting the Flap

First, the hinge should be located either nasal or superiorly. It is helpful for this to be recorded, however always consider this and try to locate the flap edge and hinge location. Then the edge of the previously cut flap must be exactly identified. There are many techniques for lifting the flap. It should be remembered that the greatest adhesion will be at the flap margin where Bowman's layer has been cut. Not all of the cut stromal surface will have strongly adhered to the bed.

Using the laser microscope, identify the shadow of the scar from the previous cut. Using an insulin needle, remove the epithelium for about 1.0 to 2.0 mm opposite the hinge along the flap edge—the edge of the flap is

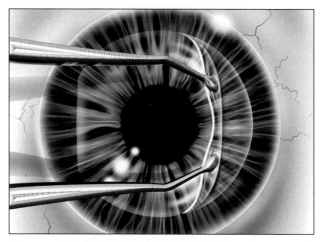

Figure 10-3. The flap is grasped with two forceps and lifted.

slightly lifted. Then, using forceps, the flap is gently peeled completely back. If this proves difficult, the epithelium should be removed for 3.0 to 4.0 mm; two forceps are then used to complete the procedure.

Another technique uses a Sinskey hook. The instrument is used to define the edge of the flap by gently dragging it toward the flap edge opposite the hinge until the edge is lifted. The surgeon proceeds along the entire circumference of the cut, the fine scar line formed in Bowman's layer is detached. Two forceps are then used to lift the flap. Rather than starting opposite the hinge, some surgeons prefer to begin lifting at 6 o'clock. Leaving the area of epithelial damage inferiorly creates less discomfort for the patient.

In another technique, a surgical pen is used to mark the edges of the flap at the slit lamp. The surgeon then proceeds under the laser with the first technique described. It may be impossible to distinguish the

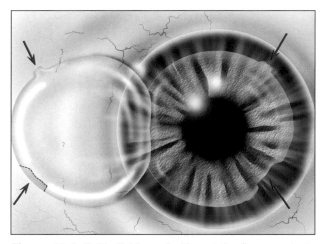

Figure 10-4. Epithelial irregularities at the flap margin in the enhancement technique.

unmarked edge with the operating microscope due to lack of tangential illumination. Again, at the slit lamp using an insulin needle, the flap edge is marked and slightly raised. Under the laser microscope, the surgeon can proceed with a Sinskey hook, blunt forceps, or a spatula.

There is a highly effective way to highlight the entire flap scar when using the operating microscope. With a damp Merocel sponge, the surgeon exerts firm pressure on the cornea. The scar will be clearly visible and, using a Sinskey hook, a semicircular area of epithelium removed corresponding to the scar. Once the entire circumference has been identified, the hook can be used to rupture the scar. The flap will peel back very easily. There are a variety of flap-lifting techniques, the technique that uses two pairs of blunt forceps is preferable. This technique avoids introducing epithelial cells into the interface. The surgeon should proceed gently, exerting slow, even, and constant traction. Care must be taken not to tear the flap edges or the flap itself. Avoid folding or twisting the flap. The flap is normally lifted from the side opposite the hinge, progressing in the same direction it was originally cut.

Another technique involves removing the epithelium at the superior edge of the hinge. A blunt spatula is then inserted under the flap until it emerges at the inferior edge opposite the hinge. The spatula is slowly and progressively moved in the direction opposite the hinge, breaking the scar and epithelium.

Lifting the flap is easy when the time between the primary operation and enhancement is short (1 to 3 months). The scar created where Bowman's layer is cut is weak and the stroma-to-stroma adhesion is minimal. After 3 to 4 months, it may prove more difficult to lift the flap. A more complicated technique may be needed.

Once the flap edge has been identified, an enhancement spatula is inserted and used to detach the entire surface of the flap from the stromal bed. Then, using one or two forceps, the flap is gently lifted. If resistance is encountered, a forcep is used to gently detach the stromal surface while lifting with another forcep. Be especially careful if the original microkeratome pass was thin. Another technique advocated by John Doane is epitheliorhexis. In this technique the edge of the flap opposite the hinge is defined and lifted with an enhancement spatula for approximately 3 clock hours. The flap is then reflected over onto itself. The epithelium is kept wet. A dry single or pair of Merocel sponges is used on the reflected stromal side of the flap to pull the flap toward the hinge in a circular capsulorhexis-type movement. This usually gives a pristine edge with minimal epithelial tags, closely approximating a fresh cut in appearance.

Once the flap is reflected, the interface and stromal surface of the flap should be carefully examined under high magnification for traces of epithelium or debris. Any epithelial cells found on the stromal bed or underside of the flap must be removed by gently scraping the area with a blunt spatula or surgical blade. The spatula or blade must be wiped clean of epithelium after every pass. If the stromal surfaces are carefully cleaned, the risk of epithelial ingrowth is reduced to no more than that associated with a primary keratectomy. Once the flap has been lifted and reflected nasally or superiorly (if down-up LASIK was performed), the ablation is performed, and finally the flap is repositioned as in a primary LASIK procedure.

Enhancement provides opportunities for not only correcting residual refractive error but also offers the opportunity to improve quality of vision. For example, if a patient requiring enhancement also complains of glare and poor night vision, a larger optic zone may be used during the enhancement ablation. If the primary ablation was not perfectly centered, the enhancement ablation can be positioned to compensate.

All of these techniques damage the epithelium, creating foreign body sensations, tearing, and burning. This increases the risk of flap displacement as a result of patients inadvertently rubbing their eyes. Nevertheless, lifting the flap for enhancement is associated with less risk than with a repeat keratectomy.

Lifting the flap for LASIK enhancement has numerous advantages:

- It is a simple surgical technique that avoids the risks associated with a second microkeratome pass
- It allows for the correction of a wide range of refractive errors and defects

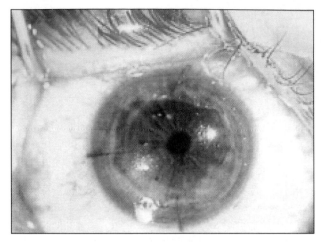

Figure 10-5. Enhancement following down-up LASIK. The operation begins with three-radius markings: two radial and one pararadial.

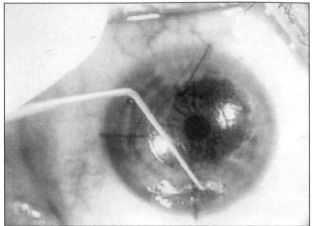

Figure 10-6. The flap is outlined with a Sinskey hook.

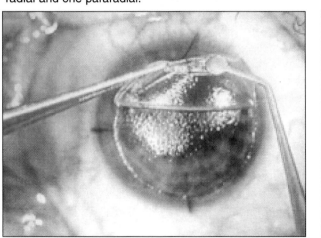

Figure 10-7. The flap is lifted from down upward with nontraumatic forceps.

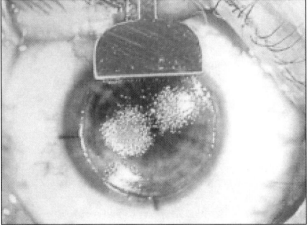

Figure 10-8. The flap is protected during photoablation.

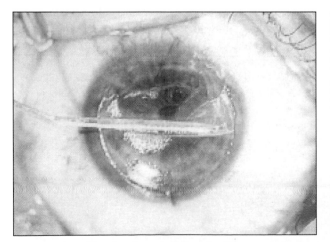

Figure 10-9. The flap is repositioned with a spatula.

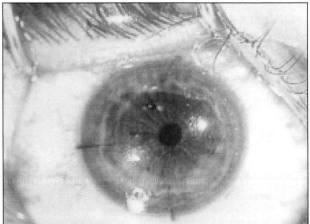

Figure 10-10. The flap has been repositioned. The interface is then washed, the flap is dried, and a striae test is performed.

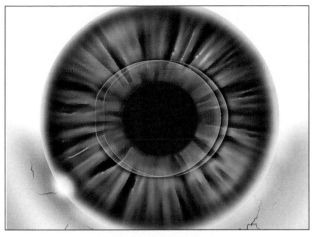

Figure 10-11. The enhancement technique with a repeat of the cut in the nasal hinge technique. The second cut normally starts more temporally.

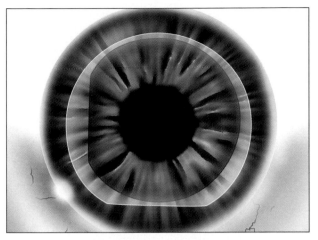

Figure 10-12. Enhancement technique with a repetition of the cut. Following the primary technique with a nasal hinge, in the repeat operation the cut is made larger, deeper, and has a superior hinge.

Table 10-1
LASIK ENHANCEMENT

Classification: Enhancement procedures can be classified according to the primary refractive procedure.
- After previous laser surgery
- Post-PRK
- Post-LASIK
- After other refractive procedures
  - Incisional surgery
  - Radial keratotomy
  - Astigmatic trapezoidal keratotomy
  - Arcuate incisions
  - Parallel incision
  - Relaxing lamellar refractive surgery
  - Lamellar keratotomy

ALK for hyperopia
- Lamellar refractive surgery with tissue removal
- Keratomileusis (freeze technique)
- In situ keratomileusis

ALK for myopia

Lamellar refractive surgery that adds tissue
- Epikeratophakia
- Keratophakia

Surgery that compresses tissue
- Circular corneal sutures
- Corneal surgery that contracts tissue
- Thermokeratoplasty

Following perforating or lamellar keratoplasty
- In aphakic or pseudophakic eyes
- Following nonrefractive surgery of the anterior or posterior segments

Following implantation of a refractive IOL (phakic IOL)

- The procedure is safe, effective, and the result is predictable

Six months or more after the primary LASIK procedure, the corneal flap is very adherent to the stromal bed. Lifting the flap is a difficult and lengthy procedure that consists of creating larger epithelial defects and distorting the flap. It is then better to cut a new flap than to try to lift the original. This is our preference, however some surgeons never cut a new flap, even after several years.

Creating a Second Flap

The advantages of recutting the flap for enhancement are:
- There are no epithelial defects to cause discomfort
- Visual rehabilitation is rapid, usually good the first postoperative day

The dynamics of enhancement are the same as for a primary LASIK procedure. The nomogram for calculating the laser ablation is unchanged. Pain and postoperative discomfort are minimized. Excessive manipulation of the flap should be avoided.

There are three disadvantages associated with a second microkeratome cut:
1. All the risks associated with a primary keratectomy still apply (thin flaps, free caps, etc).
2. The corneal profile has been altered. The central cornea is considerably flattened, often less than 40 D. This may increase the risk of free caps, perforations, etc.
3. The second microkeratome pass risks creating a free corneal wedge of tissue where the two flaps intersect (duplication of the cut). Opinions vary—many surgeons prefer to use the same plate or

273

head as used in the primary procedure with the intention of cutting at the same depth. Others prefer to use a plate or head that will produce a deeper cut and avoid cutting into the first flap. Some prefer to decenter the second cut so that it begins in virgin cornea that was not previously involved in the keratectomy. Others prefer to create a larger flap in a different position; for example, if the primary flap was 8.0 mm with a nasal hinge, for the second flap the surgeon would attempt a 9.0 to 9.5 mm flap with a superior hinge. A spatula should never be used to lift and reflect a second flap. When the spatula is inserted between the flap and stromal bed, it may detach portions of tissue cut during the primary procedure. The second flap should always be lifted and reflected using forceps. Once the flap is lifted the stromal surface should be treated with care. Sponges and cannulas should be used gently and carefully to avoid disruption of tissue involved in the first keratectomy.

LASIK FOLLOWING OTHER REFRACTIVE OR NONREFRACTIVE PROCEDURES

Preoperative Evaluation

As well as including all the elements previously discussed, the preoperative evaluation of patients that have undergone refractive procedures other than photorefractive keratectomy (PRK) or LASIK, or nonrefractive surgery with induced refractive error, should include some additional assessments. Endothelial specular microscopy is important in eyes that have undergone previous intraocular surgery (penetrating keratoplasty, cataract with intraocular lens [IOL], etc). Compromised endothelium could decrease the efficacy of the refractive procedure and affect the refractive prognosis. Surgery for cataract, retinal detachment, keratoplasty, and extensive electrocoagulation for glaucoma all create corneal hypoanesthesia with associated problems.

LASIK Following Other Refractive Procedures

LASIK Following RK

PRK following radial keratotomy (RK) carries an increased risk of haze as compared to primary PRK. Re-epithelialization is often slower, and infection and infiltrations are more likely. Finally, the refractive result is not very predictable.

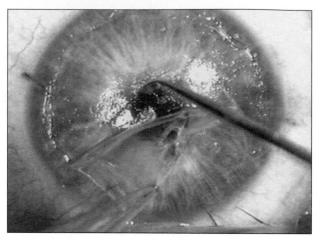

Figure 10-13. Central perforation of the flap during an attempt to lift it 11 months after the primary operation.

LASIK is more successful. It can be used in either overcorrection or undercorrection. Enhancements performed before 1 year post-RK carry a higher risk of producing a flap fragmented by open RK incisions. This risk decreases with the passage of time but is always possible. The incisions should be carefully examined preoperatively at the slit lamp. Determine the depth of the incisions, whether the scar is fibrotic, if there is any epithelium in the incision. Open incisions (with epithelial gaps) or epithelial plugs in the incisions increase the risk of epithelial ingrowth and ectasia. Measure the central optic zone (the area of central cornea free from incisions, which, following RK, is often small). Patients who complain of glare, halos, fluctuation, and poor night vision should be warned that the enhancement procedure may not improve visual quality. The surgeon faces a number of potential problems.

Rupture of the Radial Incisions

Determine the depth of the incisions made during the primary RK procedure. If these were deep and the patient is overcorrected, the incisions may open during surgery, inducing astigmatism and epithelial ingrowth. To avoid this, the flap must be handled very carefully. Lift the flap with a spatula; the spatula supports a larger area of the flap to prevent traction on one point that could cause the incisions to open. For this reason forceps should not be used. Use a plate or head that will create a deep cut (200 to 220 microns), this will reduce the risk of opening the incisions. A large flap is also advisable.

Epithelial Ingrowth in the Incisions

Using a plate or head that produces a deep cut (200 to 220 microns) will reduce the risk of distributing epithelium from inside the incisions into the interface.

We recommend that the bed and stromal surface of

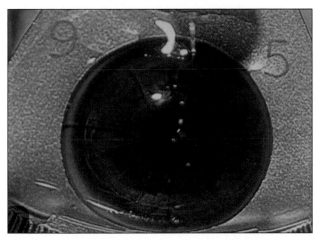

Figure 10-14. A 9.5 ring of the Hansatome and a 180-plate for the lamellar cut on an eye with previous RK.

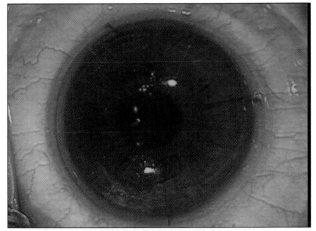

Figure 10-15. LASIK following RK with 16 cuts.

Table 10-2
COMPARISON OF PRK AND LASIK FOLLOWING RK

PRK advantages
- Possible PTK for smoothing
- No risk of incisions separating
- No problems with postoperative flap stability
- No risk of epithelial ingrowth

Disadvantages
- Haze
- Regression
- Reduced predictability
- Difficult epithelial debridement
- Prolonged re-epithelialization
- The scars respond differently to the laser energy than intact adjacent tissue

LASIK advantages
- Rapid recovery
- Reduced regression
- Possibility of higher corrections

Disadvantages
- Risk of incisions separating
- Postoperative flap instability
- Successive enhancement generally requires a new cut; lifting is not recommended

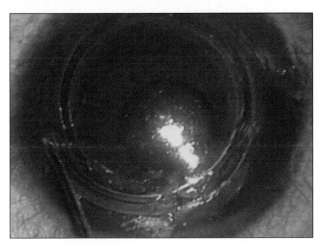

Figure 10-16. Removal of an intracorneal ring. The surgeon must wait at least 3 months before performing the lamellar cut with LASIK.

Problems with Postoperative Flap Stability

This is directly related to the RK incisions. Sutures may be necessary, especially if the flap has been fragmented. This is more likely to occur if more than eight incisions were performed or the flap is thin or small. Aligning the incisions in the bed with those in the flap provides a reliable method of repositioning the flap correctly.

LASIK Following AK

LASIK can be considered an enhancement option following astigmatic keratotomy (AK). The problems faced are similar to those encountered when enhancing RK: irregular astigmatism, possible epithelial ingrowth, possible incision rupture, etc. However, the lower number and peripheral position of the incisions reduce the risk of encountering problems. The central optic zone is uninvolved.

the flap be carefully and gently cleaned. It is important to remove any epithelial cells from the interface while avoiding any trauma to the flap.

These patients often have irregular and decentered optic zones. A topolink ablation may be useful in these cases. A laser installed with an eye tracker is indispensable.

Refractive results are sometimes unpredictable. The surgeon should explain to the patient that further enhancement may be necessary to achieve an acceptable refractive result.

Topolink may be useful if irregular astigmatism is present. As always, determine the depth of the incisions and wait for the refraction to stabilize. Generally, enhancement can be planned 5 to 6 months following primary AK.

LASIK Following Intracorneal Ring Insertion

The ring must first be removed. The surgeon then waits for complete healing of the surgical wound. Once the wound has healed and the refraction is stable, one can proceed as though performing a primary procedure.

LASIK Following LTK

LTK for the correction of hyperopia can result in overcorrection, undercorrection, or induced astigmatism. Astigmatism is usually irregular and correction will prove easier when LASIK enhancement is assisted by corneal topography. Refraction and keratometry should be stable before the enhancement is scheduled. Pachymetry measurements will determine if there is adequate corneal thickness.

LASIK Following Epikeratophakia

The surgeon should wait 1 year before considering LASIK enhancement of epikeratophakia, keratophakia, or homoplastic keratomileusis. Carefully measure the diameter of the original resection. Ideally, the second flap should have a slightly small diameter than the area where the pocket was created. The new flap should fit completely inside the scar created by the original procedure. This avoids uneven cuts and irregularities caused by the uneven surface. A 7.5 mm flap will usually satisfy this need (an applanation disk should be used to verify the planned resection diameter). The surgeon should determine the thickness of the original resection. This can be calculated with reasonable precision by examining the cornea under high magnification with a thin slit and comparing the percentage of total corneal thickness that is between the epithelium and interface of the receiving bed with the remaining cornea.

It is preferable to place the second cut within the original resection to avoid creating more than one interface. From a theoretical point of view, there could be problems of integrity if the cut is performed between the host and donor tissues. Actually, it appears that these problems are nonexistent.

Refractive predictability is good but not optimal. Response to the laser ablation is greater than expected in these eyes. Conservative treatment is therefore advisable. Due to the irregularity of the corneal surface in these eyes, topolink should be available.

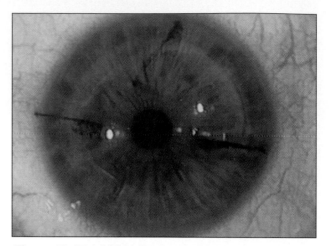

Figure 10-17. LASIK following penetrating keratoplasty.

LASIK Following PKP

Even with improvements in surgical technique, penetrating keratoplasty (PKP) is generally associated with postoperative myopia and astigmatism that is difficult to correct with spectacles (anisometropia and image distortion) or contact lenses (poorly tolerated in these eyes). Post-PKP refractive errors are generally myopic due to the accentuated corneal curvature that is created by grafting a corneal disk larger than the receiving bed. Refractive surgery is often considered.

Incisional astigmatic techniques are associated with a number of problems:

- The correction of asymmetrical astigmatism can be difficult
- Decision on placement of the incisions can be complex: should incisions extend into host tissue in a cornea thinned by keratoconus? Will incisions in the graft produce a predictable result? Should incisions be placed along the scar itself?

Persistent haze and even rejection of the graft has been seen following PRK. LASIK appears to produce a fairly predictable result with the advantages of rapid visual recovery with minimal haze and low levels of patient discomfort. The transplant must be well-healed and the sutures removed prior to considering LASIK. The refraction must have stabilized. LASIK following PKP can be planned 12 to 14 months following surgery in young patients, longer in the elderly. Sutures should be removed 4 to 6 months prior to the LASIK procedure, as they may interfere with smooth passage of the microkeratome as well as needing to wait for the refraction to stabilize following suture removal.

The Preoperative Examination

The edges of the scar must be analyzed very careful-

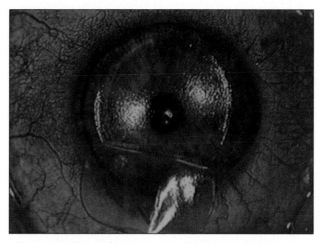

Figure 10-18. LASIK following PRK for undercorrection with haze.

ly. Defects at the edges may cause astigmatism through wound collapse. Endothelial specular microscopy is important in determining health of the endothelium and, therefore, the graft itself. Pachymetry should be performed not only on the graft, but also on the peripheral host cornea. Very thin peripheral cornea due to keratoconus is a contraindication to LASIK. The surgeon should look for alternative techniques in this case.

Problems with LASIK following PKP are associated with the effect the procedure may have on the interface between the graft and host corneas. There is a risk of wound dehiscence when the suction ring is applied and IOP elevated. A minor problem, but still a possibility, is a shift in astigmatism created with suction ring application. This could make the refractive result less predictable. Peripheral neovascularization may cause intra- or postoperative hemorrhage. Finally, one needs to consider the risk of endothelial cell loss. There is a risk of flap perforation created with the microkeratome. If the cornea is extremely steep or astigmatic, using a plate to create a thicker flap is recommended (180 microns).

Following the keratectomy, the surgeon can proceed in one of two ways:

1. The refractive ablation is performed immediately following the keratectomy (Buratto's preferred method). In the majority of cases, the refractive and functional improvement obtained will satisfy the patient. If additional refractive correction is needed, the flap can be lifted at 4 to 6 weeks postoperative and an enhancement performed.

2. The flap is not lifted and the refractive ablation is postponed. The ablation is performed 30 to 60 days following the keratectomy, after the refractive error has stabilized following any variation induced by the lamellar cut. It appears that these

variations affect approximately 50% of patients. For this reason, accurate refraction is essential.

The flap should be lifted with a spatula, not forceps. It should be larger in diameter than the transplanted graft and should be at least 160 microns thick, but 180 microns are preferable.

The graft should be well-centered and the choice of flap diameter, in the opinion of many surgeons, should correspond to the keratoplasty scar; we prefer a flap slightly larger in diameter than the graft.

If the graft is decentered, care must be taken to center both the resection and the ablation without considering the position of the graft.

Refractive results are satisfactory for the correction of myopia. They are less precise when correcting astigmatism. This is due to the generally asymmetrical or irregular nature of astigmatism in post-PKP eyes. Topolink should prove useful in these situations.

Predictability is lower than with LASIK in healthy eyes, and the patient must be informed that there is a risk of rejection, though this appears to be lower than that associated with PRK. To reduce the risk of rejection, corticosteroid drops should be used for several days prior to the procedure and continued for several weeks after surgery. Frequent monitoring will allow the surgeon to rapidly intervene in the event of rejection.

LASIK Following PRK

LASIK is the procedure of choice for enhancing PRK, as it reduces the possibility of increasing the degree of haze frequently associated with regression. Only when dense haze is present is it worthwhile proceeding with another surface, refractive treatment. This should be preceded by PTK to remove scar tissue, smooth the surface and prepare the stroma for the refractive enhancement. It is best to avoid enhancements with PRK in patients who carry a high risk of developing haze or in patients who are steroid responders (as it limits the use of steroid medications during the postoperative period). LASIK enhancement of PRK can normally be scheduled 6 months after the primary procedure. Refractive stability should be well documented.

LASIK Following Old Freeze Type Keratomileusis

Patients who have undergone keratomileusis by means of a now obsolete technique (freeze technique at the cryolathe or BKS, etc) may sometime require enhancement to correct an unsatisfactory refractive result. LASIK is the preferred technique in these cases.

However, there can be problems: the previous surgery may have left a very flat cornea or the cap may be irregular or of inappropriate diameter. A very flat cornea does not protrude through the suctions ring as much as a steeper cornea, therefore a smaller diameter of tissue is resected by the microkeratome, this increases the chance of a free cap. Some microkeratomes prevent free caps even when the cornea is very flat; nevertheless, a small flap with a small hinge can make performing the refractive ablation difficult.

These obsolete refractive techniques can easily create irregularities in the stroma and on the surface. It will not always be possible to improve the refractive and functional result.

These techniques involved cutting a fairly thick disc of tissue—there is no possibility of duplicating the cut during LASIK. There is no problem with performing the cut either inside or outside the limits of the original.

LASIK Following Nonrefractive Surgery of the Anterior Segment

Endothelial specular microscopy is important preoperatively to determine cell vitality, surgical efficacy, and refractive prognosis. Cell counts should be obtained prior to considering a laser refractive procedure on eyes having previously undergone intraocular surgery.

LASIK Following Cataract Surgery

It may happen that after cataract surgery (complicated or not), the refractive result is not as anticipated. IOL exchange can be difficult, as it involves further intraocular surgery, and it is not always easy to remove an IOL that is well-positioned in the capsular bag. It can be even more difficult if complications arose during the original procedure. There is the option of implanting a second IOL (piggyback), however, calculating lens power can be difficult and again requires further intraocular surgery.

Performing LASIK in these cases appears very attractive. The incision and refraction should be completely stable. Any sutures not inducing astigmatism should be left in situ; cutting them with the microkeratome should be avoided if at all possible. Generally, patients who have undergone phacoemulsification with a 3.5 mm tunnel incision can be scheduled for LASIK 2 to 3 months following their cataract surgery.

If there is a large conjunctival scar, it may be difficult to properly place the suction ring; in this case, PRK is preferred over LASIK. The surgeon should remember that the suction ring can induce modification of the corneal profile and anterior chamber depth. Consequently, if an anterior chamber IOL is present it could contact the corneal endothelium and cause damage.

LASIK Following Phakic IOL Implantation

LASIK has proved to be an excellent method for cor-

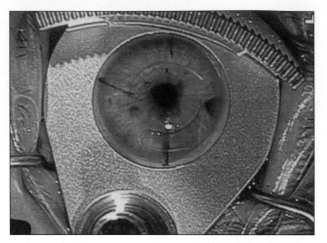

Figure 10-19. LASIK in pseudophakia with an IOL in the anterior chamber.

recting residual refractive defects, both spherical and astigmatic, following implantation of a phakic IOL, particularly when correcting severe myopia. When the refractive error is so great (ie, it cannot be completely corrected by the implant) a double procedure may be planned; first the IOL is implanted and then LASIK is used to correct the residual refractive error.

LASIK can also be used to correct refractive errors that appear over time (progression of myopia or induced astigmatism). The refraction must be stable, and the scar well healed and able to support high pressure induced by the suction ring.

If the surgeon wishes to shorten the time between implantation of the IOL and the LASIK procedure, he or she may perform the keratectomy prior to implanting the IOL (without lifting the flap or performing the laser ablation). One or 2 weeks after implanting the IOL, the flap can be lifted and the residual refractive error treated with the laser. In patients with phakic IOLs, enhancement with LASIK avoids the risk of repeat intraocular surgery for IOL exchange and allows the surgeon to use a larger optic zone than would normally be used with a single procedure.

There are three types of phakic IOLs: posterior chamber (ICL by Staar), iris-fixated (Artisan by Ophtec, Groningen, Holland), and anterior chamber (Nuvita by Bausch & Lomb). With the latter two, during LASIK the surgeon should remember that the variations in corneal profile and anterior chamber depth induced by the suction ring and microkeratome pass may bring the IOL into contact with the endothelium, causing damage as well as subjecting the IOL to considerable stress.

In eyes with a phakic IOL, the surgeon must be careful with the eye tracker. The reflecting surface of the IOL makes it difficult for the laser's video camera to capture pupil position, and may interfere with its intraoperative function, causing a suboptimal ablation. If there is any doubt about proper function, use of the eye tracker should be avoided in these cases.

LASIK Following Glaucoma Surgery

Patients who have undergone filtering surgery (with creation of a bleb) for glaucoma should wait 6 months prior to considering LASIK. The filtering bleb may interfere with placement of the suction ring especially if it is large or cystic. PRK would be the procedure of choice in these cases.

Bleb interference with good positioning of the suction ring may result in a flap that is unevenly thick, irregular, thin, superficial, or perforated. The suction ring could cause the bleb rupture, increasing the risk of infection and reducing filtration. If the bleb is flat there are usually no problems.

LASIK Following Vitrectomy or Vitreo-retinal Surgery

The surgeon must pay special attention to eyes that have previously undergone retinal surgery. Anatomical alterations in the globe may make if difficult to properly position and apply the suction ring. The surgeon should look for:

- The presence of Lincoff sponges
- The scleral hourglass from cerclage
- Hypotony from vitrectomy
- Limbal conjunctival irregularity from conjunctival peritomy

If ring placement is difficult, it may also pose problems with achieving adequate IOP elevation to proceed with the microkeratome pass. The surgeon should allow the suction ring to remain on the eye for a longer period of time than normal in order to achieve appropriate intraocular pressure. Checking IOP with the Barraquer tonometer is mandatory. If possible, suction pump power could be increased.

LASIK IN SPECIAL CASES

There are some special situations in which the LASIK may prove to be difficult. The surgeon must always be ready to face these difficulties by paying special attention to the various steps of the surgical procedure, modify the standard procedure or even abandoning the LASIK procedure altogether, steering the patient to another form of refractive surgery.

Problems may arise from the anatomy of the eye, the presence of scar tissue, and/or previous surgery; they may be patient-related or dependent on specific eye pathology.

Special Considerations

1. **Thin corneas:** please refer to the chapter on excimer laser homoplastic lamellar keratoplasty of augmented thickness.

2. **Scarred corneas:** if there is haze, small opacities or corneal scars, the surgeon should ensure that they have stabilized prior to proceeding.

- Superficial opacity: if the corneal alteration is haze that is uniform and confined to the more superficial 80 to 100 microns, the opaque tissue may be removed using PTK.

- Opacity in the middle layers: if the tissue alteration involves the slightly deeper zones (100 to 180 microns) and is fairly homogeneous, again a PTK can be used as in the previous case, followed by a cut with the microkeratome with no stop device on a donor cornea to create a disk of equal diameter and thickness; the refractive ablation is then performed on the disk, which is then sutured into position on the receiving globe.

- Deep opacities: alteration of the deeper layers, irregular opacities, or different densities within 300 to 350 microns.

In this case, a lamellar cut with the microkeratome is preferable, as this will remove all the scar tissue as described above; a plate of appropriate thickness must be used.

If there is considerable scarring, and particularly if it also involves the conjunctiva and/or sclera, the surgeon must remember that these may affect suction ring positioning and achievement of adequate IOP.

3. **Insufficient exposure:** exposure must be optimal (ie, the orbit and eye must not obstruct application of the suction ring or pass of the microkeratome during the operation). There may be some anatomical factors that make exposure more difficult. These are a prominent brow, the eyelids and the eye itself, such as sunken globe and narrow eyelid margins.

Sometimes performing a retrobulbar injection of 3 to 5 cc of balanced salt solution (BSS) mixed with 1 cc of anesthetic prior to surgery to increase exposure in sunken eyes.

It stands to reason that the surgeon must consider the inherent risks—the possibility of conjunctival edema that may prevent correct application and adhesion of the suction ring, retrobulbar hemorrhage, or perforation of the eye.

Moreover, this may induce pupil dilation that will reduce fixation ability by the patient and a risk that treatment will be decentered.

In such cases, it may be advisable to postpone treatment following the lamellar cut and perform the ablation some days later.

When the eyebrow arch is prominent, the position of the patient's head takes on major importance. The patient should have his chin slightly raised, which will help to maintain eye exposure; the two arms of the speculum must be retracted symmetrically.

The microkeratome choice is important. It must be as compact as possible. The Hansatome—an instrument that advances vertically—is more advantageous than others. The suction ring is also better and the toothed track is raised compared to other models. When using the Hansatome, the handle should be tilted to avoid the eyelid without running the risk of losing suction.

If necessary, the handle can be placed in a superior, temporal, or inferior position that will alter hinge position from the superior site.

In the most compromised cases, which may even be due to narrow eyelid margins, PRK may be preferable.

In cases of narrow palpebral fissures, a retrobulbar injection may also be considered.

The patient's head can be positioned 10° to 20° to the side (to the left side for the right eye and to the right side for the left eye). This allows the widest part of the eyelid rim to be used to its maximum advantage. This is particularly useful in the nasal hinge technique.

Alternately, a lateral canthotomy may be necessary (2.0 to 3.0 mm) following anesthesia by local infiltration. Akinesia and anesthesia of the eyelid may also be necessary.

In some cases, it may prove easier if the procedure is performed without the speculum.

If this is done, the position of the eyelids and any eyelid skin that protrudes beyond the edges of the suction ring should be carefully checked, particularly in relation to the microkeratome gears, when performing nasal hinge technique with a microkeratome fitted with gears.

Some surgeons insist on attempting to insert the suction ring between the arms of the speculum until adequate suction levels are achieved; however, this may cause corneoconjunctival alterations.

A strong speculum may be of use to open the eyelids to their maximum extension; generally, a speculum with short arms is better than one with long arms, or a speculum that can be fixed into position.

The surgeon may ask his assistant to push the speculum downward while the microkeratome is being inserted. This will distance the eyelids from the edge of the microkeratome and reduce conjunctival folds and redundancy. This may also create slight exophthalamus that may help to avoid problems during the microkeratome pass through interference with the eyelids and drape.

Alternately, the assistant can hold two speculums in position.

4. **Small and large eyes:** in both cases, the appropriate suction ring should be chosen.

With small eyes, a ring that is excessively large will not allow adequate suction to be reached.

Moreover, if the suction is inadequate, the cut will have a large diameter with the strong possibility of a free cap being produced (considering that the corneal diameter is small).

The preoperative white-to-white distance and measurement of the axial length allows the surgeon to determine the correct radius of the ring for surgery.

With small eyes and long eyelashes, the drape or Steristrips must be positioned very carefully to exclude the eyelashes from the operating field.

In the case of large eyes with large corneas, an excessively small ring will position itself on the cornea and not on the sclera. There is the possibility of obtaining a small cut with lack of hinge formation and the creation of a free cap (which is more likely to be formed with a very large cornea).

It should also be remembered that in a very large cornea, the markings may not be on the flap itself but more peripherally. As a result, they will be of little assistance for flap repositioning. Adequate marking is therefore required.

5. **Eyes with steep and flat corneas:** in steep or flat corneas, there is a risk that the flap may be thin or perforated.

A very flat cornea (mean keratometry less than 41 D) may be the reason for a free cap. A flat cornea will protrude through the suction ring to a lesser degree and will therefore present a smaller portion of the cornea to the microkeratome blade. In this case the stop device will be positioned beyond the limits of the flap.

There are suction rings that will not create a free cap on corneas of 36 D; nevertheless, a small corneal flap with a smaller hinge will be formed; this carries a greater risk of dislocation or loss.

Flat corneas will create small flaps while steep corneas (mean keratometry value in excess of 47 D) will produce large flaps with the risk of bleeding through the proximity of neovascularization. It may be useful to decenter the cut to avoid this.

A deeper plate may be used on these corneas to prevent these problems.

6. **Hypotonic eyes:** severely myopic eyes have a considerable quantity of orbital fat. These eyes will be soft, moving easily when subjected to pressure because they are not held firmly by the intra-orbital tissues. As a result, it is more diffi-

cult to fix the suction ring and microkeratome. The eye must be kept as stable as possible.

The eye is therefore prolapsed with the speculum so that the redundant conjunctiva is stretched and the globe is stabilized.

Difficulty in achieving adequate suction is also associated with the presence of vitreal syneresis (difficulty in achieving adequate intraocular pressure) and generally to the presence of a redundant conjunctiva (false adhesion of the suction ring). It is therefore necessary to check intraocular pressure with the tonometer.

For the redundant conjunctiva, the surgeon's assistant can use two Merocel sponges to stretch the conjunctiva downward and prevent aspiration by the suction ring.

Eyes with vitreal syneresis, post-cataract vitrectomy, or detached retina will generally be hypotonic. As a result, it may be difficult to achieve suitable intraocular pressure for the LASIK procedure.

If tonometry indicates a soft eye, the surgeon may increase the value of the vacuum: with the Hansatome machine, the "operate" mode is activated and the adjustment handle is turned full-circle once in a clockwise direction. However, this is not always successful and the procedure may need to be aborted.

In the event of failure, the surgeon should consider alternative surgical procedures.

7. **Poor patient cooperation:** poorly cooperative patients include patients who blink frequently and patients who have difficulty fixating.

In patients who blink frequently, it is better to use parabulbar or general anesthesia. The cut is performed under anesthesia while the ablation is performed some days later under topical anesthesia.

In patients who have difficulty fixating, once the lamellar cut has been performed when no eye tracker is available the area to be ablated is marked with fluorescein to provide continuous monitoring of ablation centration. Alternately, parabulbar anesthesia can be performed and the ablation can be performed with no fixation.

Sometimes one may keep the ring in position manually, that is with vacuum suspended, by exerting moderate downward pressure; this will help keep the eye steady; however, if the patient moves, this maneuver may result in flap damage.

In both cases, the center of the cornea can be marked, general anesthesia performed, an intentional free cap created, and finally, the refractive treatment on the cap, if certain that it is well-centered (Buratto's original technique with an ablation on the cap stroma).

8. **Accommodation spasm** with or without strabismus: in a myopic subject, if the cycloplegic

refraction reveals that there is an error and myopia is actually less than manifest, the surgeon may consider the possibility of accommodative spasm from undercorrection; if there is strabismus in a hyperopic eye, the error may be due to accommodation.

Examination with deep cycloplegia must be performed (eg, by instilling a drop of cyclopentolate three times at 10-minute intervals and then performing the test at least 30 minutes from the last instillation). Alter three times at 10-minute intervals and the test performed at least 15 minutes after the last instillation. If there are any uncertainties, atropine should be used three times a day for 5 days prior to the examination.

The examination should be performed with autorefraction, manual refraction, and retinoscopy.

With accommodative spasm, it is better to re-examine the patient when the pupil is normal using the fogging technique. If this technique confirms a level of myopia that is less than previously measured values, this will indicate accommodative spasm with myopia being less than previously reported. The operation will therefore be set according to lower myopic values.

However, if the second post-cycloplegic examination with the fogging technique does not confirm the results produced with cycloplegia, uncertainties regarding accommodative spasm will persist.

However, even in a situation of this type, the cycloplegic measurement should be used to set the parameters for the operation; that is the myopia should be considered less than it would appear to be when the normal pupil is examined. This is preferable because it is always easier to perform a repeat operation at a later stage to correct any undercorrection, rather than try to perform an enhancement for over-correction.

With hyperopia with converging strabismus of a purely accommodative nature, the correction of total hyperopia (measured following cycloplegia) must also be considered when correcting strabismus and the refractive defect.

9. **Remains of a fistulizing antiglaucoma operation:** in these cases we run the risk of not achieving appropriate suction and/or damaging the filtrating bleb with the suction ring.

If the bleb is flat, it will not pose a problem and the operation can proceed.

If the bleb is large, raised, and cystic, it is better to avoid the operation and consider other types of refractive surgery; in fact, interference by the bleb with the ring may create an unevenly thick final cut and the flaps may be irregular, thin, or perforated.

On the contrary, the suction ring may rupture some of

the cyst (ie, it may encourage infection of the bleb itself), endophthalmitis, and alter eye pressure.

If on the other hand, the glaucomatous patient still requires a trabeculectomy, the surgeon may consider the LASIK operation first, followed by antiglaucoma treatment.

Glaucoma with alterations of the visual field must encourage the surgeon to reduce the amount of time ocular pressure is high as much as possible during the LASIK procedure. Also, subsequent measurements of the eye pressure following LASIK may underestimate the values.

10. **Decentered pupil:** in these cases, the operation must be performed without the aid of the an eye tracker.

In terms of centering the ablation, it must be done by centering on the decentered pupil and not on the apex of the cornea.

The procedure must be centered along the line of vision (the line that passes through a fixed object through the center of the pupil to reach the fovea). This point may not be found at the geometrical center of the cornea. The center of the ablation is identified by marking the entrance center of the pupil when the patient fixates the coaxial light of the laser.

11. **Nystagmus:** with nystagmus, the surgeon must attempt to keep the eye steady with a Thornton ring or a Fine-Thornton ring. The assistant holds the patient's head steady with one hand and steadies the eye with the other.

The Thornton ring must be positioned perpendicular to the floor; pressure is then applied and released to ensure that the eye has not rotated when pressure is exerted. If the Thornton ring is correctly positioned, the eye will not move when the ring is released.

Sedatives are useful because nystagmus often increases under the effects of preoperative emotional stress.

The cut is performed with the microkeratome. It may also prove useful to keep the ring in position and gently push downward.

If sufficient mobility is not obtained, at this point subtenon anesthesia is performed and the ablation completed.

Contrary to retrobulbar or peribulbar anesthesia, subtenon anesthesia maintains the patient's ability to fixate while reducing or completely eliminating the nystagmus.

Again in this case, an intentional free cap can be cut with the refractive treatment performed on the cap, certain that the treatment is well centered.

Undoubtedly, the best method is when the ablation is performed with assistance of the eye tracker.

SURGICAL ATLAS
Enhancement After Down-Up LASIK Technique

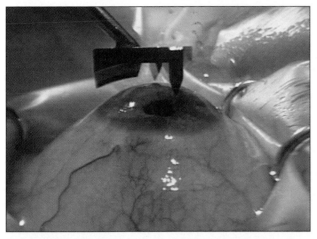

Figure A-1. The marker approaches the cornea.

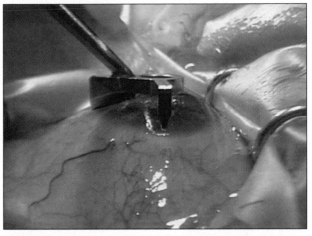

Figure A-2. The cornea is marked with slight indentation.

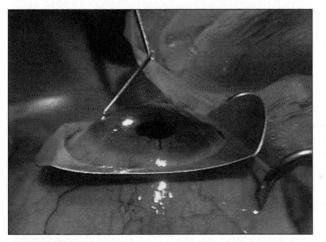

Figure A-3. The Sinskey hook delineates the edge of the flap and raises it.

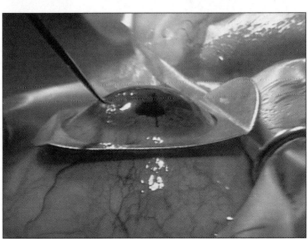

Figure A-4. An enhancement spatula peels back the cut circumference.

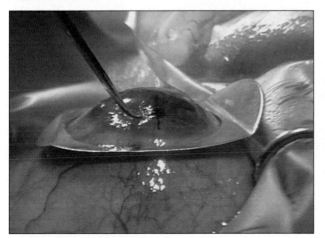

Figure A-5. The enhancement spatula proceeds toward the hinge, lifting the flap.

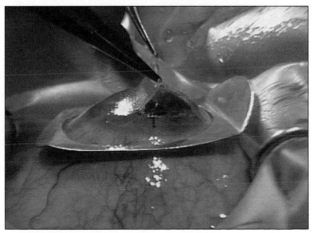

Figure A-6. The flap is lifted with two flap forceps.

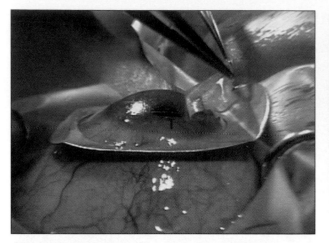

Figure A-7. The flap is placed on the positioner.

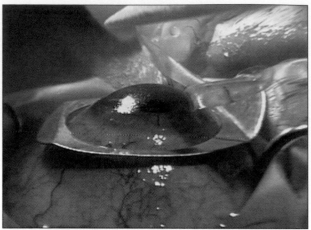

Figure A-8. The flap rests correctly on the positioner.

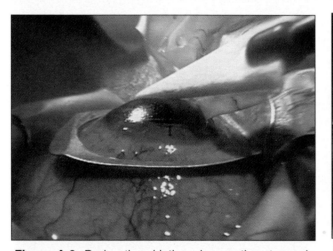

Figure A-9. During the ablation phases, the stroma is dried with a dry Merocel sponge.

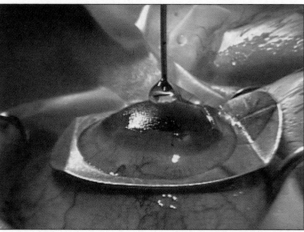

Figure A-10. After the ablation, a drop of BSS is placed on the cornea.

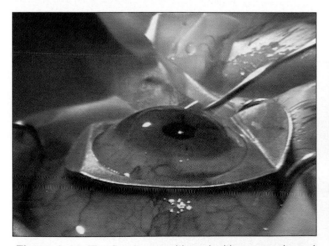

Figure A-11. The flap is repositioned with a cannula and the cornea is gently dried and massaged with a damp sponge.

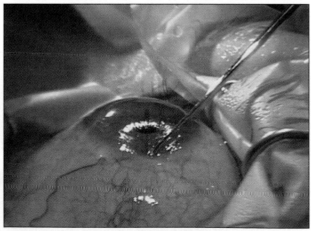

Figure A-12. The operation ends with the striae test.

Inadequate Exposure

Chan Wing Kwong, MD

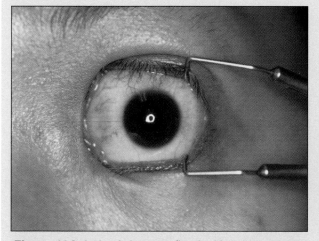

Figure 10A-1. An Asian eye fitted with a Liebermann speculum. Note the poor retraction of the eyelids that may result in inadequate exposure of the globe to fit the microkeratome suction ring.

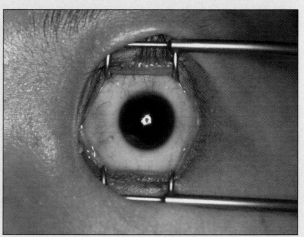

Figure 10A-2. The same eye fitted with a Murdoch speculum, which has shorter blades than the Liebermann speculum. Note the better eyelid retraction achieved with greater exposure of the globe compared to Figure 10A-1.

Adequate exposure of the eye must be achieved during LASIK surgery to allow the microkeratome's vacuum suction ring to fit. Current suction rings of most microkeratomes are of a fairly large size, which makes them difficult to apply to a globe that is inadequately exposed. Without a good fit of the suction ring, an adequate rise in intraocular pressure cannot be achieved, leading to the inability to create a consistently good quality corneal flap.

Inadequate exposure of the eye can result from the following factors:

1. Narrow palpebral aperture. A narrow palpebral aperture presents the greatest obstacle to successful application of the suction ring. This is most common in patients of Asian descent. In order to achieve a large enough palpebral opening in such cases, one should select an appropriately sized speculum with shorter blades, such as the Murdoch or Preori speculums, rather than speculums with long blades, like Liebermann speculums (Figures 10A-1 and 10A-2). The shorter blade speculums will allow a larger opening of the palpebral aperture, resulting in a proper fit of the suction ring. In other cases of extremely small palpebral apertures, a lateral canthotomy may be necessary to enlarge the palpebral aperture before the suction ring will fit. If the patient refuses a lateral canthotomy, the only other solutions are to try to apply the suction ring without the use of a lid speculum or consider performing photorefractive keratectomy.

2. Deep-set eyes. A deeply set eye can present problems with suction ring fit. This problem can be overcome by applying gentle pressure with the lid speculum in the retro-orbital direction just before the suction ring is applied. This pressure application can help to protrude a deep-set eye forward, allowing successful application of the suction ring. It is not recommended that a peribulbar injection of anesthetic be used to help protrude the eye forward, as the occurrence of conjunctival chemosis may result in blockage of the vacuum ports in the suction ring, resulting in inability of the eye to attain the necessary level of intraocular pressure for a satisfactory keratectomy. Paralysis of ocular movements will also make it impossible for the patient to self-fixate on the fixation light of the excimer laser.

3. Blepharospasm. Patients with excessive blepharospasm may cause difficulty in the application of the suction ring, even with a lid speculum in place. Excessive blepharospasm has also been known to cause an accidental loss of vacuum in the suction ring. This can occur if nonlocking speculums, such as a Barraquer speculum, are used. It is recommended that locking speculums, which cannot be overcome by a nervous patient

squeezing his or her lids, be used to ensure maximum globe exposure.

Adequate exposure of the eye is a compulsory prerequisite in all eyes undergoing LASIK surgery. Poor exposure results mainly from the patient's intrinsic orbital and eyelid characteristics and may make successful application of the suction ring difficult or impossible. Selection of an appropriate lid speculum when confronted with an eye with a narrow palpebral aperture, will help to maximize exposure of the eye without having to routinely resort to a lateral canthotomy.

LASIK in Accomodative Esotropia

Jairo E. Hoyos, MD, PhD

Donders described refractive accommodative esotropia (RAE) as occurring in patients who must accommodate to focus retinal images produced by high hyperopic refractive errors. This accommodation leads to excessive convergence, which eventually exceeds the patient's fusional divergence amplitude, resulting in esotropia. RAE patients typically have:

- High hyperopia, ranging between +3 and +10 with an average of +4.75 D.
- Moderate deviation angle, ranging between 20 and 30 prism diopters.
- Distance and near deviation within 10 prism diopters.

Treatment of RAE is based upon eliminating accommodation induced by high hyperopia, thus decreasing accommodative convergence. The standard treatment of RAE patients is optical, prescribing glasses or contact lenses for the full hyperopic refractive error, as determined under complete cycloplegia. Miotic agents have also been used, but they are controversial because of their side effects.

The main problem in RAE is the refractive error and its correction allows the correction of the esodeviation. Therefore, the surgical treatment for RAE is refractive surgery aimed at correcting the refractive error.

Our usual treatment for hyperopia since 1995 has been hyperopic LASIK. Beginning in January 1997, we began using this surgical technique in RAE patients with the following selection criteria:

1. Esotropia: accommodative refractive and mixed (after correcting the nonaccommodative component).
2. Hyperopia up to +6 D on the flattest axis.
3. Patients older than 18 years of age.

All of our RAE patients underwent a thorough ophthalmologic examination using ultrasound pachymetry and corneal topography. Those cases in which lamellar surgery was contraindicated were rejected. Visual acuity

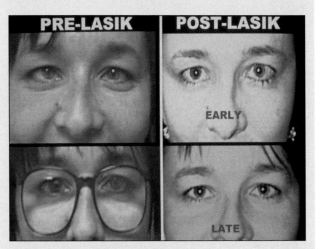

Figure 10B-1. Treatment of esotropia: pre- and post-LASIK.

and the deviation angle with and without optical correction were measured both for far and near. Cycloplegic refraction was performed and surgery was planned for total hyperopia in order to obtain orthophoria without the use of an optical correction.

The usual hyperopic LASIK technique was applied. We created a nasal flap using the Automatic Corneal Shaper microkeratome with a 160-micron plate. The suction ring was slightly decentered nasally in order to obtain a nasally displaced flap and to prevent the hinge from interfering during the ablation. In hyperopia, centering the ablation is critical because the visual axis in hyperopic eyes is nasally displaced in relation to the center of the pupil in more than 80% of cases. We always attempt to center the ablation on the patient's visual axis.

A few minutes after completing the procedure, all patients achieved orthophoria without optical correction, which has been maintained to date (2 years follow-up).

Refractive surgery is a surgical alternative in refractive accommodative esotropia and hyperopic LASIK is a good option today.

LASIK in Decentered Pupils

Michiel S. Kritzinger, MD

LASIK refractive surgery is a blessing for patients with decentered pupils. It is a constant struggle for these patients to be perfectly refracted with spectacles and/or contact lenses, especially if they have high refractive errors. It is even more distressing if they become presbyopic and must be fitted with decentered multifocal or bifocal spectacles.

The LASIK surgical technique for decentered pupils differs from the norm in that the surgeon must plan the laser ablation, obviously, to the center of the pupil and visual axis, but do not ablate the central cornea. It feels quite strange during the surgery to deliberately off-center an ablation, but it gives excellent visual results.

In my experience, all patients with decentered pupils who have been treated with LASIK thus far are ecstatic about their visual quality and quantity. The unanimous feeling is that they have never seen so well in all their lives.

IOL Calculation After LASIK

Mihai Pop, MD

Some patients, especially those who are hyperopic and corrected with H-LASIK, will slowly regress to their initial visual acuity even after a retreatment. In certain patients, a clear lens extraction with an intraocular lens implant (IOL) is a reasonable option. The major problem in IOL calculations after LASIK is the difficulty in predicting the hyperopic shift that follows implantation and evaluation of the corneal power to calculate the proper lens power.

The inability of the instruments to accurately measure corneal power after LASIK or PRK is due to the difference in radii between the front and back of the cornea, which remained untouched by the excimer laser treatment. It is expected that the measured corneal power may, in fact, be greater than the true refractive power of the cornea.[1]

Different methods exist to calculate the corneal power. These include:

1. The hard contact lens method in which the patient wears a contact lens of known corneal power. The manifest refraction is added to the corneal power of the lens. For example, if a contact lens of 44 D of curvature results in a manifest refraction of -4.50 D, the corneal power of the eye is 44 D + -4.50 D = 39.50 D.

2. Corneal videotopography at the 3.0 mm optical zone using software. The untreated optical zone should be excluded because videotopography can be inaccurate due to the difference in curvature along the LASIK optical zone and remaining untreated zone.

3. The initial topography adjusted with the intended and achieved refractions. For example, if a -4 D LASIK is performed at the corneal plane on an eye with 44 D of curvature, then the expected corneal power would be 40 D if the achieved refraction is plano. Corneal power is lower than the expected corneal power if the achieved refraction is myopic. The predicted corneal power can then be compared with the corneal power, as measured by method 1 or 2.

Although monovision is an acceptable compromise to provide near vision for patients already accustomed to such vision, it is better to aim for slight myopia in both eyes due to the potential for hyperopic shift. Two diopters are added to the highest lens power calculated by the Colenbrander/Hoffer, Hoffer Q, Holladay, SRK-T, SRK-II, or Binkhorst formula to target slight myopia. The efficiency of all formulas depends on the axial length of the eye, so it is advisable to use personalized A-constant coefficients for lens power calculation. The mean K can be used to input the formula; however, in case of a large discrepancy, the flatter of the two Ks, rather the mean K, is used. Piggybacking IOLs by implanting two lenses of approximately equal power is another option, but this usually incurs more refractive error.

Although the result of implantation may be an intended level of myopia, a slow hyperopic shift is to be expected. Patients implanted with IOLs after LASIK may present with a hyperopic shift of 1 to 2 D within the first postoperative months.

No retreatment should be done before the refraction stabilizes or before the first postoperative month. Lenses should not be exchanged for under- or overcorrections of more than 2 D; in these cases, a LASIK retreatment can be performed. LASIK retreatment post-IOL is the adjustable refractive surgery (ARS) concept.[2]

REFERENCES

1. Holladay JT. Cataract surgery in patients with previous keratorefractive surgery (RK, PRK, and LASIK). *Ophthalmic Practice.* 1997;15(6):238-44.
2. Güell J. The adjustable refractive surgery concept (ARS). *Journal of Refractive Surgery.* 1998;14:271.

Managing Small, Deep-Set and Large, Bulging Eyes

Ron Stasiuk, MD

The main goal in managing small, deep-set and large, bulging eyes with LASIK is to obtain adequate exposure and suction so that a good quality flap is formed.

Small, deep-set eyes present several problems, particularly to the novice LASIK surgeon. Good exposure of the limbus is essential. In cases of a prominent brow, the chin should be tilted up and long eyelashes draped away from the operating field. A good wire speculum, such as the Liebermann, should maximally open the eyelids. Using firm downward pressure, the globe can then be prolapsed forward. The patient should also be warned of the extra pressure and sedated more.

If the Chiron ACS is used, it is important to avoid contact with any obstruction, such as the wire speculum, eyelids, lashes, or drapes, otherwise the keratome may stop. In such a situation, the obstruction should be quickly identified, removed, and with a quick push on the reverse pedal, the keratome can proceed forward again. If using the Chiron Hansatome, tilting the handle of the Hansatome is helpful to avoid the lid margin without the risk of losing suction.

In very small, tight orbits the lid margins may be manipulated alongside the suction ring, particularly with the Hansatome microkeratome, and good suction is easy to obtain. Occasionally, the eyelid speculum can be removed altogether and the suction ring maneuvered onto the limbus for successful suction. A further option is to perform a small 2.0 to 3.0 mm lateral canthotomy, with careful postoperative observation of possible anesthetic lagophthalmos.

Different microkeratomes may be more effective than others for small, deep-set orbits. The Hansatome is excellent because of its elevated suction ring. Various base plates may be used with the manual Moria microkeratome for different keratometry and fit.

On the other hand, large, bulging eyes generally provide excellent exposure, however suction can sometimes be more difficult if the globe or orbit is

Table 10E-1

MANAGING SMALL AND LARGE EYES

Small Eyes		Large Eyes	
Problem	**Solution**	**Problem**	**Solution**
Prominent brow	Tilt chin up for better globe exposure	Soft orbit and eye	Prolapse globe firmly with speculum
Long eyelashes	Adequately drape with sterile drapes or strips	Redundant conjunctiva	Same as above
Small orbit	1. Liebermann-type speculum	Flat keratometry	Alter suction ring size or plate and prolapse globe
	2. Prolapse globe forward with speculum	Steep keratometry	Perform LASIK quickly with a moist cornea (effective with the Hansatome)
	3. Lateral canthotomy		
	4. No speculum—drape eyelids over speculum		
	5. Use different base plate with Moria manual microkeratome		
	6. Avoid microkeratome contact with speculum, drapes, lids, lashes		

very soft or if there is excessive redundant conjunctiva.

A simple solution is to firmly prolapse the globe with the wire eyelid speculum so that the conjunctiva is stretched and the globe is firm. However, if the globe is very large and the cornea is relatively flat, good contact with the suction ring at the limbus may be difficult to obtain. A different suction ring size may be the best alternative. The risk of a buttonhole developing during

LASIK with steep corneas can be avoided by performing the procedure quickly with a moist corneal surface. The Hansatome appears to be more reliable and safer than the ACS microkeratome.

If adequate suction cannot be achieved after attempting the proposed suggestions, LASIK should not be attempted and alternative refractive procedures such as PRK or lens implants should be considered.

Inadequate Exposure

Jerry Tan, MBBS, FRCS Ed, FRCOphth, FAMS

To achieve an excellent LASIK result, one of the key factors in the entire procedure is to obtain a perfect flap. The perfect flap is one that has a diameter of 8.5 to 9.5 mm in diameter, even thickness of 130 to 180 microns, with the hinge as near the limbus as possible, parallel to the negative cylinder axis in the superior or nasal half of the cornea. The cut should be as large as possible without involving the limbal blood vessels.

Inadequate exposure is one of the main causes of poor or failed flap formation.

Inadequate exposure:

1. Limits the ability of the microkeratome to move smoothly across the cornea with no obstructions.
2. Results in poor suction making it impossible to create a large, even flap.
3. Does not allow complete reflection of the flap while the laser ablation is taking place.
4. Results in inadequate drainage of fluids, causing an accumulation at the hinge and on the bed of the keratectomy.
5. Allows the lid skin and eyelashes to obstruct the microkeratome. Redundant skin and lashes can be caught in the mechanism of the microkeratome, resulting in a partial flap. The lashes also contaminate the field of surgery.

Before suction is applied, the LASIK surgeon must scan the operative field shown in the Figure 10F-1. This is best observed under medium or low magnification. Once suction is applied, there is no time to make adjustments to operative exposure, as any increase in operative time will increase the risk of other complications related to prolonged raised intraocular pressure and corneal dehydration. Excessive manipulation of the ring with the suction pressure already applied can result in sudden loss of suction and a free cap.

Adequate exposure for the LASIK procedure is very difficult in patients with the following features:

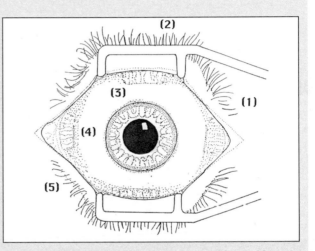

Figure 10F-1. Operative field obstructions. Key: 1. Loose skin, drapes, and orbital margin. 2. Lid speculum, drapes, and eyelashes. 3. Redundant conjunctiva. 4. Medial canthus and redundant conjuctiva. 5. Lids and orbital margin.

- Deep-set eyes
- Prominent brows
- Small internal diameter of the bony orbital rim
- Tight and short lids
- Small and narrow palpebral fissures
- Redundant conjunctiva

Fortunately, not many patients have all of these features. Most have one or two features, so adequate exposure can be achieved with various maneuvers to allow a good LASIK pass.

Many surgeons converting from PRK to LASIK, however, forget that good exposure is critical to a perfect flap. In PRK, only the cornea needs to be exposed. There is no need for the sclera to be widely exposed around the limbus. In LASIK, even an out-of-place lash or edge of plastic drape can get caught in the microkeratome track, resulting in a partial flap.

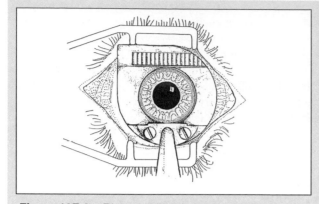

Figure 10F-2a. Ring positions in relation to the two different types of lid speculums: Barraquer speculum—large eyes, excellent exposure.

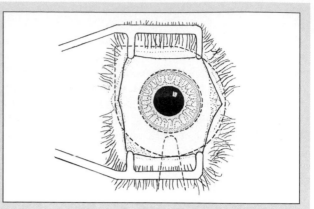

Figure 10F-2b. Ring positions in relation to the two different types of lid speculums: Barraquer speculum—small eye, inadequate exposure.

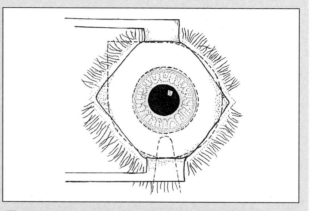

Figure 10F-2c. Ring positions in relation to the two different types of lid speculums: Cook speculum—small eye, adequate exposure.

In deep-set eyes with a prominent inferior orbital margin, the horizontal-cutting microkeratomes have an advantage. The inferior orbital rim does not interfere with the movement of the temporal-to-nasal microkeratome, whereas in the down-up cutting microkeratomes, the inferior orbital margin is a major obstruction. In the latter case, the eye may be tilted superiorly to gain a little more exposure so that the lower lid is further away and will not be cut or caught by the travelling microkeratome. If a superior orbital margin prominence coexists, it compounds the problem. Tilting the patient's head in various directions to improve exposure can be helpful. Prominent superior orbital margins can be overcome by asking the patient to extend his or her neck and lift the point of the chin superiorly. Prominent inferior and superior orbital margins are much more common in caucasian patients. Retrobulbar injections to proptose the eye can be used but are dangerous, as perforation of the long myopic globe and retrobulbar hemorrhages can occur. In addition, if conjunctival chemosis results from the injection, LASIK surgery would have to be cancelled. If one attempts LASIK in this situation, pseudosuction will occur, resulting in a thin or free cap.

In many Asian eyes, the major problem encountered is short tight lids with small palpebral fissures. This can be overcome by a lateral canthotomy, but this makes patients more anxious about pain and scarring. In general, if the distance between the medial and lateral canthus is less than 22 mm, a lateral canthotomy is required. Small palpebral fissures also prevent nasal or superior decentration of the LASIK flap. The nearer the hinge is to the pupil, the higher the possibility of irregular astigmatism after excimer laser ablation in LASIK. Irregular astigmatism is very difficult to correct; it would be best to abort the procedure and not ablate. Recut the flap after 3 to 6 months, but first make sure the cause of inadequate exposure can be corrected.

Exposure is also dependent upon the type of lid speculum used. It is best to have many types of lid speculums available and try them out preoperatively. Most surgeons will gravitate to one or two favorite speculums that work best in their patient population. The key is not to be surprised at the time of surgery, as this makes the patient and surgeon more anxious. This is a recipe for disaster.

Speculums not only provide the opening and maintenance of the palpebral aperture, they also push the redundant conjunctiva into the upper and lower fornices via its internal bar. The speculum is also essential, as the surgeon can apply downward pressure to increase intraorbital and intraocular pressure. This aids in good and complete suction. The redundant conjunctiva is dragged backward by the speculum, and the conjunctiva becomes closely applied to the globe. Unfortunately, small orbits prevent the use of this maneuver, as the speculum's downward movement is restricted by the bony orbital margin and there is no resultant proptosing of the globe. The Barraquer-type speculum is popularly used, but it must be strong enough to prevent closure of the eye while squeezing. Also, the distance between the two arms holding the upper lid and the two arms of the lower must be sufficiently separated to allow placement of the ring between its two arms both horizontally and vertically. The arm's indirect contact with the lids will also need to push redundant lid skin away from the orbital opening and microkeratome. In patients with large palpebral apertures and loose lids, the speculum must be able to open the lids maximally until the reflex and voluntary blink reflex is eliminated. There is a certain point of tension at which the patient will cease all attempts at trying to blink.

Many experienced LASIK surgeons do not use lid speculum—they tape the lids open. However, anxious patients with small palpebral fissures, short tight lids, long lashes, and severe blepharospasm have heightened chances of a failed keratectomy. A calm patient at the beginning of a procedure can be a nervous wreck at the end, squeezing the eye vigorously. Prepare for the worst case scenario and your surgery will almost always be uncomplicated.

If one is attempting speculum-free LASIK, the technique is to go below the lids and the overhanging orbital margins. Again, the most difficult cases are the lids that are tightly applied to the globe. There is no way to proptose the eye forward in this technique. Too much downward pressure will cause the conjunctiva to prolapse into the internal ring aperture as well as around the outside of the ring. The internal conjunctival prolapse can be cut during the keratectomy, while the outer prolapse can get caught in the dovetails or gears of the microkeratome. There is also a higher risk of pseudosuction when no speculum is used.

Finally, if you feel the patient's eye is not suitable because you cannot get adequate exposure for a good flap, PRK can be performed if the refractive error is low.

Manufacturers of microkeratomes have also recognized that small, gearless or gear-guarded microkeratomes are useful in many patients. In the future, surgeons will have many exposure problems solved in this group of difficult patients once these microkeratomes are available.

LASIK After a Refractive IOL Implant

Antonio Marinho, MD

INTRODUCTION

Phakic IOLs are the ideal method to surgically correct significant ametropias, because unlike corneal procedures, they do not change corneal contours and the surgical effect does not regress with time. On the other hand, although as accurate as clear lens exchange, IOLs maintain accommodation and do not appear to increase retinal risks. Based on these data, we advise the use of phakic IOLs in myopia above -12.00 and hyperopia above +5.00.

On many occasions, however, after implantation of phakic IOLs, emmetropia is not achieved. This is due to one or more of the following causes:
1. Preoperative existing astigmatism (no toric phakic IOLs available)
2. Preoperative myopia above −14.00 (Artisan 6.0 mm), -17.00 (ICL), -22.00 (Nuvita), -24.00 (Artisan 5.0 mm)
3. Induced astigmatism (suture)
4. Error in power calculations

In these cases, the refractive outcome can be enhanced with a corneal refractive procedure and the technique of choice is LASIK. The combined technique of refractive IOL and LASIK is known as bioptics.

HOW TO PERFORM BIOPTICS

There are presently two ways of performing bioptics.
1. Classical bioptics (Zaldivar): In classical bioptics, the phakic IOL is implanted as the first step and then LASIK is performed as a second step, but never before 3 months if a large incision (Nuvita or Artisan need a 5.5 or 6.5 mm incision) has been made or after 1 month if a small incision (ICL) is the case. This technique is used when bioptics is not anticipated (no extreme myopia or important preoperative astigmatism) or in situations in which there is a progression of myopia after surgery.
2. Adjustable refractive surgery (ARS): In this variant, described by Güell, the surgery is performed in three steps. In the first step, the corneal flap is created with the microkeratome, but no laser ablation is used. Afterward, the phakic IOL is implanted and laser ablation is performed as a last step. The advantage of this modality is that, as no pressure is put on the eye (suction ring), the laser ablation can be done as soon as the refractive result of the implant is stable (usually 2 weeks).

ARS is used when bioptics is anticipated or whenever a rapid final result is necessary.

RESULTS

The refractive results of bioptics are very accurate, because LASIK is performed on corneas of normal thickness and refractive errors treated with LASIK are usually below a spherical equivalent of –6.00, and in this range, accuracy and stability are very high with LASIK. Unlike LASIK retreatments for high myopia, in which regression occurs, it is rarely seen after refractive implants.

QUALITY OF VISION

Bioptics has advantages over LASIK or phakic IOLs alone, not only in the refractive outcome, but also in the quality of vision. If the ametropia is high, a small optical zone in LASIK is necessary to avoid very deep ablations. On the other hand, in extreme myopia, phakic IOLs must be used with smaller optical zones in order to remain safe for the corneal endothelium (this is why the Artisan IOL only has a 6.0 mm optic up to –14.00). This is the cause of halos and glare. Bioptics will avoid these problems and will enhance the quality of vision.

DISCUSSION

One important discussion point in bioptics (classical technique) is the fear of corneal endothelium being damaged when the suction ring is applied to the eye in order to perform the corneal flap. Studies conducted in patients implanted with anterior chamber phakic IOLs (ZB5M) and then undergoing LASIK did not show differences from implanted eyes without LASIK. The study has a follow-up of 5 years.

CONCLUSION

LASIK after phakic IOLs is an accurate and safe method to achieve emmetropia in cases of astigmatism associated with high myopia and in cases of extreme myopia. It also enables us to correct some deficiencies in IOL power calculations or surgical technique (induced astigmatism).

LASIK After LASIK

Antonio Marinho, MD

INTRODUCTION

Unlike other refractive procedures in which enhancements are difficult and, in some cases, even dangerous, LASIK has the potential for retreatment without significant complications. In this case study we will establish when and how we may perform LASIK retreatments in order to achieve an optimal result.

WHO IS A CANDIDATE FOR RETREATMENT?

LASIK retreatments should be performed when there is a significant under- or overcorrection after a primary LASIK procedure. Usually retreatment is advised when the residual ametropia is 1 D or more, but on selected cases we can even correct lower amounts.

CAN EVERY CANDIDATE BE RETREATED?

Before performing a retreatment, corneal thickness must be carefully measured. We can safely retreat only those eyes that will retain a central corneal thickness of 400 microns after the secondary ablation. This is particularly important when dealing with high myopia (regression is common), where sometimes we are left with 3 or 4 residual diopters but a corneal thickness of 400 microns. These cases should not be retreated because of danger of late corneal ectasia.

WHEN TO RETREAT

Retreatments should be performed at least 3 months after the primary procedure. Although LASIK is fairly stable, regression occurs mainly in high ametropias and sometimes progresses until the third month. A stable refraction for at least 1 month is advised before retreatment.

HOW TO RETREAT

There is always some disagreement about this question. Shall we recut (create a new flap) or lift the preexisting flap? Recutting can create important problems if we do not cut exactly in the same plane. On the other hand, lifting the flap can be easily done even 4 years after the primary procedure.

So, the rule is to lift the flap. Recutting should be considered only in the following cases:

- When it is impossible to lift the flap (strong adhesion)

- When the primary flap was not perfect (irregular flap, short flap, irregular thickness)
- When a larger flap is needed (hyperopia treatment)

When recutting, try to create a thicker and larger flap than the primary one in order to avoid problems.

HOW TO LIFT THE FLAP

Before retreatment, the patient should be observed at the slit lamp and the edges of the flap identified and marked. The patient is then brought to the laser microscope and the edge of the flap is delicately dissected with a special hook, taking special care not to disturb the epithelium. Voluntary deepithelization of the flap margins must be avoided. After dissecting the edge the flap is gently pulled with forceps. Then, the epithelium around the edge is pushed backward. The cornea must remain dry during the procedure. Laser ablation and repositioning the flap are similar to primary surgery.

REFRACTIVE RESULTS

Refractive results are usually very good. In our series, almost 80% of cases were between –0.50 and +0.50 and 100% in 1 D range, without loss of BCVA.

COMPLICATIONS

LASIK retreatment can have all the complications of a primary procedure. However, a special note must be made about epithelial ingrowth. This complication is much more frequent (14%) in retreatments than in primary cases (2.3%). This is primarily due to lifting the flap incorrectly, creating large quantities of loose epithelium. If the ingrowth is peripheral and not inducing astigmatism, it should not be disturbed. If it is central it must be removed immediately. For cases in which recurrence of epithelial ingrowth occurs, PTK on both the stromal face of the flap and the stromal bed is advised.

SUMMARY AND CONCLUSION

LASIK retreatments are a safe and accurate way to enhance the refractive result of a primary procedure as long these guidelines are followed:

- Operate only on patients with stable refractions (usually not before 3 months post primary LASIK).
- Always lift the flap (when possible) to avoid disrupting the epithelium.
- When recutting, do it larger and deeper than the primary cut.
- If central epithelial ingrowth occurs, treat it immediately.

Recutting a LASIK Flap

Marc Mullie, MD

Our preferred method for retreating an eye that has previously undergone LASIK is to recut the flap.

The technique consists of using the same keratome and depth plate. The suction ring should be positioned in such a way that the blade engages tissue at a point peripheral to the original cut. This will prevent the blade from entering at a location inside the original flap.

In a retrospective review of our first 5000 LASIK cases, 204 eyes (4%) were recut. These eyes were reoperated on at 4 to 6 months postoperatively when refractive stability had been achieved. Of these 204 eyes, 18 lost one line of BCVA, while 16 eyes gained one or more lines of BCVA. One hundred and seventy eyes neither lost nor gained BCVA. Complications included five eyes with microfolds. There were no cases of epithelial ingrowth greater than 0.5 mm.

One potential problem with recutting is tissue plane reduplication. This occurred in five eyes, but there was no loss of BCVA. These tissue "crescents" are usually peripheral. They should be left in situ when the laser is applied and the flap is carefully repositioned.

The surgical advantages of recutting are a clean edge to the flap without stripping the epithelium, or cap edge stretching and edema. This allows the flap edge to properly seal and prevent epithelial ingrowth. One recent study[1] has shown a 31% incidence of epithelial ingrowth and 11% incidence of flap edge melt by relifting post LASIK.

We strongly believe that recutting is the preferred method for retreating eyes that have had previous LASIK.

REFERENCE

1. Perez-Santonja, et al. Retreatment after laser in situ keratomileusis. *Ophthalmology.* 1999;106(1):21-28.

Laser Thermokeratoplasty

Till Anschütz, MD

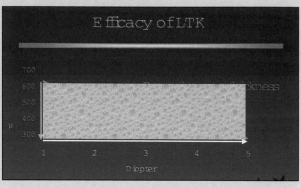

Figure 10J-1. Subjective manifest refractive change of LTK post overcorrected M-LASIK (M-PRK) in comparison to primary LTK. LTK post M-LASIK: -1.6 D (M-PRK: -1.65 D); primary LTK: -0.7 D.

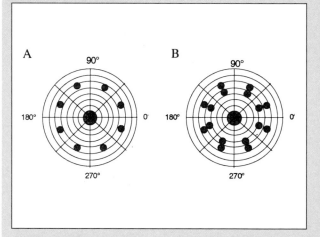

Figure 10J-3. LTK pattern. M-LASIK (M-PRK) overcorrections (1.6 D ± 0.3). A: Cornea thickness < 450 μm: one ring (6.5 mm; eight spots; 240 to 258 mJ; seven pulses). B: Cornea thickness > 450 μm and H-LASIK (H-PRK) undercorrections: two rings (6.5/7.5 mm; 16 spots; 240 to 258 mJ; seven pulses).

The nearly 100-year-old history of thermokeratoplasty, since being adopted by Lans, has been refined through the introduction of infrared lasers and simplified through noncontact procedures (Sunrise corneal shaping system).

The refractive effects, however, remain limited to a range of +0.75 to +2.5 D. Keratometry values and age influence the success of this treatment. An additional important factor is the thickness of the central cornea. Because of positive experience as a secondary procedure, LTK has gained more acceptance.

LTK post M-LASIK: We have demonstrated that

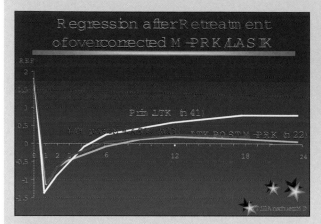

Figure 10J-2. Dependence on thickness. Thinner corneal tissues allow successful treatments of higher overcorrections post M-LASIK (or M-PRK).

LTK treatments after overcorrected M-LASIK cases (or M-PRK) provide increased efficiency and stability (Figure 10J-1). The absence of Bowman's membrane and the thinned central cornea enhance shrinkage according to the mechanical properties of the surrounding tissue. The refractive effect seems to depend on the residual tissue after ablation (Figure 10J-2).

This influences the algorithm of the treatment pattern. For an overcorrection of 1.6 D ± 0.3 and a residual pachymetry of over 450 μm, we use two rings (6.5/7.5 mm) with eight spots (240 to 256 mJ energy; seven pulses). Under 450 μm, we use only one ring (Figure 10J-3).

There are no significant differences in treatment post-overcorrected M-LASIK or M-PRK (see Figure 10J-1).

Because of the minimal approach and fast procedure time (3 seconds), we favor LTK as the alternative retreatment procedure post M-LASIK (or M-PRK). In our retreated cases, we have not found relevant vision complications such as loss of BCVA of two or more lines or adverse reactions such as retraction of the flap edges. However, retreatment after previous M-LASIK should not be performed before 6 months.

LTK post H-LASIK: The success and efficiency post previous undercorrected H-LASIK or H-PRK is not as good as post M-LASIK and post M-PRK treatments. The mean subjective manifest refractive change is similar to the results after primary LTK with mean –0.7 D. We assume the reason is the unthinned central cornea.

In contrast to other retreatment procedures like secondary H-LASIK or H-PRK with increasing complication rates (risk of apical scar), LTK seems to be a safe and easy method with very low risks. A theoretical central ablation or peripheral retraction of the flap after additional LTK steepening was not observed. Retreatment consideration should also not take place before 6 months. For all undercorrections of 1.6 D ± 0.3, we generally used two rings (6.5/7.5 mm) with eight spots (240 to 256 mJ energy; seven pulses) (see Figure 10J-3).

H-LASIK after LTK: Experience with LASIK after LTK is limited. The initial results show that LASIK after LTK is possible without negative effects. Increased wrinkling or shrinkage of the flap, or protracted healing has not been observed. Previous LTK seems to not significantly improve or decrease the refractive result. However, the flap size should overlap the previous peripheral LTK spot diameter.

Summary: As an alternative retreatment method, LTK is a promising procedure. The main advantage is its quickness and safety. The best results are obtained in treating overcorrections. The dependence on the residual tissue is obvious. A thinned, weakened central cornea and the absence of Bowman's membrane facilitates corneal steepening by secondary LTK treatments and also influence their algorithm. Improved LTK effectiveness after previously performed flaps seems to support this, as recently reported.

SECTION TWO

Lasers, Microkeratomes, Techniques, Complex Cases, and Complications Management

THE EXCIMER LASER FOR LASIK

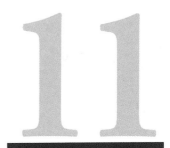

Lucio Buratto, MD and Giuseppe Perone, MD

THE EXCIMER LASER: BASIC CONCEPTS

The excimer laser belongs to a group of lasers that produce short wavelengths ranging from 150 and 300 nanometers, namely ultraviolet radiation.

The active medium of excimer lasers, or rather, the gaseous mixture that releases energy with a wavelength to interact with corneal tissue, is represented by the dimer, a reaction between a rare gas and a halogen.

The word *excimer* is a neologism created by the contraction of the two words describing the type of chemical compound (ie, excited dimer). The dimer is a molecule created by the mixture of a rare gas with a halogen; they are subjected to an electric field transforming them to an unstable state characterized by a higher energy, hence the contracted word excimer.

A certain amount of atoms and molecules (namely the gaseous mixture) can be stimulated in the presence of a strong electric field (20,000 to 40,000 volts). Supplying energy to this gas means creating a new extremely unstable condition because the atoms are energized and the electrons leave their resting state to enter orbits characterized by a higher energy; nevertheless, these electrons tend to rapidly return to their original state; this process brings about the release of energy in the form of photons. Simply put, light radiation is released. This light radiation, or simple released energy, is conveyed in the laser resonance cavity, where a system of mirrors multiplies the phenomena of atomic impact and excitation and gives rise to an amplified and monochromatic radiation with high fluence and intensity ranging from 180 and 200 mJ/cm².

In light of this, it is quite obvious that by combining rare gases with halogens in different ways, several dimers can be created, which can release different laser emissions depending on the emitted wavelength. This will be inversely proportional to the released photon energy (the greater the wavelength, the less the photon energy).

To ablate corneal tissue, the energy must be applied at high densities and the application times must be extremely short; excimer lasers presently release energy with a repetition frequency from 1, 10, to 100 Hertz.

In conclusion, excimer lasers are lasers pulsed to gas mixtures excited by electric discharges.

Which wavelength is most suitable for use in corneal surgery? The photon energy of these wavelengths has to be able to break up the corneal interatomic links, while preserving adjacent tissue as much as possible.

Among the various wavelengths studied, the most suitable was the one produced by the argon fluoride dimer (ArF), emitting 193 nm with photon energy equaling 6.42 eVolts. This choice was dictated by the fact that this wavelength is sufficiently far from the DNA absorption spectrum, so as to avoid dangerous interactions with it.

Criteria for choosing an ArF 193 nm excimer laser include:

- High photon energy
- Reduced penetration in the surrounding tissues
- Slight thermal damage
- Regular impact surface
- Absence of mutagenicity
- Strong water absorption

The C-N (carbon-nitrogen) peptic bonds show an absorption peak of about 190 nm, whereas collagen and ascorbic acid, because of their nonaromatic amino acid component, absorb some 260 nm, with a maximum of 240 nm.

Nucleic acids (absorption peak at around 250 nm) are practically confined to the epithelial layer; glycosaminoglicans, which have a very similar absorption spectrum, have a peak of around 190 nm.

The excimer photon flow released by one dimer at

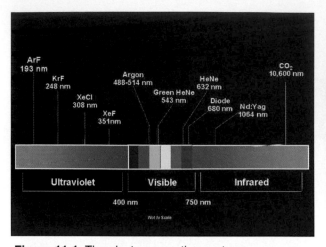

Figure 11-1. The electromagnetic spectrum.

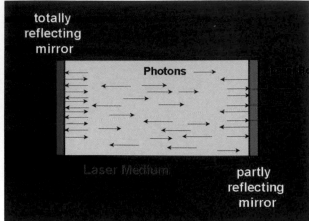

Figure 11-2. The laser principle.

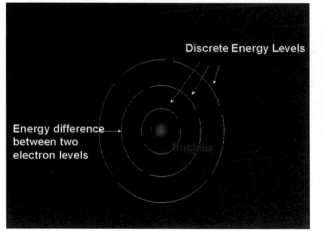

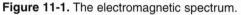

Figure 11-3. Simple diagram of an atom.

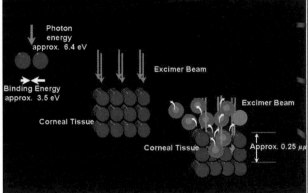

Figure 11-4. Excimer laser ablation process.

193 nm, such as the ArF, decouples the C-C (carbon-carbon) and C-N bonds of the peptic substrate of corneal proteins, whose absorption by ultraviolet light is quite high. The entity of tissue photablation is directly linked on the one hand to absorption (ie, the relationship between wavelength, energy flow, and radiation exposure time) and on the other to chromophoric characteristics of the cornea.

The tissue hit with photofragments of light molecular weight units is thus reduced; this provides an extremely precise and refined refractive treatment of tissue, with preservation of adjacent tissue: the thermal damage caused by adjacent proteins is therefore limited to about 1 micron.

Formation of ArF* molecules (*refers to the excited state) is obtained through the application of pulses characterized by an extremely high electric field acting through two effects; it energizes argon atoms and dissociates fluoride molecules by ionizing them.

The two resulting reactions are the following (where e and M are necessary partners for the reaction [neon, and helium]):

1. $Ar^* + F2 => ArF^* + F$
2. $e + F2 => F- + F$
   $F- + Ar + M => ArF^* + M$

In order for these reactions to take place efficiently, the speed of the atoms and the gas pressure must be correct; moreover, the impact probabilities and the percentage of various gases (F2, Ar, Ne, He) must be constantly monitored. When these conditions are respected the laser emits high-energy pulses lasting 15 to 20 nanoseconds (ns) (Figures 11 1 through 11-4).

STRUCTURE OF EXCIMER LASERS

From a structural viewpoint, an excimer laser is composed of:

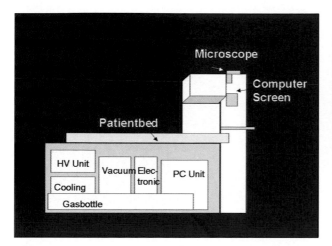

Figure 11-5. Major components of the excimer laser.

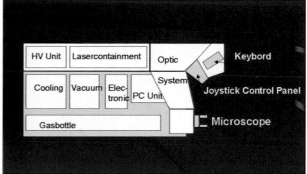

Figure 11-6. Major system components of the excimer laser.

- A laser cavity and a condenser to generate an electric discharge
- Gas reservoir (ArF)
- Optical path for transmission of the laser beam
- Computer to enter data
- Working area including an operating table, surgical microscope, and console table (Figures 11-5 and 11-6)

Cavity

The cavity houses the module where the high voltage discharge takes place and where the laser radiation is generated. It can be made of ceramic or other material, depending on the type of laser, even though most companies currently tend to use a ceramic cavity. The pressured gas mixture inside the cavity is conveyed through a fan toward the section where the electrodes are located, thus ensuring a continuous gas change.

Because fluoride is very reactive, especially during the discharge, it tends to react with the metal of the cavity, running the risk of contamination and needing frequent gas changing. This is one of the reasons why a ceramic cavity is often preferred. When the laser is equipped with a metal cavity, to overcome this drawback the electrodes supporting the discharge are mounted on a ceramic plate, which does not react with fluoride and increases the mixture life. Any impurities that could possibly form are removed through an accurate path of gas flow; by exploiting the heavier weight of contaminating materials, it conveys them toward the exterior of the cavity by centrifugal effect, eliminating them in the end through an external filter (millipore).

The laser radiation is emitted through a special window working as an outlet mirror. This is the optic bearing most of the stress, since all the laser energy created passes through it. The optic material is, of course, transparent to ultraviolet (UV) radiation and reacts poorly with the gaseous mixture in the cavity.

Gas Reservoir

Some excimer lasers are equipped with housing where the readied gaseous mixture is kept; whereas others have two distinct reservoirs containing gases to be blended later. Moreover, some excimer lasers are equipped with a bottle of nitrogen, which is conveyed along the optical path to preserve cleaning and quality of the optics lodged within. The gas bottles can be housed either inside or outside the laser frame.

Optic Path

This is the path the laser beam travels to reach the corneal tissue. Along this path, the laser beam changes in shape and homogeneity. Because the light radiation at 193 nm is absorbed and then dispersed by optical fibers, it must be transmitted by means of mirrors, lenses and prisms in an environment where the air quality interferes very little with the radiation. All this has an influence on homogeneity and on the quality of the laser beam, which must be very high if regular photoablations of the corneal surface are to be obtained.

Computer

This foundation of the whole structure is used to monitor all sorts of functions connected with the excimer laser, ranging from gas mixing, monitoring of released energy, data entry, and interfacing with external devices. Apart from the characteristics typical of any computer, a particular emphasis is given to shielding of both structures and connections, so as to avoid any possible interference with foreign equipment.

Work Area

The operating table, microscope, and console differ depending on the equipment; their use must, of course, be comfortable for the surgeon and patient. The operat-

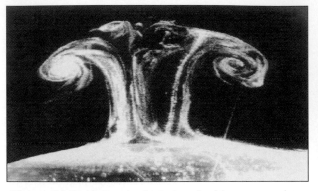

Figure 11-7. High-speed photo of wide-area excimer laser ablation of a cornea.

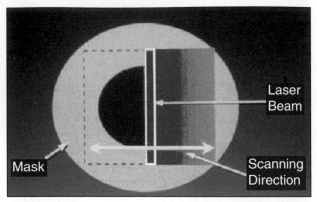

Figure 11-8. Meditec MEL 60 slit scanning ablation system.

ing table and headrest must allow the patient to lie down and comfortably remain in this position throughout the whole operation. The operating microscope must provide brightness, field depth and adequate magnifying power suitable to the surgical procedure; this is particularly important for LASIK procedures. Here, a comfortable working area is necessary to apply the suction ring and to allow any type of microkeratome without hindrance. To us, Bausch & Lomb's solution seems ideal—they added a Hansatome microkeratome central unit inside the laser itself (which was also equipped with software to monitor the microkeratome's assembly and operation).

The control panel must house the basic controls and must enable the surgeon to act easily and rapidly during various phases of the operation. The laser application times during a LASIK operation must be reduced to the minimum. It must be kept in mind that the less the time the flap is detached from the stromal bed, the better the result of the operation.

Excimer lasers are also characterized by following elements:

- Focusing system. Every laser has a particular strategy to focus the working plane. This will be discussed in more detail in the sections for each laser.
- Laser beam delivery system

Broadbeam

A broadbeam, as adopted by VISX, Summit, and the original Technolas 116, removes layers of material. The corrective effect relies on the fact that each removed layer differs in shape from the previous one, so that the thickness of overall ablated material in the center differs from that ablated in the periphery of the cornea. This technique is particularly suited to treat myopic errors since to obtain the desired effect, you simply have to send circular-shaped laser pulses, concentric with variable diameter. The same method can be used to treat

myopic astigmatism, using broadly rectangular beams of variable length. The broadbeam technique produces approximately regular and smooth surfaces and is less sensitive to eye movement. Conversely it is less flexible and requires more powerful lasers (Figure 11-7).

Scanning Slit

In excimer lasers that adopt this type of beam distribution, a particular diaphragm allows the release of a rectangular beam with changeable dimensions, which is then distributed on the cornea by means of a linear or rotation system, allowing to treat several areas of the cornea, thus avoiding excessive corneal overheating; in addition it allows ablation profiles to correct myopia, hyperopia, and astigmatism (Figure 11-8).

Flying Spot

The flying spot technique employs a small beam ablating a small "tile" of tissue with every pulse. The corrective effect is obtained by making the laser beam perform a series of excursions on the cornea, passing several times over those areas where more material must be ablated. In principle, this technique allows correction of corneas with any type of irregularity in shape and is only limited by the dimensions of the laser beam diameter (the smaller this is, the more the system can correct complex irregularities) (Figure 11-9).

EXCIMER LASER USE PARAMETERS

Wavelength

Studies carried out on this important parameter reveal that light radiation having a wavelength of 193 nm is the most suitable to create corneal ablations with regular excision edges and to limit damage to the adjacent tissue.

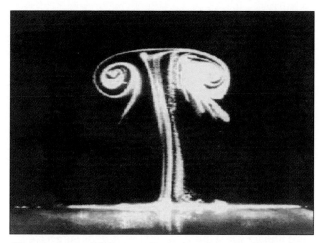

Figure 11-9. High-speed photo of a small diameter excimer laser ablation of a PMMA plate.

This is due to the chromophoric characteristics of the cornea; indeed, because of its transparency, it absorbs little energy coming from the laser beams in the visible spectrum; it should be remembered that the cornea is endowed with a delicate laminar structure which can easily be damaged by the biological effects of the laser. As a matter of fact, they can provoke an alteration in the structure of the cornea itself and of its optical and biomechanical characteristics. The interplay between cornea and laser beam follows the optical and biophysical laws regulating passage of electromagnetic radiation inside a tissue and a dioptric medium; transmission, reflection, dispersion-diffusion, and absorption phenomena depend on the characteristics of the incident radiation with reference to the chromophoric composition of the corneal tissue.

The wavelengths of the shorter ultraviolet radiation deliver stronger energies, determining a photoablation effect with reduced depth of dissipation of thermal damage.

With all these upsides resulting from the use of light radiation with a reduced wavelength, inevitably there are some downsides induced by such wavelengths. As a matter of fact 193 mm radiation prevents transmission through optic fibers with extensive damage to the optical elements of the transmission system.

Pulse Duration

This parameter is related to the fact that the excited dimer shows an extremely short half-life: from 9 to 23 ns.

Repetition Frequency

This parameter indicates the number of pulses (laser) emitted per second and is measured in hertz (Hz). Frequencies of the various lasers will be indicated in the corresponding chapters; they normally range from 10 Hz (Summit and VISX) to 200 Hz (LaserSight). Ablation of the corneal tissue does not depend on such parameters.

Theoretically, the most useful data, namely the quickest ones to perform the procedure in the shortest time, preventing corneal hydration from varying consistently, are not recommended because of the increase in the thermal effect and of the onset of damage to the optical component of the beam transmission system. However, this applies only to those lasers adopting traditional ablation programs, whereas it holds perfectly true for the newest lasers performing ablation through the flying spot technique.

Fluence

It is expressed in mJ/cm^2 and refers to the radiant exposition (ie, the energy per pulse and per surface unit of ablated tissue). Its optimal level (where efficacy of photoablative mechanism reaches its maximum for our purposes), ranges from 160 to 250 mJ/cm^2, as indicated in several studies.

The ablation threshold is usually the stage at which 193 nm radiation starts removing tissue. Measurements performed by Puliafito and Krueger report a value of around 46 to 50 mJ/cm^2; below these readings a sort of incomplete ablative photodecomposition arises, causing both irregularities and thermal effects.

The detailed study carried out by Munnerlyn and coworkers on the relationship curve between fluence and ablation depth (or efficacy) with surface treatment is quite interesting. This broadly sigmoidal curve is characterized by a flat beginning, an ascending central section corresponding to the efficient ablation region, in which 20% to 90% of incident photons are absorbed, a peak of around 200 to 230 mJ/cm^2, ending with a plateau progressively losing its ablation power. This also depends on the frequency, at least for those lasers that do not use a flying spot ablation system. The faster the pulse rate, the less time the tissue has to get rid of debris and cool down.

The main types of lasers available on the market employ fluence levels on a corneal level ranging from 160 to 250 mJ/cm^2.

Another important parameter in refractive surgery with excimer lasers is the cut rate, namely the quantity of tissue photoablated by each pulse (ablation rate).

The controversial results reported by various authors (Aron Rosa: 0.6 microns per shot; Trokel: 0.45; Rowsey: 0.12 to 0.22) can be ascribed to the following:

- Each species and the different corneal levels behave differently.
- The different hydration and depth of the cornea; these conditions can not be easily transferred to in-vivo conditions.

This is the reason why each laser had to set its own software on their optimal cut rate values:

- Summit: 0.20 microns per pulse in corrections lower than 3.00 diopters (D)
- 0.22 micron per pulse in higher errors
- VISX: from 0.21 to 0.27 microns depending on the type of treatment made and on the calibration of the instrument
- Meditec: 0.5 microns

Considering a constant cut rate, without differentiating it depending on the depth of the procedure can lead to undercorrection errors. The problem became even more evident when LASIK was adopted to correct refractive defects.

Indeed, every cornea and corneal level have their own cut rate because of the variability of conditions of tissue organization, hydration, and thickness of the individual structures. We saw that excessive stromal drying significantly increases ablation depth per pulse and can lead to overcorrection; in light of this, it is important for photoablation to remove the epithelium as quickly as possible. In this respect it is worth remembering that the epithelium is a highly heterogeneous structure, ablated with a quicker rate compared to stroma, whereas Bowman's is ablated more slowly.

Homogeneity

This important parameter indicates the homogeneity with which laser energy is distributed on the cornea; it is evident that the more homogeneous the laser beam, the more uniform the surface treated. The beam released by the resonance cavity of modern excimer lasers, apart from the latest ones with ceramic cavities and flying spot programs, is never uniform because the energy density is greater in the center compared to the periphery, and decreases with the degradation of the active medium gas. Because of the cavity conformation, the emerging beam has a broadly rectangular, hat-like configuration of 8 x 24 mm; it is delivered through a combination of mechanisms driven by a computer program, the so-called "delivery system" that distributes energy on a corneal level. These optical elements placed along the path of the laser beam are endowed with special surface treatments (magnesium fluoride or calcium stratification) to support the excimer-elevated energies. Moreover, they also play a homogenizing role (mirrors, lenses, and pivoting prisms), together with space integrators and special masks selectively eliminating the peripheral part of laser beams, transmitting the more homogeneous central part. Nevertheless, at each optic interface, a degradation of the beam occurs because of lack of power. Of the hundreds of millijoules coming out of the cavity, the overwhelming majority (up to 70% in certain machines) are lost along the optic path before reaching the corneal surface.

The quality of the beam is directly monitored before each treatment by the surgeon, who makes special ablation tests.

Number of Pulses

This parameter is checked by the surgeon. It should be kept in mind that for an established cut rate, the number of pulses determines the entity of ablation. It is automatically supplied by the computer according to the number of diopters to correct.

Eye Tracker

In order for a refractive surgery operation with an excimer laser to provide the best results, the photoablative treatment must be perfectly centered and the eye must remain still. Unfortunately, even if the surgeon centers perfectly, a patient's eye cannot remain absolutely still during the entire operation. To overcome this drawback, several systems were proposed. Some first-generation lasers used a suction ring applied to the eye; this allowed the surgeon to perform both centration and intraoperative realignment of the laser beam on the center of treatment. With the advent of photoablation strategies, employing beams with a reduced diameter and several overlapping impacts, such as PlanoScan by Chiron Technolas, such a crude centration and realignment system is practically inconceivable. There was, therefore, an urgent need to develop an eye tracking system which can recognize movements of the eye during the operation and be able to automatically realign to its new position in a very short time, so as to allow the laser beam to track the correct position.

Applications

The eye-tracking system typical of certain excimer lasers is nothing but one of the countless applications of this device in different technological fields. Indeed, these systems are widely applied outside the medical field.

During the advent of eye tracking, the war and aeronautics industries developed the eye-tracking technology; as commonly occurs, military use lead to the possibility of employing war technologies for more noble purposes.

In the optical area, ophthalmology avails itself to eye-tracking systems not only in excimer lasers, but also in cases of macular pathology, where countless potentialities can be exploited for research, to detect a fixation point, and to carry out research modalities of eye movements, with important consequences on the training of patients when looking for more functional retinal areas than those damaged by disease to the central retina. Neuropsychiatry analyzes eye movements and space orientation of eyes to gather information on behavior and reactions of patients submitted to specific tests.

The adoption of eye-tracking systems affected by the so-called "locked in syndrome," a neurological condition characterized by the inability to make movements except those of the eye, is particularly helpful. Some patients can interact with a computer that can establish the direction of their look thanks to a specific detection system; an interactive screen reacts by performing the command situated in the position of the screen toward where the patient is staring. Such an application that is extremely important for disabled people and is likely to also be applied to handicap-free people, with clear advantages.

In the field of aeronautics, the possibility to have eye-tracking systems allows both ground training of civil and military personnel, and a dramatic use in the tracking devices of military objectives. Modern warplanes are equipped with devices similar to mouse trackers; they are particular helmet-shaped instruments that can assess the direction of a look after detecting the potential delivered to special electrodes located on the scalp of the eye; the direction of the look can spot an objective, whereas a suitable stimulus (such as a more accentuated blink or a prolonged and forced opening of the eyelid) mimic the right or left click of a mouse, depending on the side in question.

The monitoring system of eye movements is also widely applied in the business field. Some large toy companies invest large capital and resources to understand reactions of their perspective customers (children) when looking at television commercials, so as to evaluate their reactions, assess the influence, and modifying their structure correspondingly, thus achieving an ideal impact.

In the industrial field, cameras and telecameras are manufactured to monitor the direction of a person's gaze and focus the instrument accordingly.

Computer science is another fascinating field in which these instruments are widely applied, with virtual reality in particular. Here too the helmet representing the interface device with the computer can detect the position of the look and follow its variations.

Technical Characteristics

Any eye-tracking system detects an eye movement and spatially with respect to a starting position. Such control is made in several ways.

Eye Movement Control Modalities

Infrared

This device is composed of:
- An LED (light emitting diode) lighting system emitting intermittent light at 950 nm (infrared) at a frequency of 2.5 Hz. This intermittent emission (chopped mode) allows not only to minimize interference by available light (distinguishing between infrared [IR] light emitted by the lighting device and this IR component in the available light), but also to increase the signal noise ratio of the reception system (the rate of incident IR light is therefore high, but the total energy is reduced).
- A reception system: phototransistors tuned in on the LED emission frequency and positioned in their proximity; the LED beam has an amplitude of 48°. The receiving transistors have an amplitude of 28°. Each unit (composed of an LED and a transistor) recognizes an eye starting position and its movements, decoding the fly back signal coming from the nose and temporal quadrants. This system can follow the rotation movement of the bulb within 30° with a resolution capacity equal to 2 minutes of arc.
- A CCD telecamera: a light-sensitive device that records color or black and white images and translates information in digital form (analogue sensors); this type of telecamera is used in excimer lasers.

DPI (Double Purkinije Image)

This system relies on continuous detection of the first and fourth Purkinije's reflex, namely that reflected by the front corneal surface and by a lens back surface. This eye tracker illuminates the eye with a collimated light beam at 930 nm (IR) and uses a combination of mirrors and lenses to follow and locate Purkinije's reflexes. The light beam is projected intermittently at a frequency of 4 Hz. Before reaching the eyeball it crosses a dichroic mirror transparent to available light. This type of ET detects eye movements at a frequency of 500 Hz, with an accuracy of 1 minute of arc.

Topolink

Topolink represents a possible alternative being studied by several manufacturing companies. The basic concept is to create a specific photoablation treatment for the cornea to be used especially in cases of highly irregular tissues. The creation of a photoablation treatment guided by the topographic traits of the cornea to be treated will enable correction of defects such as irregular astigmatism, central islands, decentralization, and to extend its use to each individual treatment, so as to achieve ablation profiles through which corneal surfaces increasingly near to the ideal cornea to be treated can be reached (Table 11-1).

Conclusions

Our extensive analysis clearly shows that there is still a long way to go before manufacturing a laser enabling us to work in the safest of ways. Eye-tracking systems

Table 11-1

EXCIMER LASER CLASSES

Medium	Wavelength (nm)	Photon energy (eVolt)
ArF	193	6.42
KrF	248	5.00
XeCl	308	4.03
XeF	351	3.50

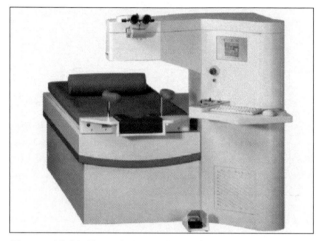

Figure 11-10. Bausch & Lomb 217C excimer laser.

Table 11-2

TECHNICAL CHARACTERISTICS OF THE BAUSCH & LOMB 217C EXCIMER LASER

Cut rate	0.25 microns per pulse
Ablation system	Flying spot
Spot diameter	2.0 mm (PlanoScan)
Cavity	Ceramic
Gas	Argon fluoride
Treatment of optical zones (max)	
Myopia	8.5 mm
Astigmatism	5.0 x 8.0 mm
Hyperopia	9.0 mm
Wavelength	193 nm
Frequency of pulses	50 Hz
Duration of pulses	18 ns
Fluence at the cornea	120 mJ/cm^2
Eye tracker	Active and passive
Topolink	Yes
Cooling	Internal, closed circuit
Microscope	Moeller-Wedel
Magnification	3.4x to 6x, 8.5x
Power supply	220 to 230 V AC/16 AC 50/60 Hz
Dimensions	Length 2.6 m width 1.5 m height 1.5 m
Weight	680 kg

The 217C has an optimal efficiency with temperature parameters of around 20°C with humidity below 45%.

must still be improved, even if certain machines, as we will see later on, already have good technology. It will be necessary to direct efforts to manufacture lasers allowing a more homogeneous refractive treatment, with optimal treatment surfaces.

THE BAUSCH & LOMB 217C EXCIMER LASER

The Bausch & Lomb excimer laser (Table 11-2), conceived and manufactured in Germany, has the latest flying spot technology. The PlanoScan ablation program is truly innovative and gives the Bausch & Lomb excimer laser advantages over some of the other laser systems currently on the market.

Features:
- A filtered air system that automatically cleans the optics each time the laser is switched on. This feature maintains efficiency and reduces the need for maintenance, prolonging the life of optical components.
- Gas integrated system. A single ArF mixture gas bottle allows between 700 and 900 treatments.
- Two mobile mirrors (wobbling mirrors) for 180° coverage, one on the X axis, the other on the Y axis, directing the photoablation by simply and automatically shifting the treating beam either through the aid of the computer or, as in some therapeutic treatments, through a joystick.
- PlanoScan ablation system. In this ablation system, the spot, which is 2.0 mm in diameter, impacts different points on the corneal surface throughout the ablation, the overlap of individual impacts outlining the chosen treatment. The main advantage is represented by reduced thermal trauma. The extremely versatile software allows for quick programming of myopic, hyperopic, and astigmatic treatments, as well as therapeutic treatments (Figures 11-10 through 11-13).

Cavity

The cavity of the 217C laser is ceramic. This material reduces the build-up of deposits from the gas mixture on the walls, increasing the number of treatments that can be performed with each gas fill. Moreover, the energy during treatments is more stable. Because the gas bottle lasts longer, maintenance costs are reduced (Figure 11-14).

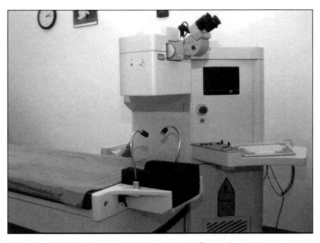

Figure 11-11. Bausch & Lomb 217C excimer laser operative area.

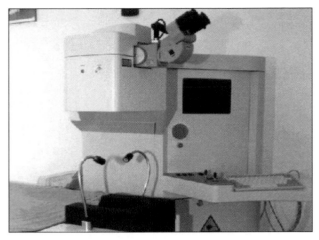

Figure 11-12. Bausch & Lomb 217C excimer laser operative area—close-up.

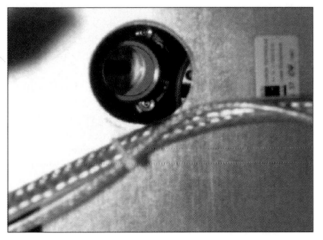

Figure 11-13. Exit window of the excimer laser ceramic beam head.

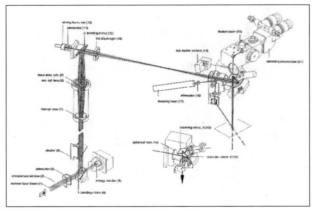

Figure 11-14. Bausch & Lomb 217C beam delivery system.

Gas Reservoir

A single gas bottle containing ArF gaseous mixture is located inside the laser housing. Its capacity allows some 700 to 900 treatments.

Optic Pathway

The laser beam reaches corneal tissue from the cavity in which it is generated by travelling along the optical path. Here it undergoes modifications that ensure correct fluence and beam homogeneity.

Once the laser beam leaves the cavity, it is redirected by a mirror through a homogenizer. The laser beam leaving the cavity has little homogeneity and is broadly rectangular in shape.

At this stage, the first He-Ne red laser is added (wavelength 635 nm), following the same direction of the excimer laser beam and acting as an aiming beam;

simply put, it makes the path covered by the 193 mm beam visible.

The two laser beams then go through a 2.0-mm diaphragm and first reach a focusing lens and then wobbling mirrors (X-Y) delivering the laser spot on to the corneal surface (Figures 11-15 and 11-16).

When the laser beam leaves the cavity, it is full of excited gas due to the influence of high-voltage discharges through an opening in one of the two reflecting walls; then it is deviated by a reflecting mirror, whose surface cannot absorb the 193 nm radiation of the excimer laser beam. The laser beam leaving the cavity is poorly homogeneous and broadly rectangular in shape; if imaged on a special photographic film it is easily noticeable that the laser beam is rectangular and extremely irregular. Before reaching the first mirror, the beam goes through two attenuators; these are special filters that let the beam they are crossed by either go through or under-

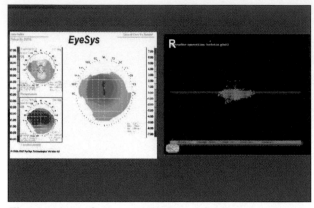

Figure 11-15. Schematic diagram of the beam delivery system.

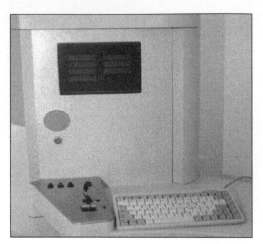

Figure 11-16. Bausch & Lomb 217C control panel.

go an attenuation, depending on the angle they have with respect to incident light.

An electrical motor controlled from the keyboard positions the attenuators using the left and right "shift" keys. When the attenuators are positioned so that the laser beam strikes at 90°, their influence and energy absorption is at peak levels; the right "shift" key turns the attenuator filter; this revolution modifies the laser beam's angle of incidence on the attenuator filter, reducing efficacy in absorbing energy.

The laser beam then goes through a homogenizer; this is a 50 cm long metal cylinder. Two highly powerful toric lenses are positioned at each end. Their axis is reciprocally orthogonal; a convergent lens is placed in the metal cylinder's distal segment. This optical system brings about a starting divergence and a subsequent convergence on orthogonal planes along the direction of the laser beam, to "blend" the laser beam itself on an impact surface after it, and to obtain an almost identical quantity of energy at all points. When leaving the homogenizer, if the light beam is well focused, has a rectangular shape, and has finally reached good homogeneity, it then reaches another reflecting mirror deviating the beam at 90°.

At this stage, the first He-Ne red laser is added (635 nm), following the same direction of the excimer laser beam and acting as an aiming beam, making the path covered by the 193 nm visible. This allows visualization where the beam impacts the target.

The two laser beams go through a 2.0-mm diaphragm and reach the focusing lens then the wobbling mirrors (X-Y), which deliver the laser spot to the corneal surface.

The wobbling mirrors are the last optic that reflects the laser beam before the cornea. Their oscillation is adjusted and optimized by the central unit and performed by two motors. Oscillation takes place along two X and Y meridians and allows positioning of the spot onto any portion of the corneal surface, thus obtaining the necessary photoablation treatment, which is programmed and optimized according to the PlanoScan algorithm. Along the optical path, the 193-nm laser beam and the aiming beam are joined by two other laser beams; a fixation mire represented by a diode laser beam (670 nm) situated in the head of the operating microscope at which it projects the fixation mire, which the patient must look at during capture by the eye tracker and the refractive ablation; a second He-Ne green laser (543 nm) is projected on the cornea from a caudal position with respect to the surgeon (it is used to focus the system on the cornea). The system is correctly focused when the green mire and aiming beam, and therefore the laser beam overlap. This procedure allows a focused treatment on the exposed corneal surface (Bowman's membrane and front stroma in PRK, central corneal stroma in LASIK) and a treatment centered on the visual axis.

Data Entry

The keyboard is easily accessible and simple to use; it is on the right side of the surgeon and built into the laser housing. In addition to software for the surgical correction of refractive defects such as myopia, hyperopia, and astigmatism, it is provided with a specific manual program for therapeutic treatments, controlled by the computer itself. The Hansatome microkeratome is also driven by the control unit. The laser can be connected with a topography unit for treatments with topolink (Figure 11-17).

Work Area

Given the reduced dimensions of the machine, the working space available for the surgeon is excellent. The choice to install the microkeratome console inside the

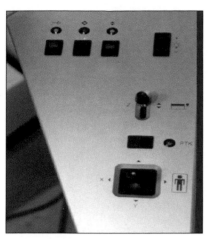

Figure 11-17. Detailed view of the Bausch & Lomb 217C control panel with joystick and switches.

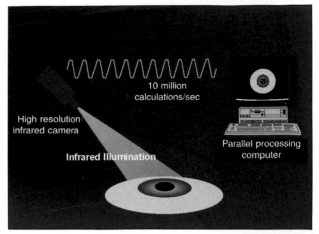

Figure 11-18. Active eye tracker.

laser housing (bridge) renders the surgical field free from any type of hindrance. The operating microscope has magnifications of 3x, 4x, 6x, and 8.5x.

Focusing System

The focusing joystick is used to overlap the green light and aiming beam's red light. During treatment, the aiming beam's red light is switched off and the fixation red light, which must always coincide with the green focusing light, is switched on (Figure 11-18).

Active and Passive Eye Tracker

This particular device, derived from the most sophisticated military tracking systems, compensates for eye micromovements without stopping the treatment. The tracking range is 1.5 mm. This means that during treatment a patient's eye movement exceeding 3.0 mm causes the ablation to stop (passive eye tracker); the treatment can start again from the point at which it was stopped when the patient resumes fixation and the eye-tracking system recognizes the memorized image. Those movements that fall within a 3.0-mm diameter trigger such a retrieval reaction by the eye-tracking system, that ablation continues in perfect alignment with the initial centering. The high resolution infrared video camera, laser scanning system, and computer jointly track the eye. Information is exchanged between these components 10 million times per second. The eye-tracking system is composed of:

- An infrared lighting system
- An infrared video camera
- A display

Infrared Lighting System

Provides optimum lighting of the operating field for

correct functioning of the eye tracker; two infrared light sources were added in model 217C to optimize functioning of the infrared video camera. They are two small light sources placed at the end of a mobile arm; the light beam they produce must be carried on the eye's surface before initialization and capturing by the eye tracker throughout the entire treatment.

Infrared Video Camera

The infrared video camera is a special video camera placed near the terminal portion of the laser output system; it can pick up the image of the anterior segment regardless of light conditions. This allows the system to detect the center of the pupil's opening and keep it aligned with the center of treatment (eye tracker). The center of the pupil's opening is calculated by recognizing the pupil's edge. Three tangents are marked on it and their median point gives rise to three perpendiculars meeting in a point identified as the center of the pupil's image.

The reckoning system foresees the adoption of 50 positions per second, with realignments every 20 milliseconds; spatial resolution (ie, the system's capability to recognize shifts of the image and to realign it accordingly) equals 25 microns. The system works in an active way (active eye tracker) for movements of ±1.5 mm from the center of the treatment (a 3.0 mm diameter). For movements beyond this range, the system stops the ablation (passive eye tracker) and restarts when the center of the image captured by the video camera falls within ± 1.5 mm from the center of treatment.

In Bausch & Lomb lasers 116 and 117, the video camera is placed laterally on the right, whereas in Bausch & Lomb 217 it is placed toward the patient's feet. Video camera position affects the way a treatment is performed; a laterally placed video camera is not hindered by the presence of instruments used to protect the hinge when nasal hinge LASIK on the right eye is performed, whereas the hinge protection maneuver in the case of nasal hinge LASIK on a left eye can block the field of the lateral infrared video camera, causing the eye tracker to go on and off, this inconvenience is resolved by using a superior hinge LASIK procedure.

In the Bausch & Lomb 217 laser, the position of the infrared video camera does not interfere with the flap protection maneuver, either in the nasal hinge procedure or superior hinge procedure.

The eye-tracker system allows more comfortable performance of surface refractive surgical procedures. This instrument is absolutely indispensable when performing LASIK because a patient cannot possibly keep fixation on a mire once the flap is raised and the laser treatment begins.

Bausch & Lomb is committed to ongoing research to further optimize the eye-tracker system, an absolutely indispensable technology in modern refractive surgery; the new eye-tracking system is called Q3 99.

Display

The laser assistant can see on the computer display the images gathered by the infrared video camera, both in the initialization screen page, in the "capturing" eye tracker page, and during treatment, along with the red/green indicator indicating the eye tracker is working.

The laser console is equipped with the following controls:

1. Four-position joystick for chair's X-Y movement.
2. Two-position joystick to obtain focus by moving the chair up and down.
3. Joystick to move the beam during phototherapeutic procedure.

   In model 217, joysticks 1 and 3 are combined: a switch allows a choice between the chair's X-Y movements or beam movements during the phototherapeutic procedure.
4. Switches (on/off) for fixation light, aiming beam, and focusing.

   In model 217, a control on the console allows the adjustment of light intensity over the operating field; whereas in models 116 and 117, this device is located on the laser housing on the surgeon's right side.

Practical Hints

Working Position

In this preliminary phase, the surgeon must determine what position (determined by a stool's height and

microscope position) is most suitable for him. It is worth remembering that the working distance in the Bausch & Lomb 217 is slightly longer than in previous models. Eyepieces should be adjusted depending on the surgeon's refractive error and on the distance between pupils. At this stage, the surgeon should also check that eyepieces are perfectly clean and set at the most suitable magnification and light intensity for the first phase of treatment.

Centering the Microscope and Focusing the Field

The first step in the procedure, when a patient is lying under the operating microscope, is to center and focus the operating field. The fixation light and green focusing light should be kept switched on. Correct centering results when the two lights are made to overlap by using the joystick. Try to center the two lights in the middle of the pupil. Check that the patient's head is properly positioned.

Eye Tracker Initialization

Initialization is a preliminary procedure before "capturing" by the eye tracker can begin. This allows the instrument to make an initial calibration in the grey range, depending on the color of the iris and diameter of the pupil. The procedure is performed after placing the lid speculum and centering and focusing using maximum magnification. This step is not influenced by light intensity.

Focusing and Centering for Eye Tracker Capture

Focusing and centering must be perfectly performed before the eye tracker capturing procedure, after epithelial removal in case of PRK, or lifting the flap in the case of LASIK (some surgeons prefer to perform this step after the keratectomy and shortly before lifting the flap). The result of the refractive ablation heavily depends on correctly performing this procedure.

1. Program the computer to capture the eye tracker. Select "treatment" from the specific menu (PRK, LASIK, or refractive) and press "X" to allow capturing of the eye tracker.
2. Switch off the fixation light and leave on both the aiming beam and focusing green light, so as to focus the system on the corneal surface and center the laser beam on the correct point.
3. Ask the patient to fixate on the red aiming beam light. The laser beam creates a reflex on the corneal surface at a point that corresponds to the visual axis.
4. With the microscope at its maximum magnification and using the X-Y joystick, center the aiming

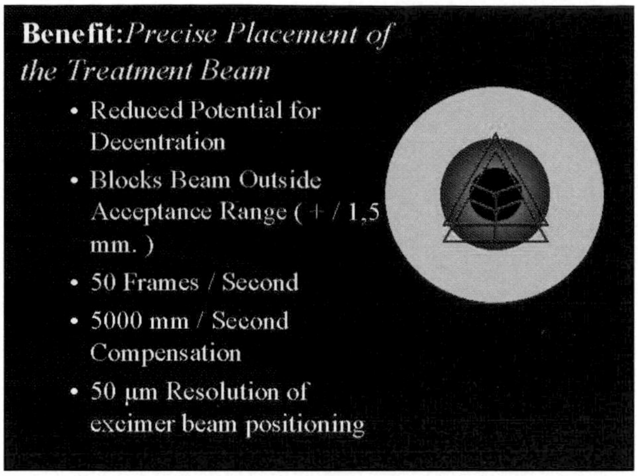

Benefit: *Precise Placement of the Treatment Beam*

- Reduced Potential for Decentration
- Blocks Beam Outside Acceptance Range (+ / 1.5 mm.)
- 50 Frames / Second
- 5000 mm / Second Compensation
- 50 μm Resolution of excimer beam positioning

Figure 11-19. Benefits of an active eye tracker.

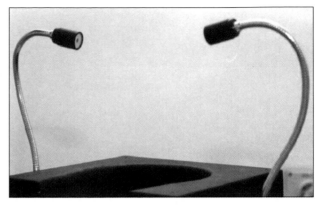

Figure 11-20. The two-neck swan-shaped infrared lights to enhance eye-tracking system sensitivity.

beam on the corneal surface with respect to the center of the intended treatment. The aiming beam, and therefore the excimer beam, are positioned in the center of the treatment zone.

5. Using the focusing joystick, make the green light overlap the red aiming beam light. The system is now correctly focused.

6. When the red aiming beam light and green focusing light are focused on the cornea in the center of the treatment zone, ask the patient to carefully fixate on the red light, press the laser pedal, and release it shortly afterward. Centering is performed and the eye tracker is captured.

7. Switch the aiming beam off and switch on the fixation light. It is better to switch the aiming beam off because the distribution modality of laser impacts in the PlanoScan system would induce search movements by the patient.

8. Check correspondence between the fixation and focusing light. This is an additional way to verify alignment; theoretically, it is superfluous if the fixation beam was correctly aligned with the aiming beam when performing the beam alignment tests.

9. Begin treatment. During treatment, the eye-tracking system allows realignment when the patient moves his or her eye within a radius of 1.5 mm. Verification takes place 50 times per second, or every 20 milliseconds; the eye tracker can recognize and correct 25-micron micromovements. In cases of a large movement of the eye, the system stops automatically and starts again when the acquired image during eye tracker capture is recognized, that is when the patient resumes fixation.

10. During treatment, the presence of the eye tracker does not relieve the surgeon of the need to con-

stantly monitor the procedure. Should you notice that the system is defocused, refocusing/centering can be accomplished by pressing the F4 key and adjusting the new position with the cursors. When the adjustment has been made, press F4 again and resume treatment.

Positioning the Model 217 Infrared Light Sources

The two infrared light sources must be positioned at a 30° angle of inclination with respect to the corneal bed and at a distance of 3.0 cm from the corneal apex.

In very light eyes, the angle of inclination should be slightly increased but never exceeding 45°.

With LASIK, positioning of the infrared light source must be made after cutting but before lifting the flap.

To ensure correct functioning of the eye tracker, the pupil's infrared image (on a computer screen) must be clear and have good contrast; the pupil must be perfectly seen and with no shadow.

The eye tracker should not be used in the following cases:

- Coloboma of the iris
- Ectopic pupil
- Infrared blurring
- Contrast problems between the iris and pupil in the infrared image. The F1 function allows exclusion of the eye tracker

What should be done when the working plane is defocused? Refocus using F4 function. When the eye tracker is used correctly patients with nystagmus can also be treated (Figures 11-19 through 11-24).

Topolink

This machine can perform treatments with the topolink option. Topography is acquired with a specific instrument provided by the manufacturer.

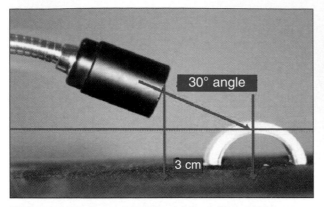

Figure 11-21. Correct position of the infrared light.

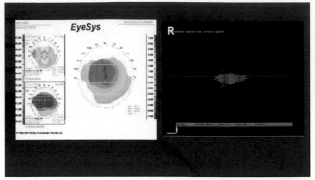

Figure 11-22. Topographic difference map (EyeSys) before and after LASIK in a patient with congenital horizontal nystagmus (left). The eye tracker realignment movements during the laser ablation are arranged along the horizontal axis (right).

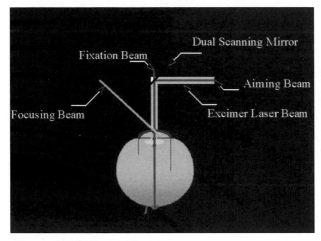

Figure 11-23. Beam alignment.

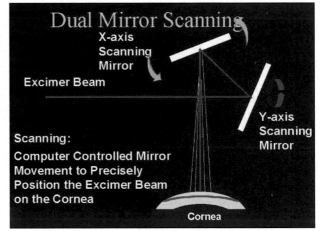

Figure 11-24. Schematic of the PlanoScan dual mirror scanning system.

PlanoScan Ablation System

Excimer laser technology has undergone a considerable evolution over the last few years. The second-generation lasers tried to overcome the major limits of these devices through the use of new ablation programs. The first ablation programs had a single optic zone treatment with a very steep gradient with resulting side effects (ie, night glare, regression, and central islands).

The multizone program was the first step forward in trying to overcome these stumbling blocks. This new concept of double or triple optical zones (multizone) like the geometric configuration of some ophthalmic lenses (aspherical) with extreme annular regions called transition regions, aimed at making passage of curvatures smoother and broaden the optical zone to reduce the incidence of aberrations introduced from the periphery.

Researchers are willing to use increasingly large optical zones; this translates into a deeper treatment, a higher quantity of tissue to ablate and represents a considerable limit in the amount of myopic refractive error that can be corrected.

Larger ablation zones mean on one hand overcoming such problems as night glare, on the other, increasing the risk of irregular surfaces, onset of central islands, and a higher incidence of haze, especially with PRK.

Removing a lot of tissue means stimulating stromal fibroplasia consistently, thus weakening the structure of the cornea.

The Bausch & Lomb 217C emits a 2.0-mm diameter, variable frequency beam that is computer guided to perform the refractive ablation. This new system is called PlanoScan.

The algorithm is optimized so that consecutive spots are not aimed at the same point, thus minimizing thermal shock to the cornea and reducing the risk of trauma or edema.

The Bausch & Lomb 217C uses a sophisticated scanning technology based on the use of wobbling mirrors that deliver the laser beam to the correct point on the corneal surface. This technology allows not only delivery

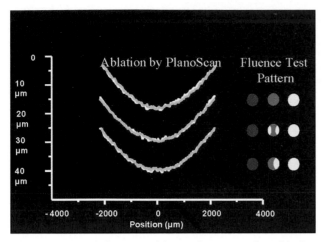

Figure 11-25. Influence of beam homogeneity with the PlanoScan.

of the laser beam to a precise point, but also to integrate an active eye tracker. This scanning technique can correct myopia, hyperopia, and myopic and hyperopic astigmatism. The biggest advantage offered by the PlanoScan algorithm compared to a multizone treatment is the much smoother ablated surface.

This is demonstrated by comparing both types of treatment on Polymethylmethacrylate. The PlanoScan profile shows a better correspondence with the theoretical calculated profile against a multizone treatment. Another advantage is that the PlanoScan technique does not create central islands.

The experience and expertise gained in the field of refractive surgery using excimer lasers and large optic zones provided the clues to search for solutions to other problems, such as the creation of central islands.

The overwhelming majority of excimer laser users and manufacturers bypassed the problem of central islands by adding additional laser pulses to the center of the treatment zone until the needed correction value was reached.

After many years of research, Bausch & Lomb discovered the reason underlying the creation of central islands and developed a new scanning algorithm to correct refractive defects: the PlanoScan system. This technique offers advantages when compared to multizone ablation methods; the first advantage (previously mentioned) is the extremely smooth corneal surface after ablation; moreover, it reduces the onset of central islands.

Each pulse of the laser beam causes 0.25 microns of corneal tissue to vaporize. After impact, a high-pressure shockwave moves away from the ablation surface. Since all the particles of the ejection material move away from the cornea at a high speed, an under-pressure zone is created between the cloud of debris and the corneal surface.

As a reaction to this differential pressure, some particles are brought back from the outside toward the inner part of this cloud of debris, filling the under-pressure zone. The speed of these mobile particles is slower than the speed of the cloud of debris moving upward. Therefore some of these particles are pushed onto the corneal surface and settle there. The resulting effect is that at each spot causes a slightly reduced quantity of tissue to be removed in the center of the treatment zone as opposed to the periphery. When comparing the picture of the cornea that has been impacted by the laser beam in a multizone treatment with a picture taken during treatment with PlanoScan, the cloud of debris in the second picture is much more subtle and concentrated. With PlanoScan, no under-pressure zones are created and there is no build-up of ejection material in the central treatment zone because all the particles can fly away and are not pushed down toward the cornea. The resulting ablated surface is much smoother.

Bausch & Lomb 217C offers three methods of performing PTK:
- Manual: the laser beam is controlled using a joystick to direct the 2.0 mm fixed spot.
- Computerized: the computer controls the spot; two parameters are entered in the computer, namely the diameter and depth of the layer to be ablated. Both parameters can be programmed and the procedure can be repeated several times.
- The active eye-tracking system can also be used.

The following is a summary of the most important benefits offered by PlanoScan:
- Low energy required
- Extreme versatility of ablation patterns (topolink)
- Reduced importance of beam homogeneity
- Absence of central islands
- Smooth treatment surfaces
- Little wear on optics
- Unlimited optic zones
- Reduced acoustic shock
- Reduced onset of haze
- Reduced trauma and corneal edema.

It is obvious that PlanoScan provides more precise and predictable ablations than possible with multizone treatment, with the capability to correct myopia, hyperopia, and astigmatism (Figures 11-25 through 11-28).

Laser 217C Fluence Test

Fluence represents the quantity of energy a laser beam has when leaving the cavity. In the Bausch & Lomb laser, is 130 mJ/cm^2.

Since alterations in fluence influence the cut rate in a directly proportional way (ablation rate), it is obvious that poor fluence of the laser beam can result in poor

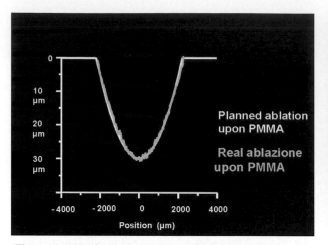

Figure 11-26. Central ablation with the PlanoScan.

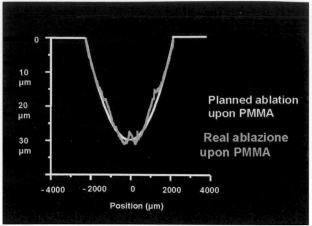

Figure 11-27. Multizone strategy of central ablation.

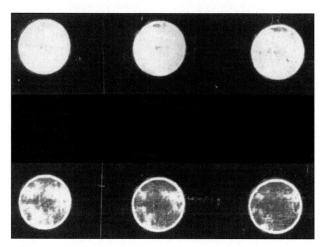

Figure 11-28. A sample ablation pattern in a fluence test.

photoablation. Moreover, when considering the origin of a laser beam and the modality with which it is delivered on the tissue, the causes underlying poor fluence are easy to detect.

With the Bausch & Lomb laser, the fluence test is performed on polymethylmethacrylate (PMMA) plate on which a subtle silver-plated foil is placed with the interposition of a layer of glue. The fluence test is performed after choosing this option in the software and after adjusting the laser beam outgoing energy. The plate is put under the microscope and the laser beam is aligned and focused on it. After enabling the fluence test by pressing "s," the footpedal delivers the 2.0 mm laser pulses on the fluence plate. The number of shots is displayed on the monitor, with a starting frequency of 50 Hz for the first shots and then with an automatic frequency of 4 Hz. The operator observes the silver-plated foil for the following events:

1. How many spots were necessary to detect red color on the PMMA?

The total number of spots necessary to obtain a complete exposure of the PMMA foil must equal 65 ± 2; this means that 63 or 67 spots can be accepted. This test is performed to make sure that the laser beam has good energy and a good cut rate.

If a number higher than 67 is necessary to expose a PMMA circle, the energy is too low and the cut rate is not sufficient; fluence must be increased by rotating one or both of the attenuators to have little or no action of the laser beam. The test is then repeated to check if values have come back within an acceptable range.

If a number of spots lower than 65 are necessary to expose a PMMA circle, this means that both energy and cut rate are too high. Fluence must be reduced rotating one or both of the attenuators to increase their action on the laser beam. The test is then repeated to check if values have come back within an acceptable range.

2. How were the superficial layers removed (foil and glue)?

Apart from monitoring the quantity of released energy conveyed by the laser beam, the fluence test allows evaluation of its homogeneity. It is very interesting to observe and understand not only how many spots but also how evenly the ablation of the superficial layers of the plate progressed.

A satisfactory homogeneity of the 2.0 mm spot ensures that the same quantity of energy is delivered on all the points of its surface. In normal conditions, there is a color change from white (the glue layer colour) and red (PMMA color) in an interval of five to six spots. A very fine and dispersed white granularity can remain; its removal with a further spot can lead to a useless energy overload.

Note: The manufacturing company considers as acceptable number of spots ranging from 63 and 67 to ensure good fluence. The white/red color change can take place in an interval of five to six spots. With a cut rate of 0.25 microns, five to six spots means an ablation of 1.25 to 1.5 microns. To correct a diopter of myopia with a 5.5-mm optical zone tissue ablation must equal 20 microns. These peculiarities should cause us to reflect on the reliability of the instrument and the extreme attention and care that must be paid when preparing and calibrating the instrument.

The edge of the red circle is a white line (the glue layer), which should be subtle and display the same characteristics 360°. It must be noted, however, that with the Bausch & Lomb 217C laser the contour of the red circle is polygonal instead of circular, as in previous models. Sometimes a noncircular test is obtained (ie, with thicker white edges). The reason for this may lay in a slight shift of the plate while the fluence test is being performed, especially if such an anomaly appears suddenly. Another possibility is bad alignment of the optics.

Any anomaly in the fluence test result causes us to seek its cause and reflect on its possible effects on treatments. All treatments should be delayed until proper fluence can be demonstrated. Anomalies in the fluence test include:

1. A red circle is obtained with the number of spots higher than 67. The energy is too low; increase energy by using the right "shift" key on the keyboard and repeat the fluence test. It the problem persists but the number of spots is lower, try to increase energy again and repeat the fluence test.

If the problem still persists, try with maximum energy (100%) and repeat the fluence test; now, if the number of spots necessary to expose the red circle falls within the expected range, treatment can be performed but the laser should be closely monitored as it is not functioning optimally. Our experience taught us to perform a gas refill when even after increasing energy, we do not achieve a considerable reduction in the number of spots to obtain ablation. After performing a gas refill, we advise the delivery of approximately 1000 pulses with energy at 100%. This maneuver allows rotation of the attenuators on the laser beam path by 90°, avoiding contamination during these pulses.

The energy is thus reduced to its minimum (the laser cavity is now full of new gas, namely with a high concentration of argon fluoride molecules available for photochemical reaction underlying the creation of the laser beam) and the fluence test is repeated.

If an excessive number of spots are still requested, the low gas quantity currently available in the cavity is

not the problem. The problem is elsewhere.

First, microclimatic conditions should be checked; high humidity, in particular (sometimes created by the presence of too many people in the laser room), can induce a sudden loss of fluence and homogeneity in the outgoing laser beam. The solution is to leave the laser room and allow the air conditioner and dehumidifier to bring environmental conditions back to normal.

The use of alcohol for epithelial removal or the presence of vaporous substances (perfumes, aftershave lotions) in the environment can have a similar effect.

Second, the quality of the gas mixture in the bottle should be checked; such a hypothesis should be tested when, after ruling out all other possibilities and after replacing the gas bottle, bad fluence is still obtained. Low repeatability of values in the following tests and discouraging results in the treatments performed.

Third, the attenuator should be checked. A fluence test should be made at this point with maximum energy (attenuators excluded) and with the attenuator at its minimum (attenuators placed orthogonally with respect to the laser beam). In ideal conditions, the "window" (ie, the difference in the number of spots necessary to expose a red circle) equals 10 spots. If this window is reduced, the attenuators are probably dirty and must be temporarily excluded or eliminated.

Lastly, if after a gas refill and ruling out the possibility of an unsuitable microclimate and eliminating an attenuator the fluence is still low, the problem may lie in the optics along the path. Simply put, the optics might be dirty, If this is the case, it will be enough to clean them properly and calibrate the instrument again. Another possibility is that one or more lenses or some mirrors along the optical path on the laser beam are deteriorated; replace them to obtain a beam with perfect homogeneity and fluence characteristics.

2. If a red circle is obtained with a number of spots higher than 67, the energy is too low. Increase it using the right "shift" key on the keyboard, then repeat the fluence test.

3. If a red circle is obtained with a number of spots lower than 62, the energy is too high. Reduce the energy using the left "shift" key on the keyboard, then repeat the fluence test.

4. If the ablation is not uniform within a 2.0-mm spot used to evaluate fluence, check the cause. Ablation defects usually appear as light-colored areas; the color of the glue layer is irregularly removed over the red PMMA plate. The following is a list of things that could occur if treatment is performed when fluence is not homogeneous.

Diffuse irregularities: These usually refer to an

uneven ablation that does not disappear after a few spots but remains for longer than 5 or 6 spots. These irregularities can be caused by the build-up of moisture, dust, or fingerprints on the silver-plated foil of the fluence plates. That is why plates should always be kept in specialized containers when they are not in use.

Localized defects: Small areas of absent ablation that stand out in the context of neighboring ablated zones. They usually appear suddenly, namely in between tests. They are normally blamed on the presence of a build-up on one of the two wobbling mirrors (X or Y) on the last segment of the optical path. They have a typical aspect and are due to a drop of liquid splashed on the mirror during treatment. To eliminate this unablated island, several spots must be emitted, usually more than five or six. This leads to unacceptable fluence values or to an over-correction. The only way to definitely solve the problem is to thoroughly check the wobbling mirrors, and remaining optics if necessary, to rule out the possibility of build-up or spots, then clean them. A localized defect can also be caused by the presence of debris on the silver-plated foil of the fluence plate.

Central defects: The term *central defect* refers to an ablation that is less powerful in the central area of the trial spot. In other words, the laser beam with a diameter of 2.0 mm is endowed with a higher energy at the periphery as against the center. This may be observed for two important reasons: first, the optics are dirty due to humidity, dust, or residuals in the central area. Second, the central area of the optics more subject to wear than the periphery. In the first case, an adequate cleaning will re-establish a correct fluence; in the latter case, the optics must be replaced. This occurs after 2000 to 2500 treatments. These conditions should be corrected as soon as possible because when considering how photoablation is performed by PlanoScan software, the results can be unpredictable.

Semilunar defects: Sometimes an incomplete ablation of the 2.0 mm spot used for the fluence test can be observed. Such a defect is shaped like a crescent moon and can enlarge to occupy almost half the spot diameter. It can be present either in the right or left half, as well as in the lower or upper half. In this case, the laser beam does not have good homogeneity because it is not properly aligned (Figure 11-29).

Treatment of Myopia, Hyperopia, and Astigmatism

The Bausch & Lomb 217C laser allows the following treatments to be performed:
- Myopia
- Hyperopia

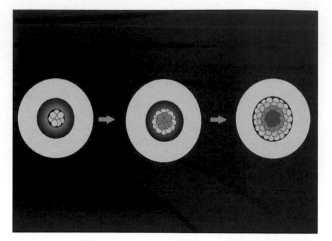

Figure 11-29. Correction of myopia with the PlanoScan.

- Myopic astigmatism
- Hyperopic astigmatism

Before starting any treatment, the laser technician must check the environmental conditions in the laser room. The laser should be switched on at least 30 minutes before use and should be tested through the fluence test; a gas refill should be done if necessary. The surgeon enters the laser room with all the patient's data that must be entered into the laser, including:
- First and last name
- Date of birth
- Desired refractive correction
- Optic zone
- Pachymetry (this data is used as an evaluation parameter)

Treatment of Myopia

After entering data, the software gives information about the ablation. The surgeon can then evaluate if refractive parameters and the optic zone should be modified depending on a patient's pachymetry.

The optic zone in the correction of myopia can reach 7.0 mm. This means transition will reach 11.5 mm because the transition zone with the new PlanoScan 2000 software is always 3.0 mm, regardless of whether the PRK or LASIK program is selected. Let us hope that in the future, different software programs for PRK and LASIK will be available because in LASIK, smaller transition zones can be used, as was the case in the 2.999 PL software.

It is worth remembering, however, that the ablation program limits the number of pulses to 4500 which, in practice, makes extremely large optic zones in cases of severe myopia impossible, even with adequate corneal thickness. The ablation profile on axes 90 and 180 can be

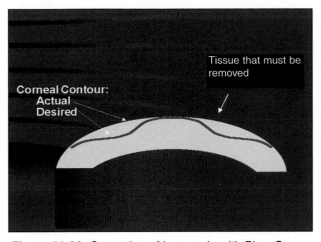

Figure 11-30. Correction of hyperopia with PlanoScan.

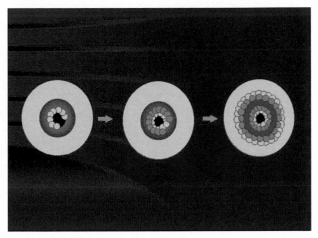

Figure 11-31. Correction of hyperopia with PlanoScan.

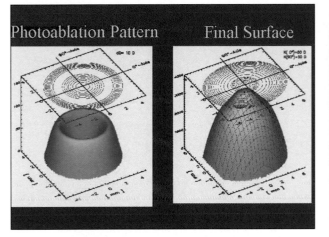

Figure 11-32. Treatment of hyperopia with PlanoScan.

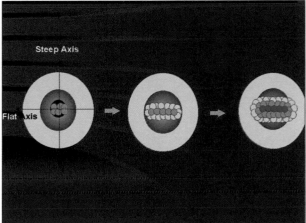

Figure 11-33. Myopic astigmatic correction with PlanoScan. The laser moves over the cornea and flattens the steepest axis.

displayed on the computer screen. The treatment is composed of four to eight phases. The eye-tracker system assists the surgeon in flawlessly centering the ablation throughout the treatment, even with extreme eye movement (Figure 11-30).

Treatment of Hyperopia

The procedure is the same as for myopia, with the recommendation that the optic zone is larger than 5.5 mm. Six millimeters is better (that is the maximum optical zone that can be used).

Hyperopia up to 10 D can be corrected (it is advisable not to exceed more than 6 D); the treatment is longer with respect to myopia, as well as the number of necessary spots. In cases of such long treatment times, an eye tracker is indispensable. The treatment is divided in four to eight phases depending on the severity of the refractive error.

Central zone blending is obtained by making an annular photoablation joined together with the adjacent

cornea according to a gentler gradient toward the optical zone, more inclined toward the periphery of the cornea, with a 3.0-mm transition zone (Figures 11-31 and 11-32).

Treatment of Myopic Astigmatism

Treatment takes place on the axis of the refractive defect. The maximum area of treatment is 5.0 x 8.5 mm. The maximum optical zone is 6.5 mm (Figures 11-33 and 11-34).

Treatment of Hyperopic Astigmatism

Treatment takes place on the sides of the axis of astigmatism. The maximum optical zone is 6.0 mm (Figures 11-35 and 11-36).

Therapeutic Treatment

It is possible to choose between a surgeon-controlled treatment and a computer-controlled treatment. In the

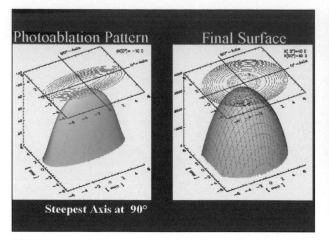

Figure 11-34. Treatment of myopic astigmatism with PlanoScan.

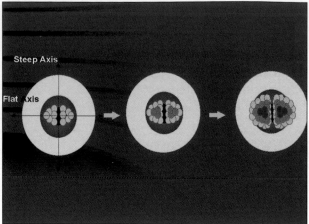

Figure 11-35. Hyperoctic astigmatism correction with PlanoScan. The laser moves over the cornea and steepens the flat axis.

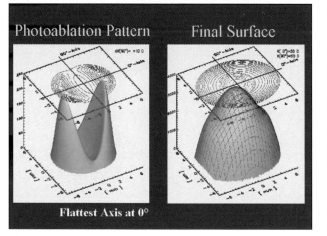

Figure 11-36. Treatment of hyperoctic astigmatism with PlanoScan.

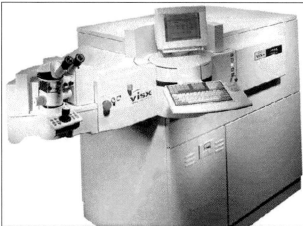

Figure 11-37. The VISX Star SmoothScan S2 excimer laser system.

former, a beam 2.0 mm in diameter is used; the beam can be conveyed on the point to be treated using the joystick. In the latter, the software allows programming of the diameter of the area to be ablated as well as the ablation depth. A special software option allows the surgeon to repeat the treatment and overlap the previous one without the need to re-enter patient data.

Conclusion

Thanks to features such as the flying spot PlanoScan ablation system, active and passive eye tracker and topolink, this laser presently represents one of the best technological choices available on the excimer laser market.

VISX STAR S2: TECHNICAL DESCRIPTION

Introduction

VISX Incorporated (Santa Clara, Calif, USA), was founded in 1986 and is a pioneering company in the field of laser refractive surgery. A VISX laser was the first used in surface ablation of a human eye (1986). In 1989, commercial distribution of the VISX 20/20 laser system began. In 1995, after 6 years of trials, this was the first laser approved for PTK by the US Food and Drug Administration (FDA). FDA approval for correction of myopia was granted in 1996. During that same year, the new VISX Star system was introduced. The new system is more compact, flexible, and more cost-effective than its predecessor. Star SmoothScan S2, the latest software version, allows for the correction of myopia and hyperopia with both mixed and compound astigmatism. VISX has approximately 500 systems installed in 40 countries, and has treated almost 1 million eyes.

The VISX Star S2 is a broadbeam laser, but differs from other broadbeam systems in two ways:

- The laser does not deliver one pulse at a time, but rather a combination of seven pulses that smooth the corneal during ablation. This technology, called SmoothScan, allows the cornea to be as smooth after ablation as it was before, favoring epithelial regrowth following PRK and adhesion of the lamellar flap in LASIK procedures.
- The VISX Star S2 differs from other broadbeam lasers in that the beam (or seven beams) can perform a scanning motion like a flying spot laser. This mixed technique allows for hyperopic and astigmatic defects to be easily treated.

Irregular corneas can be treated with the aid of a calculation algorithm called contour ablation pattern (CAP) method, which will be discussed in detail later in this chapter. The capability of scanning makes the Star S2 similar in flexibility to a flying spot laser, and the use of a beam with variable shape and dimensions instead of being fixed reduces the possibility of obtaining a mosaic effect. The overall shape of the ablated surface is obtained, even with a scanning beam, through an overlapping (either partial or complete) of ablated layers instead of an approach of using small ablations (as with the flying spot), which can never be perfect.

Cavity and Gas Reservoir

The Star S2 beam has a fluence at the corneal plane of 160 mJ/cm^2, ablating tissue at 0.25 microns per pulse. This fluence level is used because it corresponds to the value absorbed by the cornea in the most efficient and regular way. The laser software checks and modifies the various operation parameters to maintain constant fluence. The excimer laser produces a laser beam by pressurizing gas in a cavity and crossing it with a high voltage electrical discharge (25 to 30 kV). The higher the voltage, the higher the energy contained in the laser pulse. The gas comes from two bottles housed within the system: one contains a premixed combination of argon, fluoride, neon, and helium (premixed), the other contains ultra-high purity helium. Only those contained in the premix take part in the laser action. The helium contained in the second bottle is basically an inert gas used

as a buffer to keep the mixture in the laser cavity at a correct pressure—2600 mbar. An increased concentration of premix produces with equal voltage an increased energy level, whereas an increased helium concentration that dilutes the premix provokes a lower energy level. The software starts by adjusting the premix/helium levels contained in the cavity to generate the correct fluence at a voltage of 25 kV. When the laser is used, the premix slowly becomes contaminated, reducing its efficacy. If voltage is kept constant, the fluence and amount of tissue removed would gradually diminish, affecting the accuracy of treatment. The automatic control system increases the discharge voltage so as to maintain fluence at the correct level. When the required voltage reaches 30 kV, part of the contaminated gas must be replaced by a new mixture. This occurs, on average, every 10 to 20 treatments. The laser software warns that a partial gas change is necessary, calculates the exact amount to replace and delivers the "boost." The gas in the cavity is now more efficient and the discharge voltage returns to 25 kV. Many devices were added to Star to reduce gas consumption. Among them, the development of smart software that keeps the laser's history in memory, constantly adapting to the slow changes in operation caused by wear on the optics, ensuring a constantly efficient and optimized use of gas. Other devices that increase the life of the gas mixture include a recirculation system equipped with a gas purifying filter, a small cavity to reduce the quantity of gas necessary for a fill, and ceramic materials that minimally contribute to gas contamination. The overall consumption of gas depends on the number of eyes treated; if an average of 100 procedures are performed monthly, one could expect the gas bottles to have a lifespan of between 3 and 6 months. The optics of the laser are subject to wear and will need replacement after 1.5 to 3 years of use.

Optical Pathway

The excimer laser beam is created in the laser cavity and travels through an optical system that shapes and homogenizes the beam before being delivered to the patient's cornea. The beam treatment system is located in a module extending from the laser housing and acting as a support for the surgeon's console. It contains three mirrors, four lenses and other equipment necessary for shaping and sizing the laser beam. This entire module is equipped with an air purification system that functions even when the laser is off, maintaining a clean environment for the optics.

The beam is rectangular when it leaves the cavity. The first component of the beam treatment system, the integrator, homogenizes the beam, shapes it symmetrically, and divides it into seven beams. The beam-shaping component then further shapes the beam. A low-aberration lens recombines the seven beams and enables them to scan. Movement of the superimposed beams is synchronized and adjusted to obtain an extremely regular and gradual profile of the ablated surface. The seven beams, acting in concert, create an extremely smooth and precise profile (SmoothScan technology).

Computer

The optical system, its mechanical movements, and other control systems are operated directly by a computer. The laser is controlled by a second dedicated microprocessor. The surgeon's console is positioned over the surgical field and includes the microscope, video camera, positioning controls for the patient's chair, and lighting controls. Data is entered through a workstation equipped with a keyboard and monitor.

All functions in the beam treatment system are directly controlled by computer. It constantly communicates with the laser management processor, which relays operational data. It does not merely send commands to different components but constantly monitors their actions. This aspect is a part of a general philosophy on which the system was conceived; the computer, connected through a complex network of sensors to all components, can check in real time the operational state of the entire laser system.

Calibration

The user interface operates in Windows format, and provides a series of automatic procedures. The lens calibration procedure allows verification of the dioptric power generated by an ablation through a treatment simulation delivered onto a plastic card (-4 D sphere, -4 D cylinder, 0 D sphere [PTK], and +2 D sphere). SmoothScan technology performs excellent ablations on the plastic, allowing precise reading of the dioptric power generated by the ablation and fine adjustments in energy level to ensure an extremely accurate system calibration. A second automatic calibration procedure (patient energy calibration) checks the energy density and laser voltage before each treatment. If the necessary voltage exceeds the maximum allowed value, the software delivers a gas boost, then automatically repeats the calibration procedure. This procedure is extremely sophisticated because it gradually adapts itself to changes in laser operation. This makes maintenance much simpler and guarantees that the gas is used efficiently. The workstation monitor displays both the computer messages and a view of the surgical field as the surgeon sees it. During this procedure, the technician can both assist the surgeon and monitor treatment. The system provides two BNC outlets so the surgeon's view can be displayed on a monitor outside the laser suite.

Work Area

The surgeon's console, described above, is included in the work station. Here, the position of the patient is adjusted through the aid of a joystick that moves the chair along the X and Y axis and by rotation of a ring at the base of the joystick for focusing. The microscope (Lcica MS 5) has five magnification levels, allowing adjustment during various phases of the procedure according to the surgeon's personal preferences. The lamps illuminate the cornea from an oblique position, enabling an accurate view of corneal surface conditions. Beneath the microscope, a tube aspirates material ablated by the laser beam and a metallic arm supports the plastic cards during calibration. The aspiration tube can be easily shifted out of the way before and after delivery of the laser ablation. A sensor requires it to be repositioned before allowing the laser to be used. Laser delivery is controlled by a two-position footpedal: initial pressure on the pedal activates aspiration with firmer downward pressure delivering the laser.

Eye Tracker

The Star S2 does not employ eye-tracker technology. Some feel this is an obvious drawback because it increases the risk of decentered ablations. However, some feel that in broadbeam lasers eye tracking is not critical.

Topography-Guided Treatment

Introduction of the CAP method enables the laser to use information gathered from topography devices.

Focusing

Because the annular lamp is positioned near the laser down tube and produces an image of the cornea, focusing is simple. Centering is accomplished by positioning an image projected through the microscope's optics. This allows a view of the image on the cornea at any magnification.

Treatment Strategies

The software allows the following options:
- Laser removal of epithelium (transepithelial)
- Therapeutic treatment (PTK)
- Refractive treatment (PRK)
- Customized corrective treatment and for irregular CAP method)

	Table 11-3		
CAP METHOD SPECIFICATIONS			
CAP method ablation type	**Maximum**	**Minimum**	**Parameters**
Myopic surfaces			
Sphere	0 D	-30 D	
Diameter	1.2 mm	6.5 mm	
Cylinder	0 D	-15 D	
Length	4.0 mm	6.5 mm	
Width	3.0 mm	6.5 mm	
Transition zone	0.2 mm	0.6 mm	
Ellipse	0 D	-30 D (sphere)	
		-15.0 D (cylinder)	
Major axis	2.5 mm	6.5 mm	
Hyperopic surfaces			
Sphere	0 D	+6 D	
Cylinder	0 D	+4 D	
Outer diameter	6.0 mm	9.0 mm	
Inner diameter	3.0 mm	6.0 mm	
Transition zone (outer-inner)	3.0 mm	4.5 mm	
Therapeutic surfaces			
PTK slit	Length/width	0.6 mm	6.0 mm
PTK circle diameter	2.0 mm	6.0 mm	
Transition zone	0 mm	2.7 mm	

Laser Removal of Epithelium

This option is only available for myopic corrections. Because the epithelium does not have a constant thickness the number of microns to remove is programmable.

Refractive Treatments

Based on a multizone correction algorithm using a combination of spherical, cylindrical, and elliptical ablations, correction of myopia, astigmatism, hyperopia, and both mixed and compound hyperopic astigmatism are programmable (sphere from -30 D to +10 D and cylinder from -15 to +10 D).

Therapeutic Treatment

This treatment allows smoothing of the stromal surface. The extreme smoothness of the surface renders therapeutic treatment advisable only in certain cases (haze, stromal irregularities).

Personalized Corrective Treatment and the CAP Method

According to information provided by the company, this technology should allow planning of personalized multizone treatment strategies that can use spherical, cylindrical, and elliptical zones for a range similar to the standard refractive treatments. This method should provide choices with respect to power, diameter and shape of zones to be entered, adapting to any treatment strategy—from the simplest to the most complex. Moreover, irregular corneal defects may be treated. For this option, the algorithm determines the optimal treatment through the use of support software that analyzes data obtained from corneal maps. The algorithm in which the CAP method is based works as follows: starting with preoperative topography, the VISX algorithm calculates the optimal treatment and communicates this data to the topographer, which then simulates the laser treatment and displays to the surgeon the post-treatment corneal profile. The aim of the program is to completely automate the process in which the software provides an ideal treatment plan to produce a more regular and optically efficient postoperative corneal surface while leaving the surgeon the ability to program a different treatment than that proposed by the automatic system (Tables 11-3 and 11-4).

Conclusion

This machine is excellent in both control of energy and in the optical path; its latest models have introduced some innovations (CAP method). However, the lack of eye tracking still represents a limit.

NIDEK EC 5000 MODEL 2B: TECHNICAL CHARACTERISTICS

Introduction

The Nidek EC-5000 excimer laser allows the performance of photoablation treatments to correct myopia, astigmatism, hyperopia, and therapeutic photoablation. This machine has been on the market for about 6 years and is manufactured in Japan.

Cavity

The laser head is made of ceramic; this saves gas through a reduced number of gas changes. The laser's high frequency output performs quick treatments, which translates into greater patient cooperation and a reduced dehydration of corneal tissue.

Gas Reservoir

Two bottles are lodged within the laser, one charged with helium argon and neon, the other with halogen gas. A third bottle containing nitrogen is locate outside the laser. The gaseous mixture is made of fluoride argon, which can produce a beam with a 193 nm wavelength and repetition frequency up to 50 Hz; fluence accounts for 120/130 mJ/cm², with a pulse duration of 176 ns.

Optical Pathway

Once the laser beam leaves the cavity, it goes through an energy measurer and continues its journey across a series of 10 optics and mirrors until it reaches the corneal surface.

Ablation Modality

Corneal photoablation occurs by delivering a scansion beam on the cornea. Such a slit goes through the cornea on different meridians of the zone to be treated. The advantage is two-fold: it reduces tissue warming and obtains smoother and more homogeneous surfaces. Moreover, the slit diameter 9.0 mm, so the refractive and therapeutic treatments can cover a wide corneal surface.

Computer

The computer is easy to access and makes data entry simple and quick. It is positioned to the right of the surgeon. Its ablation software is particularly simple and flexible.

Work Area

The work space and focusing controls and movement of the X-Y axes are rationally and comfortably located. To ensure the surgeon's maximum comfort, the operating microscope is controlled by a special pedal. The working area is sufficiently wide to allow for use of a microkeratome.

Focusing

The focusing and alignment system recognizes a patient's correct position, not only on the X and Y axes, but also on the Z axis. Correct focusing and a precise

Table 11-4

TECHNICAL CHARACTERISTICS OF VISX STAR S2 LASER

Cut rate	0.25 microns
Cavity	Ceramic
Gas	ArF
Ablation system	Broadbeam
Optical zone	See CAP method specifications
Wavelength	193 nm
Fluence	160 mJ/cm²
Duration of pulse	15 to 20 ns
Frequency of repetition	10 Hz
Fixation	Variable, set by user
Eye tracker	No
Cooling	Internal: air and liquid nitrogen
Precalibration	Internal and on PMMA lenticles examined by a lenticle
Power supply	220 VAC stabilized single phase. 30A breakaway starting current 15A steady
Control voltage	25 to 30 kV
Dimensions	Width: 110 cm Length: 204 cm Height: 150 cm
Weight	726 kg
Room dimensions	At least 20 m² with the shortest side measuring at least 3 m

alignment are obtained when the two semicircles meet with their convexity, are symmetrically placed on the treatment area, and are crossed by the horizontal mire. This ensures that the treatment is correctly focused, centered, and aligned. An advantage is the ability of the operator to detect and correct a patient's head if its movement becomes incorrect during treatment.

Eye Tracker

The system is equipped with a good active and passive eye tracker with a frequency of 40 Hz. The realignment speed accounts for 6.0 mm/second and acts on a 5.0 mm range with an accuracy of 50 microns; reliability is good even when severe refractive errors are treated. Moreover, realignment and focusing procedures can be performed even during treatment; the telecamera shooting the image of the eye is coaxial with respect to the microscope, rather than lateral, as is the case in other systems. This avoids possible mistakes by the eye tracker when a patient moves, allowing the beam to remain perpendicular in spite of movements by the microscope.

TECHNICAL CHARACTERISTICS OF THE NIDEK EC 5000	
Cut rate	0.25 microns
Ablation system	Slit scanning (broadbeam)
Cavity	Ceramic
Gas	ArF
Maximum ablation diameter	9.0 mm
Wavelength	193 nm
Frequency	50 Hz
Duration of pulse	17 msec
Fluence	108 to 120 mJ
Eye tracker	Passive/active
Accuracy	50 micron
Range	5.0 mm
Frequency	50 Hz
Topolink	No
Microscope	Zeiss
Required power supply	220V, 50/60 Hz, 3.3 VA max
Dimensions:	
Length	0.750 m
Width	1.370 m
Height	1.516 m
Weight	650 kg
Overall dimensions	2.0 m x 2.8 m

Table 11-5

Topolink

This laser is not yet equipped with topolink.

Calibration Test

Calibration is made by PMMA plates, with immediate fluence and homogeneity tests. A 3 D photoablation is performed on a PMMA plate before the surgical treatment. The result of photoablation is then measured through a frontifocimeter and entered into the computer. To calculate the number and diameter of steps made by the diaphragm during treatment, the EC-2000 software uses the cornea/PMMA rate calculated through the laser's main nomograph, which has a value ranging from 2400 and 1765. A lower value indicates a higher correction. When the operator knows these parameters, he or she can modify the global correction of myopia and compound myopic astigmatism in a proportional way.

Treatments

Myopia and Myopic Astigmatism

Correction of myopia occurs through consecutive ablations along different corneal meridians; correction of myopic astigmatism is made by repeating ablation on the meridian of astigmatism; another method to correct astigmatism is to treat half cylinder on the flatter merid-

ian, the remaining half on the steeper, and treat the sphero-equivalent, so as to obtain a more homogeneous transition toward the nonablated corneal surface and a reduced possibility of regression.

Hyperopia and Hyperopic Astigmatism

Photoablation with revolving ablation treats hyperopia and hyperopic astigmatism. In cases of hyperopic treatment, ablation is always made with ablation on different meridians, but a ablation run is restricted to the cornea's peripheral ring, thus determining a peripheral annular ablation giving rise to a curvature of the central cornea. In cases of hyperopic astigmatism, the treatment takes place in the peripheral segment of the meridians to be treated.

In the latest model, hyperopic treatment can obtain optical zones with aspherical profile because of to the particular inclination of the peripheral incision and transition (the angle outlined by the two walls of the incision is more acute than before and the profile of the transition zone is linear).

Therapeutic Treatments

The possibility of having a 9.0 mm diameter ablation makes performing therapeutic treatments with the aid of a special masking fluid possible while obtaining excellent results in terms of quality of stromal surface (Table 11-5).

Conclusions

This machine has good reliability characteristics; and refractive and therapeutic results are excellent. On the other hand, treatment of hyperopia is a challenge for this machine as well as photoablation performed with topolink.

THE LSX LASERSIGHT EXCIMER LASER

Introduction

The LSX is a state-of-the-art compact instrument that came on the market recently. It is characterized by homogeneity of treatment and a reduced quantity of energy released for each emitted spot. Because of a sophisticated software program, it can correct myopia, astigmatism, hyperopia, as well as perform therapeutic treatments with PRK and LASIK procedures.

LSX employs a spot with variable diameter from 0.8 to 1.0 mm, using an ablation technique called flying spot. This type of ablation covers the entire treatment area 360°C, following software-guided movements depending on the type of treatment chosen, with treated zones of up to 9.0 mm in diameter. The laser has an extremely stable powered chair, with control of macrometric and micrometric movements along the X, Y, and Z axes. Software includes an autocalibration procedure, therapeutic treatments, myopia, hyperopia, astigmatism, combined treatments, LASIK treatments, and an autodiagnosis procedure (Figure 11-38).

Cavity

This instrument is equipped with a ceramic cavity designed to employ a working frequency of 200 Hz. This working principle, created to the reduced quantity of energy released per spot (0.7 to 1.2 mJ), enables the operator to use a 0.8 mm microspot with a very reduced overall intervention time or choose a 0.4 mm spot with a standard global intervention time. This extreme versatility provides a perfect combination of technological innovation to suit the operator's needs. Moreover, the synergy provided by microspot, low energy, and high treatment frequency ensures a good degree of accuracy, with perfectly smooth surfaces from the homogeneity with which energy is distributed. The use of extremely reduced energy eliminates the acoustic shock phenomenon and keeps the cornea temperature within clinically insignificant levels (2°C), even for severe corrections (up to 15 D and more). The high frequency (5 to 10 times higher than normal systems depending on the system's setting) allows for shorter operation time, such as those performed with traditional systems. Sometimes ablation times are even halved.

Gas Reservoir

The machine houses two gas bottles (ArF and He). The extremely low content of fluoride (equal to 0.19%) does not require special gas evacuation equipment. The ArF bottle has about 100 refills. Each cavity refill can perform about 40 treatments (including calibration and setting procedures). Therefore, the total possible number of operations that can be performed with two ArF and He bottles is approximately 4000.

Optical Pathway

The beam coming out of the cavity is rectangular and initially goes through an attenuator. A part of the beam is "grasped" by a beam splitter and its energy is tested; a control system regulates the attenuator inclination so that the actual energy on the corneal tissue corresponds to what was established by the fluence test. A focal lens conveys the laser beam to impact on two galvanometric lenses that are responsible for the correct direction assumed by the laser beam. Eventually a 45°-angled lens conveys the beam on the corneal tissue.

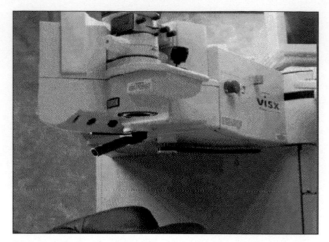

Figure 11-38. The VISX Star S2 working area.

Computer

When performing a surgical operation, the user is completely independent from the technical assistance center. As a matter of fact, the LSX has powerful software that can automatically perform everything from gas refills, to calibration and alignments. Special software called CIPTA (corneal interactive programmed topographic ablation) calculates the topography-linked ablation profile.

Work Area

Because it is compact, the machine allows the surgeon to work in a particularly comfortable environment with the computer control panel directly at hand.

Focusing System

Magnifications through the surgical microscope are 0.63x, 1.6x, 2.5x, and 4.0x. X-Y axis movement, as well as focusing, are made from a console that controls movement of the surgical chair.

Eye Tracker

The device has a fixation system with a reference target for the patient. An optional active eye tracker is also available, with laser beam realignment time accounting for 8.3 milliseconds.

Topolink

The machine is equipped to work with this technology.

Laser Beam Distribution System

The laser beam, with a variable diameter from 0.8 to 1.0 mm, is distributed on the cornea by means of a flying spot scanning technique.

Table 11-6	
TECHNICAL CHARACTERISTICS OF THE LSX LASERSIGHT	
Cut rate	0.25 microns
Ablation system:	Flying spot
Ablation modality	Software-controlled
Spot dimensions:	From 0.8 to 1.0 mm
Cavity	Ceramic
Gas	ArF
Ablation zone	From 1.0 to 9.0 mm, adjustable
Wavelength	Arf 193 nm
Pulse rate	200 Hz
Duration of pulse	10 nanoseconds
Overall fluence:	From 120 to 160 mJ/cm²
Energy per pulse at cavity outlet	From 7 to 10 mJ
Energy per pulse on the cornea	From 0.7 to 1.2 mJ
Repetition rate:	10 milliseconds
Eye tracker	Yes (optional), active
Spot realignment (ET)	8.3 milliseconds
Topolink	Yes
Cooling	Air
Power supply	Requested power: 220 V single-phase
Operation frequency	50/60 Hz
Absorption:	1.1 KVA
Dimensions	
Width	130 cm
Height	119 cm
Depth	64 cm
Weight	140 kg
Chair width	95 cm
Chair length	200 cm

Start-Up and Control Test

To start LSX automatic refill, calibration and alignment procedures must be performed. It takes about 10 minutes to perform these operations. The real length of treatment depends on the type of treatment to be performed. With an average myopia of -6 D with a 6.0 mm optical zone, approximately 30 seconds are necessary.

Treatment of Myopia, Hyperopia, Astigmatism, and Therapeutics

The machine can correct all refractive errors, as well as perform PTK treatments (Table 11-6).

Conclusion

This machine seems promising, at least in theory, given how new it is. We look forward to receiving follow-up data from users in order to make a more thorough evaluation.

MEL 70 G SCAN EXCIMER LASER

Introduction

The Mel 70 G Scan excimer laser is an Esculap Meditec third-generation laser. This machine works quickly and reliably with a spot and gaussan distribution energy beam that is 2.0 mm in diameter.

This method obtains good results in homogeneity of the treated surface. The scanning technology used by Mel 70 reduces the incidence of central islands.

Cavity

The Mel 70 G Scan laser has a ceramic cavity.

Gas Reservoir

The Mel 70 uses argon fluoride. There are two bottles of premixed gas, each with 120 refills, thus ensuring a minimum of 600 overall treatments. Cooling is guaranteed by a closed-circuit water/air inner cooler.

Optical Pathway

A series of mirrors and optics optimizes laser beam homogenization.

Work Area

The available space is suitable to perform LASIK. The hardware is controlled by a Windows 95 program, allowing extreme flexibility and the possibility of further upgrading. Data entry and postoperative control are simplified by an icon program and by use of a data bank within the system. The program is equipped with an inner assistant that guides the laser, proposing the most suitable modes as well as a manual use with nomograms directly developed by the surgeon; therefore, it does not need the support of skilled personnel.

Focusing System

The focusing and centering system is characterized by a double spot obtained from a 63 nm diode laser. The adjustable coaxial light operating microscope has five magnifications (3x, 5x, 8x, 11x, 20x, and 32x).

Eye Tracker

This laser uses an extremely fast and stable active eye tracker. The stable contrast eye-tracking system eliminates stops during treatment. The contrast stability is ensured by a clear surface of the suction ring. This ring also actively eliminates fumes and suppresses saccadic movements. Treatment is automatically interrupted in cases of horizontal and oblique movements falling outside the normal range. There is a ring for PRK and LASIK.

Topolink

This laser is equipped with connection to outer equipment and has an optional software interconnection for a corneal topographer to create bitmapped ablations.

Calibration Test

This test takes place through a fluence calibration and control test based on a two-scansion objective test on a specifically prepared support, tested by the manufacturer.

Ablation Mode

The new Mel 70 G Scan model abandoned the traditional laser beam distribution system on the cornea, typical of old-generation Meditec lasers. The new Mel 70 employs a randomized 2.0 mm diameter spot scanning.

Treatments

The Mel 70 can simultaneously correct myopia and astigmatism in a single treatment up to -12 D (myopia + astigmatism) with PRK, and up to -24 D (myopia + astigmatism) with LASIK. The optical zone can range from 4.0 to 7.0 mm with PRK and from 4.0 to 6.0 mm with LASIK. By using a 4.0-mm optical zone, corrections can be made up to -15 with PRK and -30 with LASIK.

The multizone technique also allows simultaneous correction of hyperopia and astigmatism up to +8 D with PRK (hyperopia + astigmatism), and up to + 15 D with LASIK (hyperopia + astigmatism). Correction of mixed astigmatism is also possible.

In addition, PTK with shaping or spot programs can also be performed. Meditec is also developing a program to correct presbyopia (Table 11-7).

Conclusions

This new machine offers numerous positive aspects, including eye tracking and topolink; nevertheless, this laser still needs additional testing.

SUMMIT APEX PLUS EXCIMER LASER

Introduction

The Summit Apex Plus is a broadbeam laser. Myopic correction is accomplished through adjusting the beam diameter with an expanding iris diaphragm (up to a maximum of 6.5 mm). The Summit Apex Plus is capable of correcting myopic astigmatism, hyperopia, and both compound and mixed hyperopic astigmatism through the use of an erodable laser disc that is inserted into the laser

Table 11-7	
TECHNICAL CHARACTERISTICS OF THE MEL 70 G SCAN	
Ablation system	Spot scansion
Cavity	Ceramic
Wavelength	193 nm
Repetition frequency	Adjustable from 1 to 50 Hz
Spot dimensions	2.0 mm
Duration of pulse	5 ns
Energy per pulse at the laser outlet	1200 mJ
Energy per pulse on the cornea	180 mJ/cm^2
Eye tracker	Active
Topolink	Yes
Cooling	Closed circuit water/air internal cooler
Power supply	Electrical, 230 V
Dimensions:	
Width	200 cm
Height	120 cm
Depth	250 cm
Weight	Laser unit 500 kg

down tube. The Summit Apex Plus does not need to employ eye-tracker technology.

The Summit laser consists of (Figure 11-39):
- Laser cavity and high-voltage power supply
- Hydropneumatic system to feed gas to the cavity
- Optical path and expanding diaphragm (these systems are totally integrated)

Laser cavity, Condenser for Electric Discharge, and Internal Fluence Monitoring System

Energy photons are generated in the laser cavity, which contains a high vacuum (no oxygen) excitable material (ArF gas). This cavity is fitted with an injector (to blend gases) and two electrodes through which the electric charge is produced (charge poles).

Two systems cool the cavity: a closed water cooling circuit that uses an external chiller unit and air circulated by means of an internal fan.

A negative-pressure pump system to ensure emptying and refilling of excitable gas inside the laser cavity. A valve system discharges contaminated gas.

The cavity is fed by a system of high-voltage charge condensers (20,000 to 40,000 V), and a high-efficiency charge transducer. To obtain higher voltages and a quicker discharge circuit, the condensers are placed and charged together through a second condenser, thus obtaining the so-called "pulse charge" from which the term "pulsed laser" stems.

The electric discharge, by exciting unstable dimers,

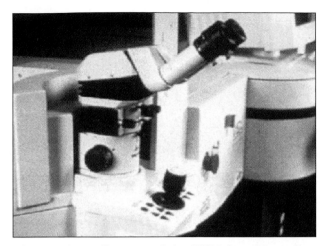

Figure 11-39. Close-up of the VISX Star S2 working area.

pollutes the gas mixture in the laser cavity, progressively degrading it. It becomes less excitable to subsequent electrical solicitations. The condensers must constantly increase voltage of the charge to obtain photon emission from residual excitable gas. In other words, the energy of a laser pulse can be kept constant for a certain period of time because of the balance between progressive degradation of excitable gas and the voltage increase at the electrodes. The gas is replaced in the cavity when voltage reaches its high limit.

The gas contained in the cavity is polluted not only by the repetition of electric discharges, but also by chemical reactions among the materials that make up the laser cavity, and to a lesser extent by molecules altered by the excitable gas and air (O_2-CO_2) present in the cavity. Because of this, Summit is testing new ceramic cavities able to bear energy exceeding 200mJ and high-voltage tension.

Fluence is constantly monitored by devices that measure ultraviolet energy, adjusting the high voltage parameter depending on the half-life of ArF mixture.

Two measuring devices monitor fluence at the cavity outlet at the end of the optical rail.

The first device (power monitor 1) is placed near the cavity outlet and provides information on the total emitted energy with values ranging at around 200 mJ, depending on the state of the excitable gas in the cavity.

The second device (power monitor 2) is placed at the end of the optical path and ensures a constant level of energy, which must be around 180 mJ.

The two systems interact to reduce or compensate all energy losses by the laser beam along the optical path.

Each time the laser is used, the surgeon and/or technician must check that the complex energy control system is providing an exact quantity of energy and it is equally distributed across the entire 6.5 mm surface (beam homogeneity test described later). Fluence and homogeneity testing should be checked periodically during the day when numerous procedures are scheduled.

The variation coefficient of the energy value on a series of 100 spots is expressed in a percentage by the computer software and must always be lower than 5% (it is normally 1% to 3%).

Gas Reservoirs

Gases used:
- Premixed argon gas premixed in a pressurized cylindrical container for 140 refills. It is placed outside the laser in some international lasers but is self-contained in most lasers.
- Fluorine gas in a cylindrical container for 140 refills. It is placed inside the laser in an airtight chamber.
- Nitrogen gas in a pressurized cylindrical container.

Optical Pathway

The laser beam optics and corresponding homogenizing lenses are kept in an airtight environment containing type PA nitrogen (99.998% pure). By releasing air from the optical rail, nitrogen preserves the overwhelming majority of the laser beam energy that would otherwise be attenuated by the presence of air; moreover, it prevents build-up of dust particles on the optics.

Computer

The computer controls are placed on the console on the surgeon's righthand side. Unfortunately, they are out of the surgeon's reach (Figure 11-40).

Working Area

The configuration of the delivery system provides a good working area, as well as plenty of room to perform LASIK.

Alignment System

The Summit laser microscope provides a coaxial view—along the same line of the excimer laser beam. The older lasers are not equipped with uninterrupted magnification through the zoom function, though the most recent lasers now have this feature as well as a standard foot-controlled X-Y movement. Focusing was traditionally accomplished by adjustment of the operating chair.

This laser centration system consists of two He-Ne beams, located at the 3 and 9 o'clock positions, converging to a point at the laser plane. Centration and focus are achieved by positioning the two diverging He-Ne beams on the pupil margins with the beams crossing at the corneal plane.

Chair controls are used to bring the eye as close as possible to the correct position; the patient's head is then repositioned until the He-Ne beams are correctly focused. This method works well.

Direct light on the operative field is provided by a series of circular lights placed around the microscope objective (and main laser axis). An oblique light source mounted on a flexible gooseneck can illuminate the field from various angles. This system can be useful in providing a very different lighting angle and is much more comfortable to the patient than bright direct illumination.

Not only do the two He-Ne beams provide centration, they also offer an absolute point in space on which the eye can be positioned according to the Z axis. As a consequence, eyepieces must be adjusted to be sure that one's own focal point coincides with the point in space at which the beams cross.

Eye Tracker

Despite considerable technological evolution in this field, this laser is not provided with an eye-tracking system. The patient is asked to maintain fixation by looking at a green light located inside an illuminated red circle. During LASIK, some surgeons rely on the suction ring kept in place after cutting at values of around 20 mm Hg to keep the eye still while the laser is working. This is not necessary, and almost all patients are able to maintain excellent fixation.

Topolink

Despite the consistent technological innovation in the field of excimer lasers, this laser is not equipped with topolink. Custom laser discs are being evaluated internationally that allow customized ablation based on topography submitted to Summit—similar to the topolink concept.

Laser Beam Delivery System

This laser employs a beam distribution system called broadbeam, which is much faster than newer lasers using the flying spot technique, though originally associated with central islands before the addition of preventative software.

Summit's beam configuration system allows treatment of myopia alone. The use of ablatable discs are necessary when treating hyperopia as well as myopic, mixed, and compound hyperopic astigmatism.

Fluence and Homogeneity Testing

Confirming the calibration of the laser system is essential to achieving accurate and consistent refractive

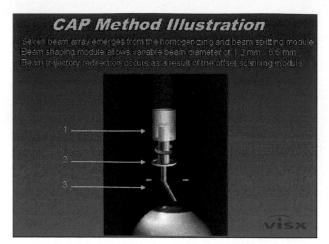

Figure 11-40. The VISX Star S2 cap method.

surgery results. If laser emission energy is too high, the laser will remove more tissue than necessary and overcorrection will result. If emission energy is too low, the laser removes less tissue, resulting in undercorrection.

Beam profile testing is performed on a mylar test card supplied by the manufacturing company. There are two steps: during the first step you should observe a 1.0 mm (black) perforation of the mylar test card between 67 to 71 shots of the laser (the number of pulses necessary to ablate a specific area is a direct measure of a laser beam's ablation power). The second part is performed with the iris diaphragm fully opened to 6.5 mm. One should observe that the first break (black) in the mylar occurs centrally and continues to evenly ablate at least 95% of the 6.5 mm circle within 30 pulses of the first break. Kodak 100-micron photo gelatine paper can be used, but it ablates at a different rate than mylar and cannot be directly substituted (wratten gelatine filter code 96 ND 100).

Ablations performed on PMMA disks are evaluated for uniformity and hot spots. The smoothness and regularity of the ablated plastic surface can be directly observed and demonstrated by the image quality of lensometer mires focused on the ablation.

Laser Start-Up

The laser chiller should be started a few minutes before starting the laser itself. Open the nitrogen and premixed argon gases. Switch the laser on. If the laser has not been used for more than 7 days, use the remaining gas in the cavity to passivate the cavity's walls (300 to 500 shots). Program a gas refill. Perform the beam homogeneity tests, as previously described.

The operator can, when requested by the laser, sends fresh gas into the cavity. This is usually required only on days of heavy use. When the instrument is refilled at start up, the laser chooses one of four energy levels depending on the efficiency of the optics along the rail, which is proportional to their wear (normally, depending on the laser beam homogenization functions they are replaced between 60,000 and 100,000 spots). The laser energy's minimum threshold accounts for 22,000 volts, below which an increased energy level must be forced. When a threshold of 24,000 is reached it is advisable to decrease the energy level because, the laser beam energy must be kept constant for a certain period of time through balance between the progressive degradation of excitable gas and the increase in voltage at the electrodes. When voltage reaches its maximum level, the gas in the cavity is replaced. Two fluoride gas microrefills (boosts) correspond to each energy level. Once the condensers reach 25,000 volt a gas boost is automatically activated to refresh the ArF mixture in the cavity with fresh gas. Consequently, the energy level drops but rises again when the laser is used. Reaching 25,000 volts triggers the use of the second gas boost. Voltage can reach 26,000 volts before a complete gas refill must be performed.

Each time a treatment is performed, the system simulates an autotest of the programmed ablation. Only when the energy level falls within a certain range will the laser allow delivery of the refractive treatment. Finally, when the laser is shut down, an automatic clearing of gas is done, as well as reconditioning of the laser cavity with a small amount of low-pressure fresh ArF gas. The nitrogen and argon premix gas bottles are turned off, followed by the chiller a few minutes later. Never disconnect the chiller from the power supply. Even when the system is off, a sucking filter inside the instrument runs to prevent nitrogen build-up around the laser cavity and to maintain a good environment for the optics.

Myopia, Hyperopia, Astigmatism, and Therapeutic Treatment

With use of the laser alone, mild, moderate, and severe myopia can be treated; to correct astigmatism and hyperopia, ablatable discs are used. By selecting "dose control" on the keyboard, a menu of available treatments is accessible. The refractive ablation can be programmed quite easily by answering the questions on the alphanumeric display. The following treatments are displayed:

- Myopia with or without pretreatment single or aspheric zone
- Myopia with astigmatism with or without pretreatment
- Hyperopia with or without astigmatism
- Phototherapeutic keratectomy

Once the procedure is selected, the "dose set" key displays a further menu of procedures.

Myopia

The refractive ablation is programmed and the laser is armed. Following the test, the laser is ready to deliver the treatment. Reduce the intensity of the operating microscope light, align the diverging red He-Ne beams at the 3 and 9 o'clock pupil margins so they intersect at the center of the cornea. The patient is asked to fix on the green blinking light inside the red circle. The computer controls the laser diaphragm, which in turn controls the distribution of laser energy on the corneal surface. Press the pedal until all shots are delivered.

The following treatments are available:

Aspheric myopic treatment: with this program there are two optic zones. The second is not a transition zone but rather a component of the treatment. The aspheric program is based on Cardano's mathematical formula. This draws a curve largely like that made when a rope is hung by its ends and subject to its own weight. Near the extremes it takes on the terminal shape of a Guassian curve. Therefore, if a transition zone must be detected, the final millimeter or so is surgeon controlled. The first zone can vary from 0.4 mm to 5.0 mm and the second from 6.0 mm to 6.5 mm. The larger program is 5.0 to 6.5 mm and the narrowest is 4.0 to 6.0 mm. With this program, corrections up to 22 D can be entered.

Aspheric myopic treatment with pretreatment: excimer lasers performing photoablation using a broad laser beam with an optic zone larger than 6.0 mm provoke the formation of central islands. The problem has been partly solved by delivering a small number of additional pulses that are without refractive consequence. The pretreatment optic zone and percentage is entered into the laser computer. I have had good results using 8% to 10% of the refractive ablation at an optic zone of 2.5 mm. Then, data is entered for an aspheric myopic ablation. The laser software performs the pretreatment and refractive ablations sequentially in a single treatment. Correction up to 22 D can be performed.

Myopic treatment with multizone program: up to three zones with increasing diameter can be chosen at will, starting from 2.0 mm up to 6.5 mm. The program creates a single curve as it passes through the three zones. The desired ablation percentage must be entered in each of the three zones. One hundred percent is usually entered in the first, 70% in the second, and 30% in the third. This program is rarely used (aspheric treatment is preferred with regular progression of the laser beam diaphragm opening) but is useful for cases of high myopia with low pachymetry because it reduces the amount of tissue removed.

Myopic treatment with a multizone program and pretreatment: the above described multizone treatment can be delivered with central island pretreatment.

Astigmatism

Treatment for astigmatism is accomplished by the using ablatable discs that are placed between the laser beam and the corneal surface. Muller began developing this concept in 1988, followed by R. Maloney and T. Seiler.

Photokeratectomy mediated by the erosion of masks was born by the concept of transferring the characteristics of a processed PMMA lenticle onto the corneal surface. They were mounted on a quartz substrate and transparent to 193 nm. This was originally placed inside a plastic shell resting on the sclera in much the same way as a suction ring. Once the device is in place, a distance of 3.5 mm is kept between the cornea and the quartz plate. A debris vacuum purification system is active. As well as a system to maintain uniform corneal hydration. Ablation is performed with the diaphragm at its maximum opening so that the beam can reach the whole disc's surface, having approximately the same cut rate of the cornea. It is then eroded first in its thinner areas, then in the thicker ones. Removal of corneal tissue mirrors the ablation of the mask starting in the anterior portions of stroma underlying the disc's thinnest zones.

The convex, concave, or toric surfaces of the discs allow ablations with micrometric precision to correct hyperopia, myopia, astigmatism, and potentially any topographic irregularity. By avoiding the "steps" created by the diaphragm's expansion, the surfaces are smoother and more uniform. These peculiarities should then translate into less epithelial stimulation and fibroblastic activation, thus reduced haze.

Problems are basically linked to the difficulty of centering a mask over the visual axis. Very often the astigmatic error is associated secondarily with average and high myopia. In this case, treatment is combined with correction of both components. These discs allow transfer of the three-dimensional geometric profile of the disc onto the cornea. They consist of a simple PMMA small disc. This is ablated by the excimer laser exactly as corneal tissue, but the laser diaphragm here is completely open to 6.5 mm. The small disc is interposed along the laser beam path and the laser energy ablates the small disc, perforating it first in its thinner part, then completely.

Once the laser beam has perforated the disc, it is allowed to reach the corneal surface, creating a negative image of the disc in the corneal stroma. The surface of the ablatable disc can take on any shape and contain either correction of a simple astigmatic defect or a more complex combination of average to high myopia and astigmatism, hyperopia, and both compound and mixed hyperopic astigmatism. Both spherical and astigmatic components can be corrected with one ablation. It is as if the shape of the disc was transferred on the surface of the cornea. This concept opens interesting technological developments, allowing at least in theory the correction of corneal asymmetries; providing discs that are custom produced to correct a particular defect (Figures 11-41 and 11-42).

Myopia with Astigmatism

The following treatment options are available:

Toric treatment: ablatable disk M is used to perform an astigmatic ablation. The ablation performed has an elliptical perimeter, with a diameter of 6.5 x 5.0 mm, although ablations of 6.5 x 6.0 are being investigated internationally. The diameter of the ablation is not adjustable. The laser beam erodes the disk over its entire 6.5 mm diameter—the iris diaphragm in the fully open position. Astigmatic corrections up to 5 D can be performed in conjunction with a myopic component of up to 10 D (we should soon be able to reach 15 D with a single programming). The ablated surface is very smooth—concentric circles typical of those created by the opening of the iris diaphragm are not visible. The principle behind these discs will soon be used to correct simple myopia. The discs are in sphere-cylinder combinations numbered from M01 to M10. The laser selects the appropriate disc during programming. They are single use.

Toric treatment with pretreatment: this allows a myopic toric correction with central island pretreatment.

Hyperopia with Astigmatism

This program uses an ablatable disc to correct both compound and mixed hyperopic astigmatism.

Hyperopia

In hyperopia, correction is obtained by increasing curvature of the central part of the cornea. Correction of hyperopia is done by first using an ablatable disc then the Axicon lens.

This hyperopic disc is thicker centrally and thinner peripherally. The peripheral area is ablated first to allow the laser to ablate corneal tissue first in the periphery and then gradually toward the visual axis. The central zone remains intact for a diameter of about 1.0 mm.

Like the astigmatic ablatable disc, the negative image of the disc's surface topography is duplicated on the corneal surface. The curvature of the cornea is thus steepened. The subsequent insertion of the axicon lens into the laser down tube creates a blend zone from the edge of the 6.5 mm refractive ablation out to 9.5 mm by deviating the beam toward the periphery.

The following program is available:

Simple hyperopia with an axicon lens: this treatment option uses the ablatable L disc followed by the Axicon

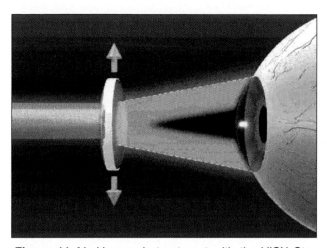

Figure 11-41. Hyperopic treatment with the VISX Star S2.

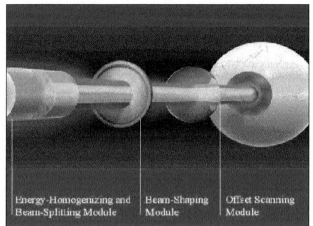

Energy-Homogenizing and Beam-Splitting Module | Beam-Shaping Module | Offset Scanning Module

Figure 11-42. Energy homogenizing and beam-shaping module.

lens to correct from +1.00 D to +6.00 D of spherical hyperopia. Central island pretreatment is unnecessary with hyperopic corrections.

Hyperopia with Astigmatism

This treatment option uses the ablatable P disc that incorporates both hyperopic and astigmatic correction, followed by the Axicon lens to correction up to +6.00 D of hyperopia combined with up to -6.00 D of astigmatism.

Therapeutics

An optic zone diameter from 2.0 mm to 6.5 mm may be selected. The anticipated number of laser pulses necessary is selected up to a maximum of 10,000. For all procedures, once programming is complete, the computer displays the chosen options, including the depth of the programmed ablation. Once the laser is armed, the laser performs an internal test and then indicates that it is ready to deliver the programmed dose. If during the test, energy levels and fluence fall outside acceptable ranges, the laser will not allow delivery of the dose. Once armed, the surgeon has 10 minutes to deliver the programmed treatment before the laser requires retesting and arming. The 3.4.1 software represents the latest version.

Conclusion

The best feature of this machine is undoubtedly energy control. The ablation strategy is no longer considered state-of-the art. All ablation patterns may be performed with the use of both standard and custom discs that allow custom ablations.

MAIN EXCIMER LASER FEATURES

Even if the different excimer lasers on the market today share many characteristics, they differ as far as parameters of the laser beam itself (duration of pulse, repetition frequency, fluence, homogeneity, and number of pulses), as well as some technological characteristics adopted for the cavity, gas reservoir, optical path, computer to enter data, work area, focusing system, and especially the laser beam distribution system (broadbeam, slit, or flying spot technique).

Most important still are some state-of-the-art technologies adopted by some manufacturing companies, such as an eye tracker and topolink.

Bausch & Lomb 217C Excimer Laser

The Bausch & Lomb 217C excimer laser belongs to the latest generation of flying spot lasers equipped with an innovative ablation program called PlanoScan. The extreme versatility of its software allows data entry of relevant to myopic, hyperopic, and astigmatic defects, as well as therapeutic treatment. This machine has a ceramic cavity for enhanced energy stability during treatments. A single bottle containing an ArF gaseous mixture performs 700 to 900 treatments. Once the laser leaves the cavity, it first goes through an homogenizer. It is then joined by a red He-Ne laser (wavelength 635 nm) following the same direction of the excimer laser beam and acting as an aiming beam; this makes visible the path travelled by the 193-nm beam. The two laser beams cross a 2.0-mm diaphragm and first reach the focusing lens, then the wobbling mirrors (X-Y), which deliver the laser spot on the needed corneal area.

The computer is easy to access and use, and is equipped with the control software for the Hansatome microkeratome. This small machine allows can install the microkeratome central unit within the laser frame (bridge) so that the operating field is free of any hindrances.

The focusing system is operated by a simple joystick. The 217C laser has an active and passive eye tracker that has been efficiency and thoroughly tested.

This laser allows the possibility to perform treatments with the topolink option. For this procedure, topographies carried out with a specific instrument supplied by the manufacturing company (orbscan topographer) are used.

In Bausch & Lomb lasers, the fluence test is performed on a PMMA plate on which a subtle silver foil is applied through a layer of glue. The test is performed after activating the software option and adjusting the laser beam output energy. The Bausch & Lomb 217C laser allows correction of myopia, hyperopia, myopic, and hypermetropic astigmatism.

Summit Apex Plus Model B Excimer Laser

The Summit laser employs a laser beam with variable diameter through a mechanical iris—a 6.5 mm broadbeam. In addition to correction of myopia by means of discs that can be ablated, hyperopia and astigmatism can also be corrected.

The laser cavity is metal (Summit is presently testing new ceramic cavities). Two energy measurers control fluence at the laser outlet at the end of the optical rail.

Three gas reservoirs are present (premixed argon gas, fluorine gas, and nitrogen). The laser beam optical path and corresponding homogenizing lenses are kept in an airtight environment containing PA-type nitrogen with a purity degree of 99.998%.

The computer controls are placed opposite the surgeon so he or she cannot possibly reach the computer during a treatment. The work area is satisfactory, as well as the conditions to perform LASIK. X, Y, and Z (focus) control functions are all positioned on a pedal activating the operating chair.

This laser is not equipped with an eye tracker system yet. The patient is asked to maintain fixation using a bright spot as a reference.

This laser employs a broadbeam laser distribution system. Having a broadbeam here makes the use of topolink technology impossible except through the use of custom discs.

The laser beam homogeneity test is performed on a test card supplied by the manufacturing company. The laser beam energy control is excellent.

Only low and average to high myopia can be corrected with the use of this laser alone. To correct astigmatism and hyperopia, ablatable discs are used.

VISX Star S2 Excimer Laser

Founded in 1986, VISX Incorporated was a pioneering company in the field of refractive surgery. It was the first to obtain approval in 1995 by the FDA for PTK. In 1996, this FDA approval was extended to the treatment of myopia.

The Star Smoothscan S2 corrects myopic and hyperopic defects, both mixed and irregular. The VISX Star S2 ablation technique can be said to belong to broadbeam lasers, even though the cornea does not receive one pulse at a time but rather a combination of seven pulses smoothing the cornea during ablation. The beam (or better the bundle of seven beams) can perform "scanning" very much like a flying spot laser. This mixed technique treats hyperopic defects (astigmatic ones too) through a calculation algorithm called the CAP method. The efficiency of this new ablation program still requires testing given its relative newness.

The cavity is made of ceramic and gases are provided by two bottles housed within the system. The beam treatment system is located in a module extending from the laser frame and serving as a support for the surgeon's console. The console, located in the intervention area, is equipped with a microscope, a telecamera, and a series of controls to move the patient's chair, modify the microscope's magnification and adjust lighting on the cornea to be treated.

Patient positioning is obtained by means of a joystick controlling the chair's vertical and horizontal movement through the X-Y axes and focusing through rotation of a ring nut at the base of the joystick. Focusing is made easier from the image on the cornea of an annular lamp positioned near the laser outlet hole.

The computer manages the different parts of the system and allows the surgeon to enter data through a workstation equipped with a keyboard and monitor.

The calibration test is performed by simulating the treatment on trial plastics (-4 D sphere, -4 D cylinder, 0 D sphere, and +2 D sphere).

This machine is not equipped with an eye tracker, which represents a serious drawback.

The introduction of the CAP method, interfacing the laser with Eyesys, Orbscan, and Technomed topographers, makes treatment with topolink possible. Given its relatively recent launch on the market, the efficiency of this technology must still be tested.

Nidek EC 5000 Model 2B Excimer Laser

This machine has been on the market for 6 years and is manufactured in Japan. The cavity is made of ceramic. The laser high-output frequency performs quick treatments.

As far as gas reservoirs are concerned, two bottles are housed within the laser: one containing helium argon, and the other containing halogen gas. A third bottle charged with nitrogen can be found outside the laser. The optical path is constituted by a series of optics and mirrors. Ablation is performed by means of slit scanning. The easily accessible computer allows quick treatment data entry.

The available work space is good. Focusing and X-Y axes movement controls are rationally positioned, thus ensuring the surgeon's maximum comfort.

The special focusing and alignment system recognizes a patient's correct position along the X, Y, and Z axes. An important upside is represented by the possibility for a surgeon to detect and correct a patient's wrong head inclination during treatment. The system is equipped with a passive and active eye tracker with 40 Hz frequency. The laser is not equipped with a topolink system.

Calibration is achieved through the use of PMMA small plates with an immediate check of fluence and homogeneity of treatment. Myopia, myopic astigmatism, hyperopia, and hyperopic astigmatism can be corrected with this laser. The possibility of a 9.0-mm-diameter scanning ablation makes this laser widely used to perform therapeutic treatments (PTK).

Coherent Schwind Keratom Excimer Laser

The first Keratom lasers were introduced in Europe in mid 1992. The laser's cavity is made of ceramic and the gas bottles containing the gases are positioned outside the frame. Once the laser beam leaves the cavity, it is deviated by a 90° mirror toward a prismatic integrator. The homogenized laser beam reaches a steel band containing special openings. The computer is on the left side of the surgeon and is easily accessible. The work space is good, so LASIK can be performed comfortably. Focusing is achieved by making the two red lateral lights (He-Ne) coincide on the corneal plane, at the center of treatment.

The Keratom is equipped with a passive eye tracker. An active eye tracker has been recently developed. The possibility of performing photoablation on the basis of a previous topographic evaluation is not yet possible with this machine. The broadbeam distribution system can be adjusted with a steel band of variable diameter. The energy leaving the cavity is monitored by a special inner device that is automatically stabilized. A second energy monitoring system is placed immediately after the integrator. To perform the fluence test, a cylinder is available. Its upper face has a slit on which a Wratten film is positioned, whereas the upper slit displays a stratified fluorescent substance. Treatments for myopia, hyperopia, and astigmatism can be performed.

Model LSX Lasersight Excimer Laser

The LSX laser ceramic cavity is characterized by a 200 Hz frequency. The machine is equipped with two gas bottles located within the laser frame, one containing Arf and the other He. The laser beam leaving the cavity first travels through an attenuator. A focal lens then delivers the beam to impact on two galvanometric lenses, ensuring that the laser beam is travelling along the right direction. Finally, a 45° angled lens conveys the beam on the corneal tissue. The extreme compactness of this machine allows the surgeon to work comfortably and directly control the computer monitor.

Special software called CIPTA (corneal interactive programmed topographic ablation) calculates the ablation profile for the topographic link. The X-Y movement, as well as focusing, are made from a console controlling movement of the operating chair. An optional active eye tracker is also available with laser beam realignment time accounting for 8.3 milliseconds. The machine is designed to work with topolink technology. The laser beam, with a variable diameter ranging from 0.8 to 1.0 mm, is distributed on the cornea according to a flying spot scansion technique.

After travelling through an attenuator, part of the beam is split and its energy tested. A second control system monitors the attenuator inclination to ensure that the actual energy on the corneal tissue corresponds to what was established by the previous fluence test. Myopia, hyperopia, and astigmatism can be corrected, in addition to therapeutic treatments.

Mel 70 G Scan Excimer Laser

The Mel 70 G Scan is an Esculap Meditec third-generation laser. This laser, equipped with a ceramic cavity, employs argon fluoride contained in two bottles. Cooling is provided by a closed circuit water/air internal cooler. The work spaces available are suitable to perform LASIK. The hardware is managed by a program running in Windows 95, providing extreme flexibility, with the possibility of further upgrading. Data entry and postoperative control are simple thanks to an "icon" program and a data bank within the system. The program is equipped with an "internal assistant" allowing both to follow the laser step by step after proposing the most suitable modes, or a manual use with nomograms directly developed the operator. Therefore, no skilled personnel are needed.

The operating microscope with adjustable coaxial light has five magnifications (3x, 5x, 8x, 11x, 20x, and 32x). This laser avails itself of an extremely rapid stable contrast active eye tracker. The machine employs topolink technology.

The new Mel 70 employs a randomized spot scansion. The spot is 2.0 mm in diameter. Moreover, it allows to correct both myopia and astigmatism in a single treatment.

BIBLIOGRAPHY

Krauss JM, Puliafito CA, Steinert RF. Laser interactions with the cornea. *Surv Ophthalmol.*1986;31:37-53.

Marshall J, Trokel SL, Rothery S, et al. A comparative study of corneal incision induced by diamond and steel knives and two ultraviolet radiations from an excimer laser. *Br J Ophthalmol.* 1986;70:482-501.

Marshall J, Trokel SL, Rothery S, et al. An ultrastructural study of corneal incision induced by an excimer laser at 193 nm. *Ophthalmology.* 1985;92:749-758.

Marshall J, Trokel SL, Rothery S, et al. Long-term healing of the central cornea after photorefractive keratectomy using an excimer laser. *Ophthalmology.* 1988;95:1411-1421.

Marshall J, Trokel S, Rothery S, et al. Photoablative reprofiling of the cornea using an excimer laser, photorefractive keratectomy. *Lasers Ophthalmol.* 1986;1:21-48.

McDonald M, Frantz JM, Klyce SD, et al. One-year refractive results of photorefractive keratotomy for myopia in non-human primate cornea. *Arch Ophthalmol.* 1990;108:40-47.

McDonald M, Kaufman HE, Frantz JM, et al: Excimer laser ablation in a human eye. *Arch Ophthalmol.* 1989;107:641-642.

Munnerlyn CR, Koons SJ, Marshall J. Photorefractive keratectomy: a technique for laser refractive surgery. *J Refract Surg.* 1988;14:46-52.

Puliafito CA, Steinert RF, Deutsch TF, et al. Excimer laser ablation of the cornea and lens. *Ophthalmology.* 1985;92:741-748.

Puliafito CA, Stem D, Krueger RR, et al. High-speed photography of excimer laser ablation of the cornea. *Arch Ophthalmol.* 1987;105:1255-1259.

Seiler T, Bende T, Trokel S, et al: Excimer laser keratectomy for correction of astigmatism. *Am J Ophthalmol.* 1988;105:117-124.

Seiler T, Kahle G, Kriegerowski M. Excimer laser (193 nm) myopic keratomiileusis in sighted and blind human eyes. *J Refract Cornal Surg.* 1990;3:97-100.

Trokel SL. The cornea and ultraviolet laser light. *Laser in der Ophthalmologie. Vol 113.* Bucherei des Augenarztes, Stuttgart: Ferdinand Enke Verlag; 1988.

Trokel SL, Srinivasan R, Braren B. Excimer laser surgery on the cornea. *Am J Ophthalmol.* 1983;96:404.

Comparing Broadbeam and Scanning Lasers

Michiel S. Kritzinger, MD

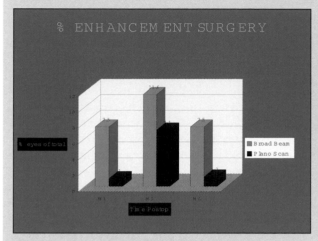

Figure 11A-1. Enhancement requirements.

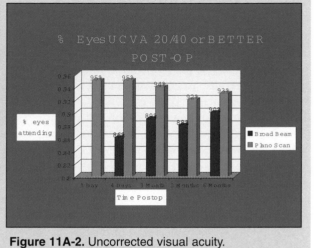

Figure 11A-2. Uncorrected visual acuity.

Excimer laser technology is like the computer industry—what you buy today is outdated tomorrow. Thus, I will only discuss the clinical visual results of different laser beams.

In 1994, LASIK was born with the second generation of ophthalmic lasers, which utilize broadbeam technology. This broadbeam is delivered to the cornea with either an expanding iris diaphragm or as a slit. The expanding iris diaphragm could be used in a single or multiple treatment zone mode.

Multizone broadbeam treatment is preferred over single-zone treatment because it creates a smoother ablation profile and causes less corneal tissue removal. Still, even the multizone treatment has its downside, which includes:

1. Creating central islands, especially without a pre-treatment program.
2. Critical fluence and homogeneity patterns that affect visual outcome.
3. Greater acoustic shockwaves on the cornea.
4. High maintenance and high energy requirements.
5. Limited ablation patterns.
6. Complex delivery system.

During early 1997, free spot scanning laser beams at 50 Hz were implemented. Patients achieved 20/20 vision sooner and had better quality and quantity of vision than broadbeam patients. Fewer visual regression and enhancement surgeries were also seen with the spot scanning lasers. Visual results improved at least 10% compared to broadbeam laser results.

Free spot scanning lasers are superior to broadbeam lasers, because:

1. Larger and more complex optical treatment ablations are possible.
2. Smoother ablation profiles, resulting in better quality and quantity of vision.
3. Less energy output, lower maintenance, fewer optics.
4. Lower beam homogeneity is necessary, with less effect on refractive results.
5. No central islands.
6. Minute shockwaves to the cornea.

The cornerstone of future excimer laser systems will be:

1. Free spot scanning for aspherical treatments.
2. Small spot size (1.0 mm).
3. Short treatment time achieved with high speed (> 200 Hz) and multiple beam ablation.
4. Super smooth surfaces.
5. Free scanning, custom ablation.

Laser technology will play a major role in future refractive surgery. As the laser technology improves, so will the visual results because the two are intimately related.

Eye Tracking and Small Beam Flying Spot Laser Technology: Platform for Customized Corneal Ablations

Marguerite B. McDonald, MD, FACS

Eye tracking is an increasingly important part of excimer laser refractive surgery. Coupled with a small flying spot beam, it provides the technology platform required to produce accurate customized ablations. Eye tracking can be active, passive, or both. An active eye tracker can detect a change in location and, as a response, move the next laser pulse. Passive tracking can detect change but merely shuts down further firing of the laser when the change exceeds a previously determined limit. The frequency with which the eye tracker samples the eye's position, as well as the speed in which the tracker responds, are both critical detection features. Though infrared camera video tracking is the simplest way to track eye movement, it is limited in its detection frequency by the frame capacity of the video camera. Eye tracking with laser radar is a more advanced method; it involves a laser-transmitted signal, which is extremely rapid because of the very high frequency pulse capacity of lasers, thereby allowing a much higher detection frequency with this system.

The Autonomous Technologies LADARVision is a new system based on laser radar technology that was used in the US military as well as NASA-sponsored research. It was used to track targets and improve weapon firing control, as well as docking space vehicles during rendezvous maneuvers. The founders of Autonomous Technologies Corporation are former NASA scientists and experts in tracking. In 1985, they began their quest to marry laser radar tracking technology to excimer laser refractive surgery.

The laser radar eye tracking system controls two axis-tracking mirrors that provide a steady line of sight to the cornea for the excimer beam. The first component of the tracker, the laser radar transmitter and sensor to measure the position of the eye, uses a 905 nm diode laser to emit a signal that measures the position of the eye and returns the information to the sensor at a rate of 4000 times per second. The second component of the tracking system is the two-axis tracking mirror assembly, which responds to position errors generated by the laser radar. The closed loop band width response time of the tracker mirror assembly allows the realignment of the mirror assembly to the eye's new position in less than 10 milliseconds or about 100 Hz. Even the most rapid saccadic eye movement (approximately 150 µm per second or 700 µm per second) can be tracked with a peak position error of only about 30 microns.[1,2]

The position of the pharmacologically dilated pupil margin is sensed by the laser radar device. Pupillary dilation provides a fixed diameter and greater surface area than the undilated pupil. A minimum pupil size of 7.0 mm is necessary for adequate tracking with the LADARVision system. The center of the undilated pupil (whose position had been previously recorded by the graphical user interface) is used as the center of the ablation area after dilation.

The graphical user interface is a Windows-based software display. The status of the tracker and the laser readiness are shown with two screens: one shows the untracked image of the eye (surgeon's view) and the other shows the eye as tracked by the laser during treatment. Despite a wide range of eye movements, the laser pulses are placed accurately with respect to the pupil margin. If an extremely large movement of the head and/or eye brings the image of the dilated pupil beyond that of the screen display, tracking is interrupted and the laser shuts itself off automatically. Once realignment and visualization of the dilated pupil are re-established, the tracker and laser are reactivated. The treatment commences at the exact place in which it had stopped.

The earliest broad beam excimer laser systems used a diaphragm to reshape the cornea, rather than a small flying spot. These first-generation lasers frequently created an irregular ablation profile on the cornea due to beam inhomogeneities or other physical/mechanical phenomena associated with the treatment process.[3] Topographic irregularities such as deep central islands, keyhole patterns, and the like have been frequently observed after PRK and LASIK with first-generation excimer lasers. These topographic anomalies result in suboptimal outcomes. Though patients often have excellent uncorrected and best-corrected Snellen acuities, they frequently complain of monocular diplopia, distortion, and poor quality of vision. Flying spot delivery systems such as the ATC LADARVision excimer laser provide corneal surfaces with little or no topographic abnormalities. Without trackers, however, flying spot lasers can actually increase the amount of topographic abnormalities. The tracker is so critical to the accurate pulse placement of the small beam flying spot laser that the ATC system shuts down ablation when the tracker is disabled. The Bausch & Lomb (Chiron/Technolas) PlanoScan laser, the Nidek EC-5000, and the LaserSight LSX laser all use different CCD or infrared camera-based tracking systems rather than laser radar. Video tracking systems can never exceed a detection frequency of 60 or 120 Hz, compared to 4000 Hz for the LADARVision system. Active tracking then responds to the detected change by moving the excimer laser servo mirrors within 10 to 25 milliseconds to the new location for the video tracking systems, compared to less than or equal to 10 milliseconds for the ATC system. The video tracking systems mentioned above are not used in the United States and are optional internationally because the video tracking detection frequency for saccadic eye movements is too slow to respond and redirect the laser before the next saccadic event occurs. Laser radar tracking will cause a repositioning response over 50 times during the saccadic event; the beam will be redirected to its appropriate location long before a new change occurs.

There is clinical evidence to support the concept that LADAR laser tracking, coupled with a small flying spot excimer laser, yields superior results. In a soon to be published article in *Ophthalmology*, uncorrected visual acuity 1 year after surgery was 20/20 or better in 72% of ATC PRK eyes (n = 229 of 318) treated for mild to moderate myopia, and refractive outcome was within ± 0.50 D of intended outcome for 76% of eyes (n = 258 of 339). The treatment of mild to moderate myopic astigmatism with PRK yielded a similar outcome: uncorrected visual acuity at 1 year was 20/20 or better in 62% of eyes (n = 72 of 116) and refractive outcome was within ±0.50 of intended in 74% of eyes (n = 88 of 119).[4]

The LADARVision system holds promise as the technology platform to provide truly customized ablations for individual eyes. Retinal physiologists and neurobiologists claim that our retinas are capable of 20/8 vision, but that we are prevented from obtaining this exquisite level of vision by our corneas. Higher order aberrations (spherical aberration, coma, etc) can be eliminated with customized ablations using wavefront sensing to guide the ablation pattern. These retinal image maps may guide the "flying spot" excimer beam to provide aberration-free vision for most patients in the new millennium.

REFERENCES

1. McDonald MB, Vanhorn LC. Autonomous T-PRK. In: Talamo JH, Krueger RR, eds. *The Excimer Manual: A Clinician's Guide To Excimer Laser Surgery.* Boston, Mass: Little, Brown & Co; 1997:355-368.
2. Boghen D, Trosst BT, Daroff RV, Dell'Osso, Birkett JE. Velocity characteristics of normal human saccades. *Invest Ophthalmol Vis Sci.* 1974;13:619-623.
3. Coorpender SJ, Klyce SD, McDonald MB, et al. Corneal topography of a small beam tracking excimer laser photorefractive keratectomy. *J Cataract Refract Surg.* In press.
4. McDonald MB, Deitz MR, Frantz JM, et al. PRK for low to moderate myopia and astigmatism with the LADARVision excimer laser system. *Ophthalmology.* In press.

Laser Environment, Fluence, and Beam Homogeneity: Why Do They Matter?

Keith Williams, FRCSC, FACS, FRCOphth

Because the excimer laser is computer controlled, there is a perception that excimer laser refractive surgery is a "point and shoot" procedure in which surgical technique and patient response are the primary factors that affect outcome. On the contrary, individual laser performance also has a material effect on clinical results. A proper laser room environment, consistent fluence, and a homogeneous beam are all important factors for ensuring consistent, quality output and high-quality, safe, and reproducible clinical results.

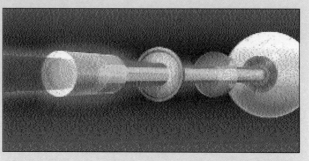

Figure 3A-1. The VISX Star S2 SmoothScan beam delivery system. Within the SmoothScan beam delivery system, seven turning beams are optically positioned to produce an ablation that has uniform energy density.

LASER ROOM ENVIRONMENT

When environmental conditions are poor, the laser's optics can become coated with debris. Even a small amount of debris will imprint a defect into the beam profile and produce an irregular ablation. The ideal laser room environment is:

- Cool (temperatures between 15° and 27°C [60° to 80°F])
- Dry (humidity < 50%)
- Free of particulate matter (barometric pressure should range from 11 to 16 psi, and the room should have a continuous, high efficiency, low particulate matter filtration system)

These conditions must be maintained 24 hours a day, every day of the year. When these conditions are maintained, excellent clinical results can be attained. With the VISX Star S2 excimer laser system, I have been able to achieve UCVA of 20/40 or better in 96% of eyes treated with LASIK for myopia or myopic astigmatism (n = 73; mean SE = -5.79 D) by the first postoperative day.

FLUENCE

Fluence is a measure of the energy directed to a specific area of the cornea with each pulse. Fluence, expressed in mJ/cm^2, determines the amount of tissue ablated per pulse. With the 193 nm excimer laser, ablation occurs after fluence reaches 50 mJ/cm^2, and most lasers operate at a specified fluence between 130 and 250 mJ/cm^2. Essentially, three clinical problems can occur when fluence levels are abnormal:

- Undercorrection. As gas levels decrease, fluence can decrease. This decreases the amount of tissue ablated.
- Overcorrection. If fluence rises above the normal operating level, each pulse will remove too much tissue and cause overcorrection and possible thermal damage.
- Corneal irregularities. Minor fluence variations from one pulse to the next can produce an irregular ablation.

Importantly, the amount of energy the optics reflect or refract determines the rate of optic degradation; optic degradation accelerates with increased fluence and frequent use of the laser.

With commercially available lasers, fluence calibration is automatic and should always be done at system start-up and before each patient treatment or test procedure. The operator should never postpone or bypass the fluence test and must always ensure an adequate gas supply.

BEAM HOMOGENEITY

Homogeneity is a measure of the distribution of energy over the entire ablation. If the beam distributes energy unevenly, the ablation will be uneven and can produce potentially severe irregular astigmatism.

When using conventional broadbeam lasers that output a single beam, manual verification of beam homogeneity with a commercially available gel/substrate material is essential. Beam homogeneity tests are not needed with technologically newer lasers, such as the VISX Star systems or scanning lasers. Slit- and spot-scanning lasers use small beams that are inherently more homogeneous. The Star laser systems contain internal image rotators and optical integrators that continuously invert, split, and reform the beam to create a composite of seven small diameter, uniform beams that move across the cornea and produce a homogenous energy profile (Figure 3A-1).

PREDICTIVE FORMULAS FOR LASIK

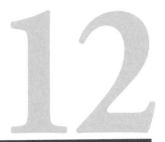

Louis E. Probst, V, MD

INTRODUCTION

The predictive formulas for laser-assisted in situ keratomileusis (LASIK) have two components: the excimer laser ablation nomogram and the adjustment factors. The excimer laser ablation nomogram controls the relative distribution of the refraction correction into one or more zones. In some of the newer excimer lasers, such as the VISX Star, the excimer ablation nomogram is controlled by the laser's computer, while in other excimer lasers, such as the Chiron Technolas 116, the ablation nomogram is fully programmable by the surgeon. The adjustment factors allow surgeons to refine the treatment protocol to reflect their particular refractive situation. In order for these formulas to be predictive, a high level of consistency must be achieved in the application of both the ablation nomograms and adjustment factors. Other extraneous variables, such as the methods of preoperative refraction, room temperature and humidity, room air quality and flow, surgical technique and time, and postoperative medications must be tightly controlled to avoid deviations from the intended correction.

It is crucial to remember that the predictive formulas (including both the excimer laser ablation nomogram and the adjustment factors) must be individualized for each surgeon. Direct extrapolations from the experience of one surgeon or one center will likely lead to an unexpected deviation of the surgical results from emmetropia. Since it is impossible to control every aspect of surgery, each surgeon must develop his or her own predictive formulas once his or her technique has become standardized and postoperative results can be analyzed. For the beginning LASIK surgeon, conservative corrections are preferable, as enhancements are easy to perform while overcorrections can be much more challenging.

Once the excimer ablation nomogram and adjustment factors have been standardized and individualized for each excimer laser surgeon, the final uncontrolled variable with LASIK is the healing pattern of the cornea. While there is a clear tendency for greater amounts of regression after LASIK for higher levels of myopia, often the degree of regression after LASIK is unpredictable. Younger patients (< 25 years) often demonstrate significant regression, while older patients (> 50 years) may not regress at all. We have observed regression of 1.0 to 2.0 diopters (D) in one eye and no regression in the other eye after bilateral simultaneous LASIK in which the excimer nomogram, adjustment factors, surgical technique, and extraneous variables were all exactly the same during the correction of both eyes. This unpredictable healing pattern of the cornea represents the limitation of corneal refractive surgery.

In order to avoid LASIK overcorrections, it is best to plan for a 10% to 20% enhancement rate for lower myopes and even higher rates with high myopes, which will allow retreatment of those patients who have regressed.

EXCIMER LASER ABLATION NOMOGRAMS FOR PRK

The excimer laser nomograms for LASIK have been developed from the excimer LASIK experience with photorefractive keratectomy (PRK). The concepts of laser pretreatment to prevent central islands and multizone ablations to decrease ablation depth and smooth the laser contour evolved as the worldwide PRK experience, as well as the increase in technological capabilities of excimer lasers.

Pretreatment Protocols

Pretreatment protocols have been added to the ablation profiles of the broad beam excimer lasers such as the VISX Star, Summit Apex Plus, and Chiron Technolas

Table 12-1															
MELBOURNE EXCIMER LASER GROUP MULTIZONE PRK TREATMENT ALGORITHM															
Diopters at Corneal Plane															
Ablation zone (mm)	-3	-4	-5	-6	-7	-8	-9	-10	-11	-12	-13	-14	-15	-16	-17	-18
4.5	-	-	-	-	-	-	-	-	-3.67	-4	-4.33	-4.67	-5	-5.33	-5.67	-6
5.0	-	-	-	-3	-3.5	-4	-4.5	-5	-3.67	-4	-4.33	-4.67	-5	-5.33	-5.67	-6
6.0	-3	-4	-5	-3	-3.5	-4	-4.5	-5	-3.67	-4	-4.33	-4.67	-5	-5.33	-5.67	-6

Table 12-2															
POP MULTIZONE PRK TREATMENT ALGORITHM															
Diopters at Corneal Plane															
Ablation zone (mm)	-3	-4	-5	-6	-7	-8	-9	-10	-11	-12	-13	-14	-15	-16	-17	-18
2.5 (pre-treatment)	-1.5	-1.5	-1.5	-1.5	-1.5	-1.5	-1.5	-1	-1	-1	-1	-1	-1	-1	-1	-1
3.5	-	-	-	-	-	-	-	-	-	-	-	-	-	-	-4	-4
4	-	-	-	-	-	-	-	-	-4	-4	-4	-4	-4	-4	-4	-4
4.5	-	-	-	-3	-4	-4	-4	-4	-2	-2	-3	-4	-3	-4	-2	-2
5	-	-2	-3	-1	-1	-2	-2	-2	-2	-2	-2	-2	-2	-2	-2	-2
5.5	-2	-1	-1	-1	-1	-1	-2	-2	-2	-2	-2	-2	-2	-2	-2	-2
6	-1	-1	-1	-1	-1	-1	-1	-2	-1	-1	-1	-2	-2	-2	-2	-2

Keracor 116 to reduce the incidence of postoperative central islands.[1] The VISX Star pretreatment is automatically calculated by the Central Island Factor (CIF) 4.01 software and incorporated into the excimer ablation protocol. Approximately 1 micron per diopter of spherical correction plus an additional 2 microns is added to each ablation protocol and is performed at 2.5 mm. The Chiron Technolas Keracor 116 pretreatment is surgeon-programmable. Generally, 1 micron per diopter plus 2 to 4 microns is added to each ablation protocol and is performed at 3.0 mm.[2] The Summit Apex Plus excimer laser allows the surgeon to choose between 0% to 10% of the total planned pulses to be delivered as part of the first ablation to the central 2.5 mm before the actual full ablation occurs. Typically, surgeons choose 8% to 10%, although some surgeons who have never experienced central islands select 0%. The newer scanning excimer laser systems, such as the Chiron Technolas 217 excimer laser, do not need pretreatment protocols, as this phenomena of undertreatment of the central cornea is avoided with these scanning laser systems.

Single and Multizone Ablations Protocols

All excimer laser refractive procedures modify the refracting power of the cornea by altering the anterior corneal curvature by the process of photoablation. Correction of myopia involves relative flattening of the central cornea compared to the peripheral cornea, which reduces the anterior corneal curvature and hence reduces the refractive power of the treated area. Because the maximal corneal stromal tissue will be photoablated from the central cornea, the thickness of the central cornea becomes important when LASIK is performed for high refractive errors with large ablation depths.

Excimer ablation techniques have evolved. The initial single-zone techniques increased from 4.0 to 6.0 mm[3,4] to improve the quality of postoperative vision and reduce the incidence of halos and regression. The multipass multizone technique was developed by Mihai Pop, MD for the VISX excimer laser,[5,6] and the multi-multizone technique was developed by Jeffery J. Machat, MD for the Chiron Technolas excimer laser.[1] These multizone techniques divide the myopic treatment into multiple zones, which decreases the ablation depth and creates a smoother ablation surface. This blending and smoothing effect of the multizone protocols has helped to reduce the incidence of post-PRK regression and haze, particularly for the treatment of high myopia.[6]

Recently, Alpins and coworkers[7] from the Melbourne Excimer Laser Group have compared the algorithms and results of three different multizones (Tables 12-1 to 12-3). PRK ablation programs were designed for the VISX 20/20 excimer laser. While each algorithm had a maximum ablation zone of 6.0 mm, they differed in the number of zones employed, the proportion of treatment assigned to each zone, and the treat-

Table 12-3

ALPINS MULTIZONE PRK TREATMENT ALGORITHM
Diopters at Corneal Plane

Ablation zone (mm)	-3	-4	-5	-6	-7	-8	-9	-10	-11	-12	-13	-14	-15	-16	-17	-18
2.5 (pre-treatment)	-1.5	-1.5	-1.5	-1.5	-1.5	-1.5	-1.5	-1	-1	-1	-1	-1	-1	-1	-1	-1
3.5	-	-	-	-	-	-	-	-	-	-	-	-	-	-2.67	-2.83	-3
4	-	-	-	-	-	-	-	-	-	-	-2.6	-2.8	-3	-2.67	-2.83	-3
4.5	-	-	-	-	-	-	-	-2.5	-2.75	-3	-2.6	-2.8	-3	-2.67	-2.83	-3
5	-	-	-	-	-2.33	-2.67	-3	-2.5	-2.75	-3	-2.6	-2.8	-3	-2.67	-2.83	-3
5.5	-	-2	-2.5	-3	-2.33	-2.67	-3	-2.5	-2.75	-3	-2.6	-2.8	-3	-2.67	-2.83	-3
6	-3	-2	-2.5	-3	-2.33	-2.67	-3	-2.5	-2.75	-3	-2.6	-2.8	-3	-2.67	-2.83	-3

ment of astigmatism. The Melbourne multizone equally divided the treatment into a maximum of three zones at 4.5, 5.0, and 6.0 mm. The Pop multizone technique utilized a pretreatment with treatment bias for the smaller zones to a maximum of six zones at 3.5, 4.0, 4.5, 5.0, 5.5, and 6.0 mm. The Alpins multizone technique also utilized a pretreatment and equally divided the treatment up to a maximum of six zones at 3.5, 4.0, 4.5, 5.0, 5.5, and 6.0 mm. Although all the algorithms were effective in reducing myopia, statistical analysis indicated that the Alpins multizone algorithm achieved better visual acuity and refractive results.

EXCIMER LASER ABLATION NOMOGRAMS FOR LASIK

The creation of the corneal flap and the routine correction of higher levels of myopia with LASIK introduced new considerations into the excimer nomograms. The depth of the ablation and the size of the ablation zones have become recognized as crucial considerations to achieve a good quality and quantity of correction while maintaining the safety of the procedure and the stability of the cornea. If all of these factors are considered, LASIK has correction limits of 10 to 15 D of myopia depending on which ablation nomogram is used.

Basic Tenets of LASIK

There are four critical values or dimensions that must be considered when performing LASIK. These are the flap thickness, the amount residual corneal stroma, the diameter of the excimer ablation, and the depth of the excimer ablation. These values determine the key concepts of LASIK—safety and stability of the procedure, and quality and quantity of the laser correction (Doane JF, Nordan LT, Baker RN, Slade SG. Basic tenets of lamellar refractive surgery. Unpublished course material).

The flap thickness must be sufficient to prevent irregular astigmatism, while not so excessive that it removes stroma potentially available for ablation. We generally use a 160 µm flap for thin corneas or large refractive corrections (> 10 D), a 180 µm flap for average corneas and moderate corrections (> 6 D), and a 200 µm flap for thick corneas and small corrections (< 6 D). Sufficient residual posterior stroma must be left after the LASIK procedure to avoid a decrease of corneal integrity and subsequent development of corneal ectasia. Since iatrogenic keratoconus has been observed after automated lamellar keratoplasty (ALK) with 200 µm of remaining posterior stromal tissue, we generally elect to leave at least 250 µm of posterior stromal tissue. The diameter of the excimer ablation should be at least 6.0 mm to create a functional postoperative optical zone of at least 4.0 mm, which will allow for sufficient quality of vision. Finally, the depth of the excimer ablation determines the quantity of myopia at can be safety treated while preserving adequate residual corneal stroma.

Ablation Depth Per Diopter

Each excimer laser ablates a different amount of stromal tissue per diopter of refractive correction because of the differences in the ablation zone diameters, amount of pretreatment, and the ablation protocols. The Munnerlyn formula[8] (depth of ablation = diopters of correction x ablation diameter^2 ÷ 3) indicates that each spherical equivalent (SE) diopter of myopic correction performed at a 6.0 mm single zone will ablate 12 microns of tissue. Pretreatment protocols added to the ablation profile of broad beam excimer lasers such as the VISX Star and Chiron Technolas Keracor 116 will increase the depth per SE diopter to 17 to 20 microns for low corrections (1 to 2 D) and 15 to 17 microns for higher corrections (3 or more diopters). The Summit Apex Plus will ablate 13 to 14 microns per SE diopter for all levels of myopia with pretreatment.

Table 12-4								
VISX STAR CORRECTION VARIABILITY								
Location	**ENH**	**Preop MR rate**	**Altitude range (-)**	**Temp**	**Humidity range**	**Drying range**	**Age adjust**	**Sphere adjust (-)**
Tulsa, Okla	21%	1.00 to 16	711	60 to 65	30 to 40	None	No	10%
Okla City, Okla	10%	1.00 to 17	1208	65 to 70	40 to 60	None	No	20%
Garden City, NY	15%	1.00 to 16	0	65 to 76	30 to 60	Subjective	Yes	Sliding: 14-18%
Seattle, Wash	5%	1.00 to 15	260	60 to 65	30 to 40	None	No	7.70%
Brea, Calif	8%	0.75 to 13.75	650	65 to 70	45 to 50	Periodic	No	8%
Indianapolis, Ind	8%	1.00 to 15	770	60 to 65	35 to 40	Periodic	Yes	20%
Denver, Colo	25%	1.00 to 20	5280	60 to 65	35 to 45	None	No	30%
Rockville, Md	15%	0.75 to 16	0	60 to 65	35 to 40	None	Yes	Sliding: 15-20%
Fairfax, Va	15%	0.75 to 16	0	60 to 65	35 to 40	None	Yes	Sliding: 15-20%
New York, NY	10%	0.50 to 22	15	65 to 68	30 to 35	None	Yes	Sliding: 10-20%
Charlotte, NC	15%	1.00 to 16	765	65 to 70	35 to 40	None	No	15%
Rockville, Md	7%	1.00 to 16	0	60 to 65	35 to 40	None	Yes	15%
Fairfax, Va	7%	1.00 to 16	0	60 to 65	35 to 40	None	Yes	15%
Greenville, SC	10%	1.00 to 16	950	65 to 70	35 to 50	Subjective	No	10%
Johnson City, Tenn	10%	1.00 to 16	1700	65 to 70	30 to 45	Subjective	No	20%

The multipass multizone ablation technique used with VISX Star "international cards" has an average stromal ablation of 12.5 microns per SE diopter. The full multi-multizone ablation technique with the ablation pattern distributed between 3.6 and 6.2 mm reduces the average stromal ablation to approximately 10 microns per SE diopter.1 While the full multi-multizone protocol significantly reduces ablation depth, it should only be used for LASIK when necessitated by a thin cornea associated with high myopia because of the compromised quality of postoperative night vision.

Correction Limits for Primary LASIK

The average central cornea thickness is approximately 550 + 100 μm.[9] Since the flap thickness during the LASIK procedure is generally 160 μm, the average cornea will have 390 microns of posterior stromal bed left after the flap creation. Therefore, the maximal myopic correction that should be performed on a patient with a 550 μm cornea using a full multi-multizone technique is generally less than 14 D while leaving a residual posterior stromal bed of 250 microns. A partial multizone ablation as performed with the Chiron Technolas 116 and the VISX Star would allow a maximal correction of approximately 12 D, and a single-zone ablation would allow a maximal myopic correction of 10 D.[10]

VISX STAR: PREDICTIVE FORMULAS FOR LASIK

The VISX Star utilizes a propriety multizone nomogram developed from the PRK multizone experience with the VISX 20/20 excimer laser. A pretreatment is combined with a multizone ablation that is not surgeon-programmable. While this limits the flexibility of the laser to adjust ablation zone size, which would be beneficial for patients with large pupils, it does reduce variation in the techniques of surgeons and therefore allows for good comparison between centers.

Early in the LASIK experience with the VISX Star excimer laser, it became clear that this laser would tend to overcorrect if the unmodified PRK correction was utilized for LASIK. Surgeons developed "adjustment factors" that were used to modify the refractive correction before it was programmed into the excimer laser in order to avoid overcorrections. These values usually involved reduction in the value of the spherical component of the refractive error by 10% to 30%.

A number of factors may contribute to the increased effectiveness of the VISX Star excimer laser when used for LASIK. The vacuum nozzle of this machine may decrease stromal hydration, increasing the effect of the excimer ablation. The slower pulse frequency may allow the cornea to dehydrate. With the new upgrade, the pulse frequency may now be increased to 10 Hz. Surgeon factors, such as the time taken to perform the procedure and the methods of drying the cornea, have also been considered.

Once several centers gained more experience with the VISX Star laser, a pattern began to emerge regarding the adjustment factors. The nomograms for 15 surgeons who have performed more than 500 LASIK procedures each with the VISX Star laser were compared (Table 12-4). The range of myopia treated and the enhancement rates were recorded to ensure that most surgeons were achieving a similar level of predictability with their pro-

Table 12-5			
PROBST LASIK NOMOGRAM FOR VISX S2 SMOOTHSCAN (10 HZ)			
	< 25 yrs	**25 to 45 yrs**	**> 45 yrs**
< 2 D myopia	90%	90%	90%
> 2 D myopia	86%	82%	80%

cedures. The room temperature and humidity range of the procedure rooms did not correlate with the adjustment factors used at each center. Most surgeons did not use drying techniques.

Altitude emerged, however, as a consistent factor that seemed to be related to the adjustment factor. When the two factors were correlated, it was found that there was a statistically significant correlation between the altitude of the refractive center and the surgeon spherical adjustment factor ($r = 0.75$, $n = 15$, $p = 0.002$, slope = 0.0032). This allows us to calculate that a city with an altitude at sea level, such as New York, should be using an adjustment factor of 12.8%, while Denver, at an altitude of 5280 feet, should have an adjustment factor of 29.7% ($12.8 + 0.0032 \times 5280$).

This variation in the effectiveness of the excimer laser at different altitudes is probably a result of changes in air density. The Ideal Gas Law solved for density is $D = P/(T \times R)$ in which D is the air density, P is the station pressure at the altitude of the refractive center, T is the temperature in Kelvin, and R is the gas constant. Increased humidity will actually decrease air density; however its effect on air density is minimal and most refractive centers have humidity control systems installed. Temperature is usually well controlled, so it is unlikely that this would introduce significant variation in results. The station pressure is the direct barometer reading. Two variables affect the barometer reading, the air pressure of the weather systems, and the altitude of the center, which will significantly decrease the air pressure at higher altitudes. While we currently adjust the spherical component of the VISX Star ablation by a constant value that seams to be related to altitude, perhaps our adjustments in the future will be based on the daily barometric reading and corresponding calculations of air density.

VISX S2 SMOOTHSCAN: PREDICTIVE FORMULAS FOR LASIK

The adjustment factors utilized for the VISX S2 SmoothScan excimer laser upgrade are very similar to those used for the VISX Star laser. Most surgeons have made only minor adjustments to their VISX Star reduction factors. Increasing the frequency of the excimer pulse to 10 Hz reduces laser time by almost 50% but does not affect the degree of refractive correction. The spherical reduction factor that we currently utilize at The Laser Center (TLC) Chicago is outlined in Table 12-5.

For hyperopic corrections, we utilize the 5.5 mm optical zone with a 9.0 mm blend zone for hyperopic LASIK with the Hansatome. For hyperopes, we add 0.5 D to the spherical refractive error to account for the greater amount of regression that occurs with hyperopia treatment.

CHIRON TECHNOLAS 116: PREDICTIVE FORMULAS FOR LASIK

With the Chiron Technolas 116, the ideal zone depth for each step of the multizone LASIK ablation was initially felt to be 15 to 20 microns to create the smoothest blended multizone ablation[2] (Table 12-6). This algorithm was similar to those used for PRK and provided a smooth blend of the myopic ablation with zones that extended from 3.6 mm to 6.2 mm for a maximum of seven zones. This full multizone ablation allowed the treatment of high levels of myopia, as the total ablation depth was minimized with the smaller zone size. Unfortunately, the smaller zone sizes resulted in a significant reduction in the effective optical zone observed on corneal topography following LASIK. High myopes treated with the full multizone algorithm demonstrated an effective optical zone that was often less than 4.0 mm. Clinically, this resulted in complaints of visual distortion and halos at night in the same manner the early small-zone PRK ablations were associated with these difficulties. Decentrations are poorly tolerated with the small-zone ablations, as the refracted light for the edge of the ablation could be in close proximity to the visual axis.

Machat has found that the size of the ablation zones should be increased so that most of the treatment is performed at a 5.5 mm or larger ablation zone.[11] This increases the depth of ablation to 30 to 40 microns per zone in the partial multi-multizone protocol, which accounts for the hydration effects of the deeper stroma and the masking effect of the corneal flap. By increasing the size and depth of ablation of each zone to 30 to 40 microns and decreasing the number of zones, the effective postoperative optical zone on videokeratography can be increased, and night vision difficulties can be minimized (Table 12-7). This partial multi-multizone ablation that we now use for LASIK ablations removes 12.5

Table 12-6

ORIGINAL MACHAT CHIRON 116 LASIK NOMOGRAM FOR HIGH MYOPIA

Important points
- No vertex distance correction
- Pretreatment 1 micron per diopter plus 2 to 4 microns total
- Depth at 3.0 mm for Chiron Technolas Keracor 116 to compensate for central island formation
- All treatment zones of equal depth (not including pretreatment step)
- All zones ideally between 15 and 20 microns
- Goal is to achieve at least 6.0 mm effective optical zone
- Compressed air is used intraoperatively to control hydration

LASIK Nomogram for -13 D Attempted Correction

Optical Zone	Dioptric Distribution	% of Treatment	Micron Depth
3.0 mm	-5.4 D	Pretreatment (1 micron/D + 3)	16
3.6 mm	-3.63 D	27.9%	17
4.2 mm	-.258 D	18.9%	17
4.8 mm	-1.90 D	14.6%	17
5.4 mm	-1.46 D	11.2%	17
5.8 mm	-1.23 D	9.5%	17
6 mm	-1.14 D	8.8%	17
6.2 mm	-1.06 D	8.15%	17

Eight zones of equal micron depth. Each zone is 0.6 mm larger than the previous zone, with two additional zones within 0.2 mm of the 6.0 mm optical zone to ensure adequate peripheral blend for reduced spherical aberration and night visual disturbances.

microns of stroma per SE diopter. While the quality of the night vision is improved with these new algorithms, the depth of ablation per diopter must be increased with the corresponding increase in zone size. This limits the quantity of myopia that can be safely corrected to approximately 15 D in an eye with an average corneal thickness.

Early in our LASIK experience with the Chiron Technolas 116, we experienced undercorrections. For PRK we had used the vertex-corrected refraction; however for LASIK, we found that the nonvertex-corrected refraction produced more accurate results. The surgical technique was modified to allow treatment of the central corneal hydration. Filtered compressed air is applied to the central stroma during pretreatment and for the first 3 seconds of each zone. An additional 3 seconds are applied during the middle of the last zone. By adhering to the partial multizone ablation nomogram and applying these techniques consistently, we have achieved very predictable results.

KRITZINGER NOMOGRAM FOR THE TECHNOLAS 217 EXCIMER LASER

The success of excellent postoperative visual results does not only depend on the nomogram, but also the following:
- Environmental factors in the operating room, such as temperature, humidity, and air drafts
- Surgical technique
- Preoperative refraction of the patient
- Postoperative medication to the patient
- The type and make of the laser in use (broadbeam/scanning)

General Rules

- Room temperature: 16° to 18°C
- Room humidity: 45 to 50%
- Exact super-imposition of red and green He-Ne beam is critical, or undercorrections will occur.
- Use 6x magnification—not larger—because you can loose your orientation to the visual axis.
- Correctly align the patient prior to lifting the flap to limit exposure time of stroma before the treatment starts. It will give you more accurate and consistent visual results.
- The Kritzinger 217 nomogram differs moderately from the Probst 217 nomogram (Table 12-8).
- Lift the flap with a Colibri. Do not use a BSS cannula, as this may introduce moisture to the bed. Do not use a spatula since foreign material (eg, epithelium) may be introduced into the interface.

Table 12-7					
TLC THE LASER CENTER CHIRON 116 NOMOGRAM					
Correction	**Pretreatment**	**%**	**Zone diameter**	**Zone depth**	**Total depth**
0 to 3.5		100	6.5		
-3.50		54.5	6.1		
		45.5	6.6		
-5.75	-3.1@3	60	5.5	41.25	
		40	6.6	42	91
-6	-3.15@ 3	60	5.5	43.25	
		40	6.6	43.75	97
-6.5	-3.35@ 3	60	5.5	46.75	
		40	6.6	47.25	104.25
-7	-3.5@3	41	5.5	34.5	
		32	6.1	34	
		27	6.6	34.5	114
-7.5	-3.65@3	41	5.5	37	
		32	6.1	36.5	
		27	6.6	36.75	121.75
-8	-3.85@3	41	5.5	39.25	
		32	6.1	38.75	
		27	6.6	39.5	129.5
-8.5	-4@3	41	5.5	41.75	
		32	6.1	41.25	
		27	6.6	41.75	137.25
		45	5	37	
		30	6.1	38.25	
		25	6.6	38.75	127
		48	4.5	31.25	
		31	5.5	31.5	
		21	6.5	31.25	106.5
-9	-4.15@3	41	5.5	44.25	
		32	6.1	43.75	
		27	6.6	44.25	145.25
		45	5	39.25	
		30	6.1	41	
		25	6.6	41	134.25
		48	4.5	33.25	
		31	5.5	33.5	
		21	6.5	33.25	113
-9.5	-4.25@3	41	5.5	46.75	
		32	6.1	46	
		27	6.6	46.75	153
		45	5	41.75	
		30	6.1	43.25	
		25	6.6	43.25	141.5
		48	4.5	35	
		31	5.5	35.25	
		21	6.5	35.25	119
-10	-4.45@3	45	5	43.5	
		30	6.1	45.5	
		25	6.6	45.5	148.5
		48	4.5	36.75	
		31		5.5	37.25
		21	6.5	37	125

345

Table 12-7, Continued

TLC THE LASER CENTER CHIRON 116 NOMOGRAM

Correction	Pretreatment	%	Zone diameter	Zone depth	Total depth
-10.5	-4.6@3	48	4.5	38.75	
		31	5.5	39	
		21	6.5	38.75	131
		40	4	25	
		25	5	25.5	
		19	6.1	30.5	
		16	6.6	30.75	126.25
-11	-4.75@3	48	4.5	40.5	
		31	5.5	41	
		21	6.5	40.75	137.25
		40	4	26	
		25	5	26.75	
		19	6.1	31.75	
		16	6.6	32	131.5
11.5	-4.9@3	48	4.5	42.25	
		31	5.5	42.75	
		21	6.5	42.5	143
		40	4	27.25	
		25	5	28	
		19	6.1	33.25	
		16	6.6	33.5	137.5
-12	-4.75@3	48	4.5	44.25	
		31	5.5	44.5	
		21	6.5	44.25	148
		40	4	28.5	
		25	5	29	
		19	6.1	34.75	
		16	6.6	35	142.25
-13	-5.1@3	48	4.5	47.75	
		31	5.5	48.25	
		21	6.5	48	160
		40	4	30.75	
		25	5	31.5	
		19	6.1	27.5	
		16	6.6	38	153.75

- Commence laser treatment, and let the assistant press the "enter" key to give continuous treatment without breaks so that you make the treatment time and stromal exposure time as short as possible.
- Avoid contact with the stromal bed. Do not wipe while lasering the stroma—this is contraindicated because it will give overcorrections with the 217 laser.
- Minimum residual cornea after ablation must be 250 microns (excluding flap thickness).
- Ideal treatment zone is 4.0 mm to 6.0 mm.
- It is advisable not to use a smaller zone diameter than 4.0 mm (night vision glaze) and a maximum zone diameter of 6.0 mm (unnecessary vertex ablation and overcorrections will result).

Kritzinger Nomograms

Myopia
For treatment of -1.0 to -13 SE diopters:
- Use subjective spectacle correction for minus spheres.
- Add 10% to sphere and cylinder
- Subtract/add the calculated cylindrical correction from/to the calculated spherical correction because:
  a. 20% hyperopic coupling shift with negative cylinders on the spherical diopters.

Table 12-8

KRITZINGER AND PROBST LASIK NOMOGRAMS FOR CHIRON TECHNOLAS 217

		Zone	Sphere	Cylinder	Comments
Myopia	Kritzinger	5.5	add 10%	add 10%	add 20% -cyl to -sph
(minus cyl)	Probst		6.0	no change	no adjustments
Hyperopia	Kritzinger	5.5	add 15%	add 10%	subtract 10% of cyl from sph
	Probst	6.0	add 10%	no change	no adjustments
Mixed	Kritzinger	5.5	add 10%	add 10%	add 1/3 +cyl to -sph
(plus cyl)	Probst	6.0	no change	no change	add 1/3 +cyl to -sph

Table 12-9

CASEBEER LASIK PERSONAL CALIBRATION NOMOGRAM
BASED ON ARIZONA'S DRY CLIMATE

The VISX Star excimer laser was used on patients with myopia and astigmatism. Pretreatment was per the laser program, ablation took place on a dry stromal bed, and there was no intraoperative wiping.

Refraction	20 to 25	26 to 30	31 to 35	36 to 40	> 40
-1	-1	-.98	-.95	- .9	-.85
-1.5	-1.5	-1.46	-1.43	-1.35	-1.28
-2	-2	-1.95	-1.9	-1.8	-1.7
-2.0	-2.5	-2.44	-2.38	-2.25	-2.13
-3	-3	-2.93	-2.85	- 2.7	-2.55
-3.5	-3.33	-3.24	-3.15	-2.98	-2.8
4	-3.8	-3.7	-3.6	-3.4	-3.2
-4.5	-4.28	-4.16	-4.05	-3.83	-3.6
-5	-4.75	-4.63	-4.5	-4.25	-4
-5.5	-5.23	-5.09	-4.95	-4.68	-4.4
-6	-5.7	-5.55	-5.4	-5.1	-4.8
-6.5	-5.85	-5.69	-5.53	-5.2	-4.88
-7	-6.3	-6.13	-5.95	-5.6	-5.25
-7.5	-6.75	-6.56	-6.38	-6.4	-6
-8.5	-7.65	-7.44	-7.23	-6.8	-6.38
-9	-8.1	-7.88	-7.65	-7.2	-6.75
-9.5	-8.08	-7.84	-7.6	-7.13	-6.65
-10	-8.5	-8.25	-8	-7.5	-7
-10.5	-8.93	-8.66	-8.4	-7.88	-7.35
-11	-9.35	-9.08	-8.8	-8.25	-7.7
-11.5	-9.78	-9.49	-9.2	-8.63	-8.05
-12	-10.2	-9.9	-9.6	-9	-8.4
-12.5	-10.63	-10.31	-10	-9.38	-8.75
-13	-11.05	-10.73	-10.4	-9.75	-9.1
-13.5	-11.48	-11.14	-10.8	-10.13	-9.45
-14	-11.9	-11.55	-11.2	-10.5	-9.8
-14.5	-12.33	-11.96	-11.6	-10.88	-10.15

b. 10% myopic coupling shift with plus cylinders on the spherical diopters.

Hyperopia

- For treatment of +1.0 to +3.0, (rarely up to +4.0) SE diopters.
- Selection of treatment program of the 217 laser (hyperopia/myopia) is dependent on the sphere and not the cylinder.
- Use subjective spectacle correction.
- Add 15% to the sphere and 10% to the cylinder.
- Subtract/add the calculated cylindrical correction from/to the calculated spherical correction because:
  a. 20% hyperopic coupling shift with negative cylinders on the spherical diopters.
  b. 10% myopic coupling shift with plus cylinders on the spherical diopters.

Information

- Hyperopic treatment regresses more than myopic treatments.
- If a patient has a high plus sphere and any strength minus cylinder, the surgeon should do a transposition to a plus cylinder (less tissue ablation, shorter treatment time, less gas consumption).
- Most plus spheres are treated in the plus cylinder prescription and a transposition is often required.

Adjustment Factors for the Refractive Correction of LASIK

Aside from the altitude of the refractive center, patient age is the other commonly considered adjustment factor. Patient age has been used in the past predominantly for the radial keratotomy and astigmatic keratotomy nomograms.[12] Age adjustments have been less consistently applied for LASIK. Since a refractive stability is achieved with LASIK by 3 to 6 months postoperatively, the hyperopic drift that occurred with radial keratotomy (RK) is not a concern with LASIK. Slight overcorrection of 0.5 D is preferable in patients under the age of 25 years, as the vision will be excellent and a small buffer is created against a future regression of effect. Middle-aged patients between 25 and 50 years are best treated with the full refractive correction unless monovision is planned in the nondominant eye. Older patients (> 50 years) are usually best undercorrected by 0.5 D, as they tend to have a greater response to the excimer ablation and are less tolerant of overcorrections.

Casebeer has described his nomogram for LASIK based on the dry climate of Arizona[13] (Table 12-9). The nomogram used at TLC Chicago makes similar adjustments on a simpler scale (see Table 12-5).

SUMMARY

LASIK is a procedure in evolution. While LASIK surgeons originally performed corrections over 20 D[14], we now limit our corrections to much lower levels of myopia to preserve the integrity of the cornea and the quality of postoperative vision. As the worldwide LASIK experience increases, the variables affecting our results are being controlled and minimized. However, each year new excimer lasers are becoming available that have different ablation nomograms and therefore will have some variation in their predictive formulas. A slow conservative initial approach to these innovations will lead to the best results for our patients.

REFERENCES

1. Machat JJ. PRK complications and their management. In: Machat JJ, ed. *Excimer Laser Refractive Surgery.* Thorofare, NJ: SLACK Incorporated; 1996.
2. Machat JJ. LASIK procedure. In: Machat JJ, ed. *Excimer Laser Refractive Surgery.* Thorofare, NJ: SLACK Incorporated; 1996.
3. Gartry DS, Kerr Muir MG, Marshall J. Photorefractive keratectomy with an argon fluoride excimer laser: a clinical study. *J Refract Corneal Surg.* 1991;7:420-435.
4. Talley AR, Hardten DR, Sher NA, et al. Results 1 year after using the 193 nm excimer laser for photorefractive keratectomy in mild to moderate myopia. *Am J Ophthalmol.* 1994;118:304-311.
5. Pop M, Aras M. Multizone/multipass photorefractive keratectomy: 6-month results. *J Cataract Refract Surg.* 1995;21:633-643.
6. Pop M. The multipass/multizone PRK technique to correct myopia and astigmatism. In: Machat JJ, ed. *Excimer Laser Refractive Surgery.* Thorofare, NJ: SLACK Incorporated; 1996.
7. Alpins NA, Taylor HR, Kent DG, Lu Y, et al. Three multizone photorefractive keratectomy algorithms for myopia. *Journal of Refractive Surgery.* 1997;13:535-544.
8. Munnerlyn CR, Koons SJ, Marshall J. Photorefractive keratectomy: a technique for laser refractive surgery. *Journal of Refractive Surgery.* 1988;14:46-52.
9. Emara B, Probst LE, Tingey D, et al. Correlation of intraocular pressure and corneal thickness in normal myopic eyes and following LASIK. *J Cataract Refract Surg.* In press.
10. Probst LE, Machat JJ. The mathematics of LASIK for high myopia. *J Cataract Refract Surg.* In press.
11. Probst LE, Machat JJ. LASIK enhancements techniques and results. In: Buratto L, Brint SF, eds. *LASIK: Principles and Techniques.* Thorofare, NJ: SLACK Incorporated; 1998.

12. Committee on Ophthalmic Procedures Assessment, American Academy of Ophthalmology. Radial keratotomy for myopia. *Ophthalmology.* 1993;100(7):1103-1115.

13. Casebeer JC. A systemized approach to LASIK. In: Buratto L, Brint SF, eds. *LASIK: Principles and Techniques.* Thorofare, NJ: SLACK Incorporated; 1998.

14. Salah T, Waring GO III, Maghraby AE, Moadel K, Grimm SB. Excimer laser in situ keratomileusis under the flap for myopia of 2 to 20 diopters. *Am J Ophthalmol.* 1996;121:143-155.

LASIK Nomograms

Jack T. Holladay, MD

Current excimer laser systems vary widely in the parameters that must be inputted into the system. One parameter that is always necessary is the programmed correction, which is the value that is used to determine the amount of pulses to be used to obtain a specific ablation depth. Unfortunately, analysis of outcomes has shown that there are many other factors that actually determine the refractive effect of the laser. Additional parameters that have been shown to be important in addition to the actual programmed amount include patient characteristics, specific surgical techniques, environmental conditions, laser model, and software version.

Patient characteristics that appear to be important include age, corneal thickness, corneal curvature, corneal astigmatism, and intraocular pressure. Important variations in surgical techniques include the time from flap to ablation, number of times the stroma dried during the ablation, hydration of the flap during the procedure, whether the flap is put down wet or dry, and how it is positioned (ie, painted, compressed, etc). Variations in flap thickness, type of keratome, and position of the hinge (nasal or superior) may all be important. Environmental conditions during the treatment, such as room temperature, humidity, barometric pressure, and elevation with respect to sea level are also important.

As a result of all of these variables, surgeons have developed nomograms that allow them to vary the programmed amount into the laser to achieve the desired refractive outcome. Current nomograms are rudimentary and usually include the patient's refraction and age. These nomograms are usually in the form of a two-dimensional table that shows the percentage the programmed amount should be reduced to get the desired effect in a specific patient. All of these nomograms reduce the programmed amount as the degree of treatment increases and the age of the patient decreases. Typically, these nomograms show as much as a 40% reduction of the programmed amount for a myopic treatment of 10 D in a patient over 65 years of age.

Software programs are now becoming available to the clinician where all of the variables mentioned above are analyzed and the nomogram becomes multifactorial, including as many as 10 variables. The additional variables improve the accuracy of the outcomes and provide patients with better vision and the surgeon with a higher degree of accuracy and confidence. At this time, the importance of each variable is not known, but the early analysis clearly shows that each surgeon should have his own personalized multifactorial nomogram. The number of variables that appear to be important range from five to 10 and their order appears to vary from site to site and surgeon to surgeon. As these nomograms are developed, our understanding of these variables will increase and, most importantly, our patient outcomes will be improved.

THE HANSATOME MICROKERATOME

Lucio Buratto, MD

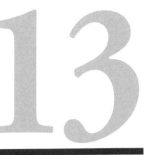

INTRODUCTION

Excimer laser-assisted in-situ keratomileusis, commonly known as LASIK, combines the lamellar surgical techniques of keratomileusis that have been under development for more than 50 years, with the more recently developed technique of photoablating the stroma in the corneal bed with the excimer laser. Myopia, hyperopia, and astigmatism can be treated with the LASIK technique with good to excellent predictability and stability. With constant refinement in the instrumentation and technique, it may be possible to match the predictability of a contact lens refractive correction with this modality by the next decade (refraction of 20/10 by the year 2010).

The Development of LASIK

During the early days of lamellar surgery, the cryolathe corneal tissue freeze and the nonfreeze planar keratomileusis techniques were complex, and the results were not predictable. In search of an improved technique, Luis Ruiz, MD of Bogota, Colombia, discontinued attempts to carve a tissue lenticule and focused on making the refractive correction by removing tissue from the stromal bed. His efforts led to the clinical development of keratomileusis in situ in which the first pass of the microkeratome allowed access to the stromal bed and the second pass removed a plano disc, the thickness of which was related to the power of the correction. Ruiz continued his efforts to improve keratomileusis and, in the late 1980s, developed an automated form of the microkeratome in which the speed and pressure on the eye were constant throughout the keratectomy because of a series of gears that automatically advanced the instrument across the cornea.[1] The instrument became known as the Automated Corneal Shaper (ACS) and the technique was called automated lamellar keratoplasty, or ALK.

With the improved microkeratome, the accuracy of the procedure increased, complications decreased, and the technique began to reach mainstream corneal surgeons. The precision of the second refractive resection, however, was still not of the level demonstrated by the excimer laser on corneal surface ablations. I addressed the disadvantages of the second refractive resection by applying excimer laser ablation to the undersurface of a free corneal cap and performed LASIK (with a free corneal cap) on a sighted human eye in 1989 and published the results in 1992.[2-4] A larger clinical study was published in 1993.[5] In experiments with blind eyes,[6] Ioannis Pallikaris, MD avoided a complete corneal cap resection and instead left the cornea attached by a flap or hinge after the microkeratome pass.

With further developments around the world, LASIK performed with the ACS reduced the risk of postoperative haze and refractive instability problems that accompanied laser corneal surface ablations, had very satisfactory results in procedures for the correction of myopia and myopic astigmatism,[7-35] hyperopia and hyperopic astigmatism,[36,37] retreatment,[38,39] and had a low incidence of complications.[40-44]

OVERVIEW OF THE HANSATOME MICROKERATOME

After input from LASIK surgeons around the world, Bausch & Lomb Surgical redesigned the Automated Corneal Shaper and introduced an easier to use, exceptionally well-built microkeratome called the Hansatome in 1997. The features incorporated into the redesigned model are shown in Table 13-1. The entire unit is now smaller and has fewer moving parts. It makes a superior hinge at the 12 o'clock position; however, a nasal flap can still be made if the surgeon so chooses. The created flap is now larger, averaging 9.5 mm, to provide a larger

Table 13-1

SIGNIFICANT FEATURES OF THE HANSATOME

Feature	Advantage
1. Creates a hinge at 12 o'clock (or at any other desired position)	• Flap realignment is easier • Blinking smooths down the flap • Flap is less likely to dislocate • Patients report less foreign body sensation
2. Creates a 9.5 mm flap (average)	• Larger area aids ablation of hyperopia and astigmatism • Flap is less likely to dislocate
3. Permanent flap thickness plate (160 or 180 µm)	• Reduces the chances of improper assembly
4. Microkeratome head pivots on a pin while cutting (does not feed into tracks)	• Smoother movement • Decreased chance of binding • Maintains a constant and uniform cutting plane
5. Only one gear and no gear track	• Simplifies use and increases durability
6. Nasally positioned, elevated, curved gear rack	• Facilitates unimpeded progression of the head
7. Faster blade oscillation, slower blade passage	• Smooth cutting action
8. Blade and blade holder are one piece	• Simpler assembly
9. Internal, preset stop	• Helps to prevent complete resection
10. Redesigned power supply	• Quiet, high output vacuum • Constant motor speed • Monitor of appropriate vacuum level
11. Back-up power supply	• Allows completion of an in-progress cut in the event of power interruption

ablation zone for the treatment of astigmatism or hyperopia. Flap realignment is easier and the chance of dislocation is decreased with the combination of a larger flap and a superior hinge position. Patients also report less foreign body sensation postoperatively.

The microkeratome head pivots on an upright pin on the suction ring, rather than feeding through tracks, and has only a single rolling gear. The motor is positioned vertically, which enables the microkeratome head to pass over the suction ring on an elevated rack, positioned nasally away from obstructions, such as eyelids, drapes, and the speculum. Loading involves merely dropping the microkeratome head onto the pin on the suction ring. Once on the pin, the head simply swivels up in an arc toward the upper lid and cuts the flap in a constant and uniform cutting plane. A left/right eye adapter that fits over the microkeratome head simplifies right or left eye surgery.

Major safety advances include a fixed and permanent thickness plate and an internal, preset stop mechanism. The redesigned power supply provides quiet, high output vacuum, a constant motor speed, cutting action that cannot be enabled without an appropriate level of vacuum, and termination of cutting if the vacuum level drops. In the event of power interruption, a backup power system allows completion of an in-progress cut.

The AccuGlide (Bausch & Lomb Surgical) disposable blade, with its affixed plastic holder that matches up with the eccentric pin on the motor, allows for convenient insertion. Blade oscillation is faster than that in the ACS and the unit moves more slowly with less resistance over the cornea, both of which aid in making a very smooth cut. This is revealed by the distinctly visible He-Ne beam red reflex dot on the cut surface of the corneal bed, just as is seen with photorefractive keratectomy (PRK)-ablated surfaces. Bleeding is less common since the superior vessels common in contact lens wearers are not cut.

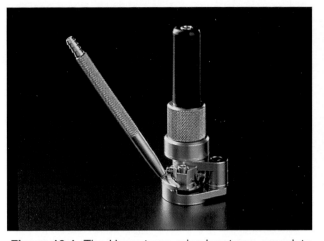

Figure 13-1. The Hansatome microkeratome, complete with suction ring, motor, and head.

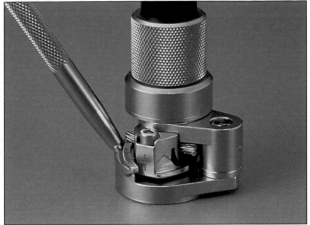

Figure 13-2. Close-up of the Hansatome microkeratome, complete with suction ring, motor, and head.

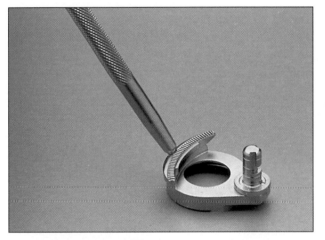
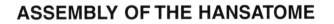

Figure 13-3. The suction ring. The Hansatome head is inserted on the pin on the right and rotates around this pin. The left side has the handle, the toothed, arc-shaped track lower, and a stop mechanism below it. The suction ring plane has no track.

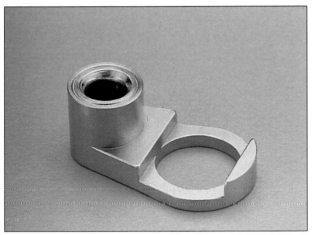

Figure 13-4. The device inserted between the head and motor that allows the motor to rotate in a clockwise direction for left eye surgery or in a counterclockwise direction for right eye surgery.

ASSEMBLY OF THE HANSATOME

Figures 13-1 to 13-8 show the parts of the Hansatome unit. There are three main steps in assembling the Hansatome. First, insert an AccuGlide disposable blade into the microkeratome head, making sure that the blade oscillates freely. Then, position the left/right eye adapter on the microkeratome head, finally, attach the motor.

Powder (talc)-free gloves should be worn during preparation and use of the microkeratome.

Preparing the Hansatome

1. Place the power/suction supply on a firm, level surface. Ensure that the main power switch on the front of the console is in the off position.

2. The receptacle for the main power cord is on the rear panel. Insert the female end of the main power cord firmly into the receptacle. Then, plug the male end of the cord into a properly grounded outlet of the appropriate voltage.

3. Turn on the main power switch on the front of the console and allow the unit to run its internal diagnostic check. The yellow light emitting diode (LED) is illuminated while the vacuum tank is being evacuated. The green LED comes on when the "ready" mode is established.

4. With no suction tubing installed, enter "operate" mode by pressing and releasing the momentary contact vacuum switch on the front panel. Set the desired patient interface vacuum using the regulator knob on the upper left side of the front panel. The reading may fluctuate a bit during the adjust-

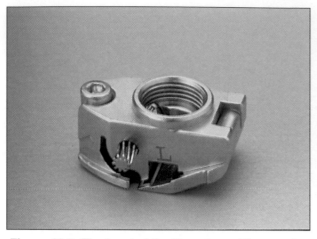

Figure 13-5. The head of the Hansatome. The opening for screwing on the motor is superiorly located. In the center lies a rolling gear that allows for the automatic progression of the motor along the toothed tracks of the suction ring.

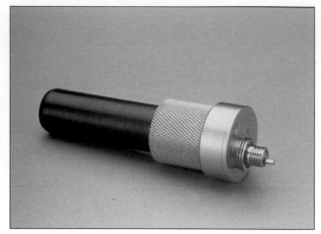

Figure 13-6. The motor of the Hansatome, which screws vertically onto the head of the microkeratome.

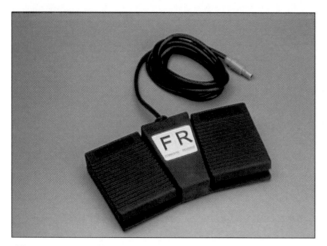

Figure 13-7. The footpedal, showing forward and reverse.

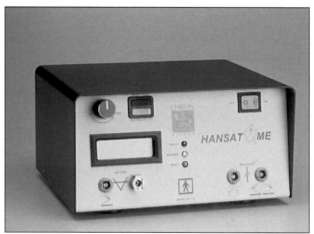

Figure 13-8. The Hansatome power supply.

ment period. To get the most accurate setting, allow several seconds for the regulator to settle as the knob is rotated.

5. Exit "operate" mode and return to "ready" mode by pressing and releasing the momentary contact vacuum switch.

6. Attach the single pedal vacuum footswitch by latching its cable connector into the appropriate port on the lower left side of the front of the panel.

7. Attach the dual motor footswitch by latching its cable connector into the appropriate port on the lower right side of the front of the panel.

8. Attach the motor/power cord by latching its cable connector into the appropriate port on the lower right side of the front panel.

9. Attach the suction tubing by depressing the suction receptacle latch on the front panel and firmly inserting the tubing connector until a positive latch is achieved. Important: if the tubing connector is not fully latched, the vacuum pump will remain occluded, and no suction will be available at the end of the tubing.

10. While both hands are free, remove the protective cap from the Hansatome motor, so it is ready to later screw the motor into the motor port of the head.

11. Remove the appropriate Hansatome head from the instrument tray. Using your thumb and forefinger, spin the rolling gear back and forth to confirm smooth movement. If the gear will not spin absolutely free of resistance, repeat the cleaning process.

12. Inspect the head to ensure that it is perfectly clean and that there is no residual debris that would inhibit the performance of the head. If residual debris is found, repeat the cleaning process.

13. Insert the AccuGlide single-use blade according to the instructions provided in each package.

14. Confirm that the blade and holder move smoothly back and forth within the cavity. If the blade does not move absolutely free of resistance, remove it and try another. If it still does not move free of resistance, remove the blade and repeat the cleaning process for the head.

15. Once the AccuGlide blade has been successfully inserted into the Hansatome head, ensure that it is centered within the cavity.

16. Carefully place the left/right eye adapter over the motor port on top of the head to correspond with the eye to be treated.

17. When preparing the device for surgery on a right eye, the adapter will effectively cover the "L" that is stamped on the head (for left), leaving the "R" (for right) in full view and indicating that the device is configured for a right-eye surgery.

18. When preparing the device for surgery on a left eye, the adapter will effectively cover the "R" that is stamped on the head (for right), leaving the "L" (for left) in full view and indicating that the device is configured for left-eye surgery.

19. The blade holder drive slot should be visible in the centered position of the motor port of the head. Remove the protective cap from the Hansatome motor and screw the motor into the motor port until it is firmly attached. Important: Push on each side edge of the blade to ensure that the blade-handling pin has engaged the blade holder slot.

20. Insert the power plug of the motor/power cord into the jack on top of the motor. Instill one drop of proparacaine into the blade cavity and run the motor in each direction for about 5 seconds. When the blade is driven, the LED should indicate an average motor current of less than 150 ma and there should be no audible or visual warnings. Visually confirm that the blade is oscillating.

   If the current exceeds 150 ma, the most likely cause is grit left in the head from inadequate cleaning. Simple dry brushing the slot often removes this grit and reduces the current to a normal level. If the blade drive pin has not been latched into the drive slot of the blade holder, the blade will not oscillate, leading to possible patient injury. Dry brush the drive end of the motor gearbox, including the drive pin and worm gear, with a dry medium-bristled toothbrush.

21. If the LED reading indicates current greater than 150 ma, the cause of excessive motor current must be resolved and corrected prior to surgical use of the device. Ordinarily, the cause is a faulty blade or unclean head. To diagnose, unscrew the motor from the head. Run the removed motor forward and backward; the current should be 35 to 55 ma. If it is higher, the motor, gearbox, or both may be at fault and service is needed. If it is normal, the problem may be with the head or blade. Cleaning of the head and/or replacing the blade should solve the problem.

22. You can proceed only if the green LED is on and normal current has been verified in a test pass. Carefully place the assembled head down, maintaining sterility and avoiding any contact with the exposed cutting edge of the blade.

23. Take the suction ring and the suction handle from the instrument tray, screw the handle onto the suction port of the suction ring until it is snug, then place the suction tubing firmly over the end of the suction handle.

24. Place the assembled Hansatome head onto the suction ring by guiding the left/right eye adapter over the pivot post of the suction ring. Align the head over the approximate starting position appropriate to the selected eye, left or right. This will allow the head/adapter assembly to drop down all the way on to the pivot post. Move the rolling gear up to the first-gear tooth of the track.

25. While lightly supporting the motor, press the forward pedal (labeled "F") of the motor footswitch to start the head across the ring. In normal operation, the head will automatically stop with two audible beeps when it has reached the mechanical stop, and the motor current will drop to zero. If this does not happen, contact your service representative. If beeps are heard and the current drops to zero at the end of the forward pass, depress the reverse pedal (labeled "R") of the motor footswitch to reverse the head back off the ring.

26. If during the forward or reverse motion the yellow LED flashes or there is an audible beep, a problem exists that must be cleared prior to surgery. The problem could be dirt or grit in the head, an obstruction in the gear rack, or a damaged spot in the gear rack.

27. Important: You may proceed with surgery only if there was no flash of the yellow LED, no audible beep, and the green LED is on. Carefully remove the head from the suction ring and place both

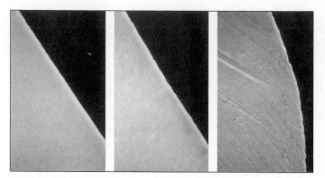

Figure 13-9. AccuGlide blade, 200x SEM micrograph. From left to right: middle, end, and corner regions show smooth blade surface.

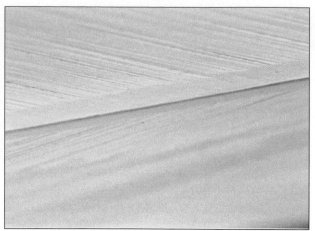

Figure 13-10. AccuGlide blade, SEM micrograph. Close-up of the cutting edge.

components down, maintaining sterility and avoiding any contact with the exposed cutting edge of the blade.

28. If the assembly and functional tests have been successfully completed and passed, the Hansatome is ready for use in a surgical procedure.

29. The Hansatome mechanical components must be cleaned immediately and thoroughly after each use. Consult your user's manual for complete cleaning and sterilizing instructions.

ACCUGLIDE BLADES

An independent third-party laboratory conducted tests evaluating the quality of microkeratome blades made by Bausch & Lomb Surgical, as well as those from several other manufacturers. Images through a scanning electron microscope (SEM) at 200x magnification are shown in Figures 13-9 to 13-17.

USER RECOMMENDATIONS FOR HANSATOME OPERATION

Since its introduction by Chiron Vision in October 1997, the Hansatome microkeratome has become widely accepted as the new gold standard. As with any precision device, there is a learning curve and period of adjustment. The following are suggestions and explanations that resulted from user feedback.

"No Salt Diet"

Salt is the worst enemy of the microkeratome motor/gearbox. Salt causes electrolytic corrosion, and, when precipitated, causes jamming of the rotating shaft. You can effectively eliminate these problems by using a technique that keeps all balanced salt solution (BSS) away from the microkeratome head and, hence, away

from the motor/gearbox. This applies to both the Hansatome and ACS. Any BSS used pre-keratectomy should be removed prior to the keratectomy. Irrigation and lubrication of the cornea in preparation for the cut may effectively be done with anesthetic drops, as described below. BSS may be used after the keratectomy, as usual. The tip of the motor must be stored with the tip down to insure that no liquid flows from the tip back into the gears and bearings of the gearbox.

Stephen Slade, MD, of Houston, Texas, offers the following, "Never let your keratome come in contact with balanced salt solution. We use proparacaine to moisten and irrigate the eye before the cut. Proparacaine has no salts, which are corrosive, but is pH balanced and contains glycerin, an excellent lubricant. After the keratome has been removed from the field, use balanced salt solution as usual. If you need to irrigate the keratome between surgeries on a bilateral case, use sterile water or proparacaine."

Blade Test

Occasionally, you may encounter a tight-fitting blade. If you electrically run a single tight blade in your microkeratome, you run the risk of galling the metal of your microkeratome head. Once galled, you will find that all blades are too tight in the damaged head, and factory service of the head will be required. Each blade should be tested in your microkeratome head prior to any electrical running. With the blade held on the blade insertion tool, manually slide the blade back and forth in the slot. If you feel resistance within the head, reject the blade. Ideally, the blade should fall out the end of the slot opposite the end of insertion under the influence of gravity alone or, at most, with a very light tap. If the blade does not pass this test, reject it. Bausch & Lomb Surgical will

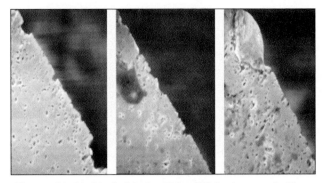

Figure 13-11. Moria blade, 200x SEM micrograph. From left to right: middle, end, and corner regions.

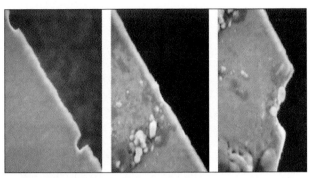

Figure 13-12. Canadian laserblade, 200x SEM micrograph. From left to right: middle, end, and corner regions.

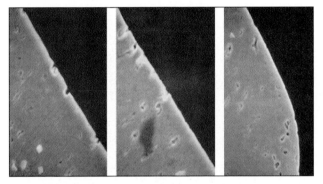

Figure 13-13. Med-Logics blade, 200x SEM micrograph. From left to right: middle, end, and corner regions.

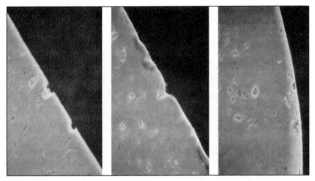

Figure 13-14. Visicare blade, 200x SEM micrograph. From left to right: middle, end, and corner regions.

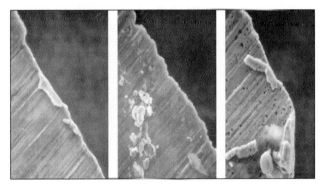

Figure 13-15. Oasis blade, 200x SEM micrograph. From left to right: middle, end, and corner regions.

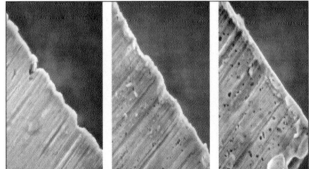

Figure 13-16. MICRO Specialties blade, 200x SEM micrograph. From left to right: middle, end, and corner regions.

exchange any AccuGlide blade that does not pass this test. Do not electrically run a dry blade in the microkeratome head for more than a few seconds at a time. Extended dry running may eventually lead to galling of the head.

Motor/Gearbox Test: Head Not Connected

Prior to attachment of the head, electrically run the motor forward and reverse. With the motor at room tem-

perature, the current should be between 15 to 30 ma. If the motor current is over 50 ma, there is a fault that must be resolved prior to surgery.

Motor/Gearbox Test: Head Connected

After verifying normal motor current, screw the motor gearbox into the head. The motor/powercord must be unplugged when turning the motor or you risk breaking the wires at the plug from repeated twisting of the cord. Tighten the motor lightly until it is "finger tight." Forced tightening may cause damage and require factory service.

Moisten and lubricate the blade by placing a few drops of proparacaine or other glycerin-containing anesthetic directly into the blade slot prior to running the blade with electrical power. Lubrication with proparacaine (or even sterile distilled water as a second choice) will generally prevent galling.

Run the blade electrically for a few seconds in forward and reverse. The motor current should indicate 50 to 80 ma. If it is over 100 ma, there is a fault that must be resolved prior to surgery.

"Warning Motor 40" Message

This indicates a motor current of over 200 ma. It is accompanied by a flash of the yellow LED and an audible beep. You should never see this warning during a cut or retraction because the motor current should be less than 100 ma during these motions. The usual cause is salt crystals impacted between the inner spinning shaft and the bearing.

Test Pass

Make the test pass with the head connected to the suction ring. The motor current should be approximately the same as in the immediately previous test. If not, there is a fault that must be resolved prior to surgery.

Cleaning the Motor Tip with Anhydrous Isopropyl Alcohol

Prior to storage at the end of each surgical day, the distal 2.0 to 3.0 mm of the motor/gearbox should be dipped in anhydrous (or 99%) isopropyl alcohol and the motor electrically driven forward and reverse for 15 to 30 seconds. Then remove the tip from the alcohol and blot on a lint and fiber-free Merocel wipe. Always compress the eccentric drive pin to help force out any liquid from behind it. If there is any discoloration on the sponge, repeat the process until the discoloration no longer appears. Continue to run the motor with the tip down for 1 minute. The motor must be stored with the tip down, which will allow any residual liquid alcohol to drip out and for the rest to evaporate.

This alcohol cleaning procedure can often be used to dissolve and remove crystalline salt and other debris from around the inner spinning shaft, which may resolve a motor overcurrent problem.

Avoid Lint and Fiber

Lint and fiber are enemies of the microkeratome. A fine piece of lint in the head has been known to come between a blade and the running surface, causing the

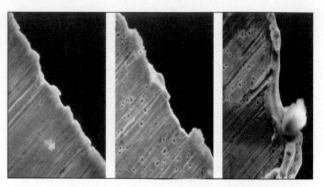

Figure 13-17. B. Graezyk blade, 200x SEM micrograph. From left to right: middle, end, and corner regions.

head to jam during a test pass. This kind of jam could easily gall a microkeratome head. Fiber has also been known to stick to a blade drive pin, jamming the it in its knife drive gear hole. Dry brushing the tip and threads of the motor should remove any existing lint or fibers. The motor tip should be wiped only with a lint and fiber-free Merocel wipe or spear.

Galling

Galling is caused by frictional hot spots from rubbing metal against metal under certain combinations of time, pressure, lack of sufficient lubrication, and speed. It could easily occur from electrically driving an improperly fitting blade. In such a case, the motor current would be above normal. Upon removal from the head, a score mark would probably be seen on the blade, and there would be a raised rough spot in an otherwise smooth and polished surface on the interior surface of the head. Thereafter, this raised rough spot would bind against perfectly good blades, scoring them in the same place as seen on the original blade. Lubrication of the blade, even with sterile distilled water, tends to minimize the frictional heating effect that causes galling. Once galled, a microkeratome head must be factory serviced to polish out the mark.

Handling a Jam During Surgery

A microkeratome that jams during surgery must be carefully managed to avoid patient injury. First, determine by visual references whether the microkeratome has traveled all the way to the mechanical stop. If not, and suction has not been broken; depress the forward pedal one or more times in an attempt to complete the flap. Never go forward/reverse/forward as that would risk transecting the flap. Once the end of the forward pass is reached, depress the reverse pedal. If the head does not immediately reverse, redepress the reverse pedal up to 10 times in succession. If that fails, release suction and carefully slide the assembled microkeratome inferiorly at a shallow angle and allow the flap to slide out of the microkeratome.

Then, away from the patient, retract the head as follows. Unscrew the motor from the head by a few degrees, no more. Apply reverse electric power. In practically all cases, the head will immediately retract. If not, try soaking the assembled motor and head in a shallow dish of isopropyl alcohol to a level no more than 3.0 mm above the bottom of the microkeratome head, and apply reverse electric power. If that does not work, repeat with the dish of alcohol in a running ultrasonic cleaner. In the extremely unlikely case that this does not work, do not continue to unscrew the motor. Instead, contact Bausch & Lomb Surgical customer service for advice. The factory can retract the head without destroying the gear rack.

Power/Suction Supply Electronic Update

In order to provide added protection against the possibility of a jam at the stopper or midcut, a change has been introduced that is now routinely applied to the Hansatome microkeratome power/suction supply when it is returned to the factory for routine cleaning, check-up, or repair. The effects of the change are as follows:

1. The overall motor current limit is increased from 400 ma to 500 ma.
2. Anytime the motor forward pedal is depressed, the full 500 ma of motor current is available for starting the motor and for overcoming isolated obstacles for 0.12 seconds after depression. Prior to the change, 400 ma was available for 3 seconds. As before, unlimited redepressions of the forward pedal can be used to overcome obstacles. The change provides the availability of a higher motor current in short impulses. The full 500 ma of motor current is available at all times when the motor reverse pedal is depressed. Prior to the change, 400 ma was available.
3. After the initial 0.12 seconds of depression of the motor forward pedal, 375 ma of motor current is available. If the motor current reaches 375 ma at any point in forward motion after that time, the motor will instantly stop and be dynamically braked. This is normal when the head reaches the stop at the completion of the forward cut. If the head is obstructed by an obstacle midcut, which causes the motor current to rise to 375 ma, the head will instantly stop, as if the stop had been reached. The normal motor current during the forward cut is 100 ma or less in properly maintained and functioning equipment. If the motor current rises to 375 ma midcut, a very serious problem exists that must be resolved prior to con-

tinued use of the equipment. It might be possible to get past the obstruction by redepression of the motor forward pedal one or more times, utilizing the high power of the resultant 0.12-second, 500-ma motor current impulses. More likely, this situation would probably require aborting the cut and following proper medical procedure for management of the complication of a partial flap.

Warning: Both prior to the change and after the change, the user should not redepress the motor forward pedal when already at the stop. If done repeatedly, this will cause undue wear on the worm and worm gear, possibly leading to wear that would require factory service. The user should always confirm full completion of the forward cut by visual landmarks and never redepress the motor forward pedal "just to be sure." Redepression of the motor forward pedal when already at the stop will generally cause a jam at the stop. Recovery from such a jam is the same as before the change. Every user must be trained in the correct method of recovery from jams in order to reduce potential patient injury and avoid serious equipment damage.

Setting the Vacuum Regulator

The Hansatome microkeratome is normally shipped with the patient-relative vacuum set at about 26 inches (in) Hg and the mark on the knob at 12 o'clock. This is the most commonly used setting at sea level, where in round figures barometric pressure is 30 in Hg. In general, the equipment will not permit operation if the patient-relative vacuum is set below 20 in Hg. The user should initially set the vacuum at about 4 in Hg below the barometric pressure indicated on the display. At sea level, this would be 26 in Hg. At higher altitudes, the value would be about 1 inch less for each 1000 feet of altitude. The vacuum level can be increased by as much as about 2 in Hg (about 1 full clockwise turn of the regulator knob) from this starting point, but at the expense of increased time lag for vacuum stabilization at entry to "operate" mode.

To increase vacuum, attach the suction tube/trap to the front panel and pinch the tubing shut at its end. Press down on the vacuum pedal and hold for a few seconds. The current patient-relative vacuum setting is displayed. Upon release of the vacuum pedal, count the number of beeps until the display shows "operate" and the green LED comes on. The average number of beeps should be four or five, which represents approximately 5 seconds. Operate the vacuum foot pedal again to exit "operate" back to "ready." The user can then turn the regulator knob clockwise about one-eighth of a turn in each trial and repeat the above test, observing the increase in beep count each time. A beep count in excess of 10 is not recommended. If the regulator knob is set too high, the beeping will continue for 30 seconds without the green LED coming on. Instead, the red LED will come on and an error message will be displayed.

By way of example, at 5500 feet altitude, the barometric pressure would be only 24.5 in Hg, a patient-relative vacuum of about 22.5 mm Hg would be achievable, and the beep count would probably be about 10. At such a high altitude, the user would probably elect the higher vacuum level, even at the expense of the longer time lag to get to "operate."

Soft Eye

In the event of a soft eye (as indicated by tonometry), the patient vacuum may be increased after entry to "operate" mode by rotating the regulator knob one full turn clockwise. That may or may not provide enough increase in patient-relative vacuum to achieve the requisite IOP to complete the case. If the tonometry reading remains questionable, do not proceed with the keratectomy. The user must remember to restore the regulator knob back the one full turn counterclockwise and recheck the patient vacuum setting before the next procedure. Failure to do so would lead to 30 seconds of beeping, following by the red LED going on, and an error message upon attempt to re-enter "operate" for the next procedure.

Cases of soft eye should generally not be treated other than at near sea level, where maximum barometric pressure is available and maximum patient-relative vacuum is thus available.

"Pump Hot" Message

This message indicates that a computer algorithm has calculated that the pump is beginning to get warm; it does not indicate equipment failure. The user is advised to complete the current case and give the equipment time to cool down with the pump not running. If the user continues use, ignoring the warning message, the pump will eventually shut itself off. In this event, the vacuum reservoir will maintain the vacuum level so that the cut can be completed in the same manner as in a power failure episode. This message will disappear if the Hansatome is left to cool down with power on and in "ready" mode. If the power/suction supply is off while the "pump hot" message is displayed, then turned back on at a later time, the "pump hot" message will again be displayed as the unit "remembers" the last display on the console. The message will eventually disappear if the unit is left on in "ready" mode. To quickly clear the message, turn the power switch off and on 10 times.

Nonrechargeable Lithium Batteries

The Hansatome microkeratome uses nonrechargeable lithium batteries for back-up, which should have enough energy and shelf life to last 10 or more years. In the event of a power failure while in "operate" mode, the batteries are used to power the microkeratome and electronics. You must exit "operate" mode, as at the end of any normal operation by pressing the vacuum pedal to promptly disconnect and preserve the batteries. Otherwise, the electronics will continue to run powered by the lithium batteries and, in less than about 30 minutes, the battery energy will be depleted to the point that the system will not permit use. Factory replacement of the batteries will be required.

CLINICAL PEARLS FROM GLOBAL REFRACTIVE SPECIALISTS

- When loading the microkeratome onto the suction ring post, it is often necessary to press down on the motor to slightly compress the cornea and thereby fully seat the left/right eye adapter before attempting engagement of the rolling gear to the gear rack. It is convenient to have the assistant visually verify closure of any gap beneath the left/right eye adapter. Also, it is often helpful to slightly tip the ring superiorly.
- Understand and visualize the endpoint of the forward pass so as not to rely solely on hearing the beep which indicates that the endpoint has been reached.
- With difficult anatomy (eg, prominent zygomatic bone), have the assistant retract the lower cheek tissue inferiorly.
- Between surgeries on a bilateral case, use a syringe to force sterile distilled water into the motor entry port of the microkeratome head. This should force out any epithelial or stromal matter left from the first eye.
- To effectively clean debris out of the microkeratome head when brushing alone was ineffective, apply Palmolive cleaning solution directly onto a blade and electrically run it in the microkeratome head.

REFERENCES

1. Ruiz L, Rowsey J. In situ keratomileusis. *Invest Ophthalmol Vis Sci.* 1988;29(suppl):392.
2. Buratto L, Ferrari M, Genisi C. Intrastromal keratomileusis

by excimer laser (193 nm): clinical results with 1-year follow-up. Presented at First Annual Congress of the Summit International Laser User Group. Geneva, Switzerland; September 1991.

3. Buratto L, Ferrari M, Rama P. Excimer laser intrastromal keratomileusis. *Am J Ophthalmol.* 1992;113:291-295.

4. Buratto L, Ferrari M. Excimer laser intrastromal keratomileusis: case reports. *J Cataract Refract Surg.* 1992;18:37-41.

5. Buratto L, Ferrari M, Genisi C. Myopic keratomileusis with the excimer laser: 1-year follow-up. *J Refract Corneal Surg.* 1993;9:12-19.

6. Pallikaris IG, Papatzanaki ME, Siganos DS, Tsilimbaris MK. A corneal flap technique for laser in situ keratomileusis. *Arch Ophthalmol.* 1991;109:1699-1702.

7. Brint SF, Ostrick DM, Fisher C, et al. Six-month results of the multicenter phase I study of excimer laser myopic keratomileusis. *J Cataract Refract Surg.* 1994;20:610-615.

8. Salah T, Waring GO, El-Maghraby A. Excimer laser keratomileusis in the corneal bed under a hinged flap: results in Saudi Arabia at the El-Maghraby Eye Hospital. In: Salz JJ, McDonnell PJ, McDonald MB, eds. *Corneal Laser Surgery.* St. Louis. Mo: Mosby-Year Book; 1995.

9. Ruiz LA, Slade SG, Updegraff SA, Doane JF, Moreno ML, Murcia A. Excimer myopic keratomileusis: Bogota experience. In: Salz JJ, McDonnell PJ, McDonald MB, eds. *Corneal Laser Surgery.* St. Louis, Mo: Mosby-Year Book; 1995.

10. Bas AM, Onnis R. Excimer laser in situ keratomileusis for myopia. *Journal of Refractive Surgery.* 1995;11(suppl): S229-S233.

11. Fiander DC, Tayfour F. Excimer laser in situ keratomileusis in 124 myopic eyes. *Journal of Refractive Surgery.* 1995;11(suppl):S234-S238.

12. Kremer FB, Dufek M. Excimer laser in situ keratomileusis. *Journal of Refractive Surgery.* 1995;11(suppl):S244-S247.

13. Kim H-M, Jung HR. Laser assisted in-situ keratomileusis for high myopia. *Ophthalmic Surgery and Lasers.* 1996;27(suppl):S508-511.

14. Knorz MC, Lierman A, Seiberth V, et al. Laser in-situ keratomileusis to correct myopia of -6.00 to -29.00 diopters. *Journal of Refractive Surgery.* 1996;12:575-584.

15. Buratto L. Down-up LASIK. Presented at the IOMSG Congress. Tangensee; September 2, 1996.

16. Buratto L. Down-up LASIK. Presented at ISRK Pre-American Academy of Ophthalmology Conference. Chicago, Ill; October 24-26, 1996.

17. Buratto L. Down-up LASIK is latest chapter in development of lamellar refractive surgery. *Ocular Surgery News.* 1996;22-23.

18. Arenas E, Maglione A. Laser in situ keratomileusis for astigmatism and myopia after penetrating keratoplasty. *Journal of Refractive Surgery.* 1997;13;27-32.

19. Perz-Santonja JJ, Bellot J, Claramonte P, et al. Laser in situ keratomileusis to correct high myopia. *J Catract Refract Surg.* 1997;23:372-385.

20. Güell JL, Muller A. Laser in-situ keratomileusis (LASIK) for myopia from -7 to -18 diopters. *Journal of Refractive Surgery.* 1996;12:222-228.

21. Marinho A, Pinto MC, Pinto R, et al. LASIK for high myopia: 1-year experience. *Ophthalmic Surgery and Lasers.* 1996; 27(suppl):S517-S520.

22. Salah T, Waring GO III, El-Maghraby A, et al. Excimer laser in situ keratomileusis under a corneal flap for myopia of 2 to 20 diopters. *Am J Ophthalmol.* 1996;121:143-155.

23. Condon PI, Mulhern M, Fulcher T, et al. Laser intrastromal keratomileusis for high myopia and myopic astigmatism. *Br J Ophthalmol.* 1997;81:199-206.

24. Blanckaert J, Sallet G. LASIK learning curve: clinical study of 300 myopic eyes. *Bull Soc Belge Ophtalmol.* 1998;268:7-12.

25. Hersh PS, Brint SF, Maloney RK, et al. Photorefractive keratectomy versus laser in situ keratomileusis for moderate to high myopia. a randomized prospective study. *Ophthalmology.* 1998;105:1512-22.

26. Farah SG, Azar DT, Gurdal C, Wong J. Laser in situ keratomileusis: literature review of a developing technique. *J Cataract Refract Surg.* 1998;24:989-1006.

27. Dulaney DD, Barnet RW, Perkins SA, Kezirian GM. Laser in situ keratomileusis for myopia and astigmatism: 6-month results. *J Cataract Refract Surg.* 1998;24:758-64.

28. Knorz MC, Wiesinger B, Liermann A, Seiberth V, Liesenhoff H. Laser in situ keratomileusis for moderate and high myopia and myopic astigmatism. *Ophthalmology.* 1998;105:932-40.

29. Lavery F. Laser in situ keratomileusis for myopia. *Journal of Refractive Surgery.* 1998;14(2suppl):S177-8.

30. Chayet AS, Magallanes R, Montes M;,Chavez S, Robledo N. Laser in situ keratomileusis for simple myopic, mixed, and simple hyperopic astigmatism. *Journal of Refractive Surgery.* 1998;14(2suppl):S175-6.

31. Waring GO III; Carr JD, Stulting RD, Thompson KP, Wiley WM. Prospective randomized comparison of simultaneous and sequential bilateral laser in situ keratomileusis for the correction of myopia. *Ophthalmology.* 1999;106:732-8.

32. Montes M, Chayet A, Gomez L, Magallanes R, Robledo N. Laser in situ keratomileusis for myopia of -1.50 to -6.00 diopters. *Journal of Refractive Surgery.* 1999;15:106-10.

33. Forseto AS, Francesconi CM, Nose RA, Nose W. Laser in situ keratomileusis to correct refractive errors after keratoplasty. *J Cataract Refract Surg.* 1999;25:479-85.

34. El-Maghraby A, Salah T, Waring GO III, Klyce S, Ibrahim O. Randomized bilateral comparison of excimer laser in situ keratomileusis and photorefractive keratectomy for 2.50 to 8.00 diopters of myopia. *Ophthalmology.* 1999;106:447-57.

35. el Danasoury MA, el Maghraby A, Klyce SD, Mehrez K. Comparison of photorefractive keratectomy with excimer laser in situ keratomileusis in correcting low myopia (from -2.00 to -5.50 diopters). A randomized study. *Ophthalmology.* 1999;106:411-20.

36. Argento CJ, Cosentino MJ. Laser in situ keratomileusis for hyperopia. *J Cataract Refract Surg.* 1998;24:1050-8.

37. Ibrahim O. Laser in situ keratomileusis for hyperopia and

hyperopic astigmatism. *Journal of Refractive Surgery.* 1998;14(2suppl):S179-82.

38. Perez-Santonja JJ, Ayala MJ, Sakla HF, Ruiz-Moreno JM, Alio JL. Retreatment after laser in situ keratomileusis. *Ophthalmology.* 1999;106:21-8.

39. Durrie DS, Aziz A. Lift-flap retreatment after laser in situ keratomileusis. *Journal of Refractive Surgery.* 1999;15:150-3.

40. Davidorf JM, Zaldivar R, Oscherow S. Results and complications of laser in situ keratomileusis by experienced surgeons. *Journal of Refractive Surgery.* 1998;14:114-22.

41. Wilson SE. LASIK: management of common complications. Laser in situ keratomileusis. *Cornea.* 1998;17:459-67.

42. Perez-Santonja JJ, Sakla HF, Cardona C, Ruiz-Moreno JM, Alio JL. Subclinical inflammation after laser in situ keratomileusis. *J Cataract Refract Surg.* 1998;24:1059-63.

43. Gimbel HV, Penno EE, van Westenbrugge JA, Ferensowicz M, Furlong MT. Incidence and management of intraoperative and early postoperative complications in 1000 consecutive laser in situ keratomileusis cases. *Ophthalmology.* 1998;105:1839-47.

44. Stulting RD, Carr JD, Thompson KP, Waring GO III, Wiley WM, Walker JG. Complications of laser in situ keratomileusis for the correction of myopia. *Ophthalmology.* 1999;106:13-20.

THE HANSATOME FOR LASIK WITH NO FLAP COMPLICATIONS

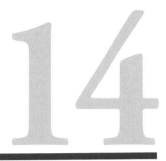

Dan Durrie, MD

INTRODUCTION

In July 1998, we began a study of our experience with LASIK procedures performed with the Hansatome and a standardized surgical technique for the correction of myopia, hyperopia, and astigmatism. Eleven surgeons from the Hunkeler Eye Centers in the Kansas City region, whose experience in microkeratome surgery ranged from high (Durrie and Cavanaugh) to those who were performing their first refractive surgery cases, participated in the study. The total of 5192 consecutive cases included every doctor's first experience with this technique.

METHODS

Overall Surgical Methodology

All surgeries were performed in a standard ambulatory surgery center, and all of the surgeons used the same standardized surgical technique (Table 14-1). Standardization is very helpful for technicians because they do not have to memorize a different technique for each of the 11 doctors. Surgeons were encouraged to use the same words in the operating room, such as "suction on" and "suction off," to eliminate staff confusion, which can lead to errors. We also monitored our results with outcome analysis to continuously improve our technique.

We used gloves and masks, but not gowns, and followed standard surgical sterilization procedures, with autoclaving and instrument cleaning between cases, as we do for cataract or other intraocular surgery. We treated each eye as a separate surgical event, using one blade and resterilizing the equipment every time. We performed surgery on one eye, had the patient leave the operating room, performed the 1-hour postoperative exam, and then had the patient return for surgery on the

second eye. The 1-hour delay was mainly for the safety of the patient.

Equipment

The flap was made using the Hansatome microkeratome and the 180-μm head only. Flaps created on eye bank and patient eyes with the 180-μm head actually measured 150 to 160 μm in thickness; thus, the 160-μm plate was not used. We used an 8.5 mm suction ring for myopia surgeries, except in cases of poor centration, and the 9.5 mm ring for hyperopia surgeries. Standard Bausch & Lomb AccuGlide blades were inserted into the microkeratome head and carefully tested before each surgery. Excimer lasers used at our center included the Apex Plus (Summit Technologies, Waltham, Mass, USA), Nidek EC-5000 (Nidek, Gamagori, Japan), and Technolas 217 (Bausch & Lomb Surgical, Claremont, Calif, USA).

Initially, central corneal thickness measurements were made by ultrasonic pachymetry, and a drop of tetracaine was applied prior to the measurement. The pachymetry readings were carefully performed to avoid causing corneal abrasions. Later in the study, the Orbscan optical diagnostic system was used for central pachymetry readings. This device evaluates the whole cornea, showing not only the anterior curvature, but also the anterior and posterior elevation and full pachymetry. However, it is important to note that the Orbscan measures tear film, epithelium, and endothelium, and thus produces a value 10% thicker than one obtained by ultrasound pachymetry. A default in the Orbscan can be set to account for this.

Performing the Surgery

An anesthetic drop was applied before the patient preparation, and the patient's eye was swabbed with Betadine. The technicians tested the blade and equipment as part of the preparation, but the surgeon always retested the equipment. We consider careful assembly and testing of the microkeratome to be the surgeon's responsibility, not the technician's. On several occasions, a blade or suction problem was detected at this stage and problems during surgery were thus avoided. Checking blade movement is important because the Hansatome can be fully assembled and not have any blade movement, and this will not be detected on other tests. Surgeon visualization is important to keep a non-moving blade from coming across the corneal surface. Surgeons also checked the suction by occluding the suction port and not the tubing. If a surgeon's thumb was not large enough to occlude the port, the palm of the hand was used.

Excess Betadine was then removed and the lashes were dried to allow the drapes to adhere. Steristrips were used to retract the upper lid lashes and evert the lower eyelids. A split 3M 1020 drape was used to hold the eyelashes out of the way. Care was taken to completely isolate the eyelashes, both in the upper eyelid and lower eyelid, without any wrinkles or folds in the drape. With the Hansatome, the most important part of the draping is on the lower lid.

A Merocel donut sponge was placed on the cornea and another drop of tetracaine was placed on the corneal surface. This sponge holds the anesthetic around the limbus and attracts oils and debris in the tear film to produce a cleaner surgical field. We attempted to minimize the number of anesthetic eyedrops, using a maximum of three. When pachymetry was done with the Orbscan, the first drop was not needed and only two were used (Figure 14-1).

The patient was carefully positioned under the laser. With a fixed or movable bed, the patient's feet, shoulders, and head should be aligned, especially when performing toric ablations. The chart should be available to allow the surgeon to check the numbers entered into the laser. Our charts were organized so that the patient's spectacle correction and manifest and cycloplegic refractions, surgical plan, and repeat manifest refractions were available on one sheet of paper. We taped the patient's topography on the laser so that the axis of ablation could be checked and the patient's name verified. I call the patient by his or her first name as a double-check. We used a standardized surgical form in the surgery center office and with the comanaging doctors. As previously mentioned, these forms have the patient's presurgery spectacle prescription, manifest, cycloplegic, and the repeat manifest refraction all on one sheet of paper, as well as the surgical plan.

While removing the Merocel sponge, we wiped it across the cornea to pick up excess oils in the tear film.

Table 14-1

STUDY METHODS
- Surgery performed in an ambulatory surgical center
- Standardized surgical technique
- One eye per surgery
- Second eye surgery 1 hour later after ocular examination of first eye
- New blade and resterilized equipment for each eye
- Hansatome microkeratome
  - 180-µm head
  - 8.5 mm suction ring for myopia, 9.5 mm for hyperopia
- AccuGlide blades
- Excimer lasers
  - Technolas 217
  - Summit Apex Plus
  - Nidek EC-5000

Then the cul-de-sac and cornea were dried with another Merocel sponge. This was done rapidly so that the cornea would not dry out, which could cause trauma to the epithelium. A rose bengal radial keratotomy (RK) marker was placed to make eight symmetrical marks on the cornea, slightly off-center to the pupil (Figure 14-2). Rose bengal was used instead of the usual gentian violet because it is less toxic and gives much finer marks for later flap alignment.

The suction ring was placed on the eye, and once the cornea was well-applanated, the surgeon asked for "suction on." The pressure was then checked on the console by the technician. For good centration, equal pressure should be placed on the handle and a second finger should be placed on the temporal part of the suction ring (Figure 14-3). Centration should now be checked and, if it is adequate, the procedure can proceed. If the centration is decentered, suction should be immediately released. It can then be retried with the same 8.5 mm ring, but if decentration is significant, I usually switch immediately to the 9.5 mm ring. The Hansatome can be reapplied and does not go back into the same groove, as the Automated Corneal Shaper unit used to do.

The pressure was checked with a Barraquer tonometer, and the cornea was wiped with a saturated Merocel sponge. Before proceeding, it is important to check the pathway from the microkeratome and be sure the drape and speculum are out of the way. If the speculum is in the way of the blade, reposition it before proceeding. I used a custom-made wire speculum by Storz, which provides adequate room and prevents the microkeratome blade from hitting the speculum. If the drape is in the way, there are three options: First, gently push the drape down just below the suction ring and then tilt the suction

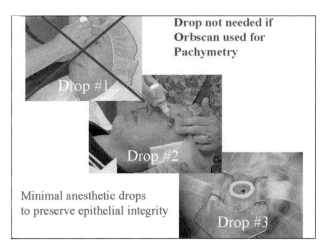

Figure 14-1. No more than three anesthetic drops should be used to preserve epithelial integrity. If pachymetry is performed with the Orbscan instead of ultrasound, the first drop is not needed.

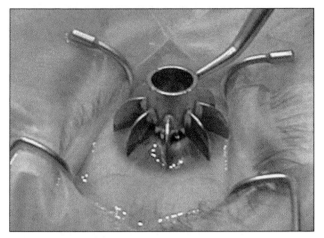

Figure 14-2. A radial keratotomy marker dipped in rose bengal stain is placed slightly off center to the pupil. Make eight symmetrical marks on the cornea to help with alignment of the flap.

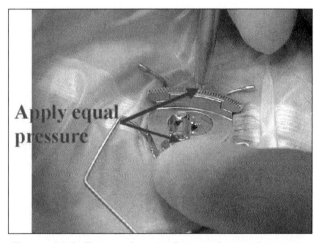

Figure 14-3. For good centration, apply equal pressure to the suction ring handle with one finger and place another finger on the temporal part of the ring.

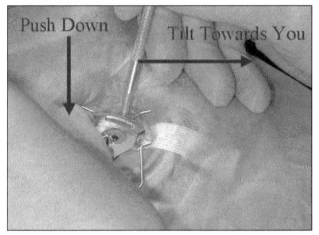

Figure 14-4. By pushing down and tilting back on the suction ring handle, the drape can be cleared in most cases.

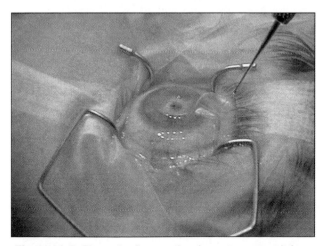

Figure 14-5. Place the flap on the drape to protect it from the upper eyelashes.

ring handle toward you (Figure 14-4). Second, the assistant can retract the drape. The third option is to redrape.

We then attached the microkeratome, told the patient we were proceeding, and performed the keratectomy. After the keratectomy, we aligned the laser using the techniques described by the manufacturer before lifting the flap. We lifted the LASIK flap with the cyclodialysis spatula and placed it on the drape to protect it from the eyelashes superiorly (Figure 14-5). The cyclodialysis spatula is then used to make one drying motion from hinge to gutter to obtain uniform drying of the stromal bed (Figure 14-6). Any fluid present around the hinge was dried by placing the tip of a dry Weckcel sponge behind the hinge so that the flap or surface of the cornea would not be touched. Then, we proceeded to perform the ablation with careful centration.

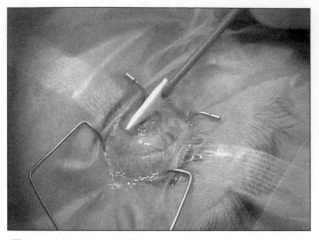

Figure 14-6. A cyclodialysis spatula makes one drying motion from hinge to gutter to obtain uniform drying of the stromal bed.

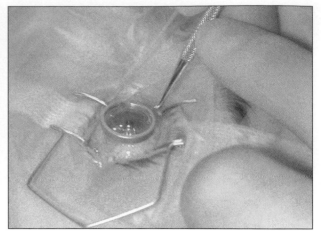

Figure 14-7. A Johnston LASIK flap applanator applanates, then rolls from hinge to gutter and off to remove excess BSS from the flap interface.

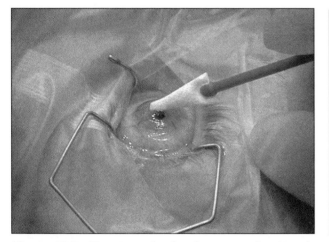

Figure 14-8a. To prevent the flap from retracting superiorly, push down at the pupil and then toward the 6 o'clock position, three to four times.

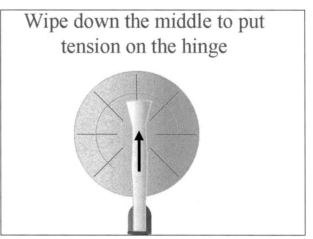

Figure 14-8b. Illustration of pushing down at the pupil and then toward 6 o'clock.

After completing the ablation, we placed the irrigator under the flap, parallel to the hinge, and in one sweeping motion, replaced the flap using a cannula. We then place the irrigator underneath the flap for minimal irrigation to align the RK marks. We did not overirrigate to prevent over-hydrating the flap and thus decreasing adherence. After moistening the tip of the sponge in the cul-de-sac, we wiped the cornea with a saturated Merocel sponge to assure perfect alignment of all of the RK marks. If there was any maladjustment at this point, the flap was re-irrigated and positioned. The same sponge was then used to remove fluid from the gutters, while taking care not to move the flap. A Johnston LASIK flap applanator is used by first applanating, then rolling from hinge to gutter and off. This serves to remove excess BSS from the flap interface (Figure 14-7). The tip of a second Merocel sponge was then moistened in the cul-de-sac and used to

push down directly at the pupil and then toward 6 o'clock three or four times (Figures 14-8a and 14-8b). The hinge made with the Hansatome has a tendency to retract the flap superiorly and needs to be pushed down.

Oxygen running at 2 liters/minute was then blown onto the cornea for no more than 5 to 10 seconds (Figure 14-9). With the previous wiping steps, very little oxygen is needed to dry the gutter, which is all that is needed to assure flap position. If Bowman's membrane wrinkles appear centrally after drying, they were stretched toward the periphery. These are common in patients with myopia of more than 6 diopters (D). I do this in virtually every case to make sure the flap is well stretched in all directions. Care should be taken not to excessively dry the cornea. Celluvisc ophthalmic lubricant (carboxymethylcellulose) was applied to the center of the flap (Figure 14-10) and smoothed out with a Weckcel sponge. The

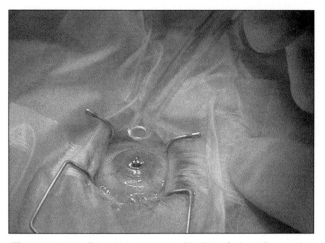

Figure 14-9. Blowing oxygen (2 liters/minute) on the cornea for 5 to 10 seconds to dry the gutter.

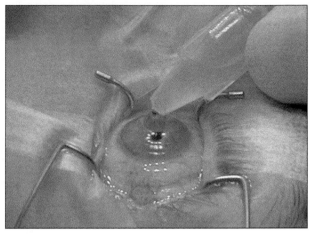

Figure 14-10. Applying Celluvisc ocular lubricant to the center of the flap.

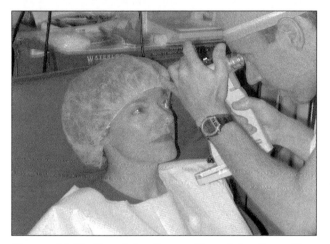

Figure 14-11. Examining the position of the flap with a portable slit lamp.

entire cornea was then irrigated with balanced salt solution.

When removing the speculum, the fingers of one hand should be used to spread the eyelids apart. Then to remove the drape, switch to the other hand and hold the eyelids apart. Neither the drape nor the speculum should ever come in contact with the flap. The blink was checked to make sure the flap stayed in good position. The fine RK marks should be clearly visible and show that the flap has not moved.

After leaving the operating room, patients were given four drops of Ocuflox (ofloxacin) and one drop of Tobradex (tobramycin and dexamethasone, Alcon,

Laboratories, Inc, Fort Worth, Texas, USA), applied 30 seconds apart. The flap was examined with a portable slit lamp (Figure 14-11). The previously placed rose bengal marks should clearly show an unshifted, well-positioned flap. The surface was also examined for any surgical debris. A drop of Celluvisc was applied and a shield was taped in place. One hour later, an examination was performed.

At the examination, uncorrected vision, manifest refraction with best-corrected vision, corneal topography, anterior segment, and fundus examinations were performed. This allowed the surgeon to check for proper function of all parts of the eye and gave patients the opportunity to discuss their vision. With this technique, most patients with myopia below 7 D have 20/50 or better vision at the 1-hour exam, and patients above 7 D range from 20/40 to 20/200. Discuss early postoperative vision with patients and explain that blurred vision at this time is normal. Patients are quite happy to be able to read an eye chart with their operated eye before having surgery on their second eye.

The examinations were performed 1 hour postoperatively for two reasons. The first is safety. We use separate equipment for each eye, and the patients like to know that the first surgery was successful before proceeding with the second eye. The second reason is for learning, and we have been able to fine-tune the technique by checking vision and the status of the flap at 1 hour. We are working toward eventually performing enhancements at the 1-hour time point. Since I first started these techniques with the 1-hour examination, I have been able to improve the average 1-hour exam vision by four lines, which has significantly improved patient satisfaction. Patients like the 1-hour delay between eye surgeries; they prefer having surgery on both eyes on the same day, but they do not want the doctor to be in a hurry.

Vision 1 Hour Postoperatively
With our technique, most patients with < 7.0 D of myopia saw 20/50 or better at the 1-hour exam, while those with > 7.0 D were in the range of 20/40 to 20/200.

INCIDENCE OF COMPLICATIONS: COMPARISON WITH THE EMORY STUDY

A study conducted by Emory University was performed on 1062 consecutive eyes by 14 surgeons in private practice who used the Automated Corneal Shaper microkeratome and the Summit Apex excimer laser current at that time (1995 and 1996).[1] The data showed 27 intraoperative complications in 2.1% of the eyes, including 10 free flaps, eight incomplete flaps, six buttonholes, one thin flap, one thick flap, and one bilevel flap. The incidence of postoperative complications was 3.1%, with 23 cases of epithelial ingrowth and 13 cases of flap slippage.

Our study included approximately the same number of surgeons but differed from the Emory study by including a larger number of eyes, and most importantly, was performed from July 1998 to March 1999 using a second-generation laser and a second-generation microkeratome (Hansatome). Our results showed none of the intraoperative complications seen in the Emory study, and although we did have three partial flap slippages that were picked up on the first day postoperatively and refloated, we had no other complications. There were no thin flaps, no incomplete flaps, no free caps, and no cases of epithelial ingrowth or lamellar keratitis.

CONCLUSION

Standardization seems to be the key to success. Both the surgeons and the staff function better with standardization, especially in paperwork and techniques, and we believe mistakes are prevented this way. We are aiming for a zero rate of flap complications and for 20/40 or better vision at 1 hour postoperatively in 100% of patients. Overall, if the incidence of complications is lowered and patient visual recovery is faster, operational costs are lowered and patient satisfaction increases. This leads to increased patient referrals and a much more satisfactory LASIK program.

REFERENCE

1. Stulting RD, Carr JD, Thompson KP, Waring GO III, Wiley WM, Walker JG. Complications of laser in situ keratomileusis for the correction of myopia. *Ophthalmology.* 1999;106:13-20.

THE ACS MICROKERATOME AND VISX STAR LASER

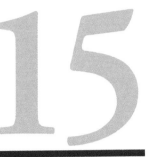

Rafael I. Barraquer, MD

INTRODUCTION

The currently preferred technique for correcting ametropia, including myopia up to the teens, regular astigmatism, and low to moderate hyperopia, is the result of two main historical developments in refractive surgery. Lamellar techniques (conceived and developed by José I. Barraquer in 1949[1-4]) and the use of lasers as refractive tools[5] converged into what we know as laser-assisted in situ keratomileusis (LASIK) or photokeratomileusis.[6-12] A discussion on the origins and rationale for this terminology can be found in the first edition of this book.[13]

The Chiron Automated Corneal Shaper (ACS) microkeratome is currently the most widely used device for the creation of the lamellar corneal flap. The VISX Star excimer laser belongs to the last generation of machines with "wide beam" delivery. The systems of this kind predominate and have the longest record in refractive surgery. This chapter reviews my current technique employing these instruments, from the preoperative phase to the surgical maneuvers and follow-up period.

PATIENT SELECTION

To the novice refractive surgeon, patient selection might appear as a rather straightforward issue. Experience shows that this is one of the most delicate aspects of the practice. It may determine success or failure, especially in terms of patient satisfaction, more than the surgical technique itself.

Most refractive surgery patients have a strong willingness to do whatever is needed to become independent of glasses and contact lenses. Many have almost made up their minds before consulting with the ophthalmologist, and some already have a considerable amount of infor-mation—misinformation as well. It is therefore essential to have a clear picture of the indications and contraindications, with all the nuances that may apply to each specific patient, in order to be able to give the right advice and to stress the most pertinent facts. It is generally unwise to try to convince a poorly motivated subject. On the contrary, we occasionally face the enthusiastic but inadequate candidate that has to be talked out of the procedure.

Indications

In our practice, we currently perform LASIK on patients from 18 years of age up to the 50s, with myopic ametropia up to -15 diopters (D) of spherical equivalent (SE). The advent of phakic intraocular lenses for high myopia has created a gray zone (-10 to -15 D) in which either procedure can be applied depending on other factors, such as age, anisometropia, profession, etc. We also treat any cylinder up to 6 D, although this can be exceeded in post-keratoplasty patients. Our current limit for hyperopia and hyperopic astigmatism is +5 D of SE under cycloplegic refraction. Chapter 13 of Buratto L, Brint SF. *LASIK: Principles and Techniques* details these indications and issues of myopia grading. They are also summarized in Table 15-1.

Contraindications

Apart from failure to comply with any of the indications, a number of conditions may contraindicate the performance of a LASIK procedure, including anatomical variations and anomalies, ocular motility and vision deficiencies, ocular diseases, general medical factors, and personal factors. In many cases, a specific condition may constitute a relative contraindication only or deserve special precautions, patient information, and preventive measures. Table 15-2 includes an updated summary of the details of these issues.

Table 15-1			
CURRENT INDICATION LIMITS FOR LASIK			
Limits	**Myopia**	**Hyperopia**	**Astigmatism**
Refraction: upper	-15 D (SE)	+ 5 D (cyclo SE)	6 D
Caveats (as the upper limit is approached)	Increased risk of visual disturbances, reduced predictability, regression		Possible undetected keratoconus, etc
Alternatives (other than spectacles or contacts)	Phakic IOL CLE + IOL	CLE + IOL Phakic IOL?	Penetrating keratoplasty
Refraction: lower	No limit (usually around 1.5 D SE, except mixed astigmatism)		
Caveats (approaching the lower limit)	Narrow risk:benefit ratio		
Age: lower	18 years		
General reasons	Progression of ametropia; legal age		
Possible exceptions	Pediatric myopic anisometropia	Pediatric accommodative esotropia	—
Age: upper	50 to 59 (rel)	50 to 59 (rel)	No limit (?)
General reasons	Medium-term risk of cataract development		
	Inaccuracy of IOL calculations in keratorefractive patients		
Possible exceptions	Significant astigmatism with low/moderate sphere and clear lens		

cyclo= cycloplegic; CLE= clear lens extraction; IOL= intraocular lens; rel= relative

Information to Patients

During the preoperative stage, the ophthalmologist should be particularly vigilant in detecting unrealistic expectations and provide adequate information. This should be delivered using clear and simple language, explaining the procedure and its realistic objectives, and include an outline of its practical steps—from preoperative studies to the surgical stage, and postoperative evolution. The known results and possible complications should be discussed in relation to the advantages and disadvantages of the remaining alternatives for correction. Table 15-3 presents the essential facts about LASIK as a positive-negative list. Above all, the patient must understand that this is surgery (indeed an elective surgery) before signing the informed consent form.

PREOPERATIVE PHASE AND INSTRUMENTS

The patient should undergo a series of exams to calculate the treatment parameters prior to the LASIK procedure and as safety baseline information. Assembling and checking the instruments and laser system, and preparation of the eyes constitute the immediate preoperative steps.

Preoperative Exams

These include refraction and the assessment of other aspects of the visual function, a complete ophthalmologic examination, several biometric measurements and other physiological tests, as listed in Table 15-4. Although some of these may not be mandatory, they provide extra baseline information and safety.

The Operating Environment

Although there may be an argument on the surgical nature of "pure" laser refractive surgery (such as PRK), this is not the case in lamellar procedures that, to begin with, include a large cut in the cornea. This implies that the general principles of ocular microsurgery must be followed, from the design of the operating room (OR) to the handling of instruments. As general conditions, we should follow the four "A's," as formulated by Barraquer[2]: asepsia, atraumia, atoxia, and amoria.

Amoria, or the avoidance of particles in the surgical field, is the one most specific of lamellar corneal refractive surgery (Figure 15-1). For this purpose, we use electronically filtered air with positive pressure, lint free OR clothing, truly powder-free gloves, and 0.22-micron microporous filters with all irrigating solutions. Sterile drapes or sterile plastic bags cover all nonsterilizable surfaces that may come in contact with the surgeon's hands or arms (Figure 15-2). All instruments are inspected under the microscope prior to being used and any particle or fiber is removed.

The ACS Microkeratome

The microkeratome is the key instrument in corneal lamellar surgery. The Chiron ACS incorporates the modifications added by Luis A. Ruiz in the 1980s to Barraquer's original microkeratome design. It contains

Table 15-2

POSSIBLE CONTRAINDICATIONS FOR LASIK

Contraindications (possible)	Comments (inform patient)	Possible solutions and recommendations
Anatomical variations		
Insufficient lid aperture (anatomical or functional: uncooperative patient)	May preclude application of suction ring. Increased risk of suction loss during lamellar cut	Reassure/increase sedation Use smaller suction ring. Screw-driven type speculum Lateral canthotomy (rarely)
Steep cornea (K > 47 D)	Correction less stable Possible keratoconus	Reanalyze topography Delay surgery
Flat cornea (K < 40 D)	Reduced applanation area Risk of free cap	Intraoperative applanometry Reduce blade excursion
Thin cornea (total thickness < 0.49 mm, estimated final bed < 0.25 mm	Risk of postoperative ectasia Possible keratoconus vs. contact lens corneal warping)	Select thinner flap gauge Intraoperative pachymetry Delay surgery
Large physiologic mydriasis (infrared pupillometry > 6 mm) Corectopia	Increased risk of postoperative halos and glare	Use largest ablation zones Use multizones or wider transition zones
Vision and ocular motility		
Convergence insufficiency with anomalous retinal correspondence	Risk of postoperative diplopia	Consult with strabismus specialist
Nystagmus	Impaired fixation	Use fixation ring
Amblyopia	BCVA will not improve	Inform patient
Large positive kappa angle	Pseudostrabimus (risk of cosmetic "surprise")	Inform patient
Ocular diseases		
Surface irregularities (pterygium, pingueculae, after retinal surgery, etc)	May prevent adherence of the suction ring	Use smaller suction ring Peritomy/resection (rarely)
Dry eyes and other epitheliopathies	Lesser concern than in PRK Risk of stem cell dysfunction in	Insure ocular surface stability before and after procedure chronic contact lens users?
Active external infection	Risk of interface infection	Treat, delay surgery
Active uveitis	Risk of exacerbation?	Treat, delay surgery
Keratoconus	Formal contraindication?	Inform patient, PK?
Other corneal dystrophies or opacities	Will not be cured by LASIK Risk of endothelial decompensation?	If superficial, PRK/PTK may be preferable
Ocular hypertension and glaucoma	Interference with flap adhesion? Increased risk of ectasia?	Check IOP preoperative and postoperative (No need for postop steroids)
Cataract (even incipient, polar, or other minor congenital opacities)	Increased risk of visual disturbances (halos, glare, reduced contrast sensitivity, night vision difficulties) that may be brought out by LASIK	Consider CLE + IOL (especially if high refraction)
Retinal dystrophies Optic nerve atrophy (even partial or incipient)	(same as for cataract)	Do fundus examination inform patient Consult retinal specialist
Myopia (especially if high)	Intrinsic risk of retinal complications (detachment, macular) with no established relation to LASIK	(same as for retinal dystrophies)

Table 15-2, Continued		
POSSIBLE CONTRAINDICATIONS FOR LASIK		
Contraindications (possible)	**Comments (inform patient)**	**Possible solutions and recommendations**
General medical factors		
Pregnancy	Myopia may progress Healing? (Less concern vs PRK)	Delay surgery?
Sjögren syndrome and other collagen diseases	Risk of surface decompensation (less concern vs PRK)	Insure ocular surface stability before and after procedure
Mental retardation and psychosis	Possible uncooperative patient	Train subject, use fixation ring
Personal factors		
Lack of a clear motivation Unrealistic expectations	LASIK is an elective procedure, etc	Thoroughly inform patient Obtain informed consent
Professional (engineers, architects, drivers, pilots, police or military corps candidates, airline crew, lawyers, etc)	Visually demanding work can make minor visual imperfections stand out Technical mentality may lead to unrealistic expectations Refractive surgery may not warrant professional success	(same as above)
Lack of informed consent	Obvious requirement	(same as above)
Uncooperative patient	Risk of suction loss, decentration, etc	Reassure, train subject Use fixation ring

K= average keratometric central corneal curvature; BCVA = best-corrected visual acuity (with spectacles); PK = penetrating keratoplasty; PRK = photorefractive keratectomy; PTK = phototherapeutic keratectomy; IOP = intraocular pressure

Table 15-3

ESSENTIAL FACTS ABOUT LASIK THAT PATIENT INFORMATION MUST INCLUDE

Positive facts	**Negative facts**
LASIK is an effective procedure for the treatment of myopia, astigmatism, and hyperopia (between certain dioptric limits).	No refractive procedure can ensure total elimination of glasses in all cases and situations. Residual refraction is common but usually of little practical relevance. Gross under- or overcorrection can be treated easily by an enhancement procedure.
It is a brief (a few minutes) outpatient procedure. It is neither painful during the surgery (under topical anesthesia) or afterward.	LASIK will not cure myopia or prevent its eventual progression, but it can be repeated.
It will improve UCVA, greatly reducing the refraction and thus the dependence on glasses.	LASIK does not aim at improving BCVA. This can actually happen after LASIK, but also a few patients may lose a line.
It requires little postoperative treatment, few postoperative visits.	Total correction of myopia will bring about a need for glasses for near vision in the presbyopic patient. Patients over 40 years of age should consider the possibility of planned undercorrection or monovision (anisometropia).
It allows a quick return to normal life (avoiding eye rubbing or exposure to trauma). The visual recovery is swift, though complete refractive stability may take up to 3 months or more.	Complications are infrequent and usually of little relevance for the refractive and visual outcome, but the possibility of visual loss cannot be completely ruled out,

Table 15-4

PREOPERATIVE EXAMINATIONS BEFORE LASIK

Refraction	Comments
(contact lens use discontinued for at least 2 weeks)	
Automated	Least useful
Manifest	UCVA, BCVA, vertex distance
Cycloplegic	Mandatory in hyperopia, usually little difference to manifest in myopia (0.5 to 1 D)
Over hard contact lens (with a reasonable dioptric fit based on manifest refraction)	Sole measure of noncorneal astigmatism Frequently greater difference with manifest (corrected to corneal plane) than cycloplegic
Other visual functions	
Glare	Bright acuity test (Mentor BAT)
Contrast sensitivity (spatial)	CSV-1000 chart (VisiTech)
Visual field (Goldmann)	(Only in cases of significant anisometropia or
Ocular motility and binocular vision	presumed amblyopia)
Ophthalmologic examination	
Anterior segment (slit lamp biomicroscopy, including photography)	Exclude external infection, dry eye, other epitheliopathy, signs of contact lens overuse, keratoconus, and other corneal pathology or existing opacities, status of anterior chamber, iris, lens, etc
Posterior segment (under mydriasis)	Document myopic macular changes, peripheral degenerations, disk status, etc
Biometrical measurements	
Corneal topography or kurtography (computer-assisted videokeratography)	As baseline data, measure corneal astigmatism, exclude keratoconus, etc
Corneal pachymetry (ultrasonic)	Central and peripheral (nine points)
Anterior-posterior axis (A-scan)	Baseline (possible progression of myopia)
Pupillometry (infrared)	In the dark and at a standard room lighting
Specular microscopy	Endothelial cell count and morphology
Other physiological tests	
Corneal sensation	Cochet-Bonnet esthesiometry
Lacrimal secretion	Schirmer test
Intraocular pressure	Goldmann applanation tonometry

gears for the automated advancement of the cutting head and, later, the stopper to create an incomplete (flap) lamellar cut.

The ACS system comprises the microkeratome handpiece with the cutting head and its motor, a suction ring, a console with the motor's power unit, and the vacuum pump for the ring. Several accessories, such as the Barraquer applanation tonometer and applanation lenses, corneal spoon and marker, and tools for assembling and checking the cutting head are also included.

The microkeratome head is composed of a main piece that contains the advancing gears and opens to accept the blade holder and blade (Figure 15-3). Once it is closed and secured by a cylindrical nut around its "neck," the applanation or gauge plate is placed and secured in its frontal aspect (Figure 15-4). The stopper can be mounted as a separate adjustable piece over the neck's nut (Figures 15-5 through 15-7). In newer models,

it is incorporated as a fixed part of the head's main piece (see Figure 15-6).

Assembly and Checking

The assembly is preferably done only by the surgeon or by the instrument technician under close scrutiny of the surgeon. Failure to properly place the stopper will lead to a free corneal cap, a minor complication compared to the intraocular penetration and possible injury to the iris and lens that will result from failure to place the applanation plate. Even "mounted," a full-thickness cut may occur if the plate has not been completely pushed into position, even by less than 1.0 mm.

Before screwing the head on the motor, the movement of the blade holder and blade is manually checked with a special tool. Any resistance indicates dirt or irregularities in the blade holder, blade holder socket, surfaces in contact with the blade, or a defective blade. Surgery

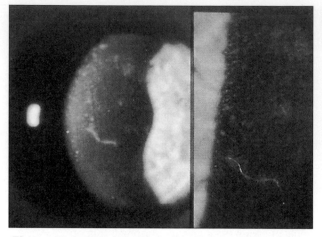

Figure 15-1. Photo showing abundant punctate and linear (lint) interface particles at 1 week postoperatively. Fortunately, these had few visual repercussions and became less apparent with time (photo used with permission from Buratto L, Brint SF. *LASIK: Principles and Techniques.* Thorofare, NJ: SLACK Incorporated; 1998).

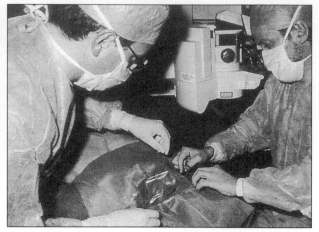

Figure 15-2. Sterile and amoric field for LASIK. The surgeon, assistant, and patient wear lint-free gowns. Sterile plastic drapes or sheets cover all surfaces that the surgeon may touch (photo used with permission from Buratto L, Brint SF. *LASIK: Principles and Techniques.* Thorofare, NJ: SLACK Incorporated; 1998).

should not be attempted until this movement is perfectly smooth, otherwise risking an incomplete flap due to an microkeratome jam.

The importance of adequate cleaning and maintenance of the microkeratome parts cannot be overstated. This should include periodic polishing to avoid build-up of a layer of debris. Especially on the lower surface of the plate, this build-up leads to shallower cuts.

The Blade

Initially, the blades were used three to four times in our practice, but intraoperative pachymetry showed that the actual cuts are centrally more shallow than the plate value, even with new blades (of two different brands), and each reuse creates a flap about 10 to 20 microns thinner. Since we started using new blades only, thin, perforated, or split flaps have become almost nonexistent.

Even with new blades, it is advisable to check the edge once it is mounted in the microkeratome under the maximum magnification of the surgical microscope (25x). Orientation of the microkeratome should be changed so the coaxial light reflects on each facet of the blade edge. The microkeratome head should never be opened with the plate on because the head of its securing screw may dent the blade (see Figure 15-6).

The Pneumatic Fixation Ring

The original ACS system included an adjustable pneumatic fixation (suction) ring with a maximum applanation diameter of 7.5 mm suited for automated lamellar keratoplasty (ALK) procedures. The newer LASIK models have a fixed ring that allows for an 8.5 mm cut. Custom rings can be made to allow for larger cuts (for

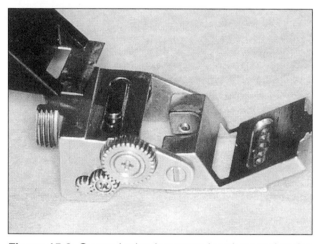

Figure 15-3. Opened microkeratome head: mounting the blade (the blade holder is already in its socket) (photo used with permission from Buratto L, Brint SF. *LASIK: Principles and Techniques.* Thorofare, NJ: SLACK Incorporated; 1998).

hyperopia) and to fit smaller eyes. It is advisable to engage the microkeratome head into the ring guides to check for its span of advance (Figure 15-8). A special lens with circular marks (Barraquer), which adapts to the base of the ring, gives an estimate of the hinge size when the blade is fully advanced. This is most useful when using an adjustable stopper and special rings.

The ring is connected to the console pump by plastic tubing that has a reservoir inserted to prevent any liquid from the surgical field reaching the pump. To check suction, occlude the ring with a thumb and feel the strength of adherence. The console manometer should indicate at least 24 cm Hg. If this value is not reached, the vacuum

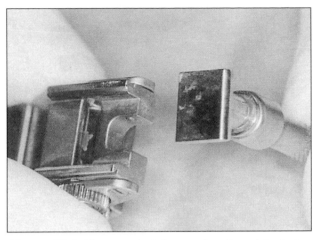

Figure 15-4. Placement of the applanation plate in the frontal part of the microkeratome head (photo used with permission from Buratto L, Brint SF. *LASIK: Principles and Techniques.* Thorofare, NJ: SLACK Incorporated; 1998).

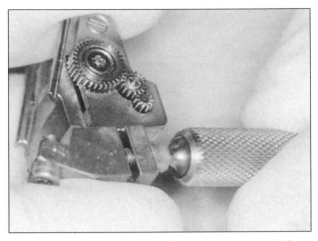

Figure 15-5. Mounting the advancement stopper. Care should be taken to ensure it is seated properly, otherwise a free cap may ensue (photo used with permission from Buratto L, Brint SF. *LASIK: Principles and Techniques.* Thorofare, NJ: SLACK Incorporated; 1998).

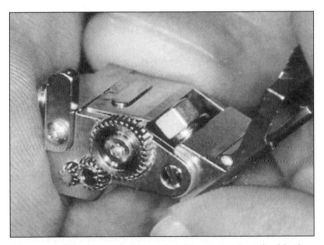

Figure 15-6. Opening the microkeratome head with the plate mounted may lead to notching of the blade (fixed stopper model) (photo used with permission from Buratto L, Brint SF. *LASIK: Principles and Techniques.* Thorofare, NJ: SLACK Incorporated; 1998).

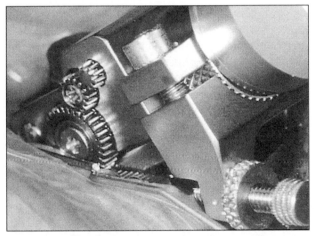

Figure 15-7. Checking the advancement of the microkeratome on the ring gears (adjustable stopper model) (photo used with permission from Buratto L, Brint SF. *LASIK: Principles and Techniques.* Thorofare, NJ: SLACK Incorporated; 1998).

pump should be checked for malfunction. However, if a conjunctival fold (or any other obstruction along the tubing or at the console valve) blocks the vacuum line, pneumatic fixation will be poor in spite of a normal manometer reading.

The VISX Star Excimer Laser

The Star excimer laser system, from VISX Inc, belongs to the third generation of wide beam and open-diaphragm ablation, ArF excimer (193 nm) laser type. It can perform central minus treatments up to 6.5 mm of diameter, either spherical (myopic), cylindrical (astigmatic), or plano (therapeutic). For hyperopic treatments, the ablation and transitional zones are rotated over the peripheral cornea reaching 9.0 mm and describing a ring (hyperopia) or double cylindrical (plus cylinder) configuration.

Its main advantages over the previous models (VISX 20/20 A and B) are, apart from the possibility of hyperopic treatments, a smaller volume, no need for liquid nitrogen, and fewer optical elements in the laser pathway. It has a longer working distance that allows the passage of the microkeratome and incorporates oblique lights in addition to the customary coaxial, which is ring-shaped. Patient fixation is assisted with a flickering red light emitting diode (LED) at the center of the objective. Centering and the limits of the ablation area can be assessed thanks to a lighted reticule with concentric

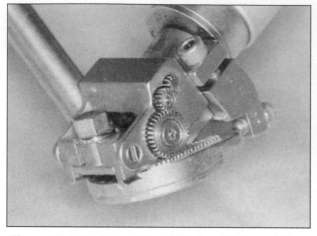

Figure 15-8. Features of the VISX Star S2 SmoothScan excimer laser delivery system (photo used with permission from Buratto L, Brint SF. *LASIK: Principles and Techniques.* Thorofare, NJ: SLACK Incorporated; 1998).

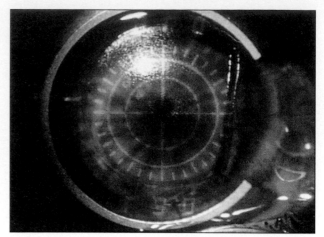

Figure 15-9. Four and 6.0-mm target-shaped mires in the optical path of the surgical microscope (a newer model includes a 9.0-mm ring) (photo used with permission from Buratto L, Brint SF. *LASIK: Principles and Techniques.* Thorofare, NJ: SLACK Incorporated; 1998).

mires (Figure 15-9) in the optical path of the operating microscope. A fine displacement of the patient chair along three coordinate axes is joystick-commanded.

The system performs a series of self-tests when it is initialized and has sensors for most of its components, so any relevant (and even possibly irrelevant) malfunction can be detected and elicit a warning message or halt. At the beginning of each session (or as needed) the centration of the beam is calibrated relative to the reticule, and the accuracy of the ablation is tested on a plastic reference plate. Fluence setting is automatically performed before each treatment. When ready, the push of a pedal first starts a blower that aspirates debris away from the operating field. A further depression of the pedal initiates the laser treatment. The process can be paused at any time by the release of the pedal (eg, if recentration or surface drying is needed) and will be resumed at the point it was left.

The latest VISX Star S2 SmoothScan model, also offered as an upgrade for existing Star systems, increases the smoothness and control of the ablation. The single wide beam output of the laser is further processed by a series of interposed modules that homogenize, split, and shape it into seven smaller beams. These can be applied together or independently in a variety of scanning patterns, resulting in a smoother ablation and the ability to perform treatment profiles unavailable in previous models, such as optical zone enlargement and customized ablations according to topography (CAP or contoured ablation pattern).

Ancillary, Retreatment, and Emergency Instruments

Apart from the microkeratome and laser, the practice of LASIK requires a series of ancillary instruments: lid speculum, markers, blunt spatulas, irrigation cannulas, surgical sponges, etc. Our preference regarding these items will be covered in the section on the surgical technique.

For retreatments, I prefer a pair of toothless, fine-tipped forceps (Barraquer) to identify the flap edge and initiate blunt dissection. A semiblunt spatula (Fukasaku, Guimaraes, etc) and "pull and tear" maneuvers (keratorhexis) follow, to lift the existing flap with minimal disturbance of the epithelium and avoid seeding cells in the interface.

In the event a complete cut is produced, atraumatic forceps may be required to extract the corneal cap from inside the microkeratome head. It then will be transferred to a plastic chamber to be stored and to avoid desiccation until the laser ablation is complete. It is also important to not overhydrate the cap.

Preparation of the Patient and the Eye

Admission and Final Interview

Although this is an ambulatory procedure, our patients are admitted to their own private room so they can relax before and after treatment. A final interview with the surgeon allows for clarification of any last minute questions or any issue to be decided, such as second eye adjustments or planned undercorrection and monovision in older patients, and is useful to calm the patient.

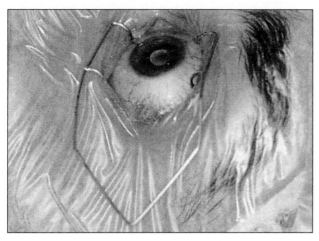

Figure 15-10. Placement of the wire speculum and plastic drapes wrapped around the lid margins and lashes (photo used with permission from Buratto L, Brint SF. *LASIK: Principles and Techniques.* Thorofare, NJ: SLACK Incorporated; 1998).

Preoperative Medications

A mild sedative (diazepam, 0.1 mg/kg) is administered 30 minutes prior to surgery. The conjunctival sac is flushed with balanced salt solution (BSS), the lid margins cleaned with a lid scrubbing lotion followed by a second saline wash, and antibiotic drops (tobramycin 0.3%) are instilled. Topical anesthetic drops (oxybuprocaine 0.2%) are given every 10 minutes starting 30 minutes prior to surgery. Excess anesthetic may lead to epithelial toxicity and even sloughing. The patient is instructed to keep his or her eyes closed to avoid desiccation of the epithelium until accompanied to the operating room (OR) (either walking or in a wheelchair and wearing a surgical lint-free gown, cap, and shoe covers). Upon entering the OR, the surgeon greets the patient, checking for identity and the eye to be operated.

Surgical Field Preparation

Once lying on the surgical chair, the patient's head is positioned and leveled with the help of a reference light in the ceiling and centering marks on the chair. The patient is stabilized by means of a deflatable cushion that adapts to the sides of the head and the back of the neck as it deflates.

A final drop of anesthetic is instilled and the surgical field is externally aseptized with 10% povidone-iodine (Betadine) and dried. A plastic drape is applied with the lids wide open, taking care to trap the lashes underneath it and allow for some excess plastic to wrap the lid margins when the speculum is placed. During this phase, the laser fluence setting program is started, which also helps the patient acclimate to the sound of the instrument.

A wire speculum is usually sufficient (Figure 15-10)

and has the advantage of being thinner and softer in case it gets in the way of the microkeratome. A stronger, screw-driven type speculum may be useful if the patient is uncooperative, but it can become an obstacle if the palpebral fissure is actually small. Centering and leveling the head is checked under the microscope; the same amount of sclera should be visible above and under the cornea. If this is not the case, the patient is instructed to raise or lower the chin accordingly, as his or her fixation is maintained on the red flickering LED of the apparatus.

SURGICAL TECHNIQUE

The LASIK procedure can be divided into three main phases: the preparation of the corneal flap by a lamellar cut, the refractive photoablation proper, and the final stage with reposition of the flap until adhesion is sufficient.

Lamellar Cut (Nonrefractive Keratotomy)

Performing the lamellar nonrefractive cut is possibly the most critical maneuver in LASIK, because most complications may originate at this moment. It is also the most surgeon-dependent step.

Corneal Marking

The placement of a mark or marks on the cornea enables a precise reposition of the corneal flap at the end of the procedure, especially in case of a total cut (free cap). This may happen either due to faulty assembly of the stopper, too small applanation area caused by a flat cornea, or suction loss resulting in a superficial, and thus of smaller diameter, cut. Longitudinal or semiradial marks are preferable; a radial mark would look the same if a free cap were inverted (epithelial face down).

It is not necessary to mark the cornea for centration purposes; there is no need to precisely center the nonrefractive cut, and it would be useless in relation to the laser beam since any superficial mark will be reflected with the flap. Several special marking instruments are available, but a gentian violet felt pen may be as effective and simpler (Figure 15-11). A first intraoperative pachymetry reading is obtained at this time.

Pneumatic Fixation

Good pneumatic fixation of the globe is essential to the production of an adequate lamellar cut. When correctly applied, it causes an immediate intraoperative pressure (IOP) rise to higher than 65 mm Hg. This gives the cornea the necessary stiffness to allow the cutting of a thin, regular lamella. Good adherence to the suction ring is a requisite for enough applanation, allowing the blade to reach the desired depth and diameter of the flap.

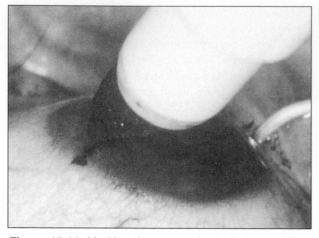

Figure 15-11. Marking the cornea for realignment reference with a semiradial line (with a gentian violet felt marker) (photo used with permission from Buratto L, Brint SF. *LASIK: Principles and Techniques.* Thorofare, NJ: SLACK Incorporated; 1998).

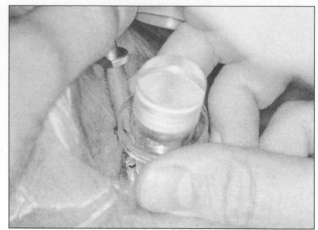

Figure 15-12. Checking IOP with the Barraquer applanation tonometer after the suction ring is in place and the vacuum pump is on (photo used with permission from Buratto L, Brint SF. *LASIK: Principles and Techniques.* Thorofare, NJ: SLACK Incorporated; 1998).

Since the microkeratome head must engage the ring's guides from the temporal side, the ring handle is usually held by the surgeon's hand opposite the patient's eye. The choice and adjustment of the speculum is crucial to ensure ring stability. In a lid-squeezing patient, the momentary discomfort caused by a tight speculum is preferable to having a complication due to suction loss. A smaller-diameter ring can also be useful, but do not forget the value of reassuring the patient or using additional sedation.

A slight (0.5 to 1.0 mm) decentration of the ring toward the nasal limbus is preferred because it results in a hinge placed further away from the ablation area. Surface irregularities such as pingueculae or pterygium may impede adhesion and have to be removed. A lax conjunctiva may occlude the vacuum hole of the ring, requiring a change in its position or even a peritomy. I have also encountered this problem in eyes with perilimbal scarring after retinal detachment surgery.

Tonometry and Applanometry

Poor ring fixation will result in a flap too thin and with an irregular bed, or a small, thin and irregular free cap. A correct reading in the console manometer does not ensure a good grip on the globe. Any block in the vacuum line may give a false impression of sufficient vacuum in spite of poor fixation. That is why several checks have to be made in every case.

The rise in IOP is the best indicator of a good grip. This is measured with the Barraquer tonometer (Figure 15-12). The applanation area (over a dry cornea) should be clearly smaller than the 65 mm Hg reference circle.

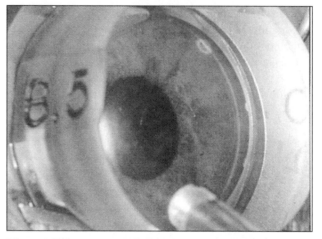

Figure 15-13. The applanation lens not only measures the diameter of the cut, but also double-checks the suction ring grip of the globe (photo used with permission from Buratto L, Brint SF. *LASIK: Principles and Techniques.* Thorofare, NJ: SLACK Incorporated; 1998).

Whenever it is about the same size, the suction is borderline and may be insufficient.

Pressing the applanation lens on the dry cornea (Figure 15-13) not only checks the size of the applanation area but also rechecks fixation in a more thorough way. While the tonometer displaces only a small volume, the applanation lens replicates the squeezing effect of the microkeratome passage. This may reveal unstable fixation. If the applanated area does not reach the reference mark of 8.5 mm, the suction grip may be inadequate or the cornea very flat. In the latter condition, the stopper might need to be adjusted for a slightly shorter blade excursion to avoid a free cap.

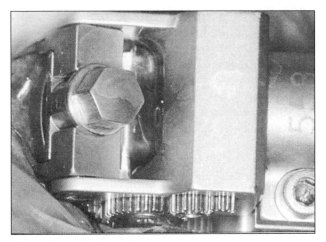

Figure 15-14. The microkeratome cut is complete. The stopper is in contact with the ring, not pinching the lids or drapes (photo used with permission from Buratto L, Brint SF. *LASIK: Principles and Techniques.* Thorofare, NJ: SLACK Incorporated; 1998).

Engagement of the Microkeratome Head

Engagement of the microkeratome head into the ring guides is a maneuver that requires some practice. These guides are unequal because the one in the gear side is a dovetail shape and the opposite one has a right-angle profile. The cutting head has the corresponding shapes in its lateral rims. To facilitate both the engagement and then the passage of the microkeratome and to avoid epithelial abrasion, the surfaces of both the cornea and the ring must be well lubricated with saline.

The microkeratome head is inserted with a slight tilt, first in the dovetail guide side and then placed down until its lower surface rests on the ring gutter, and the right-angled rim and guide also engage. The microkeratome is then slightly advanced manually until its gears approach the toothed part of the ring.

The Corneal Flap Section

Once the microkeratome head is properly engaged, performance of the lamellar keratotomy is an almost automated step. There is little room for correction and instrument function must be checked before. The 160-micron plate is commonly used. In case the stromal bed thickness is estimated to become thinner than 250-micron after the laser ablation, the 130-micron plate could be chosen (or a smaller ablation diameter). However, I have found by intraoperative pachymetry that the flaps created with the 160-micron plate are seldom thicker than 130 microns at their center.

When the pedal is depressed and the microkeratome train begins to advance, it is not necessary to hold it as during the engagement step. Instead, it should be held just slightly to prevent the cord from pulling. Pushing on

the instrument might lead to a jam. The corneal flap can be observed as it appears through the slot of the MK. Care should be taken to avoid pinching the lid skin with the stopper, particularly with the first model. If this happens, it is possible to reverse a bit, free the skin, and resume advancement. This will leave a linear mark in the stromal bed transverse to the blade movement, usually without significance. Similar marks will result whenever the MK is stopped and started again, although this maneuver may resolve a partial jam.

If the diameter of the stromal cut is not sufficient for the laser ablation, the procedure must be aborted. The flap is repositioned and the patient is informed about the complication, explaining that this will not have visual consequences and it will be possible to further attempt the procedure a few months later.

Withdrawal of the Microkeratome and Ring

When the cutting head has reached the end of its span (Figure 15-14), the motor is reversed and the head backs up to the beginning of the ring gears. At this moment, the microkeratome is manually disengaged from the ring, the vacuum pump is turned off, and the ring is removed from the eye. Ideally, the flap will remain in place, almost as if no sectioning had taken place. If the cut has been completed with no hinge, care must be taken to locate and extract the corneal cap from inside the microkeratome head and store it in the ad hoc chamber.

Laser Ablation (Refractive Photokeratectomy)

The refractive photoablation is a mainly machine-governed phase of the procedure. However, the surgeon is responsible for the selection of treatment parameters, proper handling of the flap and ablation area, and ensuring the laser beam centration.

Reflection of the Corneal Flap

The flap is gently lifted by inserting a blunt spatula under its edge and then reflected it toward the nasal side (Figure 15-15). Its thickness, useful area (relative to the position of the hinge), centering, and regularity are assessed. The flap is placed resting over the nasal conjunctiva, avoiding curling or folds. A second pachymetry reading is taken to measure the stromal bed and flap thickness. Chronic contact lens users may have a superior micropannus that bleeds at the edge. This is usually not a problem but the blood must be removed with a sponge to prevent it from interfering with the laser.

A cut that is too small but of adequate thickness (incomplete passage of the microkeratome) or small and superficial (thin and irregular due to suction loss) may

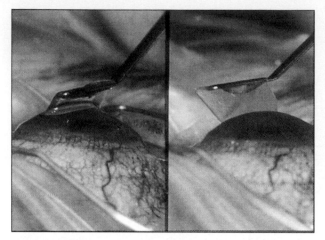

Figure 15-15. Lifting the flap with a Paton spatula at the temporal side, parallel to the hinge (photo used with permission from Buratto L, Brint SF. *LASIK: Principles and Techniques.* Thorofare, NJ: SLACK Incorporated; 1998).

become evident only at this point. If the flap is moderately thin but with sufficient area, one may decide to proceed with the treatment since this will have little influence on the refractive outcome. If the hinge slightly invades the ablation zone, especially in hyperopic cases, it should be held, retracted, and protected. A metallic instrument is preferable, since a sponge will be ablated and may spray particles on the stromal interface (LW Hirst, personal communication, May 1999). If there is not enough room for a well-centered ablation, the procedure must to be aborted.

Treatment Planning and Nomograms

The amount of correction to be attempted is a complex and critical decision that should be based on the patient's entire integrated information. Manifest and cycloplegic refraction and over-refraction with a rigid contact lens are compared, taking into account vertex distance. These values are checked for congruency with objective measurements: skiascopy, keratometry, corneal topography, and axial biometry. This also allows for an estimation of the lens power and noncorneal astigmatism. Furthermore, the differences in refraction between both eyes are compared with the results of IOL calculations based on biometric data. Of the three refraction methods (which commonly differ), the highest, lowest, or intermediate may be chosen depending on various factors, such as the degree of ametropia and age (potential for progression of myopia, presbyopia), patient's profession and preferences, and the result of the first eye, if available and stable.

The proprietary nomogram of the VISX Star, originally designed for PRK, had the tendency to hypercorrect

higher ametropias treated by LASIK. I originally used a simple adjustment scheme according to the spherical equivalent. If it was –8 D or greater (up to –15 D), 10% of the spherical equivalent was subtracted from the myopic sphere (M), as obtained by the selected refraction modality. Thus, the "intended" spherical correction (C, actually aiming for emmetropia) to be entered in the laser computer resulted as ($C = - (M - 0.10\ SE)$) (both SE and M are absolute values in this formula). In the cases between –6.00 and -7.99 D of spherical equivalent, 5% was subtracted ($C = - [M - 0.05\ SE]$). No compensation was made for lower myopias or for cylinder treatment.

To avoid the "gray zones" created by these stepped adjustments, we devised a progressive nomogram for myopic ametropias, using the spherical equivalent itself as the percent value of the spherical equivalent to be subtracted from M, thus ($C = - [M - SE^2/100]$) (Table 15-5, see page 384). In the presbyopic age, 0.1 D is also discounted each year over 39. Additional fine-tuning can be made according to the result of the first eye or in case monovision is sought.

Selection of the Ablation Zones

The relation between central ablation depth and dioptric correction achieved for a given ablation zone diameter should theoretically be constant, regardless of the laser source used (Munnerlyn's formula). However, the actual depth will be influenced by the configuration of the transition zones, which vary in each laser system. A number of operation parameters are machine-governed and cannot be altered by the surgeon. With the current software of the VISX Star, I prefer the custom program with a 10 Hz repetition rate and multiple zones for sphere, cylinder, and anti-island (APA) treatment.

For myopias up to –6 D, the maximum diameter available (6.5 mm) is used for the main spherical treatment (circular) zone. Minus cylinder is always treated as a separate, rectangle-outlined zone. To avoid excessive ablation depth, higher corrections are divided into four zones of 5.0, 5.5, 6.0, and 6.5 mm, with 25% of the spherical power in each. These diameters are reduced by 0.5 mm if the resulting stromal bed is estimated to become < 0.25 mm based on intraoperative pachymetry and theoretical ablation depth.

For each spherical zone, an anti-island treatment with 83% of the intended correction is added over a central area of 0.416 times the zone diameter. This obviates the need for specific stromal bed drying maneuvers while the ablation is carried out, except for a gross presence of liquid, usually seeping from the hinge. The ring-shaped zone used for hyperopia has 6.0-mm inner and 9.0-mm outer ablation diameter, although the transition zone reaches closer to the center.

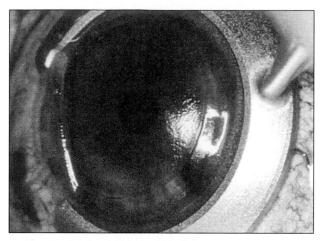

Figure 15-16. Repositioning and "painting" the flap with a marten-hair brush (photo used with permission from Buratto L, Brint SF. *LASIK: Principles and Techniques.* Thorofare, NJ: SLACK Incorporated; 1998).

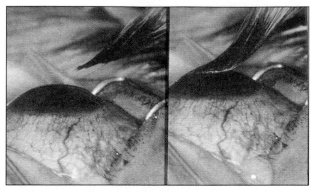

Figure 15-17. Checking for good flap adhesion by creating striae at the limbus and watching for their movement to the flap (photo used with permission from Buratto L, Brint SF. *LASIK: Principles and Techniques.* Thorofare, NJ: SLACK Incorporated; 1998).

Centering and Alignment

A decentered ablation can become an annoying and difficult complication. With the VISX Star, centering is attained by the fixation of the patient on the red flickering LED and target-shaped mires in the optical path of the microkeratome. However, improper head positioning may lead to parallax decentration in spite of having the mires apparently well centered.

Although many surgeons use the pupil center as the alignment reference, frequently it does not coincide with the actual position of the visual axis. The latter can be estimated as the center of the ring-shaped coaxial light reflection on the cornea of the fixating patient. I prefer this apparent, "real" position of the visual axis to center the laser ablation.

The visibility of the fixation LED is reduced for the patient when the flap is reflected. The intensity of the other lights may have to be diminished. When these are low, care should be taken to prevent the flap from inadvertently folding back over the corneal bed during the ablation. Some surgeons prefer self-fixation; however, an open, atraumatic ring (Katena) provides solid fixation in every case (Figure 15-16).

Before any treatment is initiated, the surgeon must recheck the accuracy of the data introduced into the laser computer according to the planned correction. During the laser application, the assistant technician announces the remaining treatment time in seconds (60, 45, 30, 15, etc) in order to inform the surgeon and calm the patient.

Final Steps

The ending phase of the procedure includes the replacement of the corneal flap, irrigation to flush any particles from the interface, and drying time to achieve initial flap adhesion, sufficient to withstand the force of lid closure and eye movements.

Flap Repositioning

To replace the corneal flap, it is simply lifted from its nasally reflected position and gently pushed back over its original bed with an irrigation cannula. A wet stromal bed is usually required to allow a final pachymetry reading, and a liquid cushion is helpful to "float" the flap back into position. Replacing the flap over a dry bed may result in malposition and distortion, causing flap folds.

I currently perform several "painting" maneuvers (after the irrigation) to ensure good extension of the flap over its bed, and to avoid any fluid getting trapped in the interface. These movements must be gentle and perpendicular to the hinge; otherwise, we risk creating folds in the flap. A wet Merocel or Keracel sponge is soft enough and does not shed particles, but the marten-hair brush is still the softest instrument for this purpose (Figure 15-17). The marks in the flap must precisely match their peripheral portions and the width of the cut edge gutter should appear constant.

Interface Irrigation

Before the flap is replaced, irrigation should be minimized, since any excess fluid will cause particles to "float in," especially if the tear film is oily. Any visible lint fragment or foreign body must be removed with fine toothless forceps. Once the flap has been repositioned, the interface is irrigated with 2 to 5 mL of filtered BSS to insure no particles, debris, or epithelial cells remain trapped. More copious irrigation may cause irregular hydration and folds in the flap.

Flap Adhesion

To ensure flap adhesion sufficient to withstand palpebral and eye movements, we wait 2 to 4 minutes from the

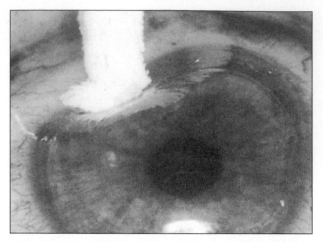

Figure 15-18. Rotation is the correct way of removing a wire speculum to avoid displacement of the flap (photo used with permission from Buratto L, Brint SF. *LASIK: Principles and Techniques.* Thorofare, NJ: SLACK Incorporated; 1998).

moment the flap appears perfectly repositioned and irrigation has ceased (longer in case of a free cap). This short-term adhesion appears to be related to the cohesive forces of the stromal proteoglycans and to the hydrostatic pressure created by the endothelial ionic pump in the presence of a rather impermeable epithelial surface. This would explain the slower adhesion of an overhydrated flap or in the presence of an epithelial defect.

After the drying time, adhesion is checked by pressing a dry surgical sponge against the limbus and watching for the formation of striae straddling the corneal periphery and into the flap (Figure 15-18). MicroSponge spears (Alcon Surgical Inc, Fort Worth, Texas, USA) are harder, and their blunt tip is better for this purpose. They also absorb more liquid—I prefer them to Merocel for removing excess fluid from the conjunctiva. However, they may shed some particles when dry, and I avoid touching the cornea with them before the flap has been replaced. Any thickened sector of the peripheral flap, indicating local edema, is suspicious of inadequate adhesion and warrants further waiting.

POSTOPERATIVE PHASE

Immediate Postoperative Period

When the flap appears to be sufficiently adherent to its bed, the speculum is removed and the patient is instructed to blink several times. The wire speculum should be rotated while its branches are compressed. To avoid engaging the flap's edge, it is safer to first extract the branch that ends at the flap hinge's side (Figure 15-19). The plastic self-adhesive drape is carefully detached and removed, and the flap is rechecked for adhesion by blinking. A single drop of an antibiotic-steroid combination is instilled. An external plastic shield is applied and the patient is instructed to keep both eyes closed during most of the first 2 to 3 hours after the procedure. An occlusive bandage is used only if an epithelial defect is present.

Early Postoperative Period

We first examine the patients 2 to 5 hours after the operation, especially checking for flap adaptation and adhesion, the presence of epithelial defects, interface debris, deposits, or folds. The patient is discharged after being instructed not to rub the eye or to lie over it, and to use spectacles (with neutral or sunglasses) and a plastic shield at night during the first month. Contact lens wear in the fellow eye can be immediately resumed. Fluorometholone-antibiotic drops are used three times a day for one week, as well as artificial tears if there is any punctate epitheliopathy.

Macroscopic epithelial defects may require an occlusive bandage until healed but usually have no consequences. If a sector of the flap is found to be displaced it may be repositioned at the slit lamp, taking care to clean the stromal bed and not to superimpose its edge over the peripheral epithelium to avoid epithelial ingrowth (Figure 15-20). Gross deposits or debris in the interface must be promptly removed under aseptic/amoric conditions. Folds can be corrected only during the first or second weeks, by lifting, rehydrating the flap, and a carefully repositioning. Their tendency to persist, even before any scarring (collagen deposition) may have taken place, could be explained by configuration changes in the stromal proteoglycans. Distilled water has the strongest hydrating power, "detangling" the proteoglycan coils and allowing the reconfiguration required for effective ironing.

Follow-up Protocol

We have established a follow-up protocol that includes a series of postoperative visits at 1 day, 1 month, 3 months, and then yearly unless other conditions require more frequent attention. The examinations scheduled for each visit are summarized in Table 15-6. Any test with abnormal results is repeated at the next exam until normalized. At the 1-year visit, patients are asked to respond to a short questionnaire on satisfaction, spectacle usage, and subjective side effects (glare, halos, etc).

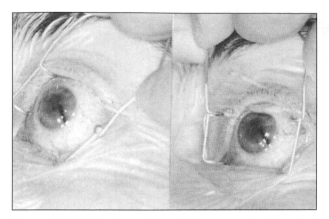

Figure 15-19. Displaced flap at the moment of the first dressing, 6 hours after treatment. It was immediately replaced with a sponge but developed interface epithelial ingrowth in 3 months. Fortunately, this was limited to the periphery and regressed 4 months later (photo used with permission from Buratto L, Brint SF. *LASIK: Principles and Techniques.* Thorofare, NJ: SLACK Incorporated; 1998).

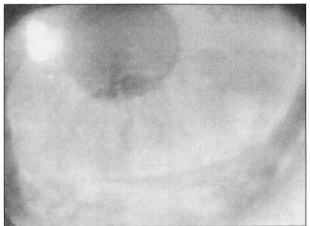

Figure 15-20. Sector of repositioned flap (photo used with permission from Buratto L, Brint SF. *LASIK: Principles and Techniques.* Thorofare, NJ: SLACK Incorporated; 1998).

Table 15-6

PREOPERATIVE AND FOLLOW-UP TEST PROTOCOL

Test	Preop	Early postop (2 to 5 hrs)	1st day	1 mo	3 mo	1 yr
Refraction (manifest)	X		X	X	X	X
Cycloplegic refraction	X				X	X
Glare test (BAT)	X			X		X
Contrast sensitivity	X			X	X	X
Corneal topography	X			X	X	X
Corneal pachymetry	X				X	X
Biometry (A-P axis)	X					X
Specular microscopy	X			X		X
Anterior segment + photos	X	X	X	X	X	X
Posterior segment	X				X	X
Lacrimal function (Schirmer)	X			X		X
Corneal sensation	X			X		X
IOP (Goldmann)	X			X		X

REFERENCES

1. Barraquer JI. Queratoplastia refractiva. *Estudios e Informaciones Oftalmol (Barc).* 1949:2:10.
2. Barraquer JI. *Cirugia Refractiva de la Cornea.* Bogota, Columbia: Instituto Barraquer de American; 1989.
3. Barraquer JI. Queratomileusis para la correcion de la myopia. *Arch Soc Amer Oftal Optom (Bogota).* 1964;5:27-48.
4. Barraquer JI. Keratmileusis. *Internat Surgury.* 1967;48:103.
5. Trokel GL, Srinivasaan R, Braren B. Excimer laser surgery of the cornea. *Am J Ophthalmol.* 1983;96:710-715.
6. Krawicz T. Lamellar Corneal Stromectomy. *Am J Ophthalmol.* 1964;57:828.
7. Pureskin NP. Weakening ocular refraction by means of partial stromectomy of cornea under experimental conditions. *Vestn Oftalmol.* 1967;80:1.
8. Ruiz LA, Rowsey JJ. In situ keratomileusis. *Invest Ophthalmol Vis Sci.* 1988;29(suppl):392.
9. Pallikaris IG. Papatzanaki ME, Stathi EZ, Frenschock O, Georgiadia A. Laser in situ keratomileusis. *Laser Surg Med.* 1990;10:463-468.
10. Buratto L, Ferrari M. Excimer laser intrastromal keratomileusis: case reports. *J Cataract Refract Surg.* 1992;18:37-41.
11. Buratto L, Ferrari M, Genisi C. Myopic keratomileusis with the excimer laser: One year follow-up. *J Refract Corneal Surg.* 1993;9:12-19.
12. Pallikaris IG, Siganos DS. Excimer laser in situ keratomileusis and photorefractive keratectomy for correction of high myopia. *J Refract Corneal Surg.* 1994;10:498-510.
13. Barraquer JI, Kargachin M, Alverez de Toledo JP. Personal technique for the correction of myopic ametropia. In: Buratto L, Brint, SL, eds. *LASIK: Principles and Techniques.* Thorofare, NJ: SLACK Incorporated; 1998.

Table 15-5

PROGRESSIVELY SPHERICAL EQUIVALENT-ADJUSTED LASIK NOMOGRAM FOR THE TREATMENT OF MYOPIC AMETROPIA WITH THE VISX STAR

S/C	-6.00	-5.75	-5.50	-5.25	-5.00	-4.75	-4.50	-4.25	-4.00	-3.75	-3.50	-3.25	-3.00	-2.75	-2.50	-2.25	-2.00	-1.75	-1.50	-1.25	-1.00	-0.75	-0.50	-0.25
-0.25	-0.14	-0.15	-0.16	-0.17	-0.17	-0.18	-0.19	-0.19	-0.20	-0.20	-0.21	-0.21	-0.22	-0.22	-0.23	-0.23	-0.23	-0.24	-0.24	-0.24	-0.24	-0.25	-0.25	-0.25
-0.50	-0.38	-0.39	-0.39	-0.40	-0.41	-0.42	-0.42	-0.43	-0.44	-0.44	-0.45	-0.45	-0.46	-0.46	-0.47	-0.47	-0.48	-0.48	-0.48	-0.49	-0.49	-0.49	-0.49	-0.50
-0.75	-0.61	-0.62	-0.63	-0.64	-0.64	-0.65	-0.66	-0.67	-0.67	-0.68	-0.69	-0.69	-0.70	-0.70	-0.71	-0.71	-0.72	-0.72	-0.73	-0.73	-0.73	-0.74	-0.74	-0.74
-1.00	-0.84	-0.85	-0.86	-0.87	-0.88	-0.89	-0.89	-0.90	-0.91	-0.92	-0.92	-0.93	-0.94	-0.94	-0.95	-0.95	-0.96	-0.96	-0.97	-0.97	-0.98	-0.98	-0.98	-0.99
-1.25	-1.07	-1.08	-1.09	-1.10	-1.11	-1.12	-1.13	-1.14	-1.14	-1.15	-1.16	-1.17	-1.17	-1.18	-1.19	-1.19	-1.20	-1.20	-1.21	-1.21	-1.22	-1.22	-1.23	-1.23
-1.50	-1.30	-1.31	-1.32	-1.33	-1.34	-1.35	-1.36	-1.37	-1.38	-1.39	-1.39	-1.40	-1.41	-1.42	-1.42	-1.43	-1.44	-1.44	-1.45	-1.45	-1.46	-1.46	-1.47	-1.47
-1.75	-1.52	-1.54	-1.55	-1.56	-1.57	-1.58	-1.59	-1.60	-1.61	-1.62	-1.63	-1.64	-1.64	-1.65	-1.66	-1.67	-1.67	-1.68	-1.69	-1.69	-1.70	-1.70	-1.71	-1.71
-2.00	-1.75	-1.76	-1.77	-1.79	-1.80	-1.81	-1.82	-1.83	-1.84	-1.85	-1.86	-1.87	-1.88	-1.89	-1.89	-1.90	-1.91	-1.92	-1.92	-1.93	-1.94	-1.94	-1.95	-1.95
-2.25	-1.97	-1.99	-2.00	-2.01	-2.02	-2.04	-2.05	-2.06	-2.07	-2.08	-2.09	-2.10	-2.11	-2.12	-2.13	-2.14	-2.14	-2.15	-2.16	-2.17	-2.17	-2.18	-2.19	-2.19
-2.50	-2.20	-2.21	-2.22	-2.24	-2.25	-2.26	-2.27	-2.29	-2.30	-2.31	-2.32	-2.33	-2.34	-2.35	-2.36	-2.37	-2.38	-2.39	-2.39	-2.40	-2.41	-2.42	-2.42	-2.43
-2.75	-2.42	-2.43	-2.45	-2.46	-2.47	-2.49	-2.50	-2.51	-2.52	-2.54	-2.55	-2.56	-2.57	-2.58	-2.59	-2.60	-2.61	-2.62	-2.63	-2.64	-2.64	-2.65	-2.66	-2.67
-3.00	-2.64	-2.65	-2.67	-2.68	-2.70	-2.71	-2.72	-2.74	-2.75	-2.76	-2.77	-2.79	-2.80	-2.81	-2.82	-2.83	-2.84	-2.85	-2.86	-2.87	-2.88	-2.89	-2.89	-2.90
-3.25	-2.86	-2.87	-2.89	-2.90	-2.92	-2.93	-2.95	-2.96	-2.97	-2.99	-3.00	-3.01	-3.02	-3.04	-3.05	-3.06	-3.07	-3.08	-3.09	-3.10	-3.11	-3.12	-3.13	-3.14
-3.50	-3.08	-3.09	-3.11	-3.12	-3.14	-3.15	-3.17	-3.18	-3.20	-3.21	-3.22	-3.24	-3.25	-3.26	-3.27	-3.29	-3.30	-3.31	-3.32	-3.33	-3.34	-3.35	-3.36	-3.37
-3.75	-3.29	-3.31	-3.33	-3.34	-3.36	-3.37	-3.39	-3.40	-3.42	-3.43	-3.45	-3.46	-3.47	-3.49	-3.50	-3.51	-3.52	-3.54	-3.55	-3.56	-3.57	-3.58	-3.59	-3.60
-4.00	-3.51	-3.53	-3.54	-3.56	-3.58	-3.59	-3.61	-3.62	-3.64	-3.65	-3.67	-3.68	-3.70	-3.71	-3.72	-3.74	-3.75	-3.76	-3.77	-3.79	-3.80	-3.81	-3.82	-3.83
-4.25	-3.72	-3.74	-3.76	-3.78	-3.79	-3.81	-3.83	-3.84	-3.86	-3.87	-3.89	-3.90	-3.92	-3.93	-3.95	-3.96	-3.97	-3.99	-4.00	-4.01	-4.02	-4.04	-4.05	-4.06
-4.50	-3.94	-3.96	-3.97	-3.99	-4.01	-4.03	-4.04	-4.06	-4.08	-4.09	-4.11	-4.12	-4.14	-4.15	-4.17	-4.18	-4.20	-4.21	-4.22	-4.24	-4.25	-4.26	-4.27	-4.29
-4.75	-4.15	-4.17	-4.19	-4.21	-4.22	-4.24	-4.26	-4.28	-4.29	-4.31	-4.33	-4.34	-4.36	-4.37	-4.39	-4.40	-4.42	-4.43	-4.45	-4.46	-4.47	-4.49	-4.50	-4.51
-5.00	-4.36	-4.38	-4.40	-4.42	-4.44	-4.46	-4.47	-4.49	-4.51	-4.53	-4.54	-4.56	-4.58	-4.59	-4.61	-4.62	-4.64	-4.65	-4.67	-4.68	-4.70	-4.71	-4.72	-4.74
-5.25	-4.57	-4.59	-4.61	-4.63	-4.65	-4.67	-4.69	-4.71	-4.72	-4.74	-4.76	-4.78	-4.79	-4.81	-4.83	-4.84	-4.86	-4.87	-4.89	-4.90	-4.92	-4.93	-4.95	-4.96
-5.50	-4.78	-4.80	-4.82	-4.84	-4.86	-4.88	-4.90	-4.92	-4.94	-4.96	-4.97	-4.99	-5.01	-5.03	-5.04	-5.06	-5.08	-5.09	-5.11	-5.12	-5.14	-5.15	-5.17	-5.18
-5.75	-4.98	-5.01	-5.03	-5.05	-5.07	-5.09	-5.11	-5.13	-5.15	-5.17	-5.19	-5.21	-5.22	-5.24	-5.26	-5.28	-5.29	-5.31	-5.33	-5.34	-5.36	-5.37	-5.39	-5.40
-6.00	-5.19	-5.21	-5.23	-5.26	-5.28	-5.30	-5.32	-5.34	-5.36	-5.38	-5.40	-5.42	-5.44	-5.46	-5.47	-5.49	-5.51	-5.53	-5.54	-5.56	-5.58	-5.59	-5.61	-5.62
-6.25	-5.39	-5.42	-5.44	-5.46	-5.48	-5.51	-5.53	-5.55	-5.57	-5.59	-5.61	-5.63	-5.65	-5.67	-5.69	-5.71	-5.72	-5.74	-5.76	-5.78	-5.79	-5.81	-5.83	-5.84
-6.50	-5.60	-5.62	-5.64	-5.67	-5.69	-5.71	-5.73	-5.76	-5.78	-5.80	-5.82	-5.84	-5.86	-5.88	-5.90	-5.92	-5.94	-5.96	-5.97	-5.99	-6.01	-6.03	-6.04	-6.06
-6.75	-5.80	-5.82	-5.85	-5.87	-5.89	-5.92	-5.94	-5.96	-5.98	-6.01	-6.03	-6.05	-6.07	-6.09	-6.11	-6.13	-6.15	-6.17	-6.19	-6.21	-6.22	-6.24	-6.26	-6.28
-7.00	-6.00	-6.02	-6.05	-6.07	-6.10	-6.12	-6.14	-6.17	-6.19	-6.21	-6.23	-6.26	-6.28	-6.30	-6.32	-6.34	-6.36	-6.38	-6.40	-6.42	-6.44	-6.46	-6.47	-6.49
-7.25	-6.20	-6.22	-6.25	-6.27	-6.30	-6.32	-6.35	-6.37	-6.39	-6.42	-6.44	-6.46	-6.48	-6.51	-6.53	-6.55	-6.57	-6.59	-6.61	-6.63	-6.65	-6.67	-6.69	-6.71
-7.50	-6.40	-6.42	-6.45	-6.47	-6.50	-6.52	-6.55	-6.57	-6.60	-6.62	-6.64	-6.67	-6.69	-6.71	-6.73	-6.76	-6.78	-6.80	-6.82	-6.84	-6.86	-6.88	-6.90	-6.92
-7.75	-6.59	-6.62	-6.65	-6.67	-6.70	-6.72	-6.75	-6.77	-6.80	-6.82	-6.85	-6.87	-6.89	-6.92	-6.94	-6.96	-6.98	-7.01	-7.03	-7.05	-7.07	-7.09	-7.11	-7.13
-8.00	-6.79	-6.82	-6.84	-6.87	-6.90	-6.92	-6.95	-6.97	-7.00	-7.02	-7.05	-7.07	-7.10	-7.12	-7.14	-7.17	-7.19	-7.21	-7.23	-7.26	-7.28	-7.30	-7.32	-7.34
-8.25	-6.98	-7.01	-7.04	-7.07	-7.09	-7.12	-7.15	-7.17	-7.20	-7.22	-7.25	-7.27	-7.30	-7.32	-7.35	-7.37	-7.39	-7.42	-7.44	-7.46	-7.48	-7.51	-7.53	-7.55
-8.50	-7.18	-7.21	-7.23	-7.26	-7.29	-7.32	-7.34	-7.37	-7.40	-7.42	-7.45	-7.47	-7.50	-7.52	-7.55	-7.57	-7.60	-7.62	-7.64	-7.67	-7.69	-7.71	-7.73	-7.76
-8.75	-7.37	-7.40	-7.43	-7.46	-7.48	-7.51	-7.54	-7.57	-7.59	-7.62	-7.65	-7.67	-7.70	-7.72	-7.75	-7.77	-7.80	-7.82	-7.85	-7.87	-7.89	-7.92	-7.94	-7.96
-9.00	-7.56	-7.59	-7.62	-7.65	-7.68	-7.71	-7.73	-7.76	-7.79	-7.82	-7.84	-7.87	-7.90	-7.92	-7.95	-7.97	-8.00	-8.02	-8.05	-8.07	-8.10	-8.12	-8.14	-8.17
-9.25	-7.75	-7.78	-7.81	-7.84	-7.87	-7.90	-7.93	-7.96	-7.98	-8.01	-8.04	-8.07	-8.09	-8.12	-8.15	-8.17	-8.20	-8.22	-8.25	-8.27	-8.30	-8.32	-8.35	-8.37
-9.50	-7.94	-7.97	-8.00	-8.03	-8.06	-8.09	-8.12	-8.15	-8.18	-8.21	-8.23	-8.26	-8.29	-8.32	-8.34	-8.37	-8.40	-8.42	-8.45	-8.47	-8.50	-8.52	-8.55	-8.57
-9.75	-8.12	-8.16	-8.19	-8.22	-8.25	-8.28	-8.31	-8.34	-8.37	-8.40	-8.43	-8.46	-8.48	-8.51	-8.54	-8.57	-8.59	-8.62	-8.65	-8.67	-8.70	-8.72	-8.75	-8.77
-10.00	-8.31	-8.34	-8.37	-8.41	-8.44	-8.47	-8.50	-8.53	-8.56	-8.59	-8.62	-8.65	-8.68	-8.71	-8.73	-8.76	-8.79	-8.82	-8.84	-8.87	-8.90	-8.92	-8.95	-8.97
-10.25	-8.49	-8.53	-8.56	-8.59	-8.62	-8.66	-8.69	-8.72	-8.75	-8.78	-8.81	-8.84	-8.87	-8.90	-8.93	-8.96	-8.98	-9.01	-9.04	-9.07	-9.09	-9.12	-9.15	-9.17
-10.50	-8.68	-8.71	-8.74	-8.78	-8.81	-8.84	-8.87	-8.91	-8.94	-8.97	-9.00	-9.03	-9.06	-9.09	-9.12	-9.15	-9.18	-9.21	-9.23	-9.26	-9.29	-9.32	-9.34	-9.37
-10.75	-8.86	-8.89	-8.93	-8.96	-8.99	-9.03	-9.06	-9.09	-9.12	-9.16	-9.19	-9.22	-9.25	-9.28	-9.31	-9.34	-9.37	-9.40	-9.43	-9.46	-9.48	-9.51	-9.54	-9.57
-11.00	-9.04	-9.07	-9.11	-9.14	-9.18	-9.21	-9.24	-9.28	-9.31	-9.34	-9.37	-9.41	-9.44	-9.47	-9.50	-9.53	-9.56	-9.59	-9.62	-9.65	-9.68	-9.71	-9.73	-9.76
-11.25	-9.22	-9.25	-9.29	-9.32	-9.36	-9.39	-9.43	-9.46	-9.49	-9.53	-9.56	-9.59	-9.62	-9.66	-9.69	-9.72	-9.75	-9.78	-9.81	-9.84	-9.87	-9.90	-9.93	-9.96
-11.50	-9.40	-9.43	-9.47	-9.50	-9.54	-9.57	-9.61	-9.64	-9.68	-9.71	-9.74	-9.78	-9.81	-9.84	-9.87	-9.91	-9.94	-9.97	-10.00	-10.03	-10.06	-10.09	-10.12	-10.15
-11.75	-9.57	-9.61	-9.65	-9.68	-9.72	-9.75	-9.79	-9.82	-9.86	-9.89	-9.93	-9.96	-9.99	-10.03	-10.06	-10.09	-10.12	-10.16	-10.19	-10.22	-10.25	-10.28	-10.31	-10.34
-12.00	-9.75	-9.79	-9.82	-9.86	-9.90	-9.93	-9.97	-10.00	-10.04	-10.07	-10.11	-10.14	-10.18	-10.21	-10.24	-10.28	-10.31	-10.34	-10.37	-10.41	-10.44	-10.47	-10.50	-10.53
-12.25	-9.92	-9.96	-10.00	-10.04	-10.07	-10.11	-10.15	-10.18	-10.22	-10.25	-10.29	-10.32	-10.36	-10.39	-10.43	-10.46	-10.49	-10.53	-10.56	-10.59	-10.62	-10.66	-10.69	-10.72
-12.50	-10.10	-10.14	-10.17	-10.21	-10.25	-10.29	-10.32	-10.36	-10.40	-10.43	-10.47	-10.50	-10.54	-10.57	-10.61	-10.64	-10.68	-10.71	-10.74	-10.78	-10.81	-10.84	-10.87	-10.91
-12.75	-10.27	-10.31	-10.35	-10.39	-10.42	-10.46	-10.50	-10.54	-10.57	-10.61	-10.65	-10.68	-10.72	-10.75	-10.79	-10.82	-10.86	-10.89	-10.93	-10.96	-10.99	-11.03	-11.06	-11.09
-13.00	-10.44	-10.48	-10.52	-10.56	-10.60	-10.64	-10.67	-10.71	-10.75	-10.79	-10.82	-10.86	-10.90	-10.93	-10.97	-11.00	-11.04	-11.07	-11.11	-11.14	-11.18	-11.21	-11.24	-11.28
-13.25	-10.61	-10.65	-10.69	-10.73	-10.77	-10.81	-10.85	-10.89	-10.92	-10.96	-11.00	-11.04	-11.07	-11.11	-11.15	-11.18	-11.22	-11.25	-11.29	-11.32	-11.36	-11.39	-11.43	-11.46
-13.50	-10.78	-10.82	-10.86	-10.90	-10.94	-10.98	-11.02	-11.06	-11.10	-11.14	-11.17	-11.21	-11.25	-11.29	-11.32	-11.36	-11.40	-11.43	-11.47	-11.50	-11.54	-11.57	-11.61	-11.64
-13.75	-10.94	-10.99	-11.03	-11.07	-11.11	-11.15	-11.19	-11.23	-11.27	-11.31	-11.35	-11.39	-11.42	-11.46	-11.50	-11.54	-11.57	-11.61	-11.65	-11.68	-11.72	-11.75	-11.79	-11.82
-14.00	-11.11	-11.15	-11.19	-11.24	-11.28	-11.32	-11.36	-11.40	-11.44	-11.48	-11.52	-11.56	-11.60	-11.64	-11.67	-11.71	-11.75	-11.79	-11.82	-11.86	-11.90	-11.93	-11.97	-12.00
-14.25	-11.27	-11.32	-11.36	-11.40	-11.44	-11.49	-11.53	-11.57	-11.61	-11.65	-11.69	-11.73	-11.77	-11.81	-11.85	-11.89	-11.92	-11.96	-12.00	-12.04	-12.07	-12.11	-12.15	-12.18
-14.50	-11.44	-11.48	-11.52	-11.57	-11.61	-11.65	-11.69	-11.74	-11.78	-11.82	-11.86	-11.90	-11.94	-11.98	-12.02	-12.06	-12.10	-12.14	-12.17	-12.21	-12.25	-12.29	-12.32	-12.36
-14.75	-11.60	-11.64	-11.69	-11.73	-11.77	-11.82	-11.86	-11.90	-11.94	-11.99	-12.03	-12.07	-12.11	-12.15	-12.19	-12.23	-12.27	-12.31	-12.35	-12.39	-12.42	-12.46	-12.50	-12.54
-15.00	-11.76	-11.80	-11.85	-11.89	-11.94	-11.98	-12.02	-12.07	-12.11	-12.15	-12.19	-12.24	-12.28	-12.32	-12.36	-12.40	-12.44	-12.48	-12.52	-12.56	-12.60	-12.64	-12.67	-12.71

THE SCMD MICROKERATOME AND SURGICAL TECHNIQUE

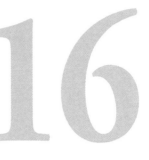

John T. LiVecchi, MD

INTRODUCTION

Laser in-situ keratomileusis (LASIK) has become virtually the most popular refractive procedure, at the time of this writing. This chapter will give the reader insight on the SCMD microkeratome used specifically for LASIK. The SCMD microkeratome was the first microkeratome made for LASIK. Its predecessor was used for keratomileusis in-situ for myopic patients (MLK-M) and hyperopic patients (MLK-H).

SCMD TURBOKERATOME SYSTEM FOR LASIK

The LASIK turbokeratome system was the first microkeratome designed specifically to produce a corneal flap in keratorefractive surgery. This system features a high-speed, high-torque nitrogen driven turbine motor that drives a reciprocating surgical blade at the ideal speed of 13,800 revolutions per minute (RPM). The turbokeratome head is a preset system to produce a corneal resection of 150 microns thick. By virtue of various factors such as intraoperative pressure (IOP), corneal hydration, and surgeon bias, the resected tissue thickness can somewhat vary. The LASIK turbokeratome system can produce flaps of four different diameters: 7.5 mm, 8.0 mm, 8.5 mm, and 9.0 mm.

POSITION OF FLAP AND HINGE

There are several factors that can influence the size of the flap and position of the hinge. Intraocular pressure should be maintained at 65 mm Hg or higher. Accurate measurements, proper suction, and sound surgical technique will provide the best results. The applanator lens confirms the diameter of the exposed cornea and produce a reference mark for the hinge position. There are four

applanator lenses provided with the turbokeratome system: 7.5 mm, 8.25 mm, 8.75 mm, and 9.25 mm. Four different vacuum fixation rings control the diameter of the cornea that is exposed above them. The rings are numbered one to four, with the number one ring being the thinnest and the number four the thickest. The number one ring allows the largest diameter of the cornea to be exposed, while the number four ring allows the smaller diameter of cornea to be exposed. The stop ring limits the travel of the LASIK turbokeratome through the vacuum fixation ring to perform a flap and hinge.

As mentioned earlier, four different diameter flaps can be produced. The flap size is indicated on each stop ring. If, for example, a 7.5 mm flap is desired, the 7.5 mm stop ring would be selected for the surgical case. The 8.25 mm applanator lens is used. The number three or four vacuum fixation ring is selected based on surgical preference. The objective is to expose a diameter of cornea that is larger than the stop ring selected. In this case, mentioned, the diameter of the cornea is confirmed with the 8.25 mm applanator lens. When a 8.25 mm diameter of cornea is exposed and the stop ring limits the travel of the turbokeratome to 7.5 mm, a flap measuring 7.5 mm will be produced with a hinge of 0.75 mm. Thus, 8.25 mm to 7.5 mm produces a hinge of 0.75 mm. The number three or four vacuum fixation ring is placed on the eye and suction is activated with the foot switch. The IOP is immediately checked with a Barraquer tonometer and must be at least 65 mm Hg. The 8.25 mm applanator lens is placed within the dovetail of the fixation ring and the meniscus of the cornea is measured with the circular scribe bar of the applanator lens. If the meniscus completely fills the scribe mark on the applanator lens, 8.25 mm Hg is exposed. The corneal exposure must exceed the size of the stop ring to produce the flap.

The thickness of the hinge is determined by how much the diameter of exposed cornea exceeds the stop ring. If the meniscus measures less than the scribe mark of the applanator lens, the vacuum fixation ring should be changed to a lower number to expose a larger diameter of cornea. The lower the number, the thinner the ring and vice versa; the thinner the ring, the more corneal exposure.

Some of the features of the "new era" LASIK turbokeratome include an innovative head design with an adjustable stop nut that can produce a 10.5 mm and larger resection. The new turbokeratome is much quieter than its predecessor. Also, no lubrication is required, as the introduction of a nonmetal durable drive-dog was instituted. The new innovative head design is one piece with a patent-pending hinge to allow proper cleaning and sterilization. Its reinforced support makes for a stronger, more reliable control and for quick and easy blade set-up. Therefore, the new keratome's unique adjustable stop nut with a hinge-design head allows greater motility and precision control.

THE LASIK NOMOGRAM

There is not one nomogram that can be used universally for LASIK. Therefore, each LASIK surgeon requires a personalized nomogram to ensure optimal results.

The LASIK Procedure: Personal Technique

Preoperative

After the patient signs the necessary informed consent, a sedative, such as valium, is offered to the patient. In my practice, 50% of patients opt for a dose of valium to eliminate preoperative anxiety. Ophthalmic solutions in the form of an anesthetic, antibiotic, and a nonsteroidal anti-inflammatory (NSAID) are given on a regular basis. My personal preference is 0.5% proparacaine times three for anesthesia; Ciloxin or Ocuflox antibiotic for prophylactic coverage; and Voltaren and NSAID drops to reduce inflammation and postoperative pain. The application of proparacaine is repeated immediately before applying the speculum. I have found that excessive doses of anesthetic can interfere with the integrity of the epithelium and weaken the adhesion between the epithelium and Bowman's membrane, causing it to be sloughed microkeratome translation.

Surgical Procedure

The patient should be prepared and draped in the usual sterile manner. I use Betadine solution to cleanse the surrounding eyelids and periocular area. The patient should be comfortably positioned on the operating chair or table. It is especially important to position the patient in the appropriate manner so laser treatment of the stroma can be performed in a timely fashion. Also important is proper positioning the patient. This will ensure an accurate ablation. This important maneuver not only makes it efficient, but also prevents excessive tissue hydration or dehydration. The microkeratome should have been assembled and pretested prior to surgery. One should also test the turbokeratome along the dovetail guides to insure a smooth translation of the microkeratome. A wire lid speculum is placed in the eye to enhance exposure. The visual axis is marked with a 2.5 mm optical zone marker. A large diameter optical zone marker specifically designed for LASIK is then centered on the visual axis. Additional marks are made across the cornea to allow accurate repositioning of the flap at the end of the procedure. This is important in the event that the flap is inadvertently amputated. A preselected vacuum fixation ring is accurately placed on the globe.

It is very important to precisely place the vacuum fixation ring on the globe, as it usually produces a slight indentation of the globe such that subsequent repositioning of the ring may not be possible. When suction is properly applied with a well-centered vacuum fixation ring, an IOP of 65 mm Hg or higher is measured with a Barraquer applanating tonometer. If the pressure is too low, adequate vacuum fixation may not have been achieved and this must be corrected in order to have an accurate corneal resection. The applanator lens is then applied to confirm the diameter of the cornea. The reference inscribed on the applanator lens will determine the intended position of the hinge. The turbokeratome head is then inserted into the dovetails of the vacuum fixation ring. The dovetails of the ring are lubricated with several drops of balanced salt solution (BSS). The passage of the turbokeratome within the dovetail guides should be performed from the surgeon's shoulder rather than from the wrist or hands. When the turbokeratome head is engaged with the dovetail guides, the turbine motor is then activated with a foot switch. The turbokeratome is then translated across the surface of the cornea in a smooth, uninterrupted fashion until the stop ring contacts with the vacuum fixation ring. A smooth, continuous passage of the turbokeratome in one hand along with a light touch holding the handle of the fixation ring in the other hand is crucial for a perfect resection. When the stop ring comes in contact with the fixation ring, stop the turbine motor while continuing to maintain suction. The turbokeratome head is then gently reversed and withdrawn from the vacuum fixation ring, allowing the corneal flap to slip through the microkeratome cutting aperture. The vacuum foot switch is last to be released and the fixation ring is then removed from the eye. If the patient is properly positioned on the operating table, laser ablation can be performed without delay in order to avoid problems associated with tissue hydration changes. While the patient fixates on the microscope fixation light, the corneal flap is reflected out of the field and laser treatment is then initiated. At determination of photoablation within the corneal bed, the flap is gently repositioned with a blunt instrument. It is repositioned accurately by virtue of the previously marked cornea. Corneal wrinkles are ironed out with a damp Merocel sponge. Compression of the central cornea enhances the removal of fluid and insures tight contact between the flap and the stroma. The cornea is then allowed to dry for approximately 3 to 5 minutes, with the microscope light out, so that the cornea holds firmly with the flap in place. The lid speculum is then removed and the patient is asked to blink the eye several times. Close observation of the corneal flap while blinking is essential to assess the stability. A topical nonsteroidal, an antibiotic drop, and a steroidal drop is instilled in the conjunctival sac. A pressure patch is contraindicated, and only a protective plastic shield is placed into position over the eye. The patient tolerates the procedure well without any reaction or complication. The patient is seen 15 minutes postoperatively to check the flap and then sent home and seen the next day for a follow-up appointment.

On the first postoperative day, the eye is examined and if all is well, the patient is instructed to use the antibiotic and steroid drop for approximately 1 week.

THE SUMMIT KRUMEICH-BARRAQUER MICROKERATOME AND SURGICAL TECHNIQUE

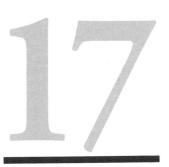

Michael Gordon, MD,
Miles Friedlander, MD, and Perry S. Binder, MD

INTRODUCTION

Rapid visual recovery and generally excellent outcomes have placed laser-assisted in-situ keratomileusis (LASIK) at the forefront of refractive surgical procedures throughout the world. In the LASIK surgical procedure, a microkeratome is used to create a lamellar flap of the anterior corneal surface that can be lifted to expose the stromal bed to excimer laser photoablation. Through variations in the depth and pattern of the ablation, the curvature of the anterior cornea can be changed, and myopia, hyperopia, or astigmatism can be corrected.[1-14]

For many years, surgeons were limited in their choice of microkeratomes since few designs were available.[15,16] However, new models have recently been introduced, including the Summit Krumeich-Barraquer Microkeratome (SKBM) (Summit Technology, Inc, Waltham, Mass, USA). This instrument is electrically powered, gearless, has a one-piece microkeratome head with a snap-on mount, multiple port suction rings, and permits full visualization of the applanated cornea. It also allows the surgeon to perform customized surgery by permitting selection of hinge and suction ring size, blade traverse distance, and advancement and oscillation speed of the blade by means of front panel settings on the control unit.

COMPONENTS OF THE SKBM

The major components of the SKBM are the control unit that includes operator controls, a microcomputer, a vacuum pump, and a back-up power supply a microkeratome handpiece that contains motors for blade oscillation and advancement a microkeratome head that has an oscillating steel cutting blade four suction rings suction ring handle and vacuum tube connector.

Technical specifications of the SKBM are shown in Table 17-1, and the assembled unit is illustrated in Figures 17-1 and 17-2.

PREPARING THE SKBM FOR USE

Step 1. Insert the blade. Use only Summit single-use, disposable steel blades with the SKBM and, to maintain cutting quality, do not allow the cutting edge of the blade to come in contact with any other surface. Carefully remove the blade from the package with powder-free gloves or sterile forceps, and insert it gently into the slot that spans the width of the microkeratome head (Figure 17-3). Keep the microkeratome head level or cover the slot openings with the thumb and index finger to prevent the blade from falling out of the slot. Confirm free movement of the blade by grasping it with forceps and moving it from side to side within the slot. If the blade moves freely, center it in the slot. If the blade sticks or resists movement, do not proceed with the procedure.

Step 2. Position the eccentric pin. At the end of the motor shaft are three small pins. The center pin is the eccentric pin, which drives the blade oscillation. Dial the eccentric pin to the 6 or 12 o'clock position to allow the motor shaft to engage correctly with the microkeratome head (Figure 17-4). If the eccentric pin is not positioned correctly, the microkeratome head will not engage with the motor shaft.

Step 3. Connect the microkeratome head to the handpiece motor shaft. Pinch the extended pins on the side of the microkeratome head and gently advance the head onto the motor shaft until it clicks. Release pinch on the pins. To ensure that the microkeratome head is connected properly, grasp the head gently between your fingers and try to move it around the shaft. If the head rotates freely or moves back and forth, it is not connected properly with the motor shaft.

Step 4. Connect the metal band to the handpiece. Perform this step only after the microkeratome head has

Table 17-1		
TECHNICAL SPECIFICATIONS OF THE SKBM		
Selectable Parameters		
Design feature	**Description**	**Comments**
Diameter of applanated cornea	0.01 mm to 10 mm	Selectable by suction ring type
Operating mode	Automatic or manual	Automatic recommended
Blade oscillation rate	0 to 20,000 RPM	User programmable
Blade advancement speed	0.1 mm to 3.0 mm/sec	User programmable
Hinge width range	0.1 mm to 9.0 mm	User programmable
Fixed Design Features		
Suction rings	Ring 21 #3 = 21 mm outer diameter,	9.0 to 9.5 mm flap diameter
	Ring 21 #4 = 21 mm outer diameter,	8.0 to 8.5 mm flap diameter
	Ring 19 #3 = 19 mm outer diameter,	9.0 to 9.5 mm flap diameter
	Ring 19 #4 = 19 mm outer diameter,	8.0 to 8.5 mm flap diameter
Flap thickness range	160 µm ± 20 µm	Precision-milled using CAD/CAM-controlled wire erosion technology
Blade type	Stainless steel	Single use, disposable
Active drive	Gearless motor drive	Computer controlled
Vacuum	0.0 to -1.0 bar	Minimum of -0.8 required for cutting a flap
Applanation window	See-through applanation plate	Has calibration markings for assessing flap diameter
Universal power supply	100 to 240 volts	Three-pin, grounded, 50-60 Hz
Back-up power	Present	Sufficient to complete one initiated procedure
Control function foot pedal or push button calibration	Self-calibrating when powered	Self-calibration continues between procedures
Accessories	Tonometer, corneal marker, sterilization tray	

been mounted to the handpiece. Note that one end of the metal band is bent at a slight angle, while the other end has a triangular eyelet and narrow slot. Starting on the side closest to the microkeratome head, slide the angled end of the metal band (with the angle extending away from the handpiece) into the tracks on the underside of the handpiece. Continue sliding the bar gently along the tracks until the round end of the narrow slot is centered over the long guidepin (located near the microkeratome head). Gently depress the slotted end of the metal band until the uppermost part of the guidepin extends through the round opening. Then, continue to slide the metal band forward until the opening at the angled end of the band connects with the short guidepin on the cable end of the microkeratome handpiece. Ensure that the long guidepin remains in the slot while you slide the band into place (Figure 17-5).

Step 5. Attach the moisture reservoir to the control unit. Insert the metal pin into the small opening on top of the control unit (directly above the vacuum port). Then attach one end of the long (2.0 m) vacuum tubing

to the angled plastic port on top of the moisture reservoir. A filter is attached to the shorter length of tubing (one side of the filter has writing on it). Attach one end of the shorter vacuum tubing (with writing on the filter facing up toward the reservoir) to the straight plastic port on the moisture reservoir and the other end to the metal vacuum port on the control unit (Figure 17-6).

Step 6. Attach the suction ring to the handle. Screw the suction ring handle onto the suction ring. Attach the open end of the 2 m vacuum tubing to the end of the suction ring handle.

Step 7. Turn the system on. Before turning the system on, be sure that all electrical cables are plugged into the control unit. Turn the system on by pressing the on/off switch on the back panel of the control unit. Allow the system to warm up for 3 to 4 minutes prior to use. This allows the back-up power supply to charge.

Step 8. Create a vacuum. When the system is turned on, the "power" light emitting diode (LED) on the front panel illuminates, and the microkeratome advancement drive automatically moves to the "reference" (start)

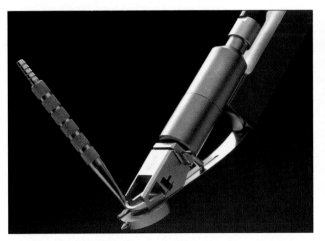

Figure 17-1. The Summit Krumeich-Barraquer microkeratome.

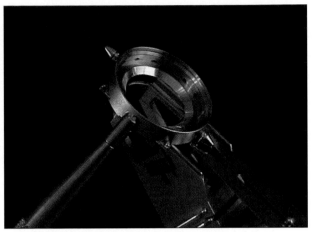

Figure 17-2. Underside view of the SKBM.

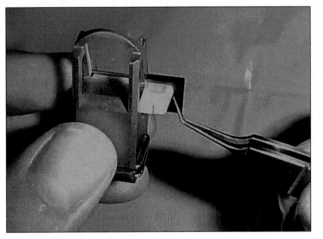

Figure 17-3. Blade insertion.

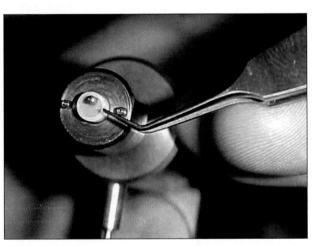

Figure 17-4. Positioning the eccentric pin.

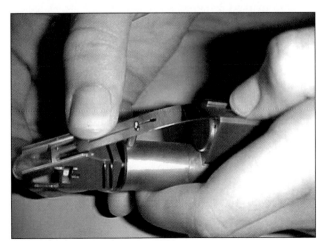

Figure 17-5. Locking the metal band.

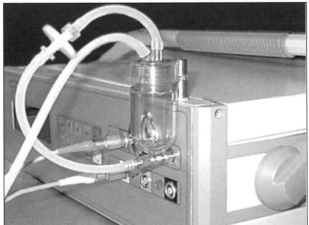

Figure 17-6. Attachment of vacuum tubing.

Table 17-2

CONTROL UNIT DISPLAY

Parameter	Display	Comments
Diameter	9.0 mm	This setting must reflect the actual diameter of the applanated cornea (ie, if applanation with the ring is 9.0 mm, set the display to 9.0 mm)
Speed	1.5 mm/sec	Advancement speed across the cornea
Cutter	14,000 RPM	Oscillation speed of the cutting blade
Hinge	0.5 mm	Width of the uncut corneal segment

Table 17-3

PARAMETERS OF SKBM SUCTION RINGS

Suction ring	Outer diameter	Diameter of created flap
21 #3	21 mm	9.0 to 9.5 mm
21 #4	21 mm	8.0 to 8.5 mm
19 #3	19 mm	9.0 to 9.5 mm
19 #4	19 mm	8.0 to 8.5 mm

The numbers used for flap size (#3 or #4) follow original Barraquer nomenclature whereby the lower the number, the larger the expected applanation.

position and the vacuum pump starts to operate. It takes approximately 30 seconds for the nominal vacuum (approximately -0.8 bar) to be reached. The microkeratome motor will not operate until this level of vacuum has been reached. For safety reasons, the vacuum pump remains on even after the nominal vacuum level has been reached.

To check the vacuum pressure, press the "vacuum" key or the vacuum foot pedal. Pinch the vacuum tubing to prevent air from entering the vacuum system. Check the vacuum gauge. The pressure should be at least -0.8 bar. If the vacuum tubing has drawn in air, the vacuum must be closed (by pinching the tubing) for about 20 seconds to rebuild vacuum pressure.

Step 9. Set the parameters on the panel. The user will be prompted to select:

- The suction ring diameter, 19 mm or 21 mm
- The mode of operation (eg, automatic [recommended] or manual)
- Cutter speed
- Hinge size

Responding to the prompts activates the operating modality, and the procedure parameters are then displayed on the control unit (Table 17-2). The parameters can be changed by moving the cursor position.

THE SUCTION RINGS

Description

A total of four suction rings are included with the SKBM: two rings with an outside diameter of 19 mm and two with an outside diameter of 21 mm. The rings must be sterilized prior to every patient procedure. The rings are also marked as either #3 or #4 to indicate expected flap size (Table 17-3 and Figure 17-7). The #3 rings will normally produce the same diameter flap on both the 19- and 21-mm rings, as will the #4 rings. The numbers used for flap size follow the original Barraquer nomenclature, whereby the lower the number, the larger the expected applanation and, therefore, the larger the flap diameter.

Suction rings marked #3 have a shallower depth, so that they sit lower on the cornea. When these rings are used during a procedure, a larger diameter of cornea is applanated and larger flaps (9.0 to 9.5 mm) are obtained. It is important to note that the 19-mm rings do not protect the eyelids and drapes to the same extent as the 21-mm rings (because the steel blade oscillates approximately 0.85 mm beyond the width of the microkeratome head). The operator should carefully monitor the progress of the steel blade during the cutting phase to

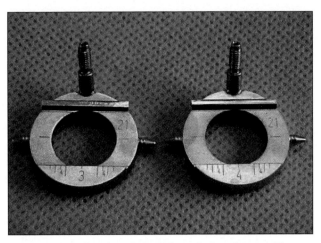

Figure 17-7. Suction rings (21 mm) showing markings.

prevent possible injury to the eyelid when using the 19-mm ring.

Suction rings marked #4 have a deeper depth, so that they sit higher on the cornea. When these rings are used during a procedure, a smaller diameter of cornea is applanated and smaller flaps (8.5 to 9.0 mm) are obtained.

In order to obtain a flap of the desired size, the meniscus of the cornea must correspond with the marking observed in the window of the microkeratome head. For example, if 8.5 mm of cornea is visibly applanated in the window and the panel setting is maintained at 9.0 mm for the cut diameter, the cut may be larger than the flap, causing a free cap. Similarly, if 9.5 mm of the cornea is visibly applanated in the window and the panel setting is maintained at 9.0 mm for the cut diameter, the cut will be smaller and the hinge larger than desired. If these do not correspond, adjust the panel settings.

Ring Selection

1. Select the appropriate suction ring and screw it onto the suction ring handle. Connect one end of the long vacuum tubing to the moisture reservoir and the other to the suction ring handle.
2. Assemble the SKBM as indicated in the section *Preparing the SKBM for Use.*
3. Use the corneal marker to mark the eye for proper placement of the suction ring.
4. Position the suction ring so that the markings on the suction ring line up with the corneal markings.
5. Activate the vacuum by pressing either the "vacuum" key on the front panel or the vacuum foot pedal. The suction ring will adhere to the eye when the vacuum is activated.

Markings on the Suction Rings

Markings on the suction rings show the center of the ring and specific distances from the center. The small vertical mark and large number (#3 or #4) in the lower part of the ring indicate both the center of the ring and the type of ring (#3 for making a 9.0 to 9.5 mm flap or #4 for making an 8.0 to 8.5 mm flap). The next two marks on the left and right of the center mark are 3.0 mm from the center; the next two, indicated by a small #4 below the mark, are 4.0 mm from the center mark; and the last two sets of marks are 5.0 and then 6.0 mm from the center.

A meniscus whose outer edges are at the 6.0-mm mark is 12 mm in diameter, one with outer edges at the 5.0-mm mark is 10 mm, one with edges at the 4.0-mm marks is 8.0 mm, and one with edges at the 3.0-mm (innermost) mark is 6.0 mm. These markings also serve to verify proper function during a test run because the blade must stop at the preselected hinge size.

OPERATION IN AUTOMATIC (RECOMMENDED) MODE

1. Prior to operation, ensure that there is no foreign matter or debris on the microkeratome head or steel blade, which can adversely affect SKBM operation. Sequelae can include bacterial contamination, interface debris, or resistance in blade movement during operation. The presence of foreign matter on the steel blade can result in injury to the corneal tissue. Increased resistance in blade mobility can also have a detrimental effect on the microkeratome motor.
2. Select the "automatic" operational mode and prepare the system for use.
3. Attach the microkeratome head and handpiece to the suction ring. Perform a test run of the SKBM before placing the suction ring on the patient's eye. The vacuum must be turned on and the vacuum tubing pinched to maintain a nominal -0.8 bar during the test run. Ensure that the steel blade oscillates freely and without resistance during the test run. Confirm that the metal band is firmly latched onto the metal band connector on the suction ring and that the microkeratome head stopped at the preselected hinge width. Remove the microkeratome head and handpiece from the suction ring.
4. Test the SKBM to ensure sufficient vacuum pressure (at least -0.8 bar). Press the "vacuum" key or the vacuum foot pedal to turn on the vacuum.

Pinch the vacuum tubing to prevent air from entering the vacuum system. Wait approximately 30 seconds. Check the reading on the vacuum gauge. The vacuum pressure should be at least -0.8 bar. If it is less, do not proceed with the procedure.

5. Place the suction ring on the operative eye. Ensure that the horizontal corneal markings line up with the horizontal lines on the suction ring. Confirm that there is no debris or loose tissue on the cornea that may interfere with the vacuum seal. Press the "vacuum" key or press the vacuum foot pedal to turn on the vacuum. The suction ring should adhere firmly to the eye if the vacuum pressure is at least -0.8 bar.

6. Use the tonometer to measure the intraocular pressure (IOP) of the applanated cornea. The IOP should be 65 mm Hg or higher. If the IOP is lower, shut off the vacuum, remove the suction ring, and repeat steps 1 to 4.

7. Position the microkeratome head and handpiece with the front guiding rail at a slight angle into the front groove of the suction ring. The rear groove of the suction ring has a spring action mechanism that guides the microkeratome head and handpiece across the cornea.

8. Gently press the microkeratome head into the rear groove until it clicks. When engaging the microkeratome head and handpiece with the suction ring, do not extend the head to cover more than one-third of the suction ring at a time. Doing so could damage the metal band of the microkeratome drive.

9. When the microkeratome head is properly engaged with the suction ring, manually push it across the suction ring until the metal band audibly latches onto the metal band connector on the ring. To ensure the metal band is firmly attached to the connector, gently pull on the microkeratome head and handpiece. The head and handpiece should not move. If they do move when pulled, the metal band is not properly attached to the connector.

10. When the cornea is applanated (flattened against the microkeratome window), it forms a meniscus (the area of the cornea touching the window). The diameter of this meniscus (as measured by the marks on the microkeratome window) determines the size of the corneal flap. Confirm that the size of the corneal meniscus (as viewed through the microkeratome window) is an even, circular shape and matches the corneal diameter that was

entered into the system. If the two diameters are not comparable, the system parameters must be changed. Also, if there is an excessive amount of fluid on the eye, the fluid can adhere to the window and cause a false meniscus reading (pseudomeniscus).

11. Confirm proper applanation by comparing the applanated cornea with the markings etched into the microkeratome window. The markings on the cornea (made with the corneal marker) should line up with the markings etched on the microkeratome window. If the markings do not line up, turn off the vacuum and remove the suction ring from the cornea. Then, turn the vacuum on again and repeat this procedure.

12. In the "automatic" mode, the entire cutting and retracting of the SKBM is administered by pressing the "start" key or footpedal. The process can be halted at any time during a procedure by again activating the "start" key or footpedal.

13. If the procedure is interrupted by pressing the motor foot pedal or the "start" key, the system will display the message "motor halted."

14. Press the "enter" key to change the parameters. The values previously entered for the procedure will appear on the display (see Table 17-2).

15. Change the parameters if necessary and press the "enter" key to confirm the changes. Press the "start" key or motor pedal to restart the cutting. The procedure will continue where it left off. It is possible to return the microkeratome head and handpiece to their original (start) position by pressing the "mode" key and moving the cursor to the "zero reference" position. Press the "enter" key to confirm.

16. After the microkeratome head and handpiece have reached the preset endpoint, they will automatically retract and go back to the "zero reference" or original (starting) position.

Zero Reference Mode

The zero reference mode is the position used to return the system to its starting position. This mode may be selected if a procedure is being interrupted and the operator wants the microkeratome head and handpiece to return to the starting position, rather than to continue from where it was stopped.

CLEANING AND STERILIZATION

The SKBM components must be cleaned with a steam cleaning unit and sterilized by autoclave before each use. Use caution when cleaning SKBM components with the steam cleaning unit to avoid burns. Do not use detergents to clean the suction rings or microkeratome head. Trace amounts of detergents on any components that come in contact with the eye can harm the corneal tissue. During the SKBM cleaning process, the components must be dried before they are autoclaved. Do not use oxygen to dry the SKBM components, as this can corrode them. The components can be dried using nitrogen gas (hospital grade, 99.9% pure) or "canned air." Drying the components prior to autoclaving will prevent water deposits from forming on the surface. The presence of residual water deposits on SKBM components may lead to resistance in blade mobility and/or decreased mobility of the microkeratome motor during operation.

The components that must be autoclaved at 121°C for at least 30 minutes are the:

- Microkeratome head (without the steel blade)
- Microkeratome metal band
- Suction rings
- Suction ring handle
- Corneal marker
- Tonometer lens

Use a sterile technique after autoclaving. Do not autoclave the microkeratome handpiece. The motors and cables may be damaged by repeated exposure to high heat. Do not immerse SKBM components in alcohol or any other solvents and do not use any lubricants, oils, etc, for cleaning purposes because they can damage the SKBM.

SUMMARY OF OPERATION
(Form 17-1)

1. Insert a new sterile blade into the sterile microkeratome head. Ensure that nothing touches the cutting edge, as this may dull the blade.
2. Connect the microkeratome head with the handpiece and confirm that it clicks and rests firmly.
3. Connect the sterile metal band with the handpiece.
4. Select suction ring #3 for a 9.0 to 9.5 mm flap, or #4 for a 8.5 to 9.0 mm flap and confirm the setting.
5. Select the operating mode and confirm settings.
6. Attach the suction ring handle to the suction ring.
7. Attach the long vacuum tubing to the moisture reservoir and suction ring handle. Attach the short vacuum tubing to the control unit and moisture reservoir.
8. Switch on the control unit power switch.

9. Mark the cornea and apply the selected suction ring according to the intended flap size. Position the ring so that the horizontal lines on the ring line up with the horizontal markings on the cornea.
10. Turn on vacuum using the front panel key or foot pedal.
11. Use a tonometer to verify that IOP is 65 mm Hg or higher.
12. Position the microkeratome head and handpiece in the front guide rail of the suction ring and gently press it into the rear groove until it clicks into place. Gently push the head along the tracks until the cornea is visible through the window on the microkeratome head.
13. Verify that the applanated corneal area is identical in size with the diameter reading (top line) on the system display. If not, change the system parameters to match the diameter of the applanated cornea.
14. Confirm that suction is adequate and the applanated area of the cornea is as desired. Check that the backup power light is lit. Start the procedure by pressing the front panel key or footpedal. Hold (do not push) the microkeratome head and handpiece, wait until it has retracted, and then release suction.

DESIGN ANALYSIS AND PERFORMANCE FEATURES IN A LABORATORY MODEL

Introduction

The proliferation of new microkeratome units necessitates evaluation of their designs for performance in creating a flap. A recent study showed that most LASIK complications were related to the flap and the surgeon's experience with the procedure.[14] Since flap quality is affected by the performance of a microkeratome, I analyzed the design features of the ideal microkeratome and compared them with the actual features of the SKBM.

In addition, we made objective corneal thickness and diameter measurements in the laboratory on cadaver eyes and compared these values to expected values intrinsic to the instrument (ie, resections 160 μm thick, 9.0 to 9.5 mm diameter, with the 21 mm #3 suction ring).

Results of Comparison to Ideal and Conclusion

The SKBM met 12 of my 13 criteria for the ideal microkeratome. The one unmet criterion was adjustabil-

SUMMIT KRUMEICH-BARRAQUER MICROKERATOME
PREPARATION FOR USE CHECKLIST
(refer to the SKBM User's Manual for complete operating instructions)

Power/suction supply and assembly

_____ a. Insert main power cord into rear of control unit

_____ b. Plug power into main power supply

_____ c. Attach vacuum footpedal

_____ d. Attach motor footpedal

_____ e. Attach suction tubing

_____ f. Attach handpiece cord

Back-up power supply/vacuum test

_____ a. Turn on power switch (ensure all cables are plugged in before turning system on)

_____ b. Check that power indicator light is illuminated

_____ c. Listen for vacuum pump to start (takes about 30 seconds)

_____ d. Initiate vacuum by pressing footpedal or vacuum key on console

_____ e. Pinch tubing to ensure minimum of -0.8 bar of vacuum

_____ f. Turn off vacuum

Microkeratome assembly

_____ a. Insert blade into microkeratome head

_____ b. Ensure blade moves freely in microkeratome head

_____ c. Ensure eccentric pin is in 6 or 12 o'clock position

_____ d. Pinch extended pins and assemble microkeratome head and handpiece

_____ e. Listen for click indicating proper assembly

_____ f. Gently pull microkeratome head and handpiece to further ensure proper assembly

_____ g. Insert metal band and ensure it is locked in place

_____ h. Instill one drop of BSS in blade slot (to lubricate blade)

Suction ring selection

_____ a. Select suction ring

_____ b. Attach handle to suction ring

_____ c. Attach suction tube to handle

Set parameters

_____ a. Set and confirm suction ring diameter

_____ b. Set and confirm mode of operation

_____ c. Set and confirm diameter of applanation

_____ d. Set and confirm speed of microkeratome head translation

_____ e. Set and confirm speed of blade oscillation

_____ f. Set and confirm hinge width

Microkeratome test

_____ a. Assemble suction ring and microkeratome head and handpiece

_____ b. Listen for click indicating proper engagement

_____ c. Pull back head and handpiece to confirm proper engagement of suction ring and metal band

_____ d. Slide microkeratome head and handpiece forward

_____ e. Pinch tubing and turn on vacuum

_____ f. Step on motor pedal

_____ g. Ensure microkeratome head travels across and back to the zero reference point

_____ h. Ensure etching on window lines up with center marking on suction ring

_____ i. Turn off vacuum

Reconfirm suction ring/diameter parameter

_____ a. Position suction ring on eye (refer to lines made by corneal marker)

_____ b. Confirm suction ring diameter matches suction ring parameters

_____ c. Turn on vacuum and instill one drop of BSS on cornea

_____ d. Attach microkeratome head and handpiece to suction ring

_____ e. Check applanation in window

_____ f. Blot excess fluid from cornea

_____ g. Confirm corneal applanation in window matches diameter parameter

_____ h. Initiate cut

Table 17-4		
RESULTS IN EYE BANK EYES		
	Corneal cap thickness (µm)	Corneal cap diameter (mm)
No of eyes	12	12
Mean (SD)	190 (17)	Horizontal 9.38 (0.32)
Range	166 to 209.0	Vertical 9.42 (0.39)

ity of vacuum level. Particularly notable is the adjustability of several features of the unit, allowing the operator to develop parameters suitable to his or her own needs and experience. Clinical data are needed to provide actual performance values from surgical cases (Table 17-4).

Corneal Measurements in Cadaver Eye Resections

Purpose

The purpose of this study was to determine, in eye bank cadaver eyes, the actual corneal thicknesses and diameters obtained when using the SKBM 160 µm microkeratome head and 21 mm #3 suction ring designed for 9.0 to 9.5 mm corneal diameters.

Methods

Twelve whole eye bank eyes, not suitable for corneal transplantation, were defrosted, inflated with balanced salt solution, and placed in a 15% sucrose solution for 40 minutes to dehydrate. All eyes had an IOP of 65 mm Hg or more. Microkeratome resections were made using the SKBM with a 160 µm head and the 21 mm #3 suction ring (designed to cut diameters of 9.0 to 9.5 mm). Cap thickness measurements were made with a mechanical measuring device (Metatoya).

Results and Conclusion

The 160 µm head produced corneal resections ranging from 166 to 209 µm, with a mean of 190 µm and a standard deviation of 17 µm. Thicker corneas have been shown to produce thicker cuts (Perry Binder, MD, personal communication), and eye bank corneas, usually

ranging from 750 to 900 µm in thickness, are thicker than the average clinical cornea of 550 µm. Thus, in this laboratory model, the SKBM produced cuts of the expected thickness and diameter without much variation (Table 17-5).

CORNEAL MEASUREMENTS IN A CLINICAL SERIES OF LASIK PERFORMED WITH THE SKBM

Purpose

The purpose of this study was to determine the ultrasonic corneal thicknesses and diameters obtained when the SKBM was used in clinical LASIK cases.

Methods

A series of flap resections were created with the SKBM as part of LASIK for correcting myopia. The 160 µm microkeratome head and suction rings 21 mm #3 or 19 mm #3 (to create a 9.0 to 9.5 mm diameter) and 21 mm #4 (to create an 8.0 to 8.5 mm diameter) were used.

The DGH ultrasonic pachymeter was used to measure the thickness of the central cornea preoperatively and the thickness of the stromal surface in the center of the entrance pupil immediately after resection. The difference between these two readings was the thickness of the flap. Flap diameter (vertical meridian) was measured monocularly (10x) with calipers to the nearest 0.5 mm.

Results and Conclusion

Corneal resection made with the 160 µm depth plate ranged from 151 to 191 µm in thickness, with a mean of 164 ± 13 µm. These values were closer to the attempted thickness (160 µm) than those obtained in over 1000 cases with the Automatic Corneal Shaper (mean = 124 ± 24 µm). Suction rings for producing flap diameters 8.0 to 9.5 mm produced diameters 8.5 to 9.5 mm. Thus, in this preliminary series, the SKBM created flaps of predictable thickness and diameter. Clinical photos of the SKBM in use are shown in Figures 17-8 to 17-11. See also Table 17-6.

Table 17-5		
DESIGN FEATURES OF THE IDEAL MICROKERATOME COMPARED WITH THE SKBM		
Ideal feature	**SKBM**	**Comments**
Machine-driven travel mechanism	Yes; automatic is recommended, but manual mode is available	Manual passage produces variations in speed that can result in hesitation marks on the stroma
Automatic drive mechanism	Yes	Gear-driven mechanisms can jam or clog and stop the passage of blade
Ability to alter size of hinge	Yes	A steep cornea can lead to too-large hinge and too large a diameter, which can induce astigmatism; a flat cornea can lead to too-small or no hinge and too small diameter
Safety features	Yes; blade stops if there is interference or loss of vacuum	
Multiple suction ports	Yes	Occlusion of a single port leads to loss of vacuum
Back-up power supply	Yes	Need battery or capacitor back-up in case of power failure
Visibility of blade as it moves	Yes	Surgeons prefer to visualize procedures
User-friendly suction rings	Yes; suction rings are easy to assemble and use Ring #21 is excellent for most eyes; Ring #19 is suitable for smaller fissures	Outer diameter should only be as large as necessary Smaller diameter rings may have less suction
Multiple suction rings	Yes; it has four suction rings Ring 21 #3 = 21 mm outer diameter, 9.0 to 9.5 mm flap diameter Ring 21 #4 = 21 mm outer diameter, 8.0 to 8.5 mm flap diameter Ring 19 #3 = 19 mm outer diameter, 9.0 to 9.5 mm flap diameter Ring 19 #4 = 19 mm outer diameter, 8.0 to 8.5 mm flap diameter	Ring that creates larger diameter flap suitable for hyperopia; ring creating smaller diameter flap suitable for myopia
Adjustable blade oscillation	Yes; SKBM unit range = 4000 to 20,000 RPM; 14,000 RPM is recommended	Industry-standardized oscillation rate is not known; unit with adjustability allows changes, as needed
Adjustable blade speed over cornea	Yes; SKBM unit range = 0.5 to 3.0 mm/sec; recommended speed is 1.5 mm/seconds	Industry-standardized blade speed is not known; unit with adjustability allows changes, as needed
Adjustable vacuum level	No	Industry-standardized pressure is not known, but higher IOP levels have produced thicker cuts Whether thickness of cut affects refractive outcome is not known
Blade quality and operation	Yes; blade is firmly attached to blade holder with screws. Blades are high-quality steel of desired length	

Table 17-6		
FLAP VALUES OBTAINED WITH THE SKBM		
Surgical case number	Corneal flap thickness (µm)	Corneal flap diameter (mm)
1	162	8.5
2	154	8.5
3	169	9.1
4	152	8.9
5	179	9.0
6	191	9.2
7	157	9.5
8	165	9.5
9	151	9.0
10	149	9.1
11	159	9.1
12	149	9.1
13	159	9.3
14	151	9.0
15	157	9.5
16	165	9.5
17	179	9.0
18	191	9.0
19	168	NA
20	152	8.9
21	162	8.5
22	154	8.5
23	188	8.8
24	166	9.1
Mean	163.7 µm	NA (#3 and #4 suction rings used)
Standard deviation	13.1 µm	NA (#3 and #4 suction rings used)
Range	51 to 191 µm	8.5 to 9.5 mm

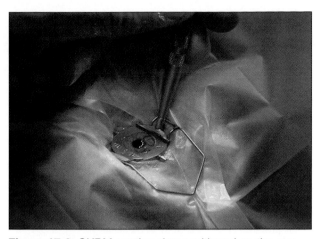

Figure 17-8. SKBM suction ring positioned on the eye.

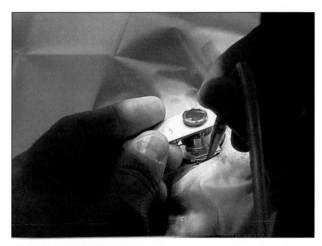

Figure 17-9. With the suction ring and suction on, a tonometer is being used to check pressure.

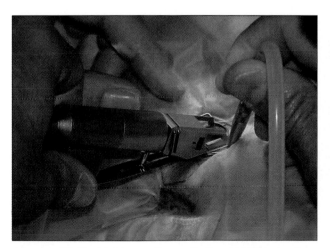

Figure 17-10. Making a flap with the SKBM microkeratome.

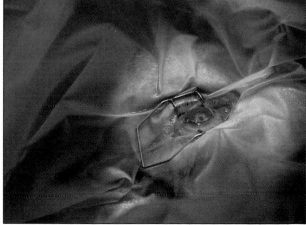

Figure 17-11. Flap reflected back, revealing a smooth corneal bed. Note: If the vacuum is allowed to draw in the air, it must be closed to rebuild vacuum pressure. This can be done by pressing the vacuum footpedal or vacuum key to shut it off, or by pinching the vacuum tubing for about 20 seconds.

REFERENCES

1. Barraquer JI. Queratoplastia. *Arch Soc Am Oftalmol Optom.* 1961;3:147-168.
2. Krumeich JH. Indications, techniques, and complications of myopic keratomileusis. In: Binder PS, ed. Refractive corneal surgery: the correction of aphakia, hyperopia, and myopia. *Intl Ophthalmol Clinics.* Boston, Mass: Little Brown & Co; 1983.
3. Ruiz L, Rowsey J. In situ keratomileusis. *Invest Ophthalmol Vis Sci.* 1988;29(suppl):392.

4. Seiler T, Kahle G, Kriegerowski M. Excimer laser (193 nm) myopic keratomileusis in sighted and blind human eyes. *J Refract Corneal Surg.* 1990;6:165-173.
5. Arenas-Archila E, Sanchez-Thorin JC, Naranjo-Uribe JP, Hernandez-Lozano A. Myopic keratomileusis in situ: a preliminary report. *J Cataract Refract Surg.* 1991;17:424-435.
6. Haimovici R, Culbertson WW. Optical lamellar keratoplasty using the Barraquer microkeratome. *J Refract Corneal Surg.* 1991;7:42-45.
7. Hanna KD, David T, Besson J, Pouliquen Y. Lamellar keratoplasty with the Barraquer microkeratome. *J Refract Corneal Surg.* 1991;7:177-180.
8. Buratto L, Ferrari M, Rama P. Excimer laser intrastromal keratomileusis. *Am J Ophthalmol.* 1992;113:291-295.

9. Buratto L, Ferrari M. Excimer laser intrastromal keratomileusis: case reports. *J Cataract Refract Surg.* 1992;18:37-41.
10. Buratto L, Ferrari M, Genisi C. Myopic keratomileusis with the excimer laser: 1-year follow-up. *J Refract Corneal Surg.* 1993;9:12-19.
11. Pallikaris IG, Papatzanaki ME, Siganos DS, Tsilimbaris MK. A corneal flap technique for laser in situ keratomileusis. *Arch Ophthalmol.* 1991;109:1699-1702.
12. Brint SF, Ostrick DM, Fisher C, et al. Six month results of the multicenter phase I study of excimer laser myopic keratomileusis. *J Cataract Refract Surg.* 1994;20:610-615.
13. Salah T, Waring GO, El-Maghraby A. Excimer laser keratomileusis in the corneal bed under a hinged flap: results in Saudi Arabia at the El-Maghraby Eye Hospital. In: Salz JJ, McDonnell PJ, McDonald MB, eds. *Corneal Laser Surgery.* St. Louis, Mo: Mosby-Year Book; 1995.
14. Stulting RD, Carr JD, Thompson KP, Waring GO, Wiley WM, Walker JG. Complications of laser in situ keratomileusis for the correction of myopia. *Ophthalmology.* 1999;106:13-20.
15. Binder PS, Akers PH, Deg JK, Zavala EY. Refractive keratoplasty: microkeratome evaluation. *Arch Ophthalmol.* 1982;100:802-806.
16. Binder PS, Moore M, Lambert RW, Seagrist DM. Comparison of two microkeratome systems. *Journal of Refractive Surgery.* 1997;13:142-153.

THE MORIA MICROKERATOME AND LASIK TECHNIQUE

Enrique Suárez, MD

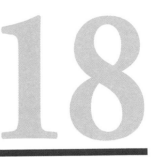

THE MORIA MICROKERATOMES

In the late 1980s, I got involved in keratomileusis in situ, using manual microkeratomes. Years later, the technology evolved to the automated models which, in my personal experience, worked adequately if the surgical volume was low.

After my transition to LASIK, and a subsequent patient volume increase, the rate of surgical complications related to microkeratome malfunction was significantly higher (close to 2%). Because of this, we began looking for a more dependable instrument. I concluded that no automated machine available at that time was capable of tolerating my routine of an average of 36 consecutive cases, per session (three times a week).

After advice from experienced high-volume surgeons, I decided to try manual microkeratomes again. This change resulted in a dramatic decrease in surgical complications.

Today, after testing more than eight different automated microkeratomes, I strongly believe that the reliability of the gas turbine-activated instrument is unparalleled. Over the last 3 years, I have performed more 9000 cases with Moria microkeratomes, the majority of them with the One version, with under 0.001% intraoperative complications.

Moria offers three different microkeratomes. In order of market introduction, they are:
- The LSK One
- The Carriazo Barraquer
- The One disposable

The Evolution II power unit operates these three microkeratomes.

The Power Unit

The new power unit (Evolution II) is designed to work with any Moria microkeratome (Figure 18-1). The versatility of this unit is particularly appealing for the surgeon who wants the option of using different types of microkeratomes.

Both the reusable and disposable One is powered by a nitrogen turbine giving high torque and speed of 15,000 revolutions per minute (RPM) or 30,000 blade oscillations per minute.

The Carriazo-Barraquer is powered by an electrical motor in the automated mode and by a nitrogen turbine in manual mode.

The power unit has two different connections for microkeratomes: one for electrical drive and the other for the pneumatic drive.

It also has several interesting features for the surgeon:
- Two powerful vacuum pumps. In normal conditions, only one pump is activated. In case of vacuum loss, the vacuum monitoring system will instantaneously activate the second pump in order to compensate the detected failure.
- The low vacuum mode. This is one of the innovative features of this unit. It permits fixation of the eye by means of the ring handle (assisted fixation) during the laser ablation without compromising retinal vascular flow. It also allows the control of peripheral bleeding in patients with peripheral corneal neovascularization.
- Audible and visual alarms. The surgeon is alerted in case of loss of vacuum, low nitrogen pressure in the tank, or low battery charge.
- Test mode. The surgeon is able to check the appropriate suction levels before the procedure.

With the rapid evolution of LASIK and the innovation of microkeratomes, one interesting aspect of this system is that it allows upgrades to newer keratomes, including the recently introduced accessories to perform LTK (lamellar therapeutic keratoplasty) with the new Moria artificial anterior chamber.

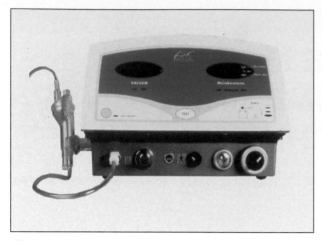

Figure 18-1. The Evolution II power unit permits the operation with manual or automated microkeratomes.

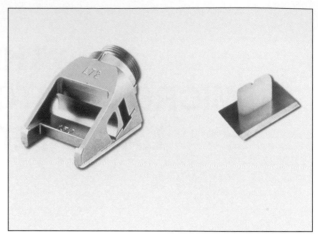

Figure 18-2. One piece head, one blade—the safest alternative.

LSK ONE

The Head

The One keratome head is based on a very simple concept: one piece, one blade. This has been a substantial simplification of the microkeratome. There are no interchangeable or adjustable plates, which is a major improvement and eliminates the potential risk associated with incorrect insertion of the plate in multipiece microkeratome heads (Figure 18-2).

The One head is made of a single piece of stainless steel, with no need for assembly or adjustment, and a built-in plate, which is integrated to set the cut depth.

Heads for different resection depths are available (from 100 microns to 180 microns) and are identified by a number engraved on the top, which represents the distance in microns between the plate and the cutting edge of the blade. The average thickness of the flap resection is a few microns greater than the head calibration. This thickness can be influenced by several parameters, such as cornea curvature and ocular pressure.

Recently, new heads have become available for lamellar transplant (ALTK) with the ability to cut up to 400 microns.

The Blade

The blade is made of stainless steel and is disposable. The blade comes attached to a plastic blade holder, which ensures its guidance and perfect oscillation in the blade housing of the microkeratome head (see Figure 18-2).

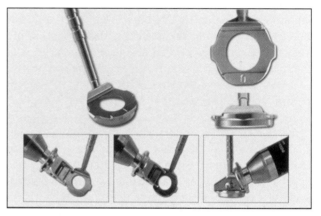

Figure 18-3. Customizing the flap is possible with the different suction rings and adjustable stop.

Turbine Motor

A high torque nitrogen turbine powers the system, which is preset at 15,000 RPM.

Suction Ring

The size of the flap is determined by the selection of one of five different suction rings: -1, 0, +1, +2, and H (Figure 18-3).

Each ring is identical in every dimension except thickness. The +2 vacuum ring is the thickest, and the –1 and the H rings are the thinnest. The H ring produces the largest flap size and is particularly indicated for hyperopia or patients with flat corneas. As the ring becomes thinner, it allows more cornea to protrude through the opening of the ring. The more cornea exposed through the ring, the larger the flap size.

Other factors can influence the resection size, such

Table 18-1					
SUCTION RING: OPTICAL ZONE NOMOGRAM*					
	+2 ring	+1 ring	0 ring	-1 ring	H ring
Cornea K > 46	8.5 mm	9.0 mm	9.5 mm	10 mm	10.5 mm
Cornea K ~ 43.5	8.0 mm	8.5 mm	9.0 mm	9.5 mm	10 mm
Cornea K ~ 42	7.5 mm	8.0 mm	8.5 mm	9.0 mm	9.5 mm
Cornea K < 40	6.5 mm	7.0 mm	7.5 mm	8.0 mm	8.5 mm

Note: For corneas smaller than 11 mm in diameter, the optical zone could increase by 0.25 mm.
For corneas larger than 12 mm, the optical zone could decrease by 0.25 mm.

The H ring may increase the optical zone by 0.25 mm compared to the –1 ring. This ring should not be used in steep corneas, and the cornea to be resected should be confirmed with applanation lenses before performing the surgery.

* This nomogram should be used only as a guide.

as the curvature and diameter of the cornea. A small eye will allow more cornea to protrude through the ring and produce a larger flap. Conversely, a large eye will reduce the amount of cornea that enters the ring and reduce the resection diameter.

The small size of the outer diameter of the ring and the variability of the desired resection diameter results in adaptability to every corneal, orbital, or interpalpebral configuration (Table 18-1).

Hinge Position and Stop Ring

The hinge position is adjustable by means of a rotating multiple stop ring that can be adjusted from 7.0 to 8.5 mm. Selection of the stop ring position can be made without disassembling the microkeratome (Figure 18-4).

Advancement of the Microkeratome

The advancement of the One keratome across the ring is manual. Manually operated microkeratomes may require an initial learning curve, but once mastered, they offer a safer approach, and they allow the surgeon to personalize the flap. The One head allows full visualization and better control during the flap resection.

Microkeratome Assembly

Assembly starts with the insertion of the blade inside the head blade housing. The second step is the coupling of the adjustable stop ring on the head. The head is then mounted on the turbine. The head and turbine are now ready and must be connected to the power unit by a flexible power cord.

The selected ring is assembled to the suction handle. The disposable tubing is attached to the handle and connected to the power unit.

Final Test

Although assembly of this system is very simple, the surgeon must do a final check before performing surgery.

For the head, the two most important points to check are the presence of the stop ring in order to avoid making a free cap, and test the blade movement by the turbine. Then, the two vacuum levels and tightness of the respective lines must be checked by activating the "test" button at the console and occluding the ring with the fingertip or by clamping the vacuum tubing just above the ring handle.

The One has been designed in an attempt to solve the weak points of other microkeratomes. This keratome is especially good for the high-volume surgeon who desires to have control of the instrument and not be controlled by the machine. Also, for those who additionally prefer to have the alternative to customize the flap for specific cases, the One allows flexibility in selecting the flap diameter and hinge size.

ONE DISPOSABLE

The One Disposable is the newer sibling of the original One. It has the same basic principles. It has a one-piece plastic molded head with one blade inserted, which, as a safety feature, cannot be removed from the head. The heads are available for cuts of 160 or 180 microns and are powered by the same turbine as the reusable One head, with an oscillation of 15,000 RPM.

Suction Rings

The rings are preassembled with the handle and aspiration tubing, and the two arms of the handle are opposite the head translation. This innovative ergonomic design improves sliding of the head and allows stabilization of the eye by opposing a force to the linear translation of the microkeratome.

The location of the stopper just above the ring, allows complete visibility of the head position in relation to the stop during the cut. This avoids false stops due to the

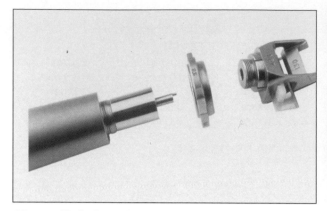

Figure 18-4. Assembling the Moria microkeratome is simple because of its design.

speculum or any other obstacle. The surgeon always knows the position of the head and can control the hinge size during the cut.

The ring has two built-in aspiration holes connected to two different aspiration lines for higher vacuum performance and safety.

Three rings sizes -1, 0, and H are available, allowing flap sizes up to 10 mm.

The hinge position is set directly on the suction ring by rotating an adjustable stop device located on the upper part of the ring, from 7.5 to 9.5 mm. The adjustment is made by means of a key, also included in the disposable pack.

Assembly

The assembly of this instrument is even simpler than the original One model. Only two steps are required:

1. Connect the head onto the turbine.
2. Connect the tubing to the vacuum line of the console.

With the same personalized resection characteristics of the ONE model, this microkeratome is an excellent alternative for surgeons with very high volume surgical practices (price sensitive), or for multi-surgeon centers because of the limited investment (just one control unit and one turbine for the disposable heads). It is also the best solution for those adverse legal environments.

LASIK PERSONAL TECHNIQUE

Patient Preparation

As any other ocular surgical procedure, LASIK should be performed in a sterile environment with appropriate filtration systems, and controlled humidity and temperature to assure the best conditions for the excimer laser performance.

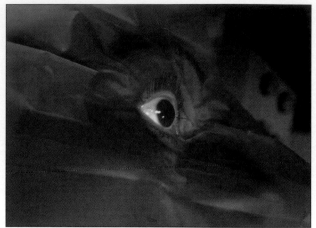

Figure 18-5. The eyelashes are retracted under the sterile drape.

The operating room should be properly prepared, and the surgeon and scrub nurse should be dressed with caps, masks, sterile special gowns and powderless gloves. Other personnel should also wear proper surgical attire.

The patient is given mild anti-anxiety medication (3 mg of Bromazepam) 2 to 3 hours before the procedure.

After arrival to the outpatient surgical facility, the patient changes into disposable clean clothes, cap, and shoe covers. He or she is then taken to the preparation room where topical anesthesia is instilled (4% lidocaine and later 0.5% proparacaine) 10 to 15 minutes prior the surgery.

In this waiting room, the patient can observe the previous patient's surgery through a monitor, and the procedure is reviewed again with a trained nurse.

The eyelids and surrounding skin are cleaned and disinfected with 5% povidone-iodine solution (Betadine) immediately before the patient is taken to the laser room. He or she is then asked to lie down on the excimer bed in such a way that there is no lateral or vertical head deviation.

A sterile self-adhesive drape (3M #1020) is placed over the eyelid margin, holding the eyelashes apart in order to isolate the surgical field and avoid interference of the eyelashes with the surgical instruments, making the globe is adequately exposed for the surgeon (Figure 18-5).

Surgical Technique

Speculum Application

The bed is moved until the patient's eye is located under the microscope field and a Barraquer wire speculum is placed to retract the eyelids with the eyelashes included under the sterile plastic drape. I prefer this speculum because it is the thinnest, lightest, and has less

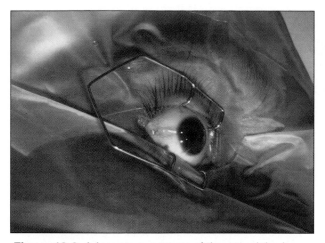

Figure 18-6. Adequate exposure of the eye globe is crucial.

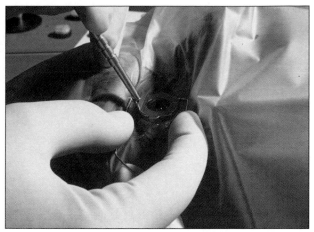

Figure 18-7. A combined maneuver to obtain eye fixation.

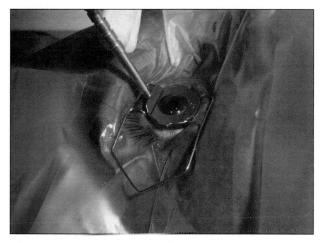

Figure 18-8. Proper pressure is confirmed.

parts that could interfere with the free microkeratome movement (Figure 18-6).

Usually a lid retractor works perfectly in large and normal eyes, but in small and deep eyes I remove the lid retractor and perform the suction ring application, flap resection, and laser ablation without a speculum in order to allow more space for the surgical instruments, replacing it later for irrigation and flap repositioning.

Epithelial Marking

I do not mark the corneal epithelium as I did in previous years while performing free cap keratomileusis in situ, since a free cap is extremely rare in our experience. If it occurs, I leave the disc in the microkeratome head until I am finished the ablation and interface cleaning, so I do not lose the cap alignment and epithelial-stromal orientation. Using a ring tip atraumatic forceps (Moria #18.225) to grasp the disc and remove it from the microkeratome head, the free cap is replaced in the original

position and carefully dried until it is totally stable. In a few cases, an interrupted 10-0 nylon suture has been placed at 12 o'clock to secure the disc in place, removing the suture two or three days after surgery.

Nevertheless, I suggest, especially for inexperienced or low-volume surgeons, marking the cornea with any of the described techniques for better flap alignment and safer handling of a free cap.

Suction Ring Application

Holding the eye speculum with one hand and pushing down gently to obtain globe proptosis and stabilization, I place the selected suction ring (according to the cornea curvature and refractive error) centered with the pupil and not with the limbus, and apply the higher suction level (70 to 80 mm Hg). (Figure 18-7).

At this time, you may notice some pupil dilation, which indirectly indicates that suction has been achieved. It is recommended to gently lift the suction ring handle in order to assure that proper vacuum was obtained (Figure 18-8). The suction level can be confirmed by the power unit vacuum gauge.

One of the great advantages of the Moria Evolution II unit is that if the appropriate suction level has not been reached; visual and audible signs let the surgeon know something is wrong. An additional safety feature is that if the optimal suction is not obtained, the pedal will sound an alarm and will not activate the motor or turbine.

It is very important to warn patients about the pressure, the transient visual loss, and the noise they will experience during this surgical step, as well as the other sensations in further stages of the LASIK procedure.

Checking Eye Pressure

Though I feel measuring the intraocular pressure after suction has been initiated is unnecessary, and I have

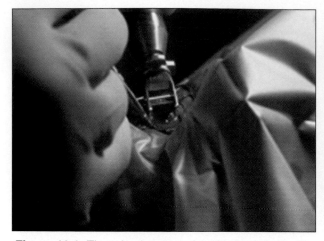

Figure 18-9. The microkeratome head is inserted in the suction ring.

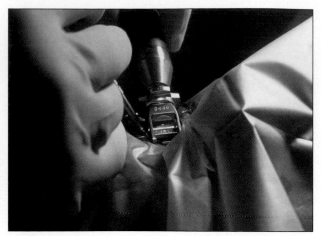

Figure 18-10. Paying attention to flap formation in the keratome head.

not done it for the last 13,500+ cases, for teaching purposes I recommend it, especially for the novice surgeon, by applying the Barraquer applanation tonometer, or any other device, to determine adequate high pressure.

Creating the Flap

I do not agree with the concept that "one size fits all." The cornea curvatures and diameters, limbal scleral curvature, high astigmatism, history of previous surgery, presence of peripheral vessels, pterygium, etc, and especially the refractive error, determine the need for a different suction ring and stop ring setting for an optimal flap resection in each particular case. The versatility of the Moria LSK One with available heads of different depth cuts, five different suction rings for diverse cornea curvatures, and a unique adjustable rotating stop ring to select the hinge width and flap disparity, gives extraordinary flexibility to "personalize" the best and safest resection every time.

Generally, I use the microkeratome head with a fixed 150-micron plate, which may provide 130-micron flaps (in flat corneas) to 180-micron flaps (in steeper corneas). If the ablation is unusually large or the cornea is thinner than average, I select heads of 130 or 100 microns to create thinner flaps and respect the 250-micron minimal stromal bed after the cornea has been ablated. Usually, we obtain larger and thicker flaps in steep corneas, and smaller and thinner flaps in flat corneas.

For every patient, I use a new sterile head with a new blade already loaded, or I use a disposable microkeratome.

Depending on the suction ring selected to obtain the intended resection (see Table 18-1) and based on the ablation diameters we choose according to the refractive error we are treating (larger in hyperopia than myopia),

the multiple stop ring is set in order to get the desired disparity (usually 0.5 or 1.0 mm) between the vertical and horizontal meridians. The ideal hinge, whenever it is possible, should be wide enough to provide excellent flap stabilization (3.0 mm or more), but at the same time leave sufficient area exposed for a good laser ablation. I am convinced that a wide hinge and thick flap are more important for flap stabilization than the hinge location.

After irrigating the corneal surface with drops of balanced salt solution (BSS) to lubricate and facilitate head translation, the microkeratome is engaged into the dovetail grooves of the suction ring. Swinging the head carefully into the ring, the surgeon confirms both rails have been properly inserted and the head is gently advanced until the blade barely passes the edge of the suction ring, feeling the free displacement of the instrument (Figure 18-9). At this moment the turbine is activated by depressing the corresponding pedal. With a uniform, firm, and constant movement, the head is moved forward through the ring, watching carefully how the flap is coming out the microkeratome head slit. The stop ring contacts the suction ring, or in some cases of flat corneas (especially with high astigmatism), and stops the resection beforehand to avoid a free cap. It is crucial to pay attention to the flap formation in the microkeratome head to avoid potential complications (Figure 18-10).

Immediately after reaching the end of the resection desired, lifting the foot of the power pedal stops the turbine, and the head is removed from the vacuum ring with a reverse movement.

It is important to hold the suction ring handle gently to avoid creating an opposite force vector to the microkeratome head movement. There are surgeons who release the handle and let the head completely guide the pass of the instrument.

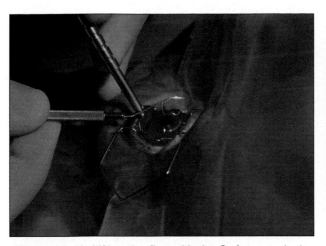

Figure 18-11. Lifting the flap with the Suárez manipulator.

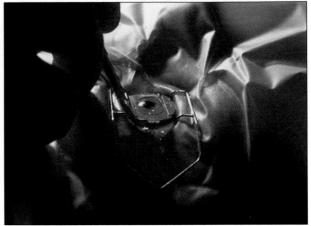

Figure 18-12. Excimer ablation under low vacuum-assisted fixation.

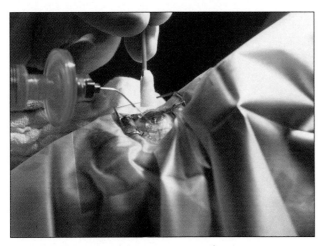

Figure 18-13. Careful interface cleaning is important.

In a case of astigmatism, the hinge should be oriented at the steepest meridian (axis of higher keratometry reading), to offer the widest exposed area to the longest ablation diameter.

With this turbine-activated unit the possibility of a resection complication related to microkeratome failure is practically nonexistent. I have used manually (turbine) operated microkeratomes in more than 11,000 cases with less than 0.001% of surgical complications, compared to 2.12% in 2067 LASIK procedures performed with electrical motor microkeratomes that I previously used.

Excimer Laser Ablation

As soon as the flap has been created, the suction is decreased to the lower level (approximately 25 mm Hg) by depressing a switch at the control unit. This new vacuum level stabilizes the globe for the fixation-assisted ablation without compromising the retinal perfusion, permitting the patient to regain vision during the laser application.

Simultaneously, the flap is lifted with a delicate spatula or flap manipulator (Moria #19044) and placed over the suction ring, which helps isolate the cap from tear debris and other foreign particles (Figure 18-11).

After checking the position of the patient's head, the laser aiming beams are focused in the center of the pupil; and under low suction-assisted fixation, the laser pedal is depressed to start the excimer ablation (Figure 18-12).

At this moment, it is advisable to alert the patient of the noise created by the laser to avoid undesired movement.

By no longer using patient self-fixation, we have practically eliminated decentration complications in our statistics. Also during the entire procedure, to assure proper alignment and pupil centration the surgical assistant constantly monitors the infrared camera's crosshair mires.

Excessive drying of the bed during ablation could lead to overcorrection, so I recommend wiping with a Merocel microsponge only when humid spots appear in the interface during the ablation. If these wet areas are not wiped, they may act as masks for the laser beam and be recognized later via postoperative topography as islands or irregular astigmatism.

Immediately after completion of the laser treatment, the vacuum foot pedal is released, the suction is broken, and the ring is removed from the eye.

Replacing the Flap

With filtered BSS (.20 microns Visitec 1030 fluid filter in a syringe), both stromal faces of the flap and corneal bed are thoroughly irrigated and cleaned with a soaked merocel sponge, eliminating the debris created during the laser ablation, as well as tear film debris and any foreign particle stuck to the interface (Figure 18-13).

Probably because of this obsessive cleaning of the

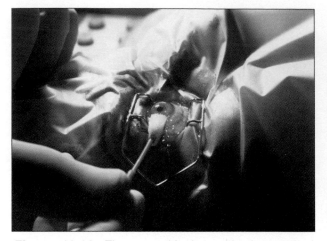

Figure 18-14. Flap repositioning with the soaked microsponge.

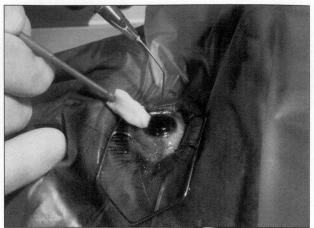

Figure 18-15. Flap adherence with the squeezed sponge and compressed air.

interface, in our clinic, we have had only four cases (out of 25,740 LASIK procedures up to April 1999) of nonspecific interface keratitis (Sands of the Sahara syndrome).

With constant irrigation, the flap is reversed to its original position with a quick maneuver of the wet sponge. The fluid trapped in the interface is then evacuated with the same hydrated merocel sponge (which will not cause epithelial damage), wiping firmly from the hinge to the opposite extreme of the flap, first with "in-out" movements (in the case of a nasal hinge) or "up-down" (in superior hinges), and later, with radial passes, starting at the hinge and following an imaginary radius that peripherally connects the center of the hinge with the flap edges (Figure 18-14). At this point, some stabilization has been achieved. Squeeze the excess fluid out of the sponge, and with the damp (not wet) Merocel sponge, repeat the same movements as before but with less pressure at the pupillary area and emphasizing the maneuver at the flap edges. At this time, I check all the edges of the flap contacting the borders of the resection so no displacement or striae are present. For me, this is a substitute for the epithelial mark alignment.

I also apply a very gentle stream of compressed air over the cornea while I am wiping with the semi dry sponge (after squeezing the excess BSS). It increases the flap adherence to the underlying stroma (Figure 18-15).

An average of 10 passes with the soaked merocel sponge are performed, and about the same number after it has been squeezed (these under air flow).

As in every surgical step of this procedure, let the patient know that you will irrigate the cornea with saline solution, as it gives some patients the sensation of bleeding.

Finishing the Procedure

After carefully checking the interface for foreign material, flap regularity, and adherence to the peripheral edges, two or three drops of Tobradex are instilled, and the eye speculum is removed. This must be a gentle maneuver, first slightly sliding the speculum nasally, then removing the superior arm of the instrument, and later the inferior one. It is advisable to hold the plastic drape firmly with two fingers of the other hand while the speculum is removed, because abrupt eyelid closure could dislocate the flap with the free edges of the drape attached to the lid margin. Use the two-finger maneuver to hold the plastic drape.

Finally, with a gentle movement, slowly remove the adhesive drape from the patient's skin to avoid squeezing, which could cause a flap dislocation.

Clear plastic eye shields are placed to protect the eyes for the first 24 hours, especially the first night, and are removed the next day at the clinic, where the patient is evaluated. Tobradex is prescribed four times a day for 2 weeks.

The follow-up visits are scheduled 3 months later if progress has been uneventful, and yearly thereafter for strict statistical controls. At each visit, a comprehensive ophthalmologic evaluation is performed, including conventional (Tomey, Alcon) and elevation (Orbscan) topographies.

Acknowledgments to Leo Reinfeld, photographer, and Kodak of Venezuela for providing the new experimental high resolution film used for the photos in this chapter.

THE CARRIAZO-BARRAQUER MICROKERATOME AND LASIK TECHNIQUE

Carmen C. Barraquer, MD
Cesar E. Carriazo, MD

INTRODUCTION

Early in 1995, we began the correction of hyperopic astigmatism, creating nasal-hinge corneal flaps. Soon after, we realized the cornea needed to be steepened in both meridians; with the help of specially designed contact lenses, we performed trials of peripheral cylindrical ablations in hyperopic astigmatism cases, and hinge ablation defects appeared as the main significant complication of this procedure. The cylindrical ablation in these cases has to be located usually in the peripheral nasal and temporal sides of the cornea.

The idea of changing the hinge position was the only way to treat these refractive errors. Thus began the quest to design a new prototype of microkeratome.

HISTORY

Prof. José Ignacio Barraquer designed the first microkeratome in 1962 to perform corneal lamellar resections of a predetermined diameter and thickness.[1] His original idea was modified and improved using different technologies that more recently became available.[2] One of the first innovations was the automation of the advance movement.

In 1972, Prof. J. Draeger presented the first automated microkeratome with a rotating blade and automated advance system.[3] He published his research, demonstrating that the regular advance movement of an automated system produces more regular cuts than manually advanced systems.[4]

We initiated a project with JI Barraquer in 1995 to develop a new microkeratome, taking benefit of the new technology available, but also of the new trends in surgery, in particular, LASIK.[5]

After a few months of experimental work, the decision was made to develop an instrument that could be driven in automated and manual modes, that could be assembled very simply, and finally that could be adaptable to every surgical lamellar technique with the least technical restrictions and the most secure parameters. In reference to the hinge, the objective was to develop a system that allowed the position of the hinge in any quadrant of the cornea.[6]

In 1996, JI Barraquer and Dr. Cesar Carriazo presented the Carriazo-Barraquer microkeratome designed for automated or manual use and for placing the hinge in any quadrant of the cornea.

THE MICROKERATOME

The microkeratome is composed of an original crown system located inside a tubular guide of the head, which engages on a pivot located on the ring; it avoids the use of external gears and tracks (Figure 19-1).

The automated advance mode has a double traction: the crown of the head engages on crowns located at the end of the pivot on the ring, different from other automated microkeratomes. The motor gives the traction to the crown and the pivot ensures the guidance of a pivoting movement.

By using rings that pivot without a crown, the head can rotate freely around the pivot; this allows the surgeon to manually rotate the microkeratome during the cut.

The Head

The head has a superior opening with an interior coil to set the motor (Figure 19-2)

It has a lateral groove that goes through and permits the introduction of the blade with the blade holder. It has a lateral curve guide that permits the sliding of the microkeratome over the suction ring and maintains its correct position.

On the other side, it has a cylindrical vertical guide that has a rotational advance system in its interior. The

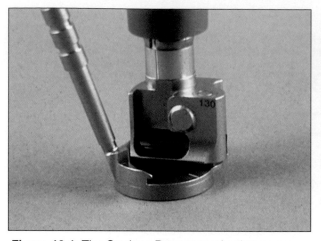

Figure 19-1. The Carriazo-Barraquer microkeratome.

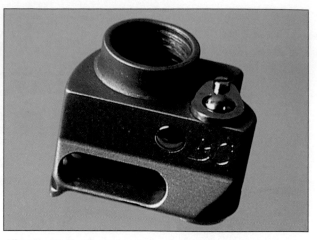

Figure 19-2. Topside view of the head: the superior opening to set the motor.

head has a fixed built-in plate located in front of the blade that applanates the cornea and determines the flap thickness.

In the center of the head is the blade housing, which is an opening that goes from side to side of the head with a 30° slope. The blade is made of stainless steel and comes sterile with a disposable blade holder. Heads are available for cuts of 130, 160, and 180 microns flap thicknesses.

The Motor

The motor (Figure 19-3) for automated advancement is electrical with two concentric shafts. The inner shaft rotates at 15,000 revolutions per minute (RPM) and activates blade oscillation. The outer shaft rotates at approximately 1000 RPM and, by means of a worm gear, connects to pinions located inside the head, which will transmit the pivot's advance movement.

A nitrogen turbine can also be used. Turbine motors have a much higher torque than electrical motors. The turbine motor has only one shaft for driving the blade oscillation at 17,000 RPM. When the turbine is used, the microkeratome is manually advanced.

The Blade

The blade (Figure 19-4) is made of stainless steel and comes sterile with a disposable blade holder. This holder has a protrusion that helps engage the blade in its housing without risk of damaging the cutting edge. The holder's special shape has been developed in order to ensure a very accurate guide into its oscillations, for an accurate and predictable cut thickness.

The Suction Rings

The rings (Figure 19-5) are very small in order to allow access to all types of eyes, including small and

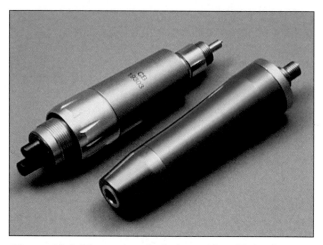

Figure 19-3. The motors. Left: the turbine. Right: (in blue) the electrical motor.

deep orbits. On the superior part of each ring, there is a pivot that serves as a guide for the rotation of the microkeratome. Rings for automated advancement have a pivot with a crown at the end; rings for manual advancement have a pivot with a flat end.

The rings have safety vacuum ports to decrease the risk of vacuum port occlusion by the conjunctiva. A preset stop is located at the base of the ring handle; this stop will limit the keratome head's travel at the end of the cut and will determine the hinge size. Every ring has a reference mark to indicate where the hinge will be positioned.

The size of the flaps can be adjusted by means of four rings of different thicknesses: +2, +1, 0, -1, and H. The +2 ring produces the smallest flap, the -1 and H ring produce larger flap diameters. The H ring is particularly designed for large flaps needed for hyperopia.

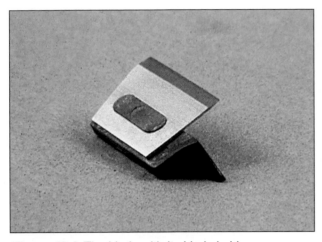

Figure 19-4. The blade with its blade holder.

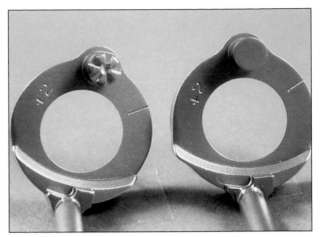

Figure 19-5. Front view of both kinds of rings.

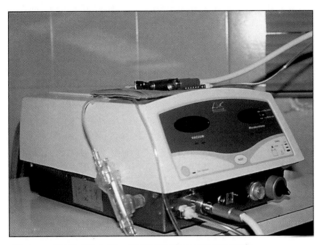

Figure 19-6. The Moria Evolution power unit.

The Power Unit

The Moria Evolution power unit (Figure 19-6) powers the Carriazo-Barraquer microkeratome. It is a battery-powered device. This unit can drive a nitrogen-powered turbine motor or an electrical motor.

The nitrogen turbine motor can only be used for manual translation of the keratome head. The automated mode requires use of the electrical motor.

Both the turbine and electrical motor are supplied with the system in order to allow the surgeon a choice of the advancement mode.

The power unit provides the vacuum for the suction ring by means of two vacuum pumps. When the vacuum is activated by the corresponding footswitch, one pump is activated. The second will act as a back-up and operates only if the control unit detects vacuum loss.

The unit has several safety devices such as alarms in case of vacuum lose, low battery charge, and deficient nitrogen pressure. It also has a low vacuum mode.

PREPARATION OF THE MICROKERATOME

Preparing the head of the microkeratome: It is assembled in three simple steps:

1. The head of the microkeratome is held presenting the lateral convex part of the microkeratome. The blade is maintained with the fingers or with delicate forceps and introduced, without touching the cutting edge, inside the blade holder.
2. The head of the microkeratome is held between the thumb and index finger to ensure the blade remains in place and will make a correct coupling with the eccentric pin of the motor shaft.
3. The head is threaded into the eccentric motor or turbine.
4. The electric cable or turbine hose is then connected to the motor and power unit.

Preparing the suction ring: The handle is part of the ring and does not need connection. The suction line is connected to the end of the handle and to the power unit.

Checking the correct function of the microkeratome and suction: The motor and head are now engaged on the pivot of the selected ring. The motor is then run forward and backward to ensure correct coupling and function. With time and experience with the system, the sound of the instrument is also a guide to how the instrument is functioning. The proper movement of the blade and free advance of the system should be checked.

Selecting the suction ring that will be used with the patient: Multiple factors can influence the size of the resected corneal disc, such as the radius of curvature, the diameter of the cornea, and the height of the suction ring.

Table 19-1

SUCTION RING: RESECTION DIAMETER NOMOGRAM

	+2 ring	+1 ring	0 ring	-1 ring
Cornea K > 46	9.0 mm	9.5 mm	10 mm	10.5 mm
Cornea K ~ 43.5	8.5 mm	9.0 mm	9.5 mm	10 mm
Cornea K ~ 42	8.0 mm	8.5 mm	9.0 mm	9.5 mm
Cornea K < 40	7.0 mm	7.5 mm	8.0 mm	8.5 mm

Note: For corneas smaller than 11 mm in diameter, the diameter could increase by 0.25 mm.
For corneas larger than 12 mm, the diameter could decrease by 0.25 mm.

The H ring may increase the diameter by 0.25 mm compared to the –1 ring. This ring should not be used in steep corneas, and the cornea to be resected should be confirmed with an applanation lens before performing the surgery.

* This nomogram should be used only as a guide.

Using the same size ring, a steep cornea will allow more tissue to be exposed through the ring and will result in a large and thicker corneal disc. A flat cornea will reduce the amount of tissue exposed and will result in a smaller and thinner corneal disc.

The small size of the outer diameter of the ring and the availability of several different height rings result in adaptability to every orbital or interpalpebral configuration and to obtaining the desired disc diameter no matter the corneal radius (Table 19-1).

H ring will increase the disc diameter by 0.25 compared to the –1 ring. H ring should be used only for flat corneas. This nomogram is suggestive only.

Hinge size: The hinge size is determined by a fixed stopper built in the ring handle, which will stop the head travel, leaving a theoretical hinge size of 4.0 mm average, depending on the diameter of the resected disc.

We believe the hinge size should be referred to as "degrees of arc" (50° to 60°), this expression would reflect the same proportion of uncut tissue (hinge) with any disc diameter.

Hinge position: In harmony with the blinking movement, the superior hinge becomes the most physiological location to avoid displacement; however, we select the best hinge position according to:

- The globe size and orbital shape: In large eyes with big orbits, the ring can be easily placed and oriented in all quadrants; but in small orbits, the ring must be positioned to allow the microkeratome to begin the cut laterally—this is the position that allows the microkeratome to be easily inserted.

    Although in many cases we can begin the cut at the vertical quadrants, the insertion at those quadrants require globe traction outside the orbit to avoid contact with the speculum and the ocular adnexa, increasing the risk of loosing suction during the cut.

- The astigmatic defect: We recommend orienting the hinge in a quadrant 90° away from the astigmatic axis to avoid a negative hinge syndrome (presented at the American Academy of Ophthalmology, Atlanta, Ga, USA 1995, by CCB) This occurs when there is ablation of the base of the hinge that induces an additive ablation effect that appears once the disc is repositioned over the cornea; topographically, it is seen as a peripheral ablated area at the base of the hinge (Figures 19-7 and 19-8) and induces irregular astigmatism that is difficult to resolve.

Initially, to solve this complication, we began to cover the base of the hinge with sponges or spatulas until we observed a few cases of induced astigmatism that showed a topographic image of elevation in red at the hinge's base. We then understood that it was produced by a nonablated area. We called it a positive hinge syndrome (Figure 19-9).

Finally, we recommend orienting the hinge 90° apart from the astigmatic axis or to program a wider diameter disc in those nasal hinges' microkeratomes (Figure 19-10).

Superior hinge lateral-up (Figure 19-11a, 19-11b, 19-12a, and 19-12b): The introduction of the microkeratome in the superior or inferior quadrants is difficult due to the anatomical orbital structure. For the purpose of obtaining a corneal superior hinge, we recommend using the nasal and temporal lateral quadrants as the microkeratome's initial position for entrance to perform the lamellar cut. On the Carriazo-Barraquer system, the corneal advance movement is performed lateral-superior, being temporal-superior for the right eye and nasal-superior for the left eye. With this approach we can obtain a superior hinge in every globe.

Manual or automatic advancement: Both systems are reliable and easy to use. The disc border, cutting surface, and resection thickness are repeatable with the

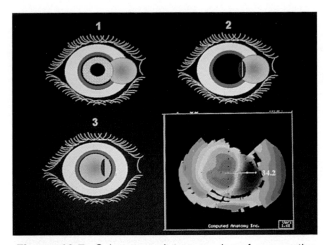

Figure 19-7. Scheme and topography of a negative hinge syndrome.

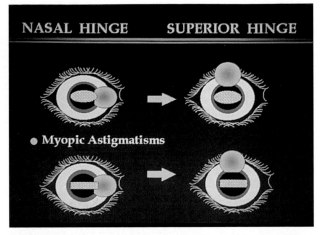

Figure 19-8. Scheme of the mechanism of hinge ablation in myopic astigmatism.

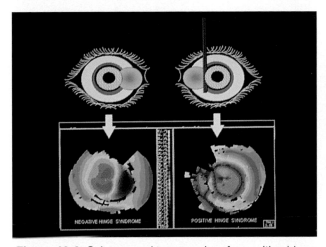

Figure 19-9. Scheme and topography of a positive hinge syndrome in comparison with the negative one in hyperopic astigmatism correction.

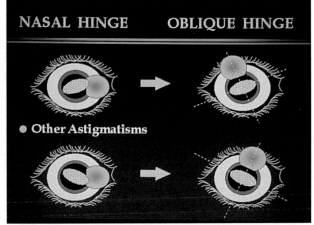

Figure 19-10. Scheme of the advantage of superior flaps to orient the hinge 90° apart from the astigmatic axis.

automatic system when a group of surgeons share it.

On the other hand, the manual system offers indirect control over the resection thickness. If the advance movement is at high speed, you will obtain a thinner disc than if the advance is performed with a slow and even movement. The turbine has a stronger torque and the blade moves at higher speed.

Right or left hand: This system has been designed to be used with the same hand in both eyes; this characteristic avoids changing the microkeratome and ring orientation and the differences in the cut quality when driven with the nondominant hand.

CLINICAL OBSERVATIONS

In the automated mode, insertion of the head in the crowned pivot of the ring is a little tricky, but we learned very quickly to turn the head inside the fingers until a perfect assembly of the crown takes place. The cut is performed smoothly, obtaining a high-quality disc in every procedure.

In the manual mode, the procedure is faster due to the easy insertion of the head in the flat-end pivot of the ring, and the rotational movement of the fingers to perform the cut gives the surgeon control of the procedure. The turbine is needed only during the cut—it is off during the reverse movement. The thickness of the disc will depend on the speed of the pass, allowing resection of different thicknesses at will; this property makes it possible for this microkeratome to be used in lamellar grafts.

In flat corneas, such as post-refractive surgery reoperations, it is possible to obtain a wide diameter and adequate thickness disc, making the cut with a slow and even movement of the fingers.

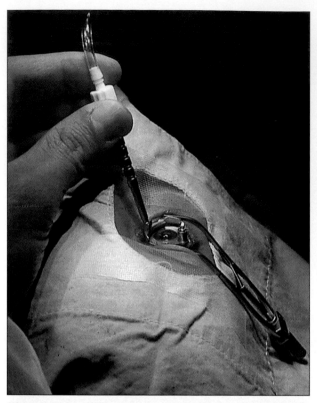

Figure 19-11a. The right eye of a patient with the ring in position.

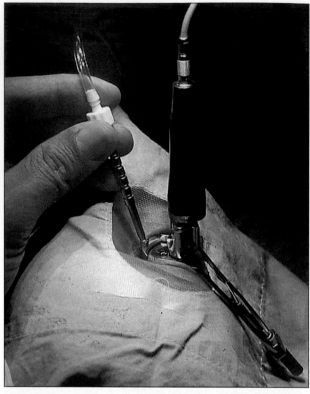

Figure 19-11b. The microkeratome has been inserted in the pivot at the temporal side of the globe.

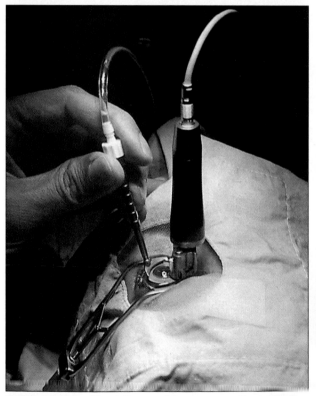

Figure 19-12a. The left eye of the same patient with the microkeratome in the nasal entrance position.

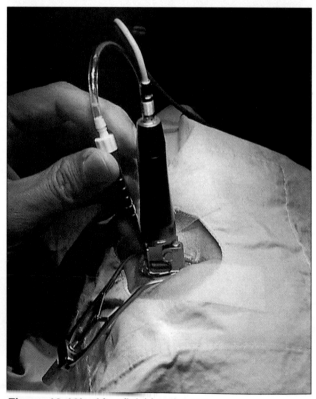

Figure 19-12b. After finishing the cut.

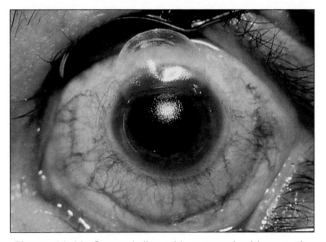

Figure 19-13. Corneal disc with a superior hinge maintained over the superior lid.

The height of the instrument makes it possible to perform the procedure without defocusing the microscope during the cut with almost every laser machine; with the VISX Star, surgeons need to lower the patient's bed in order to handle the instrument.

Handling the disc is performed with a spatula to place it over the superior lid speculum in almost a vertical position during the refractive photoablation (Figure 19-13). We do not recommend placing the disc over the conjunctiva at 12 o'clock, having found that the superior conjunctival fornix has more secretions with more debris after the laser procedure than with nasal hinge-oriented discs.

The microkeratome head must be cleaned with distilled water and alcohol before sterilization; surgical soaps might induce foam formation during the cut when the turbine motor is being used.

REFERENCES

1. Barraquer JI. Queratomileusis para la correction de la Miopia. *Arch Soc Am Oftalmol Optom.* 1964;5:27-48.
2. Barraquer C. The Microkeratome. In: Buratto L, Brint SF, eds. *LASIK: Principles and Techniques.* Thorofare, NJ: SLACK Incorporated; 1998.
3. Draeger J. Ein haulbautomatisches elektrisches keratom fur die lamellare keratoplastik. *Klin Monatsbl Augenheilkd.* 1975; 167:353-359.
4. Draeger J, Hackelbusch R. Experimentelle Untersuchungen und klinische Erfahrungen mit neun Rotatory-Instrumenten. *Ophthalmologica.* 1972;164:273-283.
5. Buratto L, Brint S, Ferrari M. Keratomileusis. In: Buratto L, Brint SF, eds. *LASIK: Principles and Techniques.* Thorofare, NJ: SLACK Incorporated; 1998.
6. Carriazo C, Barraquer JI. Bisagra superior en LASIK (nueva técnica quirúrgica). *Arch Soc Am Oftal Optom.* 1996;24:358-354.

SUGGESTED READING

Doane JF, Slade S, Updegraff S. In: Buratto L, Brint SF, eds. *LASIK: Principles and Techniques.* Thorofare, NJ: SLACK Incorporated; 1998.

Krueger R, Parolini B, Gordon E, Juhasz T. In: Pallikaris IG, Siganos DS, eds. *LASIK.* Thorofare, NJ: SLACK Incorporated; 1998.

NEW DISPOSABLE MICROKERATOMES

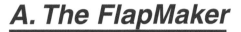

20

A. The FlapMaker

Joseph Colin, MD, Jeffrey B. Robin, MD, and Alexander Dybbs, PhD

OVERVIEW

Over the last few years, LASIK has become the predominant refractive surgical procedure worldwide. Derived from uncommonly used lamellar refractive techniques, the introduction of the excimer laser enabled LASIK to provide the benefits of lamellar procedures (minimal discomfort, rapid visual recovery, wide range of potential corrections) with the precision of this submicron laser. However, with the introduction of LASIK, it quickly became apparent that the technology for creating the flap was primitive compared to that for performing the refractive ablation. As microkeratomes that had been designed for mechanical lamellar surgery were utilized for hundreds of thousands of LASIK procedures, it was quite evident that these devices had intensive learning curves, were difficult to maintain, wore down easily, had serious safety concerns, and were expensive to purchase and operate.

With the continued explosive growth in the popularity of LASIK, developing safer, more effective, and easier to use microkeratome designs has become a major priority for refractive surgeons and the refractive surgery industry. In 1995, there was essentially one microkeratome for lamellar refractive surgeons; by 2000, there will likely be more than a dozen commercially available microkeratome designs. All of the new designs have attempted to address perceived deficiencies with traditional microkeratomes, in essence pursuing the "ideal" device.

THE IDEAL MICROKERATOME

What exactly is the "ideal" microkeratome? First, of course, it should be able to make high-quality LASIK flaps of consistent diameter, thickness and stromal bed quality. In addition, the ideal microkeratome should combine outstanding efficacy with considerations of safety, ergonomics, and economics (Tables 20-1 through 20-3).

WHY A DISPOSABLE MICROKERATOME?

We believe that a disposable microkeratome has the best opportunity to incorporate the features of the ideal microkeratome. Compared to reusable devices, disposable microkeratomes provide improvements in ease-of-use, safety and cost implications for the surgeon. Fully disposable microkeratomes by definition must have their cutting heads incorporated into suction plates, thus providing significant benefits in areas such as surgeon learning curve, staff set-up and turnover time, and surgeon use. Furthermore, blade gaps would need to be prefixed, eliminating concern regarding possible globe perforation.

With proper quality control, each disposable microkeratome would also be of the utmost quality and sterility, thus maximizing these features for each surgical case and minimizing risk to the patient and surgeon. Concerns regarding "wear and tear" and mechanical breakdown/repair would also be significantly lessened with a disposable microkeratome as opposed to a reusable device.

Disposibility eliminates the requirement for meticulous care, assembly, cleaning, and sterilization. This factor, combined with the short learning curve and ease of set-up, use, and turnover, enable the surgeon and staff to

Table 20-1
SAFETY CONSIDERATIONS OF THE IDEAL MICROKERATOME
• Fixed blade gap to eliminate the possibility of perforation of the globe
• No cutting on microkeratome reversal
• Automated translation to minimize stromal bed irregularity
• Gearless translation to minimize torque and stromal bed irregularity
• Single-use design for maximum blade quality and sterility
• Transparent to allow for visualization of the cornea

Table 20-2
ERGONOMIC CONSIDERATIONS OF THE IDEAL MICROKERATOME
• Keratome prefixed in suction ring to minimize operative manipulations and the duration of the suction onto the eye
• Automated
• Gearless to minimize the risk of obstruction and aborting the case
• Disposable to eliminate the need for device cleaning, sterilization, and maintenance

Table 20-3
ECONOMIC CONSIDERATIONS OF THE IDEAL MICROKERATOME
• Minimal initial cost
• Reasonable per case cost
• Minimal associated costs, including the need for specialized technical staffing to use and maintain the device, as well as turnover time between cases

Table 20-4
FLAPMAKER FEATURES
• Disposable
• Single use
• Transparent
• Polycarbonate design
• Automated but gearless
• Central axial cable drive locomotion
• Fixed blade gap (130, 160, 180, and 200 microns)
• Horizontal approach
• Blade rotation at 12,500 RPM
• 26° blade angle
• Available in myopic (mean 8.5 mm vertical diameter), hyperopic (mean 10.5 mm vertical diameter), and mini (for small eyes) varieties

perform more LASIK procedures in a given time period than could be done with a reusable keratome.

THE FLAPMAKER DISPOSABLE MICROKERATOME

The FlapMaker is the first clinically tested disposable microkeratome for LASIK. It was designed specifically to address well-documented concerns with traditional microkeratome designs and to meet the efficacy, safety, ergonomic, and economic considerations of the ideal microkeratome (Table 20-4). The device was designed and developed by Alexander Dybbs, PhD of Refractive Technologies, Inc (Cleveland, Ohio, USA) in 1996. It was first used clinically to perform LASIK in 1997 and has, as of 1999, been used in more than 30,000 LASIK procedures worldwide.

The FlapMaker was developed in the traditional Barraquer style (ie, a horizontal approach with a 26° blade angle). The device is transparent and made of polycarbonate. Transparency enables the surgeon to visualize the flap creation process and intervene should conditions dictate.

The FlapMaker is injection molded, which ensures repeatability and precision, and has only five component parts. Polycarbonate plastic was chosen for FlapMaker because of its strength, design flexibility, dimensional stability (±0.01%), and transparency. This state-of-the-art injection molding approach allows the FlapMaker to be delivered to the surgeon totally preassembled (with the blade inside the keratome head and with the head inserted into the suction plate/ring), thus maximizing ergonomic considerations. Safety considerations are also maximized, as the blade and gap are preset by the manufacturer. Additionally, each keratome is gamma ray sterilized to maximize sterility in this single-use device. Similarly, blade quality is also maximized via the single-use approach. Finally, the injection molding process enables the FlapMaker to be less expensive to purchase and use than reusable microkeratomes. Other economic considerations (such as a faster learning curve, decreased need for specialized staff to assemble and maintain the device, and quicker turnaround time between surgeries) make the FlapMaker even more attractive from an economic standpoint.

The polycarbonate injection molding also enables significant flexibility of the system. The manufacturer has been able to create several FlapMaker designs incorporating different blade gap depths, as well as different ring diameters and even different overall keratome diam-

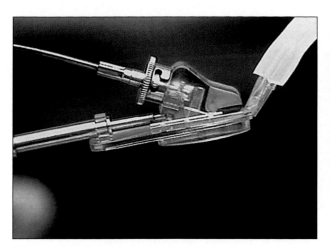

Figure 20-1. Lateral view of the FlapMaker.

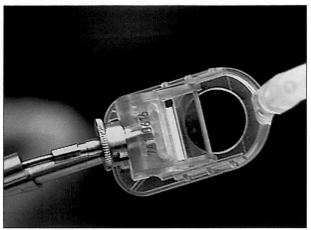

Figure 20-2. The FlapMaker is a single-use, disposable microkeratome.

eters. Presently, the FlapMaker system involves blade gap depths ranging from 130 to 200 microns, as well as ring opening diameters that can give mean flap diameters of either 8.5 mm or 10.5 mm (ideal for myopic or hyperopic cases, respectively). Furthermore, FlapMaker also comes in an overall smaller (by 2.0 mm in vertical diameter) version, colloquially referred to as the "mini" FlapMaker, which is ideal for eyes with smaller interpalpebral fissures or other similar anatomic concerns.

In order to maximize efficacy, FlapMaker designers believed that an automated microkeratome was superior to a manual device. However, the traditional approach of automating microkeratomes via gears and motors had created several problems. Prime among these included obstruction of the gears by eyelashes, eyelid skin, or debris, with risk of incomplete flap formation and case abortion. Also, gears were noted to cause torque during microkeratome translation, increasing the risk for irregularities in the stromal bed contour. Furthermore, gear propulsion systems require motors—usually hand-held devices that could be cumbersome to use. Gears and motors also contributed to overall wear and tear and maintenance concerns. Finally, recent reports regarding noninfectious interface keratitis following LASIK (Sands of the Sahara syndrome) have implicated, among other potential factors, lubricating solutions used in the hand-held motors of geared microkeratome systems.

The FlapMaker is an automated microkeratome, but it is totally gearless. Its propulsion system involves a flexible axial cable that is easily inserted into the new microkeratome head for each new procedure. The control console provides power for the axial cable, so there are no bulky handpieces, lubricants, or other potentially toxic solutions with which to contend. The control console also electronically determines and limits the exten-

sion of the axial cable so that the risk of free cap formation is minimized.

The FlapMaker blade is a high quality, surgical steel blade. It comes preset by the manufacturer in the keratome head. There is no assembly required by surgeon or staff. The blade gap is preset by the manufacturer; there are a variety of gap depths available to surgeons. The blade is powered by a second flexible cable that is easily inserted into the blade housing pin.

At the end of the surgical procedure, the entire microkeratome unit (with head, blade, and suction plate) is detached from the two cables and simply disposed. A new, sterile microkeratome unit is then removed from its sterile packing and, following simple attachment of axial and blade cables, the FlapMaker is ready for the next surgical procedure.

FLAPMAKER ASSEMBLY AND USE

The FlapMaker consists of the control/power console (Figure 20-1) and a single-use, disposal microkeratome (Figure 20-2).

The control console contains a vacuum suction pump and electronic components that connect via the flexible cables to provide translation and blade power for the disposable microkeratomes. The two cables are electronically controlled and consist of an axial cable that propels the keratome's translation and a blade oscillation cable that produces 12,500 oscillations per minute. Additionally, the power console has been electronically devised so that the blade oscillates only on forward motion of the microkeratome, thus eliminating the risk of reverse cutting (Figure 20-3). The vacuum pump simply

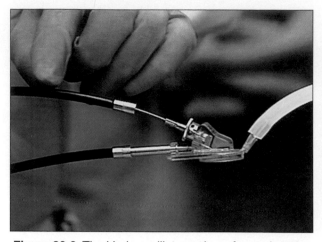

Figure 20-3. The blade oscillates only on forward motion of the microkeratome, thus eliminating the risk of reverse cutting.

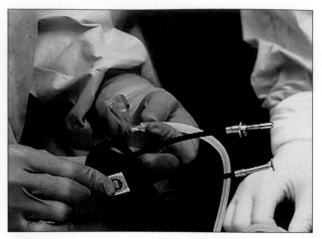

Figure 20-4. Assembly of the two cables to the microkeratome head.

connects to the suction port of the disposable microkeratome via a flexible silicone tube.

The FlapMaker microkeratome head and guide rail of the suction ring are molded as one piece; the surgeon has no need to fit the head into the dovetail of the suction ring tracks. The microkeratome unit comes totally pre-assembled (Figure 20-4) with the blade inserted in the microkeratome head and the head inserted into the suction plate/ring. There are no plates, blades, blade blocks, gap devices, stop screws, etc, for the surgeon and staff to assemble, insert, and adjust (or forget). Three simple connections (axial cable to microkeratome head, blade power cable to microkeratome head, and suction tube to suction port on microkeratome plate) ready the fixed gap microkeratome for the procedure.

The assembly of a new FlapMaker microkeratome—from removal from its sterile pack to placement on the eye—usually takes less than 1 minute. Similarly, at the end of the procedure, there are no components for the surgeon or staff to contend with. The microkeratome head is simply detached from the cables and disposed (Figure 20-5).

LASIK USING THE FLAPMAKER

The following describes a typical LASIK procedure using the FlapMaker microkeratome.

Preparation of the Patient

Prior to surgery, the patient is counseled on the steps of the procedure and what he or she can expect to experience. Although not required, many surgeons prefer to have their patients slightly sedated during the procedure. For the average adult, 5 to 10 mg of oral diazepam (or

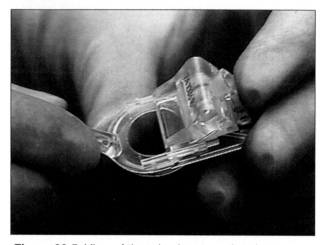

Figure 20-5. View of the microkeratome head.

equivalent) will frequently reduce patient apprehension, yet enable them to be sufficiently alert to cooperate.

Most surgeons utilize a typical preoperative regimen of cleansing the eyelid skin with Betadine solution. Many also prefer to irrigate the conjunctival fornices with saline solution to remove particulate and/or mucoid debris. Preoperative use of antibiotic and anti-inflammatory topical agents is also recommended, although care should be taken to minimize the risk of corneal epithelial toxicity resulting from these preoperative maneuvers. In this regard, it is recommended to use only the minimal amount of topical anesthetic necessary to achieve patient comfort during the procedure, as the potential epithelial toxicity of these agents is well documented. The authors use a single drop of tetracaine during preoperative preparation. No pupil-active eyedrops are necessary for routine LASIK procedures.

In the operating room, the patient is settled under the

laser microscope. The nonoperated eye is occluded with a patch to eliminate the risk of cross-fixation during the refractive treatment. Draping of the patient is then performed. There are a variety of potential draping strategies. The authors prefer a simple draping approach combining a disposable head drape (3M 1089 disposable drape) that provides a sterile field over the eyebrows and forehead, draping back over the top of the patient's head. In addition, the authors use a simple sterile, transparent adhesive dressing (Tegaderm adhesive dressing, 3M Health Care Services, St. Paul, Minn, USA) that is pre-cut to contour the eyelid margins. Tegaderm provides excellent adhesion to the lid margins and provides a sterile field over the eyelids while retracting the eyelids and eyelashes away from the ocular surface. Certainly, other strategies for draping are equally effective and the choice of strategy results from surgeon experience and preference, as well as local regulations and standards.

FlapMaker Positioning

The FlapMaker consists of the control/power console, cables, and the microkeratome unit. Generally, it is best to position the console on a stand or table immediately behind the surgeon. The cables are sufficiently long so that they can be positioned around the side of the surgeon for a particular eye (left or right). The cables are not sterile. Usually, it is sufficient to simply clean the cables with rubbing alcohol in between each case. Some surgeons have elected to wrap the cables with sterile plastic prior to each case to ensure maximal sterility.

Preparation of the Eye

Once the patient and microscope are properly positioned, the surgeon can devote attention to the process of creating the flap. The eye has been sufficiently anesthetized (see above). The area of concern for the surgeon is exposure.

Proper exposure of the ocular surface is perhaps the most important factor for successful flap creation, regardless of the keratome used. Insufficient exposure can result in a variety of problems, ranging from inability to achieve sufficient suction to the creation of thin or incomplete flaps, or even buttonholes. With a plastic microkeratome, because of its inherent light weight and flexibility, these exposure issues are even more critical. It is the authors' experience, and that of the manufacturer, that the single greatest cause of clinical problems using the FlapMaker occur because of insufficient exposure of the ocular surface.

It is critical for the surgeon to take the necessary steps and time to ensure adequate exposure. It is recommended that an adjustable lid speculum be used to achieve maximal exposure; there are a variety of these

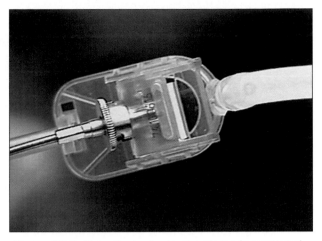

Figure 20-6. The attached microkeratome is pretested.

available, many recently introduced specifically for LASIK. Solid blade speculums are not recommended. Frequently, patients may experience some discomfort because of the speculum's pressure on the orbital rims. It is important to warn patients in advance of the procedure that this may be a source of mild discomfort. Additionally, the authors have found that a gradual expansion of the speculum is better tolerated than suddenly opening the speculum to its maximum (an analogy may be the experience with indirect ophthalmoscopy in that a gradual increase in light intensity is usually better tolerated than suddenly introducing the maximum intensity light). Throughout the process of flap creation, the surgeon must have the issue of exposure adequacy foremost in his or her mind.

Another approach to improve exposure, which is occasionally helpful in smaller eyes, is the use of a lateral canthotomy. This is a simple, low-risk procedure that when properly performed takes about 1 minute and can add sufficient exposure to allow for successful flap creation. The authors recommend that exposure issues be considered during the preoperative examination and, if it is believe that a lateral canthotomy may be necessary, this issue be fully discussed with the patient during the informed consent process.

Creating the Flap with the FlapMaker

Once adequate exposure is achieved, the surgeon can proceed with flap creation. Inked reference marks are placed on the cornea per surgeon preference. These marks are designed for proper flap realignment following ablation, as well as to enable the surgeon to properly replace and reposition a free cap should one occur.

The FlapMaker microkeratome head has previously been removed from the sterile pack and attached to the axial power cable, blade power cable, and flexible suc-

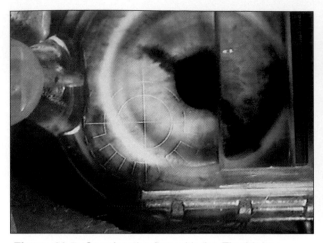

Figure 20-7. Creating the flap with the FlapMaker.

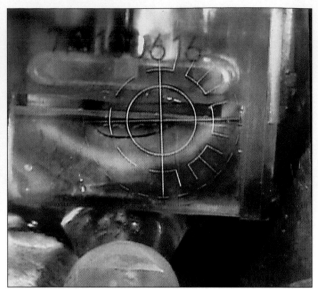

Figure 20-8. Creating the flap with the FlapMaker.

tion tube. This preparation should take less than 1 minute. It is important for the surgeon and/or staff to pretest the attached microkeratome by running it one or two times to ensure smooth translation of the keratome head across the suction plate/ring (Figure 20-6). Any perceived problem with the keratome or its translation is easily handled: the keratome is simply detached from the cables and suction tube and disposed of, and a new microkeratome head is attached and tested.

The choice of microkeratome diameter (myopic, hyperopic, mini) and corneal flap thickness are made according to the patient's refractive error and the surgeon's preference. FlapMaker surgeons usually stock a variety of microkeratomes so that individual patient considerations are easily addressed.

Once proper preparation of the eye has been achieved, the surgeon can proceed with flap creation. The transparency of the FlapMaker is very useful to facilitate proper centration of the device; a slight nasal decentration may be helpful in order to ensure sufficient stromal bed diameter for the subsequent laser ablation.

With proper centration assured, the surgeon places the FlapMaker microkeratome on the eye. In order to minimize flexing of this plastic device, it is recommended that the surgeon grasp the microkeratome head with thumb and index finger of one hand by the 12 and 6 o'clock poles of the suction plate/ring. The surgeon's other hand is used to gently support the cables (there is a support handpiece incorporating the two cables located approximately 6 inches from the insertion of the cables into the microkeratome). Gentle support of the handpiece ensures the cables will be in the proper position for maximal functioning.

The surgeon firmly places the FlapMaker microkeratome head on the eye, as previously described. Suction is then engaged by the surgical staff. There are a variety of audible and visual signs to ensure that suction has been successfully engaged; in addition, there is a suction gauge on the console. It is recommended that the suction gauge read at least 27 inches Hg to ensure a minimal level of sufficient suction to proceed with flap creation. The FlapMaker microkeratome does not have sufficient room to allow for placement of the Barraquer applanating tonometer (which will only indicate a minimal intraocular pressure of 65 mm Hg). The authors recommend the use of a Mentor pneumotonometer to give a minimal, quantitative intraocular pressure reading. However, many LASIK surgeons are comfortable with indirect clinical signs of adequate intraocular pressure, including pupil dilatation, loss of vision, and scleral blanching around the microkeratome suction ring (easily visible through the transparent plate).

With adequate suction and intraocular pressure assured, a drop of balanced salt solution is applied to the surface of the cornea. The surgeon should make a last visible check to ensure that the microkeratome translation pathway is completely free of obstructions (lid specula blades, eyelid skin, drapes, etc). The footpedal is then engaged to power both forward translation of the microkeratome head and blade oscillation. The surgeon is able to observe the cornea through the transparent head and plate; if there is any problem, the surgeon can abort the translation by simply lifting his or her foot off the pedal. Once the forward translation has been completed, the surgeon shifts foot pressure off the forward pedal and onto the reverse pedal. The blade oscillation stops and microkeratome head is pulled back to its starting position via retraction of the axial cable. Suction is then disen-

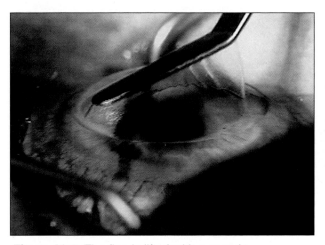

Figure 20-9. The flap is lifted with a spatula.

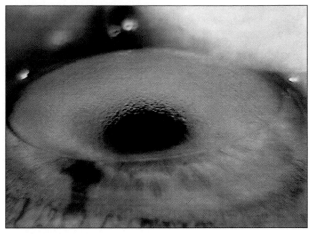

Figure 20-10. The photoablation is then performed.

gaged. The FlapMaker has an intentional slower decompression phase. It is important for the surgeon to remove the microkeratome from the eye (usually takes 5 seconds for total decompression). At this point, flap creation has been completed and the surgeon can proceed with laser ablation (Figures 20-7 and 20-8).

Completion of the Refractive Treatment

Following removal of the FlapMaker microkeratome head, the surgeon should quickly observe that the flap is intact and reference marks are well aligned. The flap can then be retracted using forceps (nontoothed), cannula, or spatula. Technique at this point is determined by surgeon preference/experience, as well as individual laser manufacturer, nomogram, and individual patient considerations. Most surgeons will protect the retracted flap/hinge with either a spatula or sponge device. Additionally, individual surgeons have preferences for drying the stromal bed during the ablation process (Figure 20-9).

The ablation is then performed per laser manufacturer and nomogram recommendations (Figure 20-10).

COMPLETION OF THE OPERATION

The flap is replaced and realigned using the previously created reference marks. Some surgeons prefer to float the flap onto a drop of balanced salt solution (BSS) or antibiotic solution on the stromal bed. Forceps, spatula or cannula can be used in flap replacement. Most surgeons will clean the interface with some degree of BSS irrigation under the replaced flap.

Following replacement of the flap and irrigation under the flap, the flap must be allowed to secure into place. This usually involves some period of drying. Some surgeons prefer to use blown air to accelerate this process. The authors recommend a simple system of allowing the repositioned flap to dry for approximately 3 minutes. In order to prevent epithelial disruption during this time, a small amount of 1% methylcellulose solution is applied to the central corneal epithelium.

At the close of the procedure, the surgeon ensures that the flap is in excellent position, the "gutter" of the wound is symmetrical throughout, and there are no visible striae or other signs of flap distortion. Any deviation from the ideal should be addressed at this point by lifting and repositioning the flap .

Antibiotic and anti-inflammatory drops are applied to the eye (the authors prefer ofloxacin and prednisolone acetate 0.1%), the speculum is gently removed, and the eye drapes are removed. At this point, proper flap adherence is ensured by having the patient blink several times and viewing the flap for any change in position. The surgeon may then proceed to the second eye (if performing a bilateral same-session procedure) or discharge the patient to the recovery area. If the surgeon proceeds to perform LASIK on the second eye, it is recommended that a new FlapMaker microkeratome be used.

Although the LASIK procedure is technically complete at this point, it is very helpful to ensure that the flap remains in excellent position prior to discharging the patient from the surgical facility, as it has been recognized that early flap slippage is a not uncommon problem. Many surgeons now prefer to check the patient at the slit lamp 15 to 45 minutes after surgery in order to ensure proper flap positioning and appearance. Any problems with the flap can then be immediately addressed by returning the patient to the operating room.

PREVENTION OF LASIK COMPLICATIONS

It is beyond the scope of this chapter to fully address all possible LASIK complications. However, it is appropriate to discuss commonly seen complications, particularly those that can be affected (positively or negatively) via the use of the FlapMaker microkeratome.

The following are LASIK complications that can be minimized by proper use of the FlapMaker :

- Decentration: the transparency of the FlapMaker head is very helpful to obtain a good centration on the corneal limbus.
- Inadequate exposure: the greatest source of problems with any keratome, but perhaps more so with the FlapMaker. Use of an expanding open-blade lid speculum is critical. In some cases, this needs to be combined with lateral canthotomy. Finally, use of the mini FlapMaker, which is 2.0 mm shorter in vertical diameter than the regular FlapMaker (or the Chiron Automated Corneal Shaper) is helpful in smaller eyes.
- Inadequate suction: the suction gauge on the FlapMaker console should read a minimum of 27 inches Hg in order to ensure adequate suction. Anything less should render the case aborted and may indicate vacuum pump problems. As noted above, the use of indirect clinical signs and – more preferably, a pneumotonometer should give the surgeon a sufficient IOP reading in order to ensure an optimal flap.
- Loss of suction: it is very unusual for the FlapMaker, once suction is successfully engaged, to lose suction during the procedure. Possible causes include improper manipulation of the keratome head during translation and, more likely, inadequate exposure of the globe, enabling the speculum blades to get under the keratome plate and disrupt suction. Again, good exposure is critical. Additionally, the authors have found that running the keratome by the patient's ear prior to the actual procedure acclimates the patient to the sound of the keratome and minimizes the risk that he or she will have a startle response once the keratome blade oscillation is engaged. Also, once the keratome suction is engaged, the surgeon should remove his hand from the keratome head and simply maintain the keratome's proper position by gently supporting the cable handpiece (as described above). This will eliminate the risk of the surgeon inadvertently causing problems with the keratome or plate during keratome translation.

FLAPMAKER KEYS TO SUCCESS

The clinical keys to success using the FlapMaker microkeratome are:

- Excellent exposure of the globe
- Excellent suction and intraocular pressure
- Preoperative mean keratometries between 41 and 48 diopters (corneas not too flat or too steep)
- Press suction ring directly on eye, as previously described
- Ensure that the cables remain in their natural position during translation of the keratome
- Test run the keratome to ensure optimal translation and blade movement

Dr. Robin is a paid consultant to Refractive Technologies, Inc. Dr. Dybbs is owner and president of Refractive Technologies, Inc. Dr. Colin has no financial or proprietary interest in the products or companies described in this chapter.

B. The Unishaper

J. Charles Casebeer, MD

THE SINGLE-USE UNISHAPER DISPOSABLE KERATOME

Laser-assisted in situ keratomileusis (LASIK) is an excellent procedure when used within its limits and performed well. It produces excellent results for refractive errors to approximately 14 diopters (D) of myopia, 4 D of hyperopia, and 4 to 6 D of astigmatism depending on the brand of laser used. In the CRS (Clinical Research, Inc) Food and Drug Administration (FDA)-sanctioned study of LASIK[1] patient satisfaction is extremely high. In these data, which are pending FDA approval of LASIK with the VISX Star and Summit Apex Plus in the United States, lasers show that the traditionally recognized side effects of LASIK (glare, ghosting, halos, starbursts, trouble driving at night, etc) are not any worse after surgery than they were before. Approximately 95% of patients achieved 20/40 or better at 3 months without enhancement. Loss of two lines of acuity is 1% and consecutive hyperopia is very rare (< 1%) in patients being treated for 1 to 7 D of myopia and up to 4 D of astigmatism. Even patients with greater than 7 to 14 D of myopia have excellent results, albeit less than the lower diopter group. Results like this earn the respect of the public as well as the eye surgeon, and LASIK has established itself as a valuable, desirable surgery for many people with refractive errors.

Above these limits, side effects can become problematic. Corneal ectasia becomes an increasing risk as the amount of myopia to be treated increases, especially in thinner corneas.

I believe any well-motivated and well-trained ophthalmologist can perform this procedure. However, in order to add this procedure to a general ophthalmology practice, safety must be paramount, along with a demonstrably high degree of predictability. Neither the public nor the doctor should be exposed to a significant degree of risk, and the surgeons and their staffs should not have to be virtual experts in technology in order to perform the surgery safely.

Although there is a myriad of potential complications, with the exception of the rare endophthalmitis, one thing that can cause loss of an eye is the microkeratome. Other problems, either surgical or equipment related, do not threaten the physical integrity of the eye. The keratome must be simple to use and highly reliable. In fact, it is my experience that fear of the keratome is almost universally the thing keeping most eye surgeons from performing LASIK.

The Automated Corneal Shaper (ACS)[2] brought keratomileusis to ophthalmology because of specific design features that made it superior to the earlier Barraquer keratomes. Specifically, these features include an automated passage and a stopper, generally relieving the surgeon of specific skill related to passage of the keratome and therefore quality of the keratotomy. It also introduced the ability to make a hinge while not having to deal with free tissue in most cases beginning in the Spring of 1993. However, the ACS introduced a number of new problems and is a very user-unfriendly instrument.[3] Specifically, it is a very complex instrument that requires great skill in disassembly, cleaning, inspection, blade insertion, reassembly, and checking function. Unfortunately, errors in this process can cause complications ranging from poor or no keratotomy to loss of the eye. The removable plate to select gap can be left out or improperly installed and may lead to entrance into the eye and essentially evisceration of the globe. In retrospect, this fatal flaw has caused considerable misery to patients and LASIK surgeons. Complications of this magnitude are not tolerable in this totally elective procedure.

Newer reusable keratome designs address the problem of the removable plate by having the gap set at the factory, but they still retain considerable complexity and require attention to detail and skill by the technical staff

and surgeon to avoid keratome—induced complications. In addition to improper cleaning or assembly leading to malfunction, the continued use of the instrument and the maintenance associated with it inexorably lead to gradual deterioration of the metal parts and can propagate errors from user to user until a failure finally results.

In 1996, I visited Dr. Luis Ruiz, the designer of the ACS, in Bogota, Colombia and he showed me a disposable keratome based on the design of the ACS but addressing, in my opinion, all of its problems. The thought of disposibility had occurred to me and, probably many other people, but it seemed technically impossible to achieve. In fact, he had operated on more than 100 eyes with excellent results using a hand-made polycarbonate keratome. The possibility of no cleaning, no blade insertion, and no assembly was very exciting, and the implications for safety in using a preassembled keratome/suction ring unit that could be thrown away at the end of the case were obvious. Of course, it would require great skill in manufacturing to assure proper preassembly, blade insertion, and tolerances; but if feasible, it could create a revolution in keratome safety and attitudes regarding them.

Such skill is possible in the injection molding industry and has been demonstrated in other disposable medical devices (and recently, this keratome). The development of molds made of the right specifications is difficult, but once accomplished, it leads to a very high reproducibility of the product. Following a series of sometimes painful revisions and laboratory and clinical studies, such a keratome is now available. The Ruiz disposable is now manufactured as the Unishaper by LaserSight Technologies of Orlando, Fla, USA.

Although this is classified as a plastic keratome, it is made of new, very hard and durable plastics called Lexan and Ultem. These plastics are polycarbonate-based polymers with very different physical characteristics from the soft, pliable plastics to which we are more accustomed. Injection molding allows production of keratomes that are virtually identical to each other, creating a very desirable "sameness" from unit to unit. The good features of the ACS (eg, constant speed of passage and excellent suction) have been retained, although improvements have been made even in these features. The drawbacks of the ACS (eg, inserting the keratome into the suction ring just before the keratotomy, the removable plate, and disassembly problems, cleaning, and reassembly) have been obviated.

The gear drive is on both sides of the keratome and is shielded by plastic skirts, allowing more symmetrical passage of the keratotomy and essentially eliminating the possibility of incarcerating material, such as cilia,

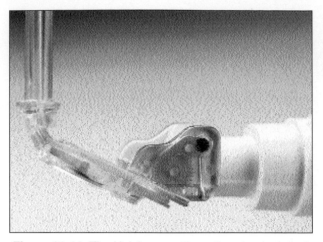

Figure 20-11. The Unishaper with suction ring installed.

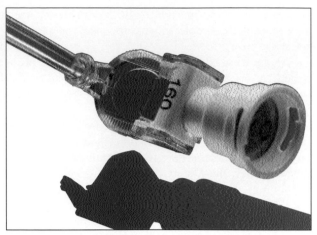

Figure 20-12. The Unishaper.

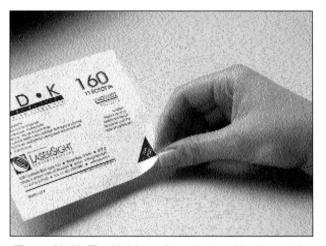

Figure 20-13. The Unishaper's sealed peel-back container.

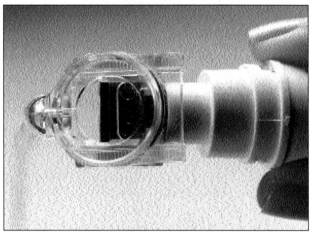

Figure 20-14. The entire Unishaper is discarded after use.

drapes, etc, into the gear drive. The keratome is installed in the suction ring at the factory to eliminate the awkward maneuver of putting the keratome in the suction ring with the suction ring already on the eye (Figure 20-11) The blade angle is 25° in keeping with José Barraquer's tediously worked out principals. The suction ring has an aperture diameter of .488 inches and an outside diameter of .772 inches (Figure 20-12). Because of a reduction transmission into which the motor is inserted, the gear drive runs at 5.5 mm per second and the blade oscillation speed is 7500 RPM. The keratome head is assembled at the factory, including installation of a high quality, high power inspected blade. The blade is stainless steel and manufactured using an EDM process. The suction handle serves as the highly visible stopper for the keratome. Every unit is checked for suction ring function before shipment. The assembled keratome suction ring unit is packaged in a plastic container, sterilized

by gamma radiation, and labeled as to gap specifications (Figure 20-13).

With this keratome, the procedure can be done with the help of any technician, even without specific keratome training. Preparation consists of removing the pre-assembled unit, hooking up the suction tube, installing the motor, and checking passage of the head. Compared to the ACS, it reduces the number of steps in this process from 18 to four and the time of preparation from approximately 45 minutes to approximately 2 minutes. When the procedure is completed, the entire unit is discarded (Figure 20-14).

Clinical use of the unit is very simple. The power console can be read in five languages and inhibits the keratome from working if suction in the pump is below the preset, safe limits and disables the keratome in the event suction begins to decline or fails during passage of the keratome. It has an easily seen backlit display that

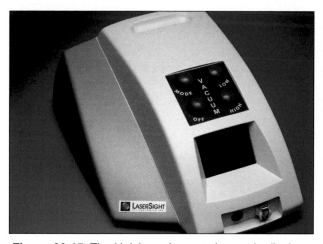

Figure 20-15. The Unishaper's control console display.

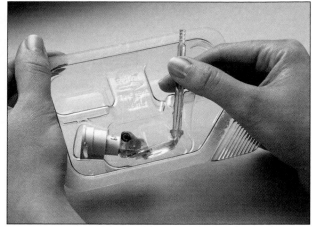

Figure 20-16. The preassembled Unishaper is removed from its package.

continuously shows the suction level in the pump and an elapsed timer to track the amount of time the patient is under high suction (Figure 20-15). It is 110 volts and 60 Hz. The dimensions are 5 x 9 x 4 inches and weighs 3 pounds.

The tear-off top of the package is removed using sterile technique, and the preassembled unit is removed from the package (Figure 20-16). The suction tubing is attached to the suction handle and the motor clicked into the transmission housing on the keratome head. With that, the unit is ready to go. It is good practice to put the thumb or finger into the aperture and assure continuity of suction from the console to the suction ring, and pass the keratome to the stop and back to verify proper operation.

A solid blade, spring lid speculum (eg, the Barraquer "paper clip") is used to cover the cilia; no drape is used. Since the keratome is already mounted in the suction ring, the entire unit is placed on the eye. The keratome unit is very small in outside dimensions and placement is usually very easy. Visibility is excellent. After centration is accomplished using the limbus as a guide, the suction is turned on and the intraocular pressure rises. Proof of the patient having no light perception or measuring the pressure with the Mentor pneumotonometer verifies suction in the eye is very high (greater than 100 mm Hg), as we now know is necessary. If the suction is not above safe levels in the pump, the keratome will not operate. It is very important to wet the cornea and the anterior applanation surface with balanced salt solution (BSS) to lubricate passage over the cornea. The polycarbonate plastics exert more friction than metal, so lubrication is very important. If BSS is used, passage will be very smooth. The field is checked to make sure there are no obstacles and the foot pedal is depressed, driving the keratome across the suction ring and causing it to bump into

the suction handle opposite it then stop. The flap can be seen externalized on the front surface of the keratome head. The surgeon can easily see that the passage has been completed. It is then backed up, the suction released, and the keratome suction ring unit removed. With keratometry of 43.50 D the cap will be approximately 9.2 mm in diameter. While it is in the retracted position the blade is covered by the suction ring and therefore protected from accidental damage.

The flap is turned back by the "flop" method onto the conjunctiva, the bed is inspected and treated with the laser well-centered, and the cap is returned by "flopping" it onto the wet stromal bed, inspecting it for alignment and lack of cap deformities, then seated with the painting technique using an expanded, squeezed out Merocel sponge. No waiting is necessary, the lid speculum is removed, and the patient is asked to blink to assure no movement or deformities of the cap. Tobradex drops are instilled and a transparent eye cover is applied to protect the eye from external trauma.

If the fellow eye is to operated on, the keratome unit is secured by the technician, and following satisfactory completion of the first eye, the second eye is treated in the same manner.

Contributing to versatility of its use. the hinge can be placed in any position on a great majority of eyes by putting the easily placed, small suction ring on the eye horizontally and rotating it to the desired hinge position while under suction (eg, superior if the surgeon prefers it, performing the keratotomy and removing the suction ring). The horizontal nasal hinge is still preferred, as management of the flap is easier and more sterile because of more room and lack of cilia and lid margins.

Clinical results and ease of use has been excellent. Future designs will likely allow selection of units with differing suction ring heights and aperture diameters to allow custom flaps of desired diameter and thickness to match the characteristics of the photablation and degree of refractive error.

In summary, this new technology will allow LASIK to become a simpler, safer procedure, allowing more surgeons to perform it and the public to have more access to it.

REFERENCES

1. The CRS Study of LASIK. FDA Protocol. Scottsdale, Ariz: CRS Clinical Research; 1996-1998.
2. Cascbeer JC, Ruiz L, Slade S. *Lamellar Refractive Surgery.* Thorofare, NJ: SLACK Incorporated; 1996.
3. Casebeer JC, Slade S. A comprehensive system of refractive surgery. *Course Manual.* Irvine, California: Chiron Vision; 1995.

SUGGESTED READING

Buratto L, Brint S, eds. *LASIK: Principles and Techniques.* Thorofare, NJ: SLACK Incorporated; 1998.

Casebeer JC. A systematized approach to LASIK. Course Manual. Scottsdale, Ariz: Casebeer Education Foundation; 1998.

Casebeer JC. A systematized approach to LASIK. Course Manual. Scottsdale, Ariz: Casebeer Education Foundation; 1999.

Elander R, Rich LF, Robin JB. *Principles and Practice of Refractive Surgery.* Philadelphia, Pa: WB Saunders Co; 1997.

Machat JJ, Slade SG, Probst LE, eds. *The Art of LASIK, 2nd Edition.* Thorofare, NJ: SLACK Incorporated; 1999.

Pallikaris IG, Siganos D. LASIK. Thorofare, NJ: SLACK Incorporated; 1998.

THE MICROJET KERATOME

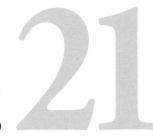

Stephen Brint, MD and Eugene I. Gordon, PhD

INTRODUCTION

Modern refractive surgery has various forms of expression. The most popular is LASIK. A key element of the LASIK procedure is the blade-based microkeratome (BBM) to produce the hinged flap. The number and variety of commercially available BBMs is truly impressive. Performance in the hands of an experienced surgeon is quite adequate and the safety is beginning to approach acceptable levels. Currently, it is difficult to single out any one device as standing well above the others. Moreover, knowledge of the behavior of BBMs is limited and anecdotal. Its actual behavior during cutting is not well known or understood. What seems clear is that the potential for significant improvement in the capability of the BBM is limited. This chapter is dedicated to providing the background of a new microkeratome principle that has the potential for making major improvements.

Here is a partial list of microkeratome performance parameters for which data on the BBM are limited or not available:

1. Reproducibility and accuracy of achieved flap thickness
2. Uniformity of flap thickness
3. Flap roundness and reproducibility of achieved diameter
4. Quality of the flap edge
5. Width of the hinge
6. Nature of the cut surface
7. Intraocular pressure (IOP) before and during the cut

BLADE-BASED MICROKERATOMES

The blade of any BBM is at least 100 µm in thickness and 1.0 mm in width. Strength of the blade material is its main limitation. The oscillating blade exerts considerable force on the corneal tissue as it cuts, hence the level of tissue distortion is high. For a typical BBM, setting the desired flap thickness to 160 µm may produce a flap with a thickness in the range of 120 to 200 µm. However, flap thickness control may be important for LASIK. The stroma is not uniform with depth. Consequently, it is likely that the photoablation rate depends on the depth of the exposed stromal surface. If so, the uncontrolled thickness of the flap influences the achieved correction and induces statistical error.

If the flap is too thick, it may limit the extent of available correction. The potential for keratoectasia sets a lower limit on the remaining stromal bed thickness of about 250 µm. A 200 µm flap brings the overall corneal minimum to 450 µm. This limits tissue removal to about 100 µm for a nominal corneal thickness of 550 µm, less for a thin cornea. Hence, the maximum safe correction is about 8 diopters (D) for an average thickness cornea.[1]

Flap uniformity presents a major problem. When the flap is a buttonhole or a two-part flap, the procedure is aborted. While the incidence of such extreme events is low, they are simply the pathological upper limit of an out-of-control nonuniformity. If the nonuniform flap is reestablished in precisely the same position, it may not produce refractive error, but the circumstance is typically not evaluated or reported. Nonuniformity of the cut may also induce irregular astigmatism. When the flap edge is tapered, the flap may not be round. Epithelial ingrowth is a potential consequence. Hence, items three and four in the above list are related.

Modern microkeratomes are designed to produce hinges of a predetermined width. However, short or long cuts still occur and often cause postponement of the procedure.

The exposed surface following a lamellar cut with an oscillating blade microkeratome exhibits a field of dev-

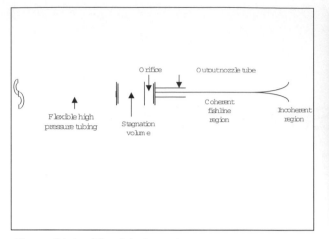

Figure 21-1a. Microjet elements.

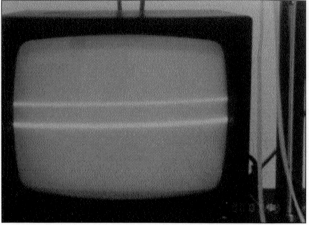

Figure 21-1b. Photograph of the beam, as seen from the side.

astation and destruction when viewed under high magnification (300x) scanning electron microscope (SEM). Each surface lamella is cut and shredded. The shredded boundary of a cut lamella is fused, presumably from blade friction associated with use of a high-speed blade. All keratocytes at the surface are lost. Cut surfaces are rarely observed at such high magnification and "smoothness" is not viewed as an issue, just a marketing opportunity. However, the nonuniformity and irregularity of the actual surface cannot help the quality of photoablation.

Even the sharpest blades require tissue resistance to cut. Hence, for successful use of a BBM, the IOP must be elevated to achieve cutting. The use of the scleral chuck or globe fixation device affords the opportunity to elevate IOP. The minimum useful IOP is 65 mm Hg. However, greater values improve the quality of the cut, and some surgeons report use of 100 mm Hg (Chayet). Applanation during the cut increases the IOP by roughly another 20 mm Hg.[2] Hence, the actual IOP associated with the creation of the flap is at best marginally safe. Possible outcomes include glaucoma, detached retina, and ischemia.

THE MICROJET MICROKERATOME

The use of microjet cutting associated with a microkeratome overcomes the noted deficiencies of a blade-based device. In what follows, we describe the microjet-based device, how it operates, and what can be achieved.

We define the microjet arbitrarily as a coherent, high-speed waterjet beam with a beam diameter of under 50 μm. Although many of the properties of the microjet have been described in other literature[3,4] they are reviewed briefly here. Figure 21-1a schematically illustrates the elements of microjet beam formation.

The microjet system operates at a stagnation pressure of about 20 to 25 Kpsi (kilopounds per square inch) (1360 to 1700 atmospheres). The high-pressure tubing is flexible and thin, yet strong enough to support the high pressure fluid. The shape and size of the stagnation volume geometry plays a key role in producing a coherent beam. The fabrication of the circular orifice, made of ruby, is critical to proper beam formation. The resulting beam diameter is about 87% of the orifice diameter. A typical beam diameter is 33 μm, although beam diameters as low as 20 μm have been used. There is a trade-off between stagnation pressure and beam diameter. The smaller the beam diameter, the greater the required stagnation pressure to achieve effective cutting. A stagnation pressure of 25 Kpsi is relatively straightforward. Higher pressures increase the size and cost of the system. The output nozzle plays a role in stabilizing the beam but is not essential.

Figures 21-2a and 21-2b illustrate the result of a microjet cut across the apex of a human cornea. This is a cut without applanation—the so-called "free cut." Note that the beam cuts across the epithelium, then across the Bowman's layer, and then finally through the stroma. What is striking about the circumstances is although the beam traveled in a plane, the cut boundary was clearly not in the same plane. Unambiguously, the beam moved tissue laterally and found the path of least resistance to tissue separation. Hence, it cut along interfaces between layers rather than across layers until at the last instant the tissue resisted further displacement and then the beam cut across a layer. Clearly, the beam exerts transverse force on the tissue and moves it.

In Figure 21-3, the cornea is depicted as applanated

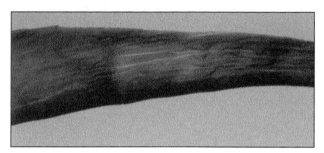

Figure 21-2a. A free cut.

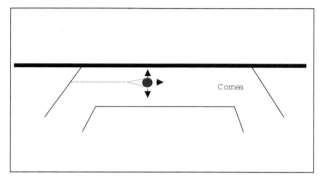

Figure 21-3. Origin of tissue separation forces.

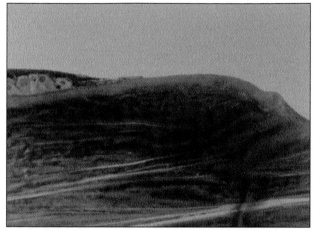

Figure 21-2b. Magnified view of the same cut.

during the cut. The direction of the microjet is right to left and it is scanning from left to right. The microjet is able to exert transverse forces on the tissue and cause separation. The origins of the transverse force are small-angle collisions of the high speed water with the tissue at the perimetric boundary of the beam. The water at the perimetric boundary is deflected to the trailing edge of the beam and this produces a reactive transverse force on the tissue. A detailed experimental study of beam forces during the cut has been carried out using an elegant experimental technique. It illustrates the loss in beam power as it cuts across the tissue (Gordon and Madden, personal communication, 1999). As a result of the collisions, the water breaks sections of intact lamella layers away from the stroma as demonstrated later. Hence, cutting is usually accompanied by ablation or erosion. Ablation never involves loss of partial thickness lamellar layers or keratocytes. The lamellar layers are carried away by the spent water.

By virtue of the applanation, internal hoop forces develop in the cornea and tend to push the cornea back to its normal position. Thus, there is a tendency for the cornea to move upward toward the microjet beam in the stromal bed beneath the beam. This enhances the rate of erosion. That tendency is not reflected in the flap region above the beam, which tends to move away from the beam. Thus the stromal bed experiences more erosion than the underside of the flap. The important conclusion

from this model is that the greater the scan speed of the microjet beam, the less time there is for erosion to occur and the smaller the amount of eroded tissue. Another important conclusion is that the greater the amount of applanation, the greater the rate of erosion. These two characteristics allow shaping merely by waterjet cutting, as noted next.

Figure 21-4 illustrates the stromal bed of a human cadaver cornea that has been cut with a microjet under the following conditions. The high scan rate reduces the erosion rate to a negligible value. One clearly sees the resulting step increase in the height of the cornea, about 60 μm in this case, at the center. The magnitude of the step increase diminishes toward the entrance and exit boundaries of the cut, reaching zero in the regions where the applanation is zero. There is also a mirror image of the step in the underside of the flap, except that the step increase is reduced by about half.

This is an elegant demonstration of the erosion and its dependence on scan rate and degree of applanation. It follows that producing a flap without erosion should be done at high scan rate and with the minimal amount of applanation. One minimizes the amount of applanation by using a flat vacuum applanator or template and extending the anterior surface so as to produce extension in the cornea rather than compression. This will be discussed in more detail later.

Figure 21-5 shows the stromal bed as viewed with SEM at a magnification of 1000x. It is clear that there are no cut lamellae and the keratocytes remain in their normal positions. Figure 21-6 is a high magnification TEM (transmission electron microscope) photo of the cornea cross-section. It is clear that tissue is removed one lamellar layer at a time. The lamellae are cut cleanly across, so that sections of lamellae are removed. In Figure 21-7, one sees the same type of removal with excimer laser

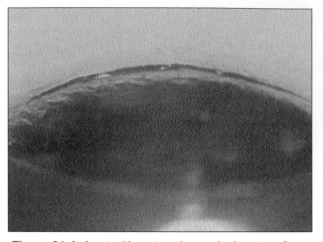

Figure 21-4. A cut with a step change in the rate of erosion.

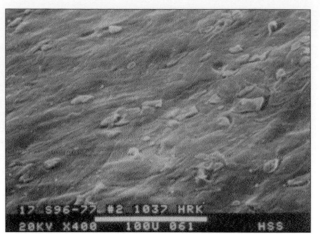

Figure 21-5. Scanning electron micrograph of the stromal bed with a microjet cut.

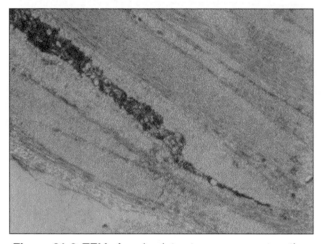

Figure 21-6. TEM of a microjet cut cornea cross-section.

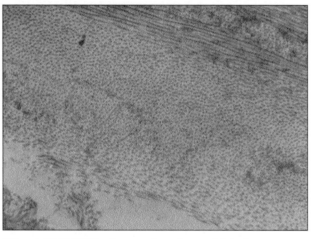

Figure 21-7. TEM of an excimer laser ablated cross-section.

ablation, except that the boundaries of the cut lamellae are fused and folded back producing a large solid mass of collagen. One also sees a change in the fibril spacing near the surface. This is a thermal effect not seen with microjet ablation. Both phenomena produce back-scattering of light (ie, haze).

The design of a scleral chuck for use in a microjet keratome is unexceptional (Figure 21-8). The goal is to achieve adequate holding and resistance to motion of the globe without increasing the IOP. Hence, one must avoid distortion of the globe. Typical base IOP values are about 25 mm Hg. The increase in IOP during the cut is about 10 mm Hg. An essential element of the scleral chuck is the beam block shown schematically in Figure 21-8. The edge of the beam block intercepts the microjet beam and directs it away from the cornea. Hence, the tissue in the shadow region of the beam block is not cut, leaving a hinge. Note that the geometry guarantees the position of the hinge relative to the boundary of the flap. The hinge is positioned superiorly. With the microjet cut there is never a short or long cut.

Figure 21-9 illustrates the geometry of the applanator. The key feature is the flat applanator consisting of contiguous spaces serving as micro vacuum channels. When the cornea is applanated against this surface, the total holding force is substantial, perhaps 500 gram weight. However, the cornea will readily peel away from the surface. The guard cylinder plays a vital role. It defines the circle of the cut with great precision and reproducibility, and guards against peeling by virtue of strong holding forces at the boundary. Notice in the figure that while the cornea is held flat against the applanator, the cornea is extended above its normal position. This virtually eliminates erosion around the boundary. It also sets the angle of the tissue at about 45° relative to the plane of the microjet scan. The overall effect is that the

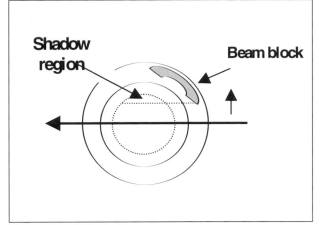

Figure 21-8. Scleral chuck with beam block.

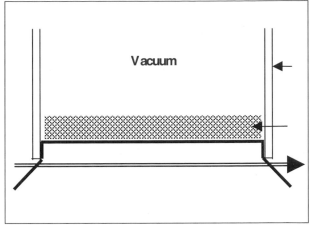

Figure 21-9. Schematic of an applanator configuration.

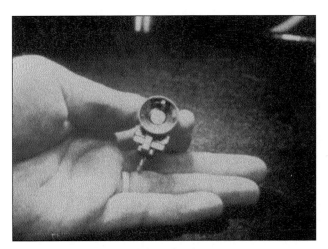

Figure 21-10. Photo of the microkeratome.

Figure 21-10 shows an experimental version of the microjet microkeratome.

SUMMARY

The important principles and elements of a microjet microkeratome have be described. The features of blade-based microkeratomes, which potentially reduce the capability of LASIK are eliminated by the new device. These improvements include accurate thickness control and uniformity of the flap, perfectly round flaps of a pre-scribed diameter, and flaps with a square edge. Hinge width is accurately controlled. The cut is made at normal IOP. The new device has the potential to make a major contribution to this growing field.

REFERENCES

1. Seiler T, Koufala K, Richter G. Iatrogenic keratasia after laser in situ keratomileusis. *Journal of Refractive Surgery.* 1998;14:312-317.
2. Rozakis GW. *Refractive Lamellar Keratoplasty.* Thorofare, NJ: SLACK Incorporated; 1998; 93-105.
3. Gorgon E, Parolini B, Abelson M. Principles and micro-scopic confirmation of surface quality of two new waterjet-based microkeratomes. *Journal of Refractive Surgery.* 1998;14:338-345.
4. Pallikaris IG, Siganos DS. *LASIK.* Thorofare, NJ: SLACK Incorporated; 1994; 27.

circular boundary of the flap is virtually perpendicular to its surface. It resembles a manhole cover. There is no taper. The shape of the flap is circular at precisely the diameter of the guard cylinder.

The vacuum applanator also holds the cornea firmly in position during the cut. Mechanical vibration and displacement of the anterior corneal surface are minimized. Thus, production of surface artifacts such as striations is controlled. The cut surface is remarkably clean.

Measured flap thickness is 157 ± 2 microns every-where on the flap, every time. The flap thickness is meas-ured with a Mitotoyu micrometer. The observed variation is partly the error range of the micrometer.

TREATMENT OF ASTIGMATISM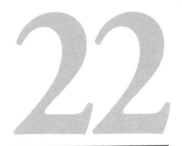

Stephen G. Slade, MD and John F. Doane, MD

TREATMENT OF ASTIGMATISM

Our understanding of astigmatism lags behind our facility's with myopia and even hyperopia. Moreover, with more accurate ways to treat spherical refractive errors, our patients are achieving better and better results. They are now expecting to see 20/20 without glasses. Any residual refractive error, even as low as 0.75 diopters (D) of astigmatism, can create a disappointed patient. This paradox of refractive surgery is that the better results we are now able to achieve create ever higher expectations from both the patient population and the provider. This means we must be able to address the millions of people worldwide, for example, that have astigmatism alone.

Whereas the treatment of spherical refractive errors, myopia, and hyperopia have progressed with our understanding the treatment of astigmatism has lagged behind. One can look at the many different treatments to correct astigmatism and, as with anterior chamber intraocular lenses (IOLs), realize that no one technique is perfect. Perhaps the key to treating astigmatism is realizing the diversity of the condition and understanding the resultant refractive error to be able to create and plan treatments specifically for each individual cornea. In this chapter, classification of astigmatism will be briefly covered, with the bulk of the material given to treatment. We will review the types of astigmatism, the available treatments, planning a treatment, technique, and results. Finally, we will try to evaluate where we may see improvements in the treatment of astigmatism (Figure 22-1).

ASTIGMATISM IN THE POPULATION

Patients with astigmatism cannot accommodate or "correct" for it as patients with hyperopia. They may complain of ghost images or even diplopia. Patients with with-the-rule astigmatism complain less, as most letters and objects in our environment are vertically elongated. The amount of astigmatism that is troublesome to a patient is variable but usually around 0.5 D. Spectacle lenses are poorly suited for astigmatism correction, as they may cause anisekonia, especially for newly corrected astigmatism patients. As refractive surgery can change the asphericity or "forgiveness" of the cornea, astigmatism may be better treated with surgery than spectacles.

THE EYE AS AN OPTICAL SYSTEM

The form of the normal cornea can be described by saying that there is a central optical zone where the curvature is approximately spherical and which extends horizontally about 4.0 mm, and somewhat less than this vertically and is decentered outward and usually also a little downward: and that the peripheral parts are considerably flattened, decidedly more so on the nasal side than the temporal and usually more so upward than downward. —Helmholtz 1896

Astigmatism is best understood from the optics of the cornea and then through the different ways we can treat the problem. In this section we will review the pathology of astigmatism, the eye as an optical system, look at the various ways of treating it with the excimer laser, and then present specific techniques and rationale for planning actual treatments.

We have known about the aspherical nature of the cornea for well over 100 years. In the "spherical" asphere the cornea has a constancy of curve so that there are no meridians of differing curvature. In the spherical emmetropic patient the converging power of the cornea is matched with the need to focus parallel rays that strike the cornea to the retina.

Astigmatism can be described as the two major axes of curvature over this asphere, 90° apart. This is regular astigmatism, and the two major axes on the cornea can be corrected by spectacles to give 20/20 best-corrected vision. Regular astigmatism can also be treated with various techniques, including conventional excimer laser ablative patterns used as part of photorefractive keratoplasty and LASIK.

Astigmatism must be properly diagnosed before treatment. Any irregular astigmatism must be identified. Irregular astigmatism can be best diagnosed by hard contact lenses or viewing the rings of a photokeratoscope or the mires of a manual keratometer for distortion or irregularity. If a patient sees better with a hard contact lens than with spectacles irregular astigmatism must be suspected. Transmissive defects or opacities must also be ruled out as a cause of lost best-corrected visual acuity.

Irregular astigmatism can be "regular irregular" or "irregular irregular." Regular irregular astigmatism means there are prime meridians of curvature, but they are not 90° apart (sometimes called nonorthogonal) or they are asymmetrical in power across the visual axis. Irregular irregular astigmatism is nonmeasurable fluctuations to the surface so that no spectacle lens can compensate. Astigmatism that fits within these definitions can be treated and diagnosed by a hard contact lens. The conventional broadbeam laser treatments we have for astigmatism are spherical or symmetrical and therefore cannot eliminate irregular astigmatism (Figure 22-2a through 22-2e).

Simple Hyperopic Astigmatism

Here, the meridian of maximum power is emmetropic; therefore, it forms a line image of a point on the retina. If that meridian is at 90°, the astigmatism is with-the-rule and the line focused on the retinal is horizontal. The meridian of minimum power is hyperopic. It will form a vertical line image behind the retina. The interval of Sturm extends from the retina to beyond it. Spectacle correction would be with a plus-cylinder lens.

Compound Hyperopic Astigmatism

Here, both maximum and minimum axes are reflectively hyperopic and focus beyond the retina. One axis is beyond the other. In the figure, with-the-rule astigmatism is demonstrated. A plus cylinder spectacle lens combined with a plus sphere is needed.

Simple Myopic Astigmatism

With simple myopic astigmatism, the eye is emmetropic in one meridian. A far point is imaged on the

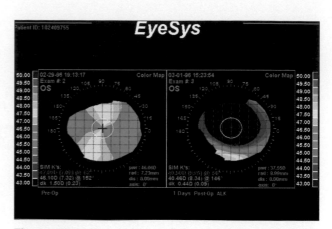

Figure 22-1. Pre and post (left and right respectively) topographies of corneal astigmatism treated with excimer laser ablation.

retina by this meridian and in the vitreous by the other major meridian, 90° opposite. A minus cylinder lens is used to correct this condition.

Compound Myopic Astigmatism

Both meridians of the cornea are too strong and focus in the vitreous. In the figure the axis at 90° is even stronger than the one at 180°, with-the-rule. A minus cylinder lens, along with a minus spectacle lens, is needed.

Mixed Astigmatism

Here there is a hyperopic and myopic component. One line is focused in the vitreous and the other is beyond the retina.

Irregular Astigmatism

When the astigmatism can be measured but the axes are not 90° apart, the astigmatism is regular irregular, or nonorthogonal. Irregular astigmatism can occur as a result of trauma, keratoconus, corneal disease, or be congenital. This type of astigmatism can also be shown on corneal topography when one half of the bow tie is larger than the other. This is asymmetrical astigmatism. These types of astigmatism are not optimally corrected by spectacle lenses because the eye does not always look through the same point on the lens as it moves. A rigid contact lens or refractive surgery is potentially a better choice. In asymmetrical astigmatism, a symmetrical treatment can leave a central peninsula (Figures 22-3a and 22-3b). An asymmetrical design of operation is needed.

THEORY OF TREATMENT

One can compare regular astigmatism with a toric

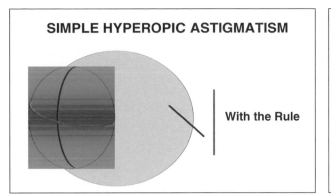

Figure 22-2a. The vertical meridian of the cornea is the steepest (of maximum power) and focuses on the retina. The flatter horizontal meridian is hyperopic and focuses behind the retina.

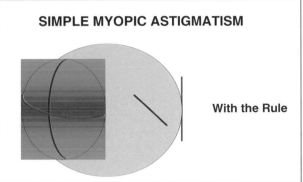

Figure 22-2b. The vertical meridian of the cornea is the steepest (of maximum power) and focuses a horizontal line in front of the retina. The flatter horizontal meridian is emmetropic and focuses on the retina.

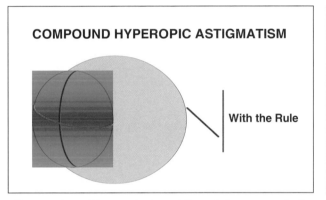

Figure 22-2c. The vertical meridian of the cornea is the steepest and focuses a horizontal line in back of the retina. The flatter horizontal meridian is more hyperopic and focuses further beyond the retina.

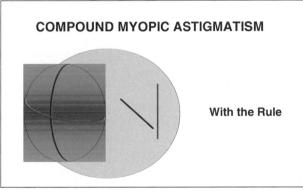

Figure 22-2d. The vertical meridian of the cornea is steepest (of maximum power) and so focuses a horizontal line in front of the retina. The flatter horizontal meridian is still steep and also focuses in front of the retina.

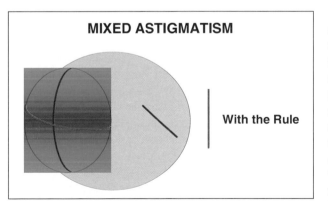

Figure 22-2e. The vertical meridian of the cornea is the steepest (of maximum power) and focuses a horizontal line in front of the retina. The flatter horizontal meridian is too flat and focuses behind the retina.

shape to that of the back of a spoon with one axis steeper than the opposite axis. The goal of treatment is to even up the axis, collapse the differing focal lines in the eye, and bring focus to the retina. One way this may be accomplished is by flattening the steep axis. This is the traditional approach of astigmatic keratotomy—cuts on the steep axis flatten the meridian and move the focal line away from the cornea as the converging power of the meridian is reduced. Lasers have accomplished this with moving blades and scanning spots by removing more tissue across a central band aligned along the meridian and then progressively less tissue as the band widens perpendicularly from the meridian (Figures 22-4a and 22-4b). This flattens the steep meridian. This flattening moves the most forward-focused axis back toward the retina. The overall effect on refraction is flattening or inducement of hyperopia. Obviously this would not be desirable in a patient with pre-existing hyperopia. If a patient with hyperopic astigmatism was treated with this negative cylinder approach, moving one axis backward first to collapse the focal lines, then one must move both lines, including the one that was just moved back, forward to focus the pair on the retina. This is a redundant ablation.

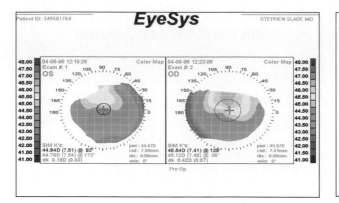

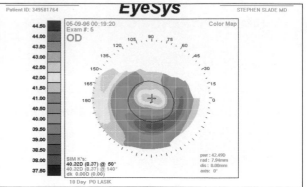

Figure 22-3a. Right and left eyes preoperatively. Note areas of congenital superior asymmetric astigmatism.

Figure 22-3b. Right eye after symmetrical superior laser ablation. Note remaining pensile of untreated cornea in the area of preoperative superior asymmetric astigmatism.

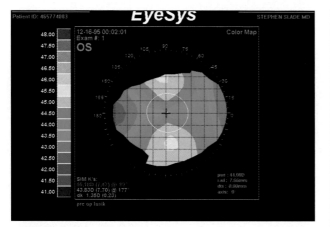

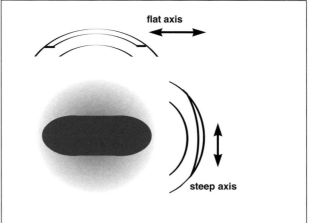

Figure 22-4a. Topography of with-the-rule astigmatism (steep at 90° meridian).

Figure 22-4b. Correction of astigmatism. The steeper axis is flattened, and the flatter axis is unchanged.

Alternatively, the rear focus line can be brought forward via steepening the flat axis by removing more tissue from the mid periphery like the ablation for hyperopia. This is especially advantageous in hyperopic astigmatism as only steepening or rearward movement of the focus lines occur and no redundant ablation is necessary.

In clinical practice, we have therefore learned that the most predictable way to treat a specific astigmatic correction is to remove the least amount of tissue by using the cylinder technique that is most direct and avoids redundancy. For compound myopic astigmatism, this is the minus cylinder format because we will first flatten the steep meridian to create a spherical surface, which will then be flattened to the desired flatter spherical corneal power. In compound hyperopic astigmatism, we have found it most advantageous to use the plus cylinder ablation format (as noted above) to first steepen the flat meridian, creating a spherical surface that will then be steepened to the desired higher spherical corneal power.

Mixed astigmatism allows for three possible treatment plans: minus cylinder format, plus cylinder format, or crossed cylinder format. Again, the option that removes the least amount of tissue is likely to be the most predictable format to create the desired refraction and visual outcome. As it turns out, the crossed cylinder format removes the least tissue in mixed astigmatism treatments and is likely to be the best option. In crossed cylinder format, the myopic focal plane in front of the retina is moved rearward toward the retina with the minus cylinder ablation, and the hyperopic focal plane is move frontward toward the retina with plus cylinder ablation. No spherical (myopic or hyperopic) ablation is required. On average a plus cylinder ablation of mixed astigmatism requires three times, and a minus cylinder ablation requires two times, as much time as a crossed cylinder ablation for a given refraction. Additionally, the overall depth of ablation for the major and minor meridians is greatest for the plus cylinder ablation, intermediate for

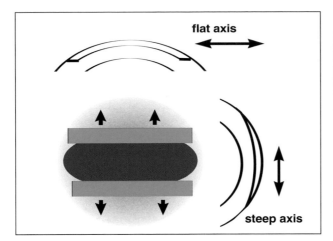

Figure 22-5. The blades move apart as the ablation is laid down to allow more treatment to be applied to the central horizontal meridian.

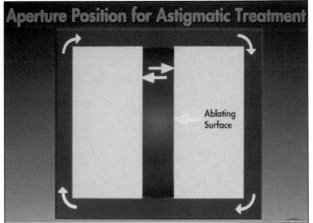

Figure 22-6. VISX Star Parallel Plates for Astigmatic Treatment.

the minus cylinder ablation, and least for the crossed cylinder ablation.

Coupling

While the main purpose of the ablation is to alter the treated meridian, usually the steep axis, the effect on the opposite meridian must be known. With keratotomy incisions over a steep axis, the opposite axis is steepened as the steep axis is flattened. This secondary effect changes the spherical component and is termed "coupling." Excimer ablations that are asymmetrical over the steep axis do not, in theory, affect the flat meridian. Tissue is removed, but in a similar depth across the axis. Theoretically, the radius of curvature is reduced as the axis is "lowered" toward the retina and is then actually minutely steeper.

METHODS OF EXCIMER AND NONEXCIMER TREATMENT OF ASTIGMATISM

Excimer Astigmatism Treatment

There are several conventional ways of applying an excimer treatment to the cornea to treat astigmatism. All incorporate a typically symmetrical beam and achieve a graded treatment by masking or covering portions of the beam in some way. Because of this starting point in design, they are not designed to treat astigmatism that varies in magnitude across the visual axis or where the axes are not perpendicular to one another. However, the majority of astigmatism can be treated with good results using these techniques.

Opening Blades

The most conventional way to treat astigmatism is to flatten the flat axis by layering bands of ablation across the axis with opening blades. The central band of tissue that is aligned along the initial slit receives all the treatment, and the treatment diminishes as the blades open. This is a symmetrical ablation and, in theory, does not affect the opposite meridian.

Mask

The idea of patterning an ablation onto the stromal surface is used in the Summit Technology mask system for treating astigmatism. The mask is made of a material with a known ablation rate, which is shaped to deliver a graded ablation to the cornea with the "steeper" area of the corneal surface receiving more treatment to flatten that area. The mask is thinner over such areas and melts away, while the flatter areas are still protected from ablation by the thicker portions of the mask. The mask must be ordered for each patient, as it is the reverse image of the individual patient's refraction. Initial results with an early hand-held variety have been surpassed with a new system that is mounted in the optical pathway of the laser itself.

Rotating Circle

Another way to deliver a graded ablation is by a rotating circular diaphragm. An oval ablation, delivered through a nonmoving mask, does not necessarily affect the astigmatism. However, if the mask rotates, the effect is very much like a set of blades. Such a mask is also capable of performing the diaphragm's function at the same time (Figure 22-7).

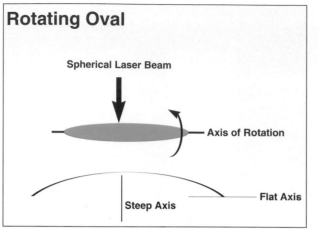

Figure 22-7. The oval aperture is aligned with the long dimension in the axis of the flat meridian. The oval is then rotated as the ablation is performed so the steep axis is flattened and the flat axis is unaffected.

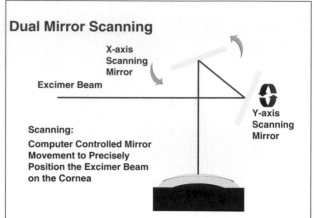

Figure 22-8. Dual mirror scanning allows computer-controlled mirror movement to precisely position the excimer beam on the cornea.

Scanning Variable Diameter Spots

Early scanning lasers have used variable diameter spots to treat astigmatism. The Technolas 116 laser is an example. The beam in a scanning laser is directed to two scanning mirrors that control and turn the beam toward the cornea. The mirrors are connected to servo-mechanisms and are controlled by the computer. Various files are written and available for each combination of spherical error and astigmatism. The ablation is started with a small diameter spot scanning along the flat axis. After one or more passes have been laid down, the spot increases in diameter and continues. This process allows more treatment to be placed along the strip of cornea that is perpendicular to the steep axis with a tapered, graded pattern extending out along the steep axis. Looking along the steep axis, more treatment is placed centrally than peripherally as in myopia and the axis is flattened. In theory the flat meridian is only reduced to a smaller concentric circle and actually steepened a minute amount as it moves to a very slightly smaller radius of curvature (Figures 22-8 and 22-9).

PlanoScan

More advanced scanning lasers use a fixed diameter spot to rapidly pattern the cornea as determined by the computer. The beam is directed to "hit" the steep areas more and avoid the flat areas to reshape the myopic astigmatic patient, for example. These lasers, such as the Technolas PlanoScan must use a higher rate of fire as each shot removes less tissue than a large diameter beam. In myopia treatment, the rate of fire must be around four times that of a broadbeam laser to take the same amount of total ablation time. The length of time of the ablation is important, as irregular drying during a prolonged abla-

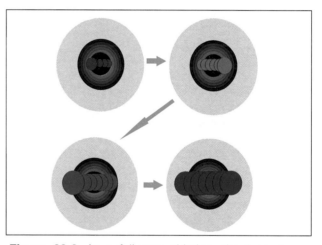

Figure 22-9. In a full-area ablation, the laser beam moves along the axes of the astigmatism with increasing beam diameter.

tion can result in an irregular ablation. Advanced laser with ceramic tubes capable of firing 50 or more times a second are used.

There are several advantages with such scanning lasers. The beam is blended and overlaid many times and does not have to be of the same high quality as a broadbeam. Therefore, the optical system may be made simpler and with fewer lenses. Because the beam does not require as much power, the laser itself can be smaller. The chance of central islands is minimal, as clearance of the ablated material from the smaller spot pattern is easier.

A main advantage, in regard to astigmatism, is the ability to steepen as well as flatten an axis. The cornea can be addressed in positive as well as negative cylinder. This is particularly useful with hyperopic patients with

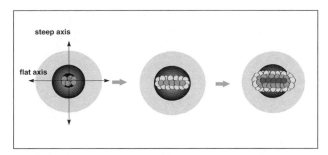

Figure 22-10. Excimer laser correction of myopic astigmatism.

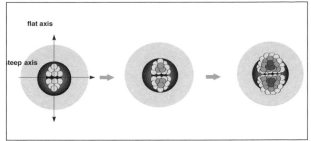

Figure 22-11. Excimer laser correction of hyperopic astigmatism. The laser beam moves over the cornea and steepens the flat axis.

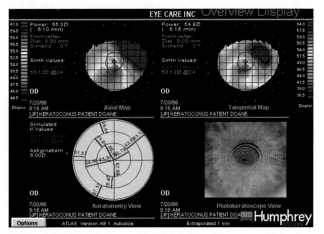

Figure 22-12. Topography of keratoconus eye. Note the inferior steepening and irregularity of the mires on photokeratoscopy (lower right).

astigmatism. All axes can be steepened, rather than flattening the steep axis then steeping the entire cornea, as would be done in minus cylinder ablations (Figures 22-10 and 22-11).

NONEXCIMER LASER METHODS OF ASTIGMATISM TREATMENT

Keratotomy

Keratectomies work in a different way from excimer ablations for astigmatism. Any incision flattens the cornea immediately adjacent to it and at the meridian that is perpendicular to the cut itself. The other meridian, unlike an excimer ablation, is also affected. While the steep axis perpendicular to the cuts is flattened, the flat meridian is slightly steepened. This is the coupling effect. In a patient with a hyperopic opposite meridian, this is obviously beneficial. An example would be a patient with +1.00 -3.00 at 180°. This patient could be treated effectively with astigmatic keratectomy since the coupling principle would correct the 1 D of hyperopia.

Holmium Laser

As in small degrees of spherical error, holmium laser keratoplasty can be useful in treating astigmatism. There will be an initial overcorrection, but the ease of surgery and rapid functional recovery are attractive for lower ranges of astigmatism.

TREATMENT PLANS FOR ASTIGMATISM

Designing a treatment for astigmatism has most elements of any refractive surgery, along with a few specific choices due to the specific shape of the cornea.

Patient Examination

In general, follow good practice with patient education and informed consent to create realistic expectations. Currently, results are not as good with astigmatism as with spherical errors, and the patient should be aware of the expected outcome. Specific corneal pathology often found in these patients (such as keratoconus) must be identified (Figure 22-12). Make sure the identified astigmatism is corneal. Correlate the refractive astigmatism cylinder with the topographical astigmatism. Lasers can only treat corneal astigmatism. Treating the cornea for lenticular astigmatism or residual ocular (noncorneal astigmatism) by ablating a crossed cylinder on the cornea may make the patient's condition worse, especially when he or she develops a cataract and the lenticular component of the astigmatism is removed.

Measuring

The treatment plan for astigmatism will differ depending on the type of astigmatism. Topographical mapping, keratometry, and refraction are all important and must be considered. A patient in contact lenses must discontinue wear long enough for any corneal warpage and induced astigmatism to settle to the baseline. For long-term wearers of rigid lenses, this may take weeks or even months until repeat stable readings are obtained. Figure 22-13 is an example of postoperative irregular astigmatism due to flap striae after LASIK. Note the irregular mires on photokeratoscopy in the lower right-hand corner of the display.

SURGICAL TREATMENT OF ASTIGMATISM

Check and recheck the refraction. Correlate it to the keratometry. Make sure it is stable. Have the patient out of glasses or contacts until stable readings are acquired. This may take weeks or even months in long-term contact lenses wearers. Identify the component of decreased vision in the patient by a cylinder-only refraction. If the sphere is only sufficient, consider leaving the astigmatism untreated.

Determine a surgical plan. In general, plan to slightly overcorrect against-the-rule astigmatism (steep at 90°), and undercorrect with-the-rule corneal astigmatism. Patients with with-the-rule astigmatism often have a better range and depth of vision than spherical patients. Also, make sure the fellow eye consider the fellow eye. If the fellow eye has astigmatism, especially oblique astigmatism that the patient likes and you do not plan to treat, consider leaving matching oblique astigmatism untreated.

Surgical Steps for Excimer Astigmatic Ablation

The keratectomy is made in the usual LASIK fashion but with regard to the axis of astigmatism. With most patients' with-the-rule astigmatism, a flap placed in the superior position, as suggested by Buratto, is best. Otherwise, be sure to decenter the flap enough nasally to allow for the treatment.

The ablation is carried out, being careful to protect the underside of the flap from ablation in large-dimension scanning techniques. Also the accumulation of fluid during the ablation must be monitored to avoid irregular build-ups that could mask parts of the bed and cause irregular ablations. The axis of the cylinder should be verified with a mark during the ablation as described below.

Replace the flap as usual, then the remainder of the case is carried out in the standard fashion. If an epithelial abrasion results from the mark, the patient should be warned of a higher likelihood of pain for the first few hours postoperatively.

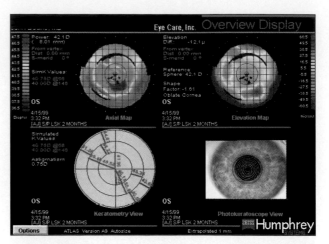

Figure 22-13. An example of postoperative irregular astigmatism due to flap striae after LASIK. Note the irregular mires on photokeratoscopy in the lower righthand corner.

Surgical Steps for Keratotomy Combined With Excimer

1. Mark the axis. This may be done at the slit lamp immediately prior to surgery or in the operating room. The surgeon may use a landmark, such as a scleral vessel or pterygium. Be careful about using iris landmarks, as they may be difficult to see through the bed of a LASIK keratectomy. Also, small vessels may be obscured by the edema of the suction ring or hyperemia. I prefer to place a reference mark on the patient's eye just prior to the patient lying down. Place a drop of topical anesthetic in the eye and instruct the patient to look at a distant point. Avoid letting the patient fixate at a near object, possibly inducing accommodative esotropia. Use a surgical felt tip marker to place one small dot at 6 o'clock at the limbus. Try to avoid disrupting the corneal epithelium. Use this mark during the ablation by aligning it with the microscope reticule.

2. Perform the ablation in the usual fashion first, before the t-cuts. Measuring the pachymetry of the cornea and doing the keratotomy can indent the cornea and create an irregular surface that could produce irregular astigmatism if ablated.

3. Preset the depth of the diamond knife to the preoperative thickness minus 160 microns. After the ablation, recheck the depth directly at the site of the planned keratotomy. Adjust the knife for any difference. Always place the arcuate keratotomy at 7.0 mm. Any closer will increase the effect but can induce irregular astigmatism.

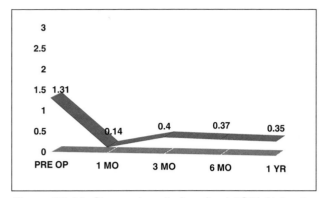

Figure 22-14. Change in cylinder after LASIK. Note stabilization by 3 months.

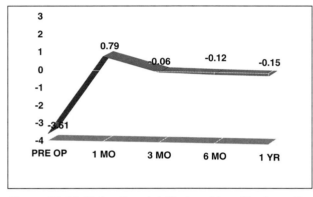

Figure 22-16. Refractive stability is achieved by 3 months with LASIK.

4. Replace the flap.
5. Alternatively, the surgeon may wait until after the operation to see if the astigmatism has changed. This is a good idea if the amount of astigmatism is small. The ablation itself can induce or alter the pre-existing astigmatism. If the cuts are made within a few months, place them outside of the flap at an 8.0-mm zone or greater depending on the diameter of the flap. If 4 or more months have passed, the flap can usually be safely cut, in which case keratotomies at 7.0 mm should be performed.

LASIK ASTIGMATISM RESULTS

The efficacy of using variable spot scanning to treat astigmatism associated with myopia is shown in the Ruiz/Slade study. Here 171 eyes in 88 patients were treated. The group with astigmatism consisted of 91 eyes. The range of astigmatism was 0.00 D to 8.00 D pre-operatively. At 1-year follow-up, the mean astigmatism was reduced from 1.31 to .35 D (Figure 22-14). Ninty-four percent of the eyes saw 20/40 or better uncorrected,

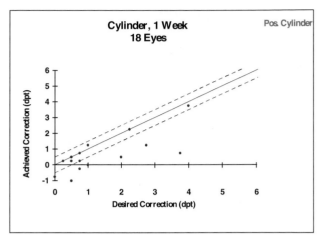

Figure 22-15. Scattergram of hyperopic astigmatic results. Moderate undercorrection noted at all levels of treatment.

and 65% saw 20/20 or better uncorrected. Only two patients lost two lines of best-corrected vision.

Early results with PlanoScan for astigmatism associated with hyperopic patients are shown in the Arbelaez study (Figure 22-15). Here, 1-month results are given on 18 eyes. The scattergram shows moderate undercorrection across the entire range up to 4 D of attempted correction. This method, although in evolution, seems to hold promise for astigmatism, especially hyperopic astigmatism.

RETREATMENTS

Retreatments should be timed to allow for accurate corneal stability. Long-term LASIK results have shown the operation to be reasonably stable at 3 months. Figure 22-16 shows this finding from the Ruiz/Slade LASIK study. With large undercorrections, the flap may be lifted earlier and the stroma ablated. In most cases, a recut flap after 4 months is preferable as a smoother surface is created and the risk of epithelial ingrowth is reduced.

FUTURE ASTIGMATISM TREATMENTS: TOPOGRAPHICAL AND WAVEFRONT ANALYSIS-ASSISTED LASERS

Our treatment of astigmatism has lagged behind our treatment of more easily addressed spherical errors. The many different methods, while helpful to the clinician, point out the need for one proven superior technique.

The future of laser astigmatism correction is almost completely dependent on further increasing sophistica-

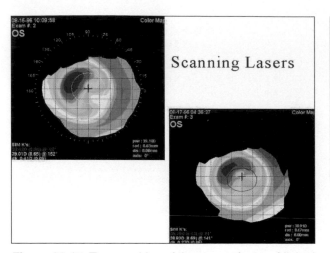

Figure 22-17. Topographies of the two surfaces of linked ablation.

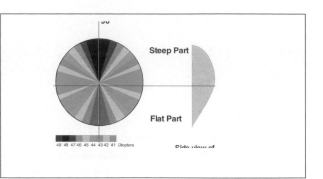

Figure 22-18a. Irregular astigmatism. Preoperative topography of a with-the-rule negative astigmatism at 180°.

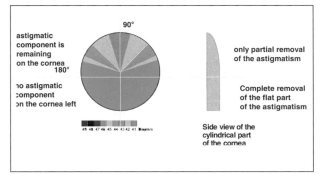

Figure 22-18b. Irregular astigmatism without topographic assistance. Postoperative topography after a normal astigmatic treatment. There is a remaining part of the astigmatism on the steep half that could not be removed with a normal regular astigmatic treatment.

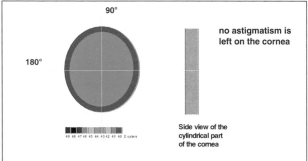
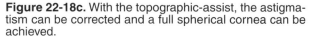

Figure 22-18c. With the topographic-assist, the astigmatism can be corrected and a full spherical cornea can be achieved.

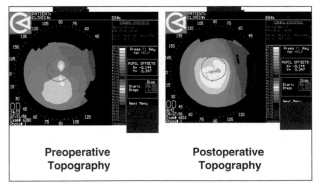

Figure 22-19. Pre- and postoperative topographies of customized treatment of an irregular astigmatism.

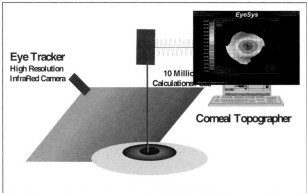

Figure 22-20. Diagram illustrating a topographically driven LASIK procedure.

tion of laser design and ways to measure the cornea. Then, these two components must be linked together so that the laser is directed in its ablation to whatever is presented to it by the topographer, or wavefront analysis. The laser should be capable of producing any ablation pattern without the current symmetrical bias created by circular diaphragm-controlled broadbeam lasers. Intuitively, it would seem the most desirable combination would be a real-time feedback loop between the laser and the device that measures the progress of the ablation and directs the laser. With further meditation of this idea, LASIK may not be the appropriate solution. The reason for this comment is that on creating a lamellar flap, there will be minute irregularities of the stromal bed created by the microkeratome that any analyzing system may try to "smooth out" in addition to the pre-existing asymmetries of the cornea. On repositing the flap, the under surface will have minute irregularities from the microkeratome that have not been "smoothed" by the laser ablation. As it is without active linking, the two surfaces fit back together like a jigsaw puzzle, (ie, the elevation of one surface fits into a depression on the other). With linked ablations, the two surfaces may be less compatible when placed back together and lead to a less desirable visual effect Figure 22-17).

The linking of corneal and ocular analysis (wavefront analysis) to guide laser ablation is under frenzied investigation. These lasers would have the ability to treat irregular astigmatism, as well as offer the most efficient system for regular astigmatism. The current process involves obtaining two distinct sets of information. The first involves a static picture of the cornea via corneal topography. This can include analysis of the anterior and posterior corneal surfaces, as with the Orbscan system. In addition, wavefront analysis is completed for the ocular system in which the path of light from the anterior corneal surface to the retina is evaluated. The data from wavefront analysis is used to create the best optical image on the macula. The future ablation process will include a formula combining data from both the corneal analysis and the wavefront analysis to direct the laser ablation to produce the best corneal optic for maximizing visual function (Figures 22-18a through 22-18c).

The promise of these more accurate lasers driven exactly to the shape of the target eye should have the flexibility to provide one best system for all astigmatic errors (Figures 22-19 and 22-20).

BIBLIOGRAPHY

Arenas-Archila E, Sanchez-Thorin JC, Naranjo-Uribe JP, Hernandez-Lozano A. Myopic keratomileusis in situ: a preliminary report. *J Cataract Refract Surg.* 1991;17:424-35.

Arrowsmith PN, Sanders DR, Marks RG. Visual, refractive and keratometric results of radial keratotomy. *Arch Ophthalmol.* 1983;101:873-81.

Barraquer C, Guitierrez A, Espinoza A. Myopic keratomileusis: short-term results. *J Refract Corneal Surg.* 1989;5:307-13.

Barraquer JI. Keratomileusis. *Int Surg.* 1967;48:103-117.

Barraquer JI. Method for cutting lamellar grafts in frozen corneas: New orientations for refractive surgery. *Arch Soc Am Ophthalmol.* 1958;1:237.

Barraquer JI. Oueratoplastia refractiva. *Estudios Inform Oftal Inst Barraquer.* 1949;10:2-21.

Barraquer JI. Results of myopic keratomileusis. *Journal of Refractive Surgery.* 1987;3:98-101.

Bores L. Lamellar refractive surgery. In: Bores L., ed. *Refractive Eye Surgery.* Boston, Mass: Blackwell Scientific Publications; 1993.

Brint SF, Ostrick DM, Fisher C, Slade SG, et al. Six-month results of the multicenter phase I study of excimer laser myopic keratomileusis. *J Cataract Refract Surg.* 1994;20;610-5.

Buratto L, Ferrari M, Genisi C. Myopic keratomileusis with the excimer laser: 1-year follow-up. *J Refract Corneal Surg.* 1993;9:12-19.

Carson CA, Taylor HR. Melbourne excimer laser and research group. *Arch Ophthalmol.* 1995;113:431-6.

DelPero RA, Gigstad JE, Roberts AD, et al. A refractive and histopathological study of excimer laser keratectomy in primates. *Am J Ophthalmol.* 1990;109:419-29.

Ditzen K, Anschuetz T, Shroeder E. Photorefractive keratectomy to treat low, medium and high myopia: a multicenter study. *J Cataract Refract Surg.* 1994;20(suppl):234-8.

Dougherty PJ, Wellish KL, Maloney RK. Excimer laser ablation rate and corneal hydration. *Am J Ophthalmol.* 1994;118:169-76.

Duane TD. *Clinical Ophthalmology.* Volume 1. Hagerstown. Md: Harper and Row; 1979.

Epstein D, Fagerholm P, Hamberg-Nystrom H, Tengroth B. Twenty-four-month follow-up of excimer laser photorefractive keratectomy for myopia. *Ophthalmology.* 1994;101:1558-64.

Fagerholm P, Hamberg-Nystrom H, Tengroth B. Wound healing and myopic regression following photorefractive keratectomy. *ACTA Ophthalmologica.* 1994;72:229-34.

Gartry DS, Kerr Muir MG, Marshall J. Excimer laser photorefractive keratectomy: 18 month follow-up. *Ophthalmology.* 1991;99:1209-19.

Heitzmann J, Binder PS, Kassar BS, Nordan LT. The correction of high myopia using the excimer laser. *Arch Ophthalmol.* 1993;111:1627-34.

Kaufman HE. The correction of aphakia. *Am J Ophthalmol.* 1980;89:1-10.

Krwawicz T. Lamellar corneal stromectomy. *Am J Ophthalmol.* 1964;57:828-33.

Liu JC, McDonald MB, Varnell R, Andrade HA. Myopic excimer laser photorefractive keratectomy: an analysis of clinical correlations. *J Refract Corneal Surg.* 1990;6:321-8.

Littman H. Optic of Barraquer's keratomileusis. *Arch Oftal Optom.* 1966;6:1.

Lohmann CP, Fitzke F, O'Bart D, et al. Corneal light scattering and visual performance in myopic individuals with spectacles, contact lenses, or excimer laser photorefractive keratectomy. *Am J Ophthalmol.* 1993;115:444-53.

Maguire LJ, Klyce SD, Sawelson H, et al. Visual distortion after myopic keratomileusis: computer analysis of keratoscope photographs. *Ophthalmic Surg.* 1987;18:352-6.

Marshall J, Trokel SL, Rothery S, et al. Long term healing of the central cornea after photorefractive keratectomy using an excimer laser. Ophthalmology. 1988;95:1411-21.

Nordan LT. Keratomileusis. *Int Ophthalmol Clin.* 1991;31:7-12.

Nordan LT, Fallor MK. Myopic keratomileusis: 74 consecutive nonamblyopic case with 1-year of follow-up. *Journal of Refractive Surgery.* 1986;2:124-128.

Pureskin N. Weakening ocular refraction by means of partial stromectomy of cornea under experimental conditions. *Vestnik Oftalmologii.* 1967;80:19-24.

Ruiz LA, Slade SG, Updegraff SA, Doane JF, Moreno ML, Murcia A. A single center study to evaluate the efficacy, safety and stability of laser in situ keratomileusis for low, moderate, and high myopia with and without astigmatism. In preparation.

Salah T, Waring GO, El-Maghraby A. Excimer laser keratomileusis in the corneal bed under a hinged flap: results in Saudi Arabia at the El-Maghraby Eye Hospital. In: Salz JJ, McDonnel PJ, McDonald MB, eds. *Corneal Laser Surgery.* St. Louis, Mo: Mosby-Year Book; 1995.

Seiler T, Derse M, Pham T. Repeated excimer laser treatment after photorefractive keratectomy. *Arch Ophthalmol.* 1992;110:1230-3.

Seiler T, Holschbach A, Derse M, et al. Complications of myopic photorefractive keratectomy with the excimer laser. *Ophthalmology.* 1994;101:153-60.

Seiler T, Kahle G, Kriegerowski M. Excimer Laser (193 nm) myopic keratomileusis in sighted and blind human eyes. *J Refract Corneal Surg.* 1990;6:165-73.

Seiler T, Wollensak J. Myopic photorefractive keratectomy with the excimer laser. One-year follow-up. *Ophthalmology.* 1991;98:1156-63.

Serdarevic O, Vinciguerra P, Bottoni F, Zenoni S, DeMolfetta V. Excimer laser photorefractive keratectomy for high myopia. ARVO Abstracts. *Invest Ophthalmol Vis Sci.* 1992;33(4suppl):763.

Sher NA, Barak M, Daya S, et al. Excimer laser photorefractive keratectomy in high myopia. *Arch Ophthalmol.* 1992;110:935-43.

Sher NA, Hardten DR, Fundingsland B, et al. 193 nm excimer photorefractive keratectomy in high myopia. *Ophthalmology.* 1994;101:1575-82.

Slade SG, Doane JF, Dishler JG, et al. A prospective multicenter clinical trial to evaluate automated lamellar keratoplasty (ALK) for the correction of myopia. In preparation.

Swinger CA, Barker BA. Prospective evaluation of myopic keratomileusis. *Ophthalmology.* 1984;91:785-792.

Tuft SJ, Zabel RW, Marshall J. Corneal repair following keratectomy. *Invest Ophthalmol Vis Sci.* 1989;30:1769-77.

Correction of Astigmatism with a Cross Cylinder Ablation

Paolo Vinciguerra, MD

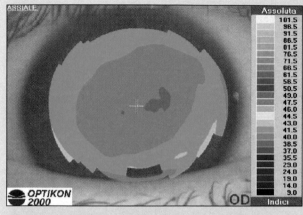

Figure 22A-1. Postoperative topography shape of a +1 -3 cyl. Note the persistence of a postoperative prolate shape instead of the commonly seen oblate postoperative pattern.

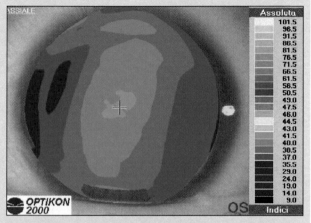

Figure 22A-2. A -5 -2 cylinder. No remaining astigmatism was found.

Regression, corneal haze, and functional symptoms often complicate the excimer laser correction of astigmatism. One of the main causes of these complications is poor transition to the nonablated peripheral cornea induced by most of the commonly used ablation strategies.

A new ablation strategy, combining ablation along the steep and flat meridian to correct astigmatism with the excimer laser, may allow the avoidance of these complications and be more effective in avoiding these complications. In fact, regular astigmatism is characterized by two main orthogonal meridians (the flattest and the steepest) and by countless intermediate meridians with increasing curvature from one to the other.

The common ablation strategies allow a perfect correction only along the main meridian, while the oblique meridians are overcorrected; this induces an irregular "four-leaf" astigmatism.

The ablation strategy used is the following:

1. Ablation of half the power of the cylinder along the steepest meridian with a 5.5 mm optical zone size and 3.5 mm transition zone size.
2. Ablation of the remaining cylinder along the flattest meridian with optical zone size from 5.5 mm to 6.5 mm, depending on the dioptric correction, and a transition zone size of 2.0 mm.
3. Correction of the entire spherical equivalent with a 5.5 mm to 6.5 mm optical zone and a 1.5 mm transition zone.
4. At the end of the refractive ablation steps, PTK-

style smoothing is performed with 9.0 mm of optical zone, 10 Hz frequency, applying masking fluid on the cornea.

Examples of cross-cylinder ablation:

Preoperative refraction: -3.00 D = -6.00 D/180°. Ablation steps.

1. +3.00 D/90°
2. -3.00 D/180°
3. -6.00 D (SE)

Preoperative refraction: +2.00 D = -5.00 D/165°. Ablation strategy:

1. +2.50 D/75°
2. -2.50 D/165°
3. -0.50 (SE)

Preoperative refraction: +4.00D = -8.00D/90°. Ablation steps: 1. +4.00 D/180°; 2.-4.00 D/90°; 3. None

The first results of this technique are very promising: we treated 33 eyes of 22 patients, with the following preoperative refraction data: mean sphere -2.5 ± 4.9 D (-12 to 3.5 D); mean cylinder -3.2 ± 1.3 D (-1.3 to -6 D); mean spherical equivalent of -4.1 ± 4.8 D (-12 to 1.5 D).

The 33 PRK procedures were performed using a Nidek EC 5000. Mean spectacle-corrected visual acuity improved from 0.75 ± 0.22 to 0.86 ± 0.13 at 6 months (p = 0.001); no eyes lost two or more lines of BSCVA at the end of follow-up, and only two eyes (9.1%) lost one line. On the contrary, seven eyes gained two or three lines of BSCVA (31.8%) and four gained one line (18.2%).

The refractive data at the end of the 6-month period was: mean sphere 0.15 D ± 0.54 D; mean cylinder -0.44

D ± 0.36 D; mean spherical equivalent of -0.07 D ± 0.87 D (all three series were statistically significant with p < 0.0016).

CONCLUSION

Unlike other ablation strategies, the cross-cylinder method creates a smooth transition (low dioptric gradi-ent) between the treated and untreated cornea. This is achieved by first treating the cylinder and then the spherical equivalent on a corneal surface that has become spherical.

The advantage of this technique: more physiologic postoperative corneal shape (as illustrated in the postoperative corneal topography on the previous page), sparing tissue, and not overcorrecting the oblique meridians.

LASIK Treatment on a Flatter Astigmatic Axis

Arturo Maldonado-Bas, MD

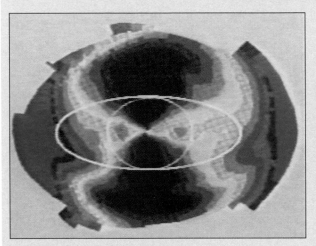

Figure 22B-1. Toric ablation induces hyperopic shifts in both axes.

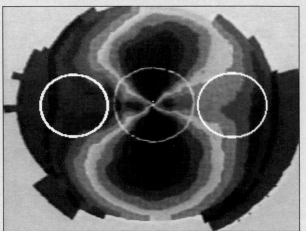

Figure 22B-2. Peripheral ablations steepen the flatter axis and, by the coupling effect, the steeper one is flattened.

Barraquer's thickness laws are not only used to correct spherical ametropia but also astigmatism.

Equal dioptric power in both corneal axis can be achieved by means of central ablation on the steeper axis, which will flatten it, or by means of symmetrical peripheral ablations on the flatter axis, which will steepen it.

Presently, most traditional treatments for astigmatism vary depending on whether the astigmatism is myopic or hyperopic.

Toric ablation is useful to correct compound myopic astigmatism with a myopic spherical component equal to or higher than 1 D, since even when the steeper axis is flattened, the flatter axis is also ablated with a consequent spherical hyperopic shift of between 0.25 and 0.30 D for each astigmatic diopter corrected.

In hyperopia, symmetrical peripheral ablations are performed on the flatter axis. Using these ablations with myopic PRK software, 4.0 mm in diameter will induce a coupling effect of 50% of the refractive error, similar to the one produced by an arcuate incision 90° in length.

Considering all the previous concepts, we will now consider the possibility of treating all types of astigmatism using peripheral ablations combined with the corresponding spherical treatment.

For a clearer understanding, we will use five examples with different refractive errors: simple, compound hyperopia, mixed, simple, and compound myopia.

In all the cases, the 90° vertical axis will be 46 D and the 0° horizontal axis will be 40 D.

In all the cases we will consider a symmetrical ablation in the horizontal axis using myopic PRK software with 4.0 mm of optical zone diameter and –6 D in each ablation.

The result will approximately be a steepening of the flat axis by 3 D and a consequent flattening of the steep axis by 3 D as well.

1. In the case of simple hyperopic astigmatism, the example is a patient with +6 at 90°, keratometry 46 in 90° x 40 at 0°.

   The emmetropic vertical axis is 46 D at 90°, while the hyperopic is 40 D at 0°.

   Performing peripheral symmetrical ablations of

–6 D, with PRK software, 4.0 mm in diameter in the flatter axis, the astigmatism will be corrected and turned into a +3 D sphere.

The hyperopic error will be later corrected with hyperopic software.

2. In the case of a compound hyperopic astigmatism with a patient with +2 + 6 at 90° and the keratometry of 46 D at 90° and 40 D at 0°, the vertical axis is hyperopic by +2, while the horizontal one is +8 D.

PRK ablations of –6 D, 4.0 mm in diameter, will correct the astigmatism leaving +5 D of hyperopia that will be corrected using the hyperopic software.

3. In the case of a mixed astigmatism +3 -6 at 0° and a keratometry of 46 at 90° x 40 in 0°, the 90° axis is steeper by 3 D and the 0° axis flatter by 3 D than what is needed for emmetropia.

Performing a peripheral symmetric ablation over the 0° axis of –6 D, 4.0 mm in diameter, we steepen the flat axis by 3 D and, due to the coupling effect, the steeper axis is flattened by 3 D, leaving the cornea spherically neutral.

4. In the case of simple myopic astigmatism in a patient of –6 at 0° and keratometry of 46 at 90° x 40 at 0°, the myopic axis is 90° while the emmetropic axis is 0°.

Performing two symmetrical PRK –6 D, 4.0 mm in diameter on the 0° axis, we steepen the emmetropic axis and make it myopic by 3 D and flatten the myopic axis making it hyperopic by 3

D, thus leaving a spherical myopia of –3 D, which will be treated with the corresponding software for myopic ablation.

5. In the case of compound myopic astigmatism of –2 – 6 at 0° and keratometry of 46 D at 90° x 40 at 0°, the latter will be –2 D myopic, while the 90° axis will be –8 D myopic.

Performing two symmetrical peripheral ablations, 4.0 mm in diameter and –6 D on the flattest axis, this will be steepened by 3 D and the 90° axis will be flattened 3 D, turning the refractive error into a spherical myopia of –5, which will be treated with the corresponding software for myopic ablation.

In this way, any astigmatic error may be treated by steepening the flatter axis. The advantages of this technique are:

- The range of errors that can be treated is greater.
- Less tissue is ablated in the visual axis in cases of simple and compound astigmatism. Thus, in the fifth case, with a toric mask we would ablate 2 D in the horizontal axis and –8 D in the vertical axis within the pupillary area.

By peripherally ablating on the flatter axis, central treatment would be –5 D, thus saving tissue. In hyperopic astigmatism, peripheral ablation is the best option. In mixed cases, we do not ablate tissue over the visual axis. The surgeon must remain aware that he or she is changing the corneal surface, and therefore, keratometric measures should be remembered.

TREATMENT OF HYPEROPIC ASTIGMATISM

Carlos J. Argento, MD
María José Cosentino, MD

23

LASIK (laser-assisted in situ keratomileusis) has been the technique used for the correction of myopia, compound myopic astigmatism, myopic and hyperopic astigmatism, and hyperopia. Myopia and compound myopic astigmatism results have reached acceptable predictability and safety levels.[1,2,3,4]

Other surgical techniques have been used for the treatment of simple and compound hyperopic astigmatism and, even though they have demonstrated good results at the beginning, a certain degree of instability, or regression, in their evolution frequently occurs.[5,6,7,8] In mixed astigmatism (and particularly in those cases in which the spherical equivalent was equal to zero), incisional techniques have attained rather satisfactory results.[9,10]

Until recently, treatment of astigmatism has been performed on the steepest meridian, either by means of incision or with a laser. With laser treatment, it involves ablation along the entire steep meridian. Therefore, this ablation includes a small part of the flattest meridian (Figure 23-1). In this manner, all treatments (no matter which technique is used) produce a hyperopic refractive change at the opposite meridian, which consequently becomes hyperopic.

We prefer using LASIK to perform the treatment of positive cylinder at the flattest meridian. An ablation of tissue perpendicular to the flattest meridian is performed according to Barraquer's thickness rule, thus increasing the optical power of this meridian (Figure 23-2).

The aim of this chapter is to analyze the predictability, safety, and stability of results in the treatment of simple hyperopic astigmatism, compound hyperopic astigmatism, and mixed astigmatism, with the LASIK technique steepening the flattest meridian using the PlanoScan program.

OUR EXPERIENCE

We treated 65 cases of simple hyperopic astigmatism, 278 compound hyperopic astigmatism, and 155 mixed astigmatism.

All patients had a stable refractive history before the procedure. The risks and benefits of the LASIK technique, as well as its therapeutic alternatives, were explained to the patients before their consent was obtained.

Patients were studied under the same preoperative protocol: uncorrected distance and near visual acuity, best-corrected far and near visual acuity, subjective correction with and without cycloplegia, biomicroscopy, tonometry, funduscopy, pachymetry, keratometry, and corneal topography.

Those patients who had any kind of superficial corneal pathology, corneal ectasia, significant refractive media alterations, or collagen diseases were excluded.

Preoperative patient preparation consisted of the topical instillation of ofloxacin 0.3% eyedrops four times daily, 48 hours before the procedure. Anesthesia was achieved 1 hour before surgery with topical eyedrops of lidocaine 4% and proparacaine hydrochloride 0.5%, supplemented with oral sedation (diazepam 5 mg). The operating room was kept within the same temperature—between 18° and 21°C and humidity between 38% and 45%—conditions in all cases. Air ultrafiltration and ultraviolet light exposure of the laser device and of the environment were performed 24 hours before the day of surgery.

The patients were continuously instructed to maintain optimal fixation in relation to the laser beam, and they were familiarized with the noise produced by the laser shots before the procedure. They were also warned

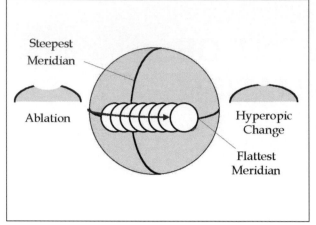

Figure 23-1. Laser treatment for astigmatism at the steepest meridian.

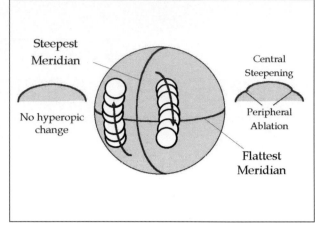

Figure 23-2. Treatment with the PlanoScan for single hyperopic astigmatism at the flattest meridian.

of transient vision loss during suction in order to prevent any surprise.

The Technolas Keracor 116, 117C, and 217 excimer laser was used in all cases, with the PlanoScan versions 2.4 and V2.422 for hyperopias. The ablation in the PlanoScan algorithm is based on a 2.0 mm flying spot with pseudorandom positioning. This ablation is performed as two opposite semi-ring ablations (two opposite D-shaped ablations), each one at either side of the steepest meridian; thus producing a steepening of the flattest meridian, almost without intervention on the other meridian (Figure 23-3a).

The distance between the deepest point of the two ablations yields the diameter of the optical zone; it can be varied between 4.2 mm and 5.5 mm. This gives a transition zone (a nonoptical zone designed to blend the optically ablated zone with the untreated area of the cornea) of approximately 2.0 mm from the deepest spot to the unablated cornea on each side, with a consequent total ablation diameter ranging between 8.1 and 9.5 mm (Figure 23-3b). The central zone between both semi-ring ablations is an unablated zone, thus minimizing the axial crossover (Figure 23-3c).

Each shot removes 0.25 microns of tissue, then the proper overlapping of successive accurately positioned shots act as a sculptor's chisel, removing chips, to finally give the final shape of the corneal stroma.

The exact coordinates of each shot to achieve the required curvature is precalculated by the software before surgery and then arranged in its sequence to minimize overlap frequencies greater than 12.5 Hz (times per second); this prevents overheating. The small size of the beam makes the ablation smooth, provides independence from the beam's homogeneity and does not give sharp edges to the ablation. This is coupled with the

advantageous possibility of easily changing the shape of the ablation just by changing the algorithm.

The laser fluence was checked before each procedure by verifying the homogeneity and symmetry of the pulses according to optimal values of 65 shots ± one. The keratectomies were performed using the Automated Corneal Shaper and Hansatome microkeratomes.

In all cases, the eyelashes were removed from the surgical field with adhesive tape and a lid speculum was used. The cornea was then marked with three asymmetric guides prepared with a 3.0 mm marker stained with gentian violet so as to achieve a better apposition of the corneal flap (whether the hinge of the flap was maintained or not).

After this, the suction ring was placed and decentered nasally according to the power of the keratectomy: those values below 41 diopters (D) remained almost centrated, while those over 42 D were decentered by 1.0 mm or more depending on the astigmatism. The microkeratome was then passed after checking its performance before each procedure. Viscoelastic substance was applied on the perilimbal bulbar conjunctiva near the hinge in order to create a viscous bed protecting the corneal epithelium when it comes into contact with the conjunctiva.

We usually create the flap with a nasal hinge, but when the astigmatism is with-the-rule and the flattest meridian is less than 40.5 D, the section is created with the microkeratome from down upward. A superior hinge is thus achieved, preventing the laser ablation from hitting the hinge.

With our nomogram, we first used optical zones of 4.4 mm, 4.6 mm, and 4.8 mm; now we are using an optical zone of 5.8 mm. In those cases in which cycloplegic refraction was not significantly different, we used sub-

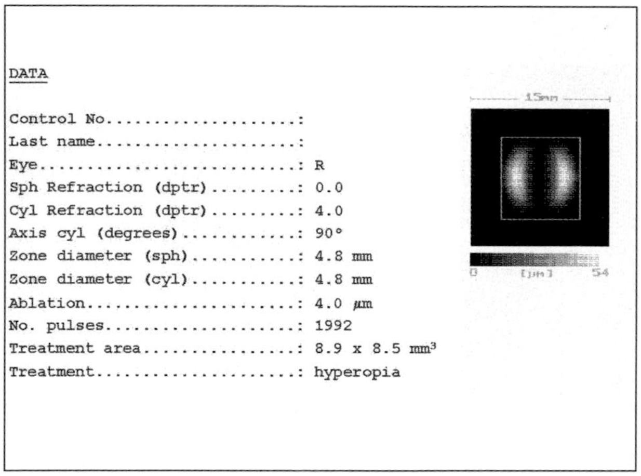

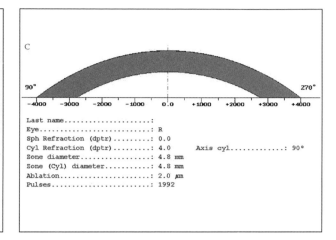

Figure 23-3a. Performance of the excimer laser with PlanoScan software.

Figure 23-3b. Performance of the excimer laser with PlanoScan software.

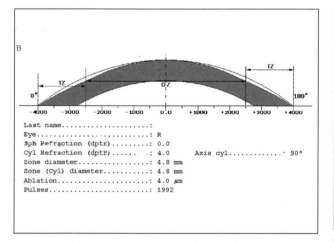

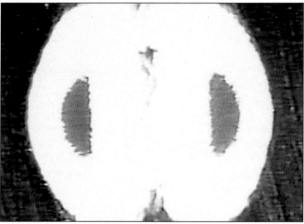

Figure 23-3c. Performance of the excimer laser with PlanoScan software.

Figure 23-4. Treatment with PlanoScan for simple hyperopic astigmatism.

jective refraction values, but when it was significant, refraction was considered the average between the subjective and cycloplegic refraction. For hyperopic spherical values less than or equal to +2 D, 65% was added to the correction; for hyperopic spherical values higher than +3 D, a 75% increase was added.

Patient age was another factor taken into account. In patients under 40 years of age, a 25% increase was used; in those between 40 and 60, we made a 30% addition, and in those over 69, the increase was 35%. For the correction of hyperopic astigmatism, an increase of 70% was added to the cylindrical correction in those cylinders lower than or equal to +1 D, while the increase ranged from 60% to 70% in cylinders between +1 and +2 D; this increase was 50% in cylinders higher than +2 D. For example, according to our nomogram, in a 50-year-old patient with a refraction of +2.0 sph +2.0 cyl at 90°, a 65% increase in the spherical correction was performed

based on the amount of hyperopia, and a further 30% was added according to his age (ie, a total of 95% addition was made to the spherical refraction value, while a 50% addition was made on the cylindrical refraction). Therefore, the final intended refraction for this patient was sph +4 cyl +3 at 90°.

Patient were encouraged to maintain fixation. For the treatment of simple hyperopic astigmatism, a peripheral ablation parallel to the steepest meridian was performed with the laser. This peripheral ablation caused an incurvation on the flattest meridian (treatment for hyperopic astigmatism) with no modification at the steepest meridian (see Figure 23-2). Figure 23-4 shows the laser treatment for simple hyperopic astigmatism performed on a check plate. In compound hyperopic astigmatism, the laser performed an ablation peripherally, thus incurvating both meridians (treatment for hyperopia). Furthermore, two peripheral hemiablations were per-

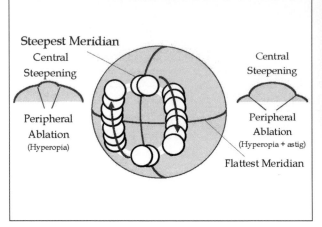

Figure 23-5. Treatment with PlanoScan for compound hyperopic astigmatism at the flattest meridian.

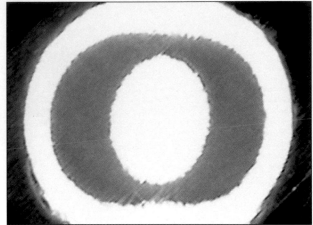

Figure 23-6. Treatment with PlanoScan for compound hyperopic astigmatism on the check plate.

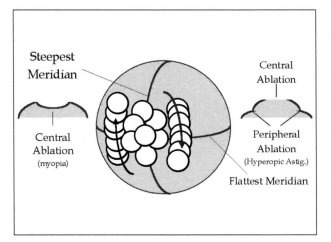

Figure 23-7. Treatment with PlanoScan for mixed astigmatism at the flattest meridian.

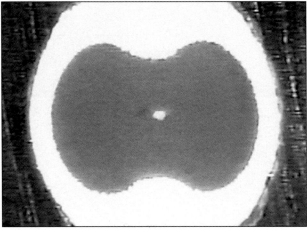

Figure 23-8. Treatment with PlanoScan for mixed astigmatism on the check plate.

formed with the laser on the flattest meridian (treatment for hyperopic astigmatism). Therefore, a peripheral ablation perpendicular to the steepest meridian, as treatment for hyperopia, and another peripheral but deeper ablation perpendicular to the flattest meridian for the treatment of hyperopia plus hyperopic astigmatism was carried out (Figure 23-5). Figure 23-6 shows the laser treatment for compound hyperopic astigmatism performed on a check plate. The treatment for mixed astigmatism consisted of a central ablation at the steepest meridian in order to flatten it (treatment for myopia). At the flattest meridian, in addition to the central ablation, a peripheral ablation leading to a relative incurvation of the central flattened area was performed (treatment for myopia and hyperopic astigmatism) (Figure 23-7). Figure 23-8 shows the laser treatment for mixed astigmatism on the check plate.

The bed was systematically dried with oxygen gas (2 ml/minute) between each phase of treatment. The flap

was replaced after its hydration with three drops of balanced salt solution (BSS) on the stromal side. A 27-gauge cannula was placed under the hinge, tangential to the limbus, and the flap was repositioned by means of a quick and safe maneuver toward the temporal side ("maneuver of the samurai," as it resembles a Japanese warrior's spade blow).

The interface was then washed with BSS by means of the same 27-gauge cannula introduced from the superior edge, and irrigation was initiated when it reached the central 2.0 mm of the section.

Once irrigation was completed, the correct position of the flap in relation to the marks was verified. Following this, expression of the remaining liquid under the flap proceeded with the same irrigation cannula. As a first step, expression was performed from the hinge toward the temporal side, passing through the pupil (Figure 23-9[a]), then from the pupil upward and down-

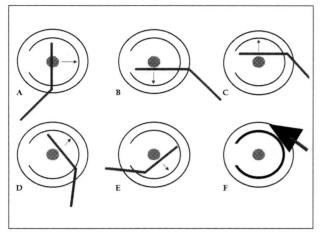

Figure 23-9. Expression of the liquid from the interface.

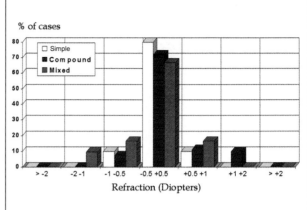

Figure 23-10. Distribution of spherical equivalent corrections at the sixth postoperative month.

Table 23-1				
POSTOPERATIVE EVOLUTION OF SIMPLE HYPEROPIC ASTIGMATISM AT THE FIRST, THIRD, SIXTH, AND 12TH MONTH				
Control	BSCVA	Refraction (sph eq)	Vectorial Change (cyl)	Number
Preop	0.64 ± 0.32	+1.96 ± 0.61	+3.75 ± 1.51	65
1 month	0.83 ± 0.10	-1.12 ± 0.22	4.26 ± 1.40	53
3 months	0.82 ± 0.09	+ 0.15 ± 0.81	3.69 ± 1.23	41
6 months	0.83 ± 0.13	+0.19 ± 0.77	3.42 ± 0.75	34
12 months	0.82 ± 0.17	+0.31 ± 0.55	3.12 ± 0.68	17

ward (Figures 23-9[b] and 23-9[c]); the last step involved the intermediate sectors (Figures 23-9[d] and 23-9[e]).

After expressing the liquid, the area was dried with Merocel sponges until a sulcus was formed in the periphery of the flap (Figure 23-9[f]).

After completing the drying stage, the speculum was removed with the utmost care, trying to prevent the flap from being dislodged by the patient's blinking.

Postoperative treatment with topical instillation of tobramycin 0.3% and dexamethasone 0.1% four times daily for a week and once daily for another week, was used.

The following check-ups were performed: first day, first week, second week, first month, third month, sixth month, first year, and second year. The parameters examined at each visit were: uncorrected visual acuity, best-corrected visual acuity, subjective correction, biomicroscopy, tonometry, keratometry, and corneal topography.

For easier analysis, the population studied was divided into three groups according to type of preoperative astigmatism (simple hyperopic astigmatism, compound hyperopic astigmatism, mixed astigmatism).[11,12]

SIMPLE HYPEROPIC ASTIGMATISM

Of the 65 cases studied, 17 (26.3%) were males and 48 (73.7 %) were females. Thirty cases (46.2 %) were under 40 years of age and 35 cases (53.8 %) were older than 40. The follow-up period was 3 months in 63.1% of cases, 6 months in 52.3%, and 12 months in 26.2%.

Preoperative best-corrected visual acuity was 0.64 ± 0.32, spherical equivalent was +1.96 ± 0.61 (range: +1.00 to +2.50), and cylinder was +3.75 ± 1.51 (range: +2.0 to +5.0).

Table 23-1 shows the evolution of the postoperative correction values (spherical equivalent and cylinder) and best-corrected visual acuity at the postoperative first, third, sixth, and twelfth months. In regard to cylindrical correction, there was a trend of overcorrection in the immediate postoperative period with a later undercorrection in the intermediate postoperative period. In most cases, this undercorrection was proportional to the amount of preoperative hyperopic astigmatism.

Figure 23-10 shows the distribution of corrections according to the spherical equivalent at 6 months postop-

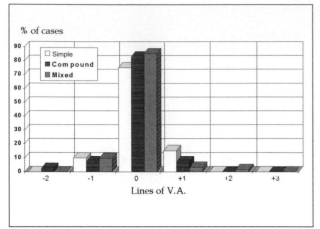

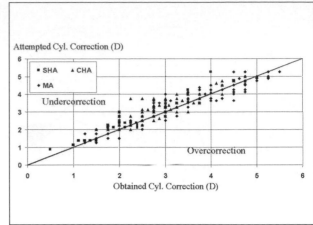

Figure 23-11. Gained and lost lines of visual acuity at the sixth postoperative month.

Figure 23-12. Attempted cylinder correction versus post-operative cylinder correction at the sixth month.

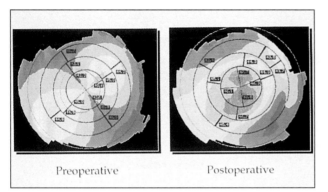

Figure 23-13. Preoperative and sixth postoperative month corneal topographies in simple hyperopic astigmatism.

eratively. Eighty percent of the cases were ±0.5 D; and 100% were ±1 D.

Cases with an uncorrected visual acuity of 20/40 or better were 92.3% at 6 months postoperatively. Uncorrected visual acuity of 20/20 or 20/25 was 81.5% at the sixth month. A satisfactory improvement in uncorrected visual acuity was observed between the first and sixth months postoperatively.

In regard to safety, Figure 23-11 presents the number of lines of best-corrected visual acuity gained and lost 6 months after the procedure. The total number of cases fell between zero ± one line of visual acuity; a predominance of preoperative lines of visual acuity retained can be clearly observed. Seventy-five percent of cases retained the preoperative best-spectacle visual acuity; 10% lost one line, and 15% gained one line.

Figure 23-12 presents the relationship between the attempted cylinder correction and the obtained cylinder correction at the postoperative sixth month. It shows a trend in undercorrection.

Figure 23-13 shows preoperative and postoperative sixth-month corneal topographies of a case with simple hyperopic astigmatism.

COMPOUND HYPEROPIC ASTIGMATISM

Of the 278 cases studied, 52 (18.7%) were males and 136 (81.3%), females. One hundred and thirty-six cases (48.9%) were under 40 years of age and 118 (51.1%) were older. About 70.5% of cases were followed for 3 months; 57% for 6 months, and 41.3% for 12 months. The preoperative values for best-corrected visual acuity were 0.76 ± 0.13, the spherical equivalent was +3.58 ± 0.81 (range: + 2.50 to +4.25), and cylinder was +3.28 ± 1.23 (range: +2.00 to +5.75).

Regarding postoperative uncorrected visual acuities, it is important to realize that in some cases the target correction was low myopia. Table 23-2 shows the evolution of the postoperative correction values (spherical equivalent and cylinder) and best-corrected visual acuity at postoperative first, third, and sixth months. With the cylindrical correction, there was a slight trend in overcorrection in the immediate postoperative period with a later regression in the intermediate postoperative period, the total cylindrical correction remained unchanged at the sixth postoperative month. In regard to the spherical equivalent, very satisfactory correction levels with great stability were attained (it should be kept in mind that there were some cases with high correction values).

Figure 23-10 shows the distribution of corrections as to the spherical equivalent 6 months after the procedure. About 71.9% of cases were ± 0.5 D, 90.2% were ± 1 D; and 100% were ± 2 D.

The cases with an uncorrected visual acuity of 20/40

Table 23-2				
POSTOPERATIVE EVOLUTION OF COMPOUND HYPEROPIC ASTIGMATISM AT THE FIRST, THIRD, SIXTH, AND 12TH MONTH				
Control	BSCVA	Refraction (sph eq)	Vectorial Change (cyl)	Number
Preop	0.76 ± 0.13	+3.58 ± 0.81	+3.28 ± 1.23	278
1 month	0.77 ± 0.22	-0.56 ± 0.42	3.34 ± 1.22	236
3 months	0.76 ± 0.18	+ 0.24 ± 0.34	3.26 ± 1.16	196
6 months	0.75 ± 0.18	+ 0.35 ± 0.49	3.14 ± 0.43	158
12 months	0.74 ± 0.31	+0.56 ± 0.64	3.09 ± 0.95	115

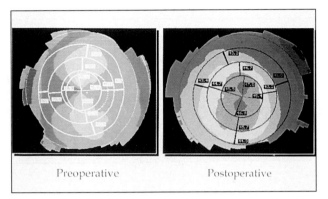

Preoperative   Postoperative

Figure 23-14. Preoperative and sixth postoperative month corneal topographies in compound hyperopic astigmatism.

or better accounted for 86.4% at 6 months postoperatively. Uncorrected visual acuity of 20/20 or 20/25 accounted for 74.1% at the sixth month after the procedure.

In regard to safety, Figure 23-11 presents the number of lines of best-corrected visual acuity gained and lost at 6 months after the procedure. As shown in Table 23-2, 82.9% retained the preoperative lines of visual acuity, 7.3% gained one line of visual acuity, 7.3% lost one line of visual acuity, and 2.5% lost two lines of visual acuity.

Figure 23-12 represents the relationship between the attempted cylinder correction and the obtained cylinder correction at the sixth postoperative month.

Figure 23-14 shows preoperative and postoperative sixth-month corneal topographies of a case with compound hyperopic astigmatism.

MIXED ASTIGMATISM

A total of 155 cases were studied, of which 80 (52%) males and 75 (48%) females were treated. Ages were under 40 years in 75 cases (48.7%) and over 40 years in 80 (51.3%). Follow-up was in 85.2% was 3 months; 52.2% at 6 months, and 27.1% at 12 months. The preoperative values for best-corrected visual acuity was 0.88 ± 0.22, spherical equivalent was +0.28 ± 1.38 (range: –1.12

to +4.25), and cylinder was +3.33 ± 1.62 (range: +0.50 to +7.25).

Table 23-3 shows the evolution of the postoperative correction values (spherical equivalent and cylinder) and best-corrected visual acuity at the first, third and sixth postoperative months. In regard to cylindrical correction, there was a mild trend in overcorrection in the immediate postoperative period. This overcorrection regressed, though not completely, in the intermediate postoperative period. The total cylindrical correction was thus maintained 6 months after the procedure. Changes in the spherical equivalent demonstrated averages very close to zero. This is obvious since we are dealing with mixed astigmatism.

Figure 23-10 shows the distribution of corrections, according to the spherical equivalent, at the sixth postoperative month. About 66.7% of the cases were ± 0.5 D and almost 100% were ± 1 D. The cases with an uncorrected visual acuity of 20/40 or better accounted for 95.4% at the postoperative sixth month. Uncorrected visual acuity of 20/25 or better accounted for 77.4% at the sixth month after procedure.

In regard to safety, Figure 23-11 presents the number of lines of best-corrected visual acuity gained and lost 6 months after the procedure. About 85.2% of the cases retained lines of visual acuity; 3.3% gained one line, and 1.6% gained two lines. There were no lost lines of visual acuity.

Figure 23-12 represents the relationship between the attempted cylinder correction and the obtained cylinder correction at the sixth postoperative month. It shows low under- and overcorrections. Figure 23-15 shows preoperative and postoperative sixth-month corneal topographies of a case with mixed astigmatism. Finally, Tables 23-4 and 23-5 show the complications, classified into intra- and postoperative, for each type of astigmatism.

OUR CONSIDERATIONS

In modern refractive surgery, the treatment for simple and compound hyperopic astigmatism has always yield-

Table 23-3				
POSTOPERATIVE EVOLUTION OF MIXED ASTIGMATISM AT THE FIRST, THIRD, SIXTH, AND 12TH MONTH				
Control	BSCVA	Refraction (sph eq)	Vectorial Change (cyl)	Number
Preop	0.88 ± 0.22	+0.28 ± 1.38	+3.33 ± 1.62	155
1 month	0.85 ± 0.31	-0.36 ± 0.56	4.22 ± 0.71	139
3 months	0.88 ± 0.23	- 0.19 ± 0.61	4.05 ± 1.12	132
6 months	0.89 ± 0.19	+ 0.05 ± 0.51	3.58 ± 1.20	82
12 months	0.87 ± 0.31	+0.08 ± 0.45	3.41 ± 0.88	42

Table 23-4			
INTRAOPERATIVE COMPLICATIONS			
	SHA	CHA	MA
Suction loss	0% (0/65)	1.8% (5/278)	1.9% (3/155)
Free cap	0% (0/65)	1.8% (5/278)	0% (0/155)
Flap incomplete	0% (0/65)	0% (0/278)	0% (0/155)
Flap perforation	0% (0/65)	0% (0/278)	0% (0/155)

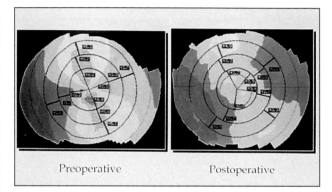

Figure 23-15. Preoperative and sixth postoperative month corneal topographies in mixed astigmatism.

ed poorer results than the treatment of spherical errors.[13,14,15,16]

Since the advent of the excimer laser, in combination with keratomileusis, new possibilities have been available for the treatment of these astigmatisms.

We have been using the Technolas Keracor 116, 117C, and 217 laser with broadbeam and PlanoScan programs. When we started to work with this equipment in January 1995 at our first center (Tucumán, Argentina), we only performed treatment for myopic astigmatism. The ablation was performed at the steepest meridian, thus inducing a certain degree of hyperopia at the other meridian. From our experience, for every 1.25 astigmatism diopters ablated, 0.25 positive diopters are induced at the other meridian.

In November 1995, when we began using the PlanoScan program, we started using it for the treatment of astigmatism by incurvating the flattest meridian. Before this time, we had sporadically used the noncontact holmium laser in order to incurve the flattest meridian. The results were unsuccessful since regression occurred even in combination with the treatment for hyperopia (unpublished data). Therefore, we gave up this modality for the treatment of simple and compound hyperopic astigmatism.

In regard to mixed astigmatism with a spherical equivalent close to zero, results have proven to be very

satisfactory with arcuate incisions.[17] The desired result is achieved by the coupling phenomenon: flattening of the steepest meridian and incurvation of the flattest meridian due to the offsetting effect.[18]

Treatment for mixed astigmatism using LASIK has been an actual challenge, since we already had a method capable of managing the problem with real efficacy. We did a comparison between the predictability and safety in LASIK versus arcuate keratotomy.[19] In simple hyperopic astigmatism, the results obtained have been satisfactory, though undercorrected. In one-third of cases, preoperative uncorrected visual acuity was 20/40 or better; 6 months after the procedure, this percentage rose to 90.1%. Uncorrected visual acuity of 20/25 or better was in 63.7%. In compound hyperopic astigmatism, the spherical and cylindrical corrections at 6 months have been very satisfactory (see Table 23-2). Uncorrected visual acuities of 20/40 or better were not present in any case preoperatively, while these values were found in 86.4% of cases at 6 months postoperatively. Uncorrected visual acuity 20/25 or better was reported in 77.4%

In mixed astigmatism, the results were outstandingly good. The preoperative uncorrected visual acuities were 20/40 or better in 38% of cases; 6 months after the procedure, this percentage rose to 95.4%. Uncorrected visu-

Table 23-5

POSTOPERATIVE COMPLICATIONS

	SHA	CHA	MA
Epithelial ulcer	4.6% (3/65)	2.9% (8/278)	1.3% (2/155)
Infiltrates	0% (0/65)	3.2% (9/278)	0% (0/155)
Folds	4.6% (3/65)	1.1% (3/278)	2.6% (4/155)
Decentration	0% (0/65)	1.1% (3/278)	0% (0/155)
Infection	0% (0/65)	0% (0/278)	0% (0/155)

al acuity of 20/25 or better was reported in 77.4%. Furthermore, the results of spherical and cylindrical corrections were very pleasing.

In regard to induction at the other meridian, despite the low number of simple hyperopic astigmatism cases studied, the spherical equivalent was +0.19 ± 0.772 at 6 months postoperatively. This spherical equivalent value comes from the cylindrical undercorrection obtained. No spherical equivalent rise, per se, was thus produced, as may have occurred if induction had been performed at the other meridian in order to turn it hyperopic.

In compound hyperopic astigmatism, residual hyperopia 6 months after the procedure was +0.35 ± 0.49, as expected according to the undercorrection characteristics of the method. In our paper *Hyperopic LASIK*, of an updated number of 679 cases, spherical equivalent of hyperopic cases with no astigmatic component was close to the spherical equivalent of compound hyperopic astigmatism without.[20] From this, we may infer that the treatment for hyperopic astigmatism did not produce any variation in the spherical component of the refractive error.

The same occurred with mixed astigmatism in which the spherical equivalent did not vary, or it did mildly (from +0.88 ± 0.22 to +0.04 ± 0.52 at 6 months postoperatively).

These observations have led us to presume that the variation at the other meridian in all three types of astigmatism is negligible.

In the three types of astigmatism, predictability was good. In decreasing order, it was substantially better in mixed astigmatism, then in simple astigmatism, and lastly in compound astigmatism (probably due to the fact that they were highly hyperopic).

The ceramic head and the eye tracker, which were added to our laser, enabled us to reduce the duration of the procedure and to have a more stable energy supply and better fixation control. We assume that these changes contributed to improvement in our results. Another advance we recently incorporated is the Topolink, giving us the possibility of performing treatment according to the intraoperative corneal topography. This will undoubtedly be very useful for the treatment of asymmetric astigmatism.

We think that the LASIK technique, in combination with the PlanoScan program of the Technolas Keracor excimer laser, has proven to be very useful for the treatment of simple hyperopic astigmatism, compound hyperopic astigmatism, and mixed astigmatism at the flattest meridian, with no induction of correction at the other meridian.

REFERENCES

1. Kremer F, Dufek M. Excimer laser in situ keratomileusis. *Journal of Refractive Surgery*. 1995;11:244-7.
2. Gimbel H, Surenda B, Kaye G, Ferensowicz M. Experience during the learning curve of laser in situ keratomileusis. *J Cataract Refract Surg*. 1996;22:542-550.
3. Bas A, Onnis R. Excimer laser in situ keratomileusis for myopia. *Journal of Refractive Surgery*. 1995;11:229-33.
4. Salah T, Waring G, El Maghraby A, Moadel K, et al. Excimer laser in situ keratomileusis under a corneal flap for myopia of 2 to 20 diopters. *Am J Ophthalmol*. 1996;121:143-55.
5. Grandon S, Sanders D, Anello R, Jacobs D, et al. Clinical evaluation of hexagonal keratotomy for the treatment of primary hyperopia. *J Cataract Refract Surg*. 1995;21:109-10.
6. Durrie D, Schumer D, Cavanaugh T. Holmium:YAG laser thermokeratoplasty for hyperopia. *J Refract Corneal Surg*. 1994;10:277-80.
7. Anschütz T. Laser correction of hyperopia and presbyopia. *Int Ophthalmol Clin*. 1994; 34:107-37.
8. Gloor B, Rol P, Fankhauser F, Hoppeler T, et al. Kritische gedanken zur heutigen laserchirurgie der kornea. *Ophthalmologe*. 1995;92:389-96.
9. Pulaski, JP. Transverse incisions for mixed and myopic idiopatic astigmatism. *J Cataract Refract Surg*. 1996;22:307-312.
10. Duffey R, Jain V, Tchah H, Hofmann R, et al. Paired arcuate keratotomy. A surgical approach to mixed and myopic astigmatism. *Arch Ophthalmol*. 1988;106:1130-1135.
11. Spiegel M. *Teoría y Problemas de Estadística*. Bogotá: Ed Andes; 1982.
12. Jaffe N. *Cataract Surgery and its Complications*. St. Louis, Mo: Mosby-Year Book; 1976.
13. Nordan L, Maxwell W. Hexagonal keratotomy. *J Refract Corneal Surg*. 1993;9:228-9.
14. Werblin T. Critique of hexagonal keratotomy raises a ruckus (letter). *J Refract Corneal Surg*. 1992;8:408.
15. Thompson V. The surgical correction of myopic and hyperopic astigmatism. *Int Ophthalmol Clin*. 1994;34:87-96.
16. Dausch D, Klein R, Landesz M, Schroder E. Photorefractive keratectomy to correct astigmatism with

myopia or hyperopia. *J Cataract Refract Surg.* 1994;20(suppl):252-257

17. Chavez S, Chayet A, Celikkol L, Parker J, et al. Analysis of astigmatic keratotomy with a 5.0 mm optical clear zone. *Am J Ophthalmol.* 1996;121(1):65-76.

18. Hanna K, Jouve F, Waring G, Ciarlet P. Computer simulation of arcuate keratotomy for astigmatism. In: Waring G. *Refractive Keratotomy.* St. Louis, Mo: Mosby-Year Book; 1992.

19. Argento C, Fernandez Mendy J, Cosentino MJ. LASIK versus arcuate keratotomy for to treat astigmatism. *J Cataract Refract Surg.* 1999;25: 74-382.

20. Argento C, Cosentino MJ. LASIK in situ keratomileusis for hyperopia. *J Cataract Refract Surg.* 1998;24:1050-1058.

HYPEROPIC LASIK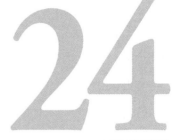

Maria Clara Arbelaez, MD
Michael C. Knorz, MD

INTRODUCTION

Several techniques, including hexagonal keratotomy, automated lamellar keratoplasty (ALK), thermal keratoplasty, holmium: YAG laser thermal keratoplasty (LTK), and photorefractive keratectomy (PRK) have been used to correct hyperopia.[1,2,3,4,5] All procedures showed significant regression and poor predictability, and we are still searching for a reliable keratorefractive procedure for the correction of hyperopia.[6] LASIK is showing promise in the correction of myopia-could it be as good for hyperopia?

Possible limitations of LASIK in hyperopia include the use of a comparatively small optical zone, which is theoretically more critical to decentration, may cause night driving problems, and could lead to refractive instability with change in pupil size.

SURGICAL TECHNIQUE

In this series, LASIK hyperopic surgery was performed at the Clinica de Oftalmologica de Cali, Cali, Colombia, by one surgeon (Arbelaez) using topical anesthesia (proparacaine 0.4%). For the keratectomy, the Automated Corneal Shaper (ACS) equipped with a mechanical stop and modified suction ring, was used to cut a 9.0-mm hinged flap. The suction ring was manufactured for the ALK-E unit No. 670 by Gusor Ltd, Bogota, Colombia.

It has a 0.5 mm larger diameter to create a larger flap, which is required because of the large ablation zone in hyperopic corrections. When the standard suction ring is used, it should be decentered nasally by about 0.5 mm to accommodate the large ablation zone required .

A flap size smaller than the ablation zone will cause partial blockage of the ablation, resulting in either irregular astigmatism or scarring at the edge of the cut where

Bowman's layer is ablated. The preset flap thickness was 160 µm in all eyes, but actual thickness was not measured to avoid possible contamination of the surgical field. After the cut, suction was released, but the suction ring was left on the eye. The corneal flap was carefully displaced nasally using a spatula, and the laser was centered over the middle of the entrance pupil. The oblique lights were slightly dimmed during the ablation to maintain a pupil size of approximately 3.0 to 4.0 mm to facilitate fixation control by the surgeon. The ablation was subjectively centered over the middle of the entrance pupil by the surgeon using the suction ring (without suction).

The stromal bed was neither irrigated nor dried to avoid changes in hydration. Fluid accumulation at the hinge during the ablation was removed with a Merocel. After the ablation, a drop of balanced salt solution (BSS) was placed on the stromal bed, and the flap was replaced. We then irrigated the interface to float the flap and remove debris. The flap was then painted into position with a wet, soft Merocel sponge. Once the flap was aligned, we waited 2 minutes to ensure proper adhesion.

After surgery, tobramycin and dexamethasone eyedrops (Tobradex) were administered and the eye was covered with a hard shield for the first night. Topical treatment with Tobradex (one drop three times daily) was continued for 5 days and then discontinued.

ABLATION PARAMETERS

Ablation was performed using the Keracor 117C excimer laser using software version V 2.7, which is designed for LASIK and PRK. No changes were made to convert PRK dosing to LASIK. The hyperopia software uses a scanning 2.0-mm beam to create an annular ablation profile. By ablating an annular zone of the paracentral cornea, the central cornea is steepened, and the refractive power of the central cornea is increased. The planned central optical zone was between 4.5 to 5.5 mm.

Table 24-1			
REOPERATIONS			
Group	# eyes operated	# (%) eyes at 12 mos postop	# (%) eyes retreated (overall)
Spherical hyperopia	192	60 (31%)	14 (7%)
SE 1 to 3 D	88	24 (27%)	2 (2%)
SE 3.1 to 5 D	57	20 (35%)	2 (4%)
SE 5.1 to 9 D	47	16 (34%)	16 (21%)
Toric hyperopia	164	50 (30%)	24 (15%)
SE 1 to 3 D	109	23 (21%)	12 (11%)
SE 3.1 to 5 D	29	14 (48%)	4 (14%)
SE 5.1 to 9.5 D	26	13 (50%)	8 (31%)

A 4.5 mm zone was used in five eyes (hyperopia more than 5 diopters [D]) and a 5.5-mm zone in 14 eyes (hyperopia up to 5 D). In all other eyes, a 5.0-mm zone was used. To achieve a planned optical zone of 5.0 to 5.5 mm, an 8.0-mm zone was ablated. The term planned optical zone is used here as the final optically active portion of the cornea, which may somewhat differ due to epithelial remodeling. In group 2, an additional astigmatism correction was performed. The astigmatism was corrected using the plus cylinder by steepening the flat corneal meridian. Steepening is achieved by ablating the mid-periphery of the cornea in the flat meridian.

PATIENT POPULATION

The number operated was 356 hyperopic eyes (223 patients) between March 1995 and March 1997. Exclusion criteria included age under 18 years, chronic eye diseases such as cataract, glaucoma, uveitis, keratoconus, diabetes, and autoimmune diseases. All patients were informed of the nature of the study, and written consent was obtained. Most treated patients came from outside of Cali and had to travel for treatment and each follow-up visit. This may have contributed to the high number of eyes lost during follow-up. In addition, many patients declined to come even for a free follow-up visit when they were called for the 12-month visit, stating that they liked the result and were unwilling to come again. Thus, only 120 eyes were available for follow-up at 12 months postoperatively. In 10 of these eyes, monovision correction had been performed for reading, and these eyes were excluded. Patients were divided into two: spherical and toric. The spherical group included hyperopia of +1 to +9 D and corneal astigmatism of less than 1 D. The toric group included hyperopia of +1 to +9.5 D and corneal astigmatism of 1 to 7.5 D. The average age in the spherical group was 42 ± 9.1 years (range: 20 to 60 years). The average age in the toric group was

38 ± 9.3 years (range: 19 to 56 years). Both groups were subdivided into three subgroups to analyze the outcome in reference to the preoperative spherical equivalent (low hyperopia: +1 to +3 D; moderate hyperopia: +3.1 to +5 D; high hyperopia: +5.1 to +9.5 D). The number of eyes in each group and subgroup is given in Table 24-1.

In 23 patients in group 1 and in 19 patients in group 2, both eyes were treated. The time interval between treatments was 1 day in most cases, but in some cases it ranged up to 14 days.

Patients were examined preoperatively and 1 day, 1 week, 3 months, and 12 months postoperatively. We measured subjective spectacle refraction (fogging technique). In addition, cycloplegic refraction (cyclopentolate) was performed preoperatively, and attempted correction was based on cycloplegic refraction. We always used the manifest cycloplegic refraction to compensate for the effects of accommodation. All refractions given are spectacle refractions.

Uncorrected and spectacle-corrected visual acuity were tested using the Mentor B-VAT II-SG system. Visual loss was calculated as the difference in line number on a logarithmic scale (eg, a drop from 20/20 to 20/40 or from 20/100 to 20/200 both represent a three-line loss). Contact lenses were discontinued at least 3 weeks (hard lenses) or 2 weeks (soft lenses) prior to examination.

RETREATMENTS

Retreatments were usually performed 3 months after surgery. If patients were not emmetropic and not satisfied with the result at the 3-month follow-up, a retreatment was offered. In all retreatments, the flap was lifted using a blunt spatula (Arbelaez LASIK spatula, Asico). The overall rate of retreatments due to under- or overcorrections was calculated for each subgroup. The results presented in this chapter include retreatments.

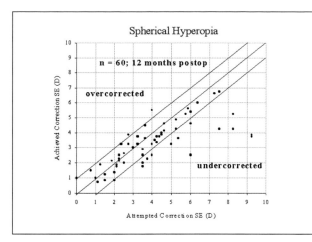

Figure 24-1a. Scattergram of attempted versus achieved correction after spherical hyperopic LASIK.

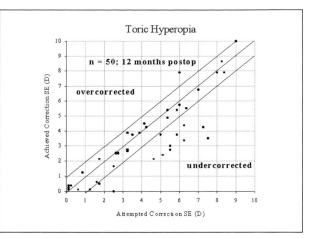

Figure 24-1b. Scattergram of attempted versus achieved correction after toric hyperopic LASIK.

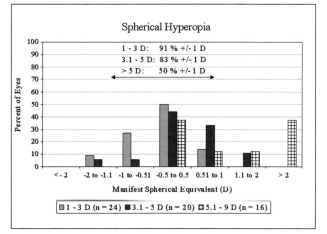

Figure 24-2a. Scattergram of refractive error after spherical hyperopic LASIK.

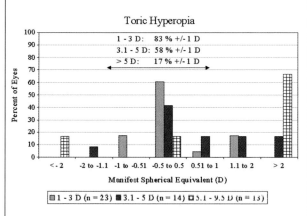

Figure 24-2b. Scattergram of refractive error after toric hyperopic LASIK.

REFRACTION

The scattergrams of attempted versus achieved correction for both groups are shown in Figures 24-1a and 24-1b.

Considerable undercorrection is evident in high hyperopia. Refractive error at 12 months is shown in Figures 24-2a and 24-2b. In low spherical hyperopia, 13 eyes (55%) were within ± 0.5 D, while in low toric hyperopia, 14 eyes (61%) were within ± 0.5 D. In moderate spherical hyperopia, nine eyes (44%) were within ± 0.5 D, while in moderate toric hyperopia five eyes (36%) were within ± 0.5 D. In high spherical hyperopia, six eyes (38%) were within ± 0.5 D while in high toric hypcropia 4 eyes (31%) were within ± 0.5 D. Predictability was usually higher in the spherical subgroups than in the respective toric subgroups, and differences both between the moderate and high hyperopia subgroups were statistically significant (moderate hyperopia, p = 0.04; high hyperopia, p = 0.005). Comparing subgroups within each group, predictability was lower with the higher the hyperopia, both in the spherical and in the toric groups. Differences between low and high hyperopia subgroups were statistically significant (spherical group, p = 0.001; toric group, p = 0.005). In the low spherical hyperopia group, two eyes (8%) were overcorrected by more than 1 D while none were undercorrected by more than 1 D. In the moderate spherical hyperopia group, one eye (5%) was overcorrected by more than 1 D while two eyes (10%) were undercorrected by more than 1 D. In the high spherical hyperopia group, none of the eyes were overcorrected by more than 1 D, while eight eyes (50%) were undercorrected by more than 1 D. In the low toric hyperopia group, none of the eyes were overcorrected by more than 1 D while four eyes (17%) were undercorrected by more than 1 D. In the moderate toric

463

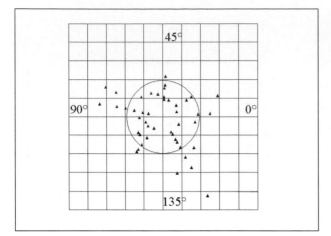

Figure 24-3a. Double-angle plot of astigmatism of the toric groups: preoperative astigmatism.

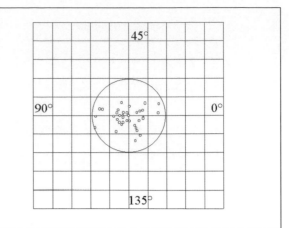

Figure 24-3b. Double-angle plot of astigmatism of the toric groups: postoperative astigmatism.

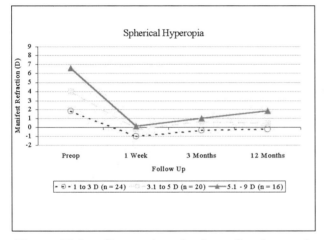

Figure 24-4a. Change in refraction after hyperopic LASIK: spherical group.

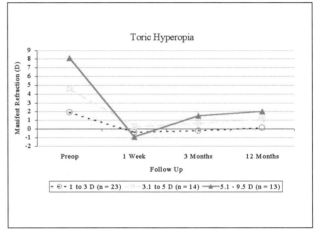

Figure 24-4b. Change in refraction after hyperopic LASIK: toric group.

hyperopia group, one eye (7%) was overcorrected by more than 1 D, while five eyes (36%) were undercorrected by more than 1 D. In the high toric hyperopia group, two eyes (15%) were overcorrected by more than 1 D, while nine eyes (69%) were undercorrected by more than 1 D (see Figure 24-1b).

Double-angle plots of preoperative and postoperative astigmatism are shown in Figures 24-3a and 24-3b. Astigmatism was reduced in all eyes, and the postoperative plot showed no trend toward a certain axis.

Change of refraction is shown in Figures 24-4a and 24-4b. Refraction was stable in low and moderate hyperopia, but about 2 D (spherical group) to 3 D (toric group) of regression occurred in high hyperopia.

VISUAL ACUITY

Uncorrected visual acuity at 12 months postopera-

tively is shown in Figures 24-5a and 24-5b. In general, uncorrected visual acuity was better in the spherical group than in the toric group. In both groups, efficacy was acceptable in low and moderate hyperopia but poor in high hyperopia. Uncorrected visual acuity was 20/20 or better in 10 eyes (42%) of the low spherical hyperopia group and in three eyes (13%) of the low toric hyperopia group. Uncorrected visual acuity was 20/20 or better in five eyes (25%) of the moderate spherical hyperopia group and in one eye (7%) of the moderate toric hyperopia group. None of the eyes in the high hyperopia subgroups achieved an uncorrected visual acuity of 20/20 or better.

Change in spectacle-corrected visual acuity is shown in Figures 24-6a and 24-6b. In low and moderate spherical hyperopia, none of the eyes lost two or more lines. However, in high spherical hyperopia, two eyes (13%) lost two or more lines. In low toric hyperopia, none of the

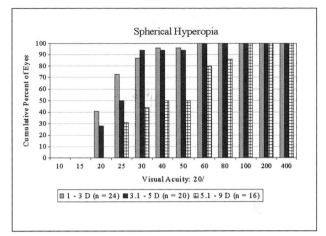

Figure 24-5a. Cumulative bar graph of uncorrected visual acuity after spherical hyperopic LASIK.

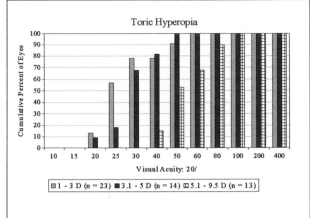

Figure 24-5b. Cumulative bar graph of uncorrected visual acuity after toric hyperopic LASIK.

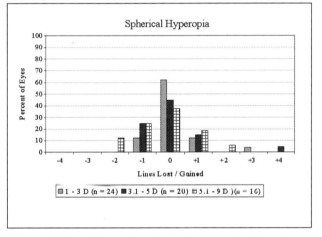

Figure 24-6a. Change in spectacle-corrected visual acuity after spherical hyperopic LASIK.

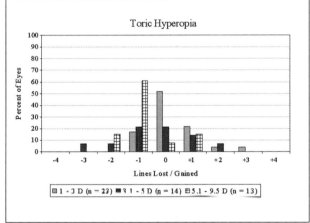

Figure 24-6b. Change in spectacle-corrected visual acuity after toric hyperopic LASIK.

eyes lost two or more lines. In moderate toric hyperopia, two eyes (14%) lost two or more lines, and in high toric hyperopia, two eyes (15%) lost two or more lines.

RETREATMENT

Of the 356 eyes operated, we performed 38 retreatments (11%), due to undercorrection. The number of retreatments for each group is included in Table 24-1.

COMPLICATIONS

Of the 356 eyes in the study, a free cap occurred in two eyes (0.6%). The cap was replaced after ablation, and the postoperative course was uneventful. In another two eyes (0.6%), presumed sterile keratitis occurred 2 days after surgery and was treated using prednisolone 1% eyedrops. In one of these eyes, a slight corneal scar,

similar to grade 1 haze persisted, but no visual loss occurred. In the other eye (0.3%), epithelial ingrowth developed 4 weeks after surgery, and the flap was lifted to remove the epithelium. The postoperative course was uneventful thereafter. One patient (both eyes operated, 7 D correction for spherical hyperopia, 4.5 mm planned optical zone) reported severe fluctuation of vision despite unchanged spectacle-corrected visual acuity. No other intra- or postoperative complications were observed.

PREDICTABILITY

In low spherical hyperopia, 13 eyes (55%) were within 0.5 D and 22 eyes (91%) were within 1 D of target refraction, while in moderate spherical hyperopia, nine eyes (44%) were within 0.5 D and 17 eyes (85%) were within 1 D (see Figure 24-1b). Thus, predictability seemed to be somewhat lower than in myopic LASIK.[7,8]

After LASIK, six eyes (38%) were within 0.5 D and eight eyes (50%) within 1 D in high hyperopia, while four eyes (31%) were within 0.5 D and six eyes (46%) within 1 D in high hyperopic astigmatism in our series.

Differences in predictability between the high hyperopia groups and the low and moderate hyperopia groups were statistically significant (see Figure 24-1b).

Comparing spherical and toric groups, predictability was significantly higher after spherical corrections. A lower predictability of toric corrections was also observed after LASIK for myopia.[7] The most likely reason for the lower predictability of toric corrections seems to be an axis misalignment. A 10° error in axis may result in an undercorrection of 30%. The double-angle plot of postoperative astigmatism confirms the scatter observed but indicates no trend toward a certain axis (see Figure 24-2a).

STABILITY

We observed little change in manifest refraction between 1 week and 12 months in low and moderate hyperopia. After PRK in hyperopia up to +6.50 D, continuing regression was observed at 6 months[9] and at 1 year.[11] In high spherical and toric hyperopia, we also observed a regression of about 2 D (spherical group) to 3 D (toric group) (see Figure 24-2b).

EFFICACY

Uncorrected visual acuity was 20/20 or better in 10 eyes (42%) of the low spherical hyperopia group in our study,[10] Uncorrected visual acuity was 20/40 or better in more than 90% of eyes in low and moderate spherical hyperopia and about 80% in low to moderate toric hyperopia. In high spherical hyperopia and in high toric hyperopia, only 50% and 17%, respectively, had an uncorrected visual acuity of 20/40 or better (see Figure 24-3a).

REOPERATIONS

Overall, 14 eyes (7%) of the spherical groups and 24 eyes of the toric groups (15%) required reoperation due to undercorrection. The retreatment rate was very low in low and moderate spherical hyperopia but high in high hyperopia. Retreatments were more frequent in toric hyperopia (Table 24-1).

SAFETY

Regarding the safety of LASIK, we must consider intraoperative and postoperative complications and visual loss. Two free flaps (0.6%) occurred, two eyes (0.6%) developed presumed sterile keratitis early postoperatively, and one eye (0.3%) required reoperation because of epithelial ingrowth. The US Food and Drug Administration (FDA) panel on excimer laser PRK for myopia has published guidelines stating that loss of best-corrected visual acuity should be limited to 5% of eyes losing two or more lines.[13] In our study, a loss of two or more lines of spectacle-corrected visual acuity did not occur in low and moderate spherical hyperopia and in low toric hyperopia. In moderate toric hyperopia, two eyes (14%) lost two or more lines, while in high hyperopia, two eyes (13%) of the spherical group and two eyes (15%) of the toric group lost two or more lines (see Figure 24-3b).

While interpreting visual loss, we have to consider that all measurements were performed with spectacle correction. Correcting hyperopia at the corneal plane instead of the spectacle plane will cause minification of the retinal image.[14] As the change in image size is about 2% per diopter only, it will be significant in high hyperopia only and cannot explain the loss of spectacle-corrected visual acuity observed. More likely, the loss of spectacle-corrected visual acuity in high hyperopia is due to image degradation by significant optical aberrations caused by the new corneal surface. These aberrations become more significant the higher the amount of correction.

We are aware of several limitations of our study. The most important is the low follow-up rate. Only 120 of the 356 eyes (34%) were available at 12 months. We also evaluated manifest refraction instead of cycloplegic refraction postoperatively, which has the advantage reflecting a real-life scenario. However, hyperopia might be underestimated. Cycloplegic refraction has the advantage that no accommodation occurs, but the dilated pupil makes it difficult to measure corneal refraction, especially postoperatively. A multifocal effect is created by the annular ablation profile, which makes it even more difficult to reliably refract these eyes. In addition, we would expect an apparent undercorrection as part of the incoming light is refracted by an annular zone of the cornea of lower refractive power, surrounding the central, fully corrected zone.

We did not use an artificial pupil in our study. To

evaluate the accuracy and stability, we relied on manifest refraction. We also observed a lower predictability of toric corrections and residual astigmatism in a significant number of cases. The most likely reason is axis misalignment. As the treated astigmatism was high (up to 7.50 D), even a slight misalignment of the axis could lead to significant undercorrections, considering an undercorrection of approximately 30% per 10° axis shift.[12]

The results show that LASIK is safe and effective in low and moderate spherical hyperopia. Results are less accurate in low and moderate toric hyperopia. For high hyperopia and high hyperopic astigmatism, visual acuity, predictability, and safety were sufficiently poor, advising against LASIK in these groups.

REFERENCES

1. Grandon SC, Sanders DR, Anello RD, Jacobs D, Biscaro M. Clinical evaluation of hexagonal keratotomy for the treatment of primary hyperopia. *J Cataract Refract Surg.* 1995;21:140-149.
2. Kezirian GM, Gremillion CM. Automated lamellar keratoplasty for the correction of hyperopia. *J Cataract Refract Surg.* 1995;21:386-392.
3. Manche EE, Judge A, Maloney RK. Lamellar keratoplasty for hyperopia. *Journal of Refractive Surgery.* 1996;12:42-49.
4. Koch DD, Kohnen T, McDonnell PJ, Menefee R, Berry M. Hyperopia correction by noncontact holmium: YAG laser thermal keratoplasty. *Ophthalmology.* 1997;104:1938-1947.
5. Dausch D, Klein R, Schroder E. Excimer laser photorefractive keratectomy for hyperopia. *J Refract Corneal Surg.* 1993;9:20-28.
6. Waring GO. Evaluating new refractive surgical procedures: free market madness versus regulatory rigor mortis. *Journal of Refractive Surgery.* 1995;11:335-339.
7. Knorz MC, Wiesinger B, Liermann A, Seiberth V, Liesenhoff H. LASIK for moderate and high myopia and myopic astigmatism. *Ophthalmology.* 1998;105:932-940.
8. Daya SM, Tappouni FR, Habib NE. Photorefractive keratectomy for hyperopia. *Ophthalmology.* 1997;104:1952-1958.
9. Jackson WB, Casson E, Hodge WG, Mintsioulis G, Agapitos PJ. Laser vision correction for low hyperopia. *Ophthalmology.* 1998;105:1727-1738.
10. Vinciguerra P, Epstein D, Radice P, Azzolini M. Long-term results of photorefractive keratectomy for hyperopia and hyperopic astigmatism. *Journal of Refractive Surgery.* 1998;14(suppl):S183-185.
11. Pietilä J, Mäkinen P, Pajari S, Uusitalo H. Excimer laser photorefractive keratectomy for hyperopia. *Journal of Refractive Surgery.* 1997;13:504-510.
12. Knorz MC, Koch DD, Martinez-Franco C, Lorger CV. Effect of pupil size and astigmatism on contrast acuity with monofocal and bifocal intraocular lenses. *J Cataract Refract Surg.* 1994;20:26-33.
13. McDonnell PJ. Excimer laser photorefractive keratectomy-the food and drug administration panel speaks. *Arch Ophthalmol.* 1995;113:858-859.
14. Applegate RA, Howland HC. Magnification and visual acuity in refractive surgery. *Arch Ophthalmol.* 1993;111:1335-1342.

Treating Hyperopia
Till Anschütz, MD

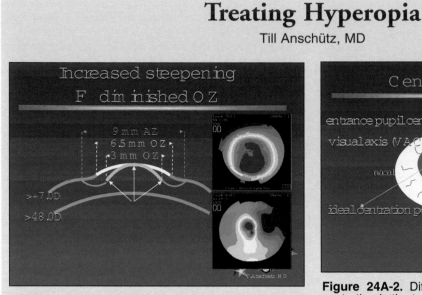

Figure 24A-1. K-readings over 48 D significantly reduce optical zone sizes.

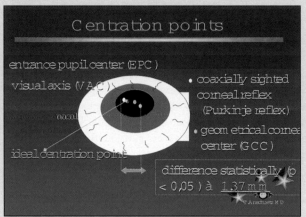

Figure 24A-2. Different centration points. The ideal centration is the temporal border of the Purkinje reflex.

LASIK treatment of hyperopia is the logical evolution of this technique considering the success of myopic LASIK. However, central steepening of the cornea makes the planned correction of the hyperopic eye more difficult compared to the treatment of myopia. Numerous attempts have been described.

What are the elements of successful treatments?

K-reading: Obviously, biomechanical and corneal structure limits exaggerated corneal steepening. K-readings over 48 D increase the complication rate dramatically for H-LASIK and H-PRK and reduce the effective optical zone. Optical zones of 6.0 mm will be diminished to less than 4.0 mm in H-LASIK (or H-PRK) treatments if the preoperative refraction is more than +6 D (Figure 24A-1).

Frequently, retreatments (H-LASIK and H-PRK) with increased corneal steepening provoke a kind of biomechanical central corneal reaction like a pseudo-Salzman nodule. We call this an apical scar.

Optical zone: The influence of the optical zone in successful hyperopic treatment is more important than in myopic treatments. Our own experience demonstrates that optical zones greater than 5.5 mm improve the refractive outcome of hyperopic treatments. Optical zones less than 5.5 mm increase the complication risks due to a high loss of BCVA.

Flap size: A large optical zone of 6.0 mm requires an ablation zone of 8.5 to 9.0 mm and a flap size for H-LASIK of 9.3 mm. New microkeratomes allow this flap size. The concern with small optical zones is the increased dependence on perfect centration. An optical zone of 5.0 mm is minimized to 3.0 mm after a decentration of only 1.0 mm.

If the flap size is smaller than 9.0 mm, the peripheral ablation may compromise the hinge and reduce the LASIK-specific induced smaller optical zone.

Centration and fixation: Correct centration and fixation are other important aspects of treating hyperopia.

After examining more than 1000 hyperopic eyes, we demonstrated that nearly 90% of all hyperopic eyes fixate nasally and mostly superonasally. In comparison, myopic eyes fixate mostly centrally (77%). This is an important difference for the centration procedure in treating hyperopia. There are four possible points of centration (Figure 24A-2):

1. The entrance pupil center (EPC), incorrectly considered as the corneal intercept of the line of sight.
2. The geometrical corneal center (GCC).
3. The Purkinje reflex (coaxially sighted corneal reflex) as the corneal intercept of the fixation line to the corneal apex.
4. The visual axis center (VAC).

Statistically, (p < 0.005) the line between these external centration points is 1.4 mm. For centration, this amounts to a big difference with a significant influence on visual outcome. What is the ideal centration point?

Ideal centration point: Our experience shows that the VAC is the correct point for centration. This is the real line of sight—the line between fixation and focal point.

This VAC is situated near to the Purkinje reflex on

the line between the EPC and the coaxially sighted corneal reflex (Purkinje reflex). Because the statistical difference between the Purkinje reflex and VAC amounts to only 0.1 to 0.3 mm, we recommend,as a technically easy and safe way of marking, the temporal border of the Purkinje reflex as the ideal centration point (see Figure 24A-1).

Summary: Treating hyperopia is different from treating myopia and much more difficult (biomechanically different in smaller eyes). Treating hyperopia is limited (+5 D), requires a larger flap size (9.5 mm), and requires exact centration (VAC). Complications include the increased risk of decentration and poor postoperative refractive outcome (loss of BCVA). Additionally, optimized optical and transition zone profiles will help avoid high regression and establish H-LASIK as a safe and effective procedure.

LASIK for Hyperopia

Thomas Kohnen, MD

While the surgical correction of myopia and astigmatism has been of great interest in the last two decades, the surgical correction of hyperopia has remained an elusive goal. In most of our patients, hyperopia does not exceed +3.0 D. The refraction rarely falls in the range of +6.0 to +8.0 D. In comparison to myopic corneal correction in which the main objective is to flatten the central cornea, in hyperopia the central cornea has to be steepened to gain corneal power. To achieve central corneal steepening by photoablation using the excimer laser, stromal tissue must be removed in a ring-shaped fashion around the corneal center. The ablation profile typically consists of a refractive central untreated zone or optical zone (OZ) and a peripheral ablation zone. Historically, the first hyperopic treatments using the excimer laser were performed with photorefractive keratectomy (PRK) using a refractive zone between 4.0 to 5.0 mm. The central 1.0 to 2.0 mm were untreated; at the periphery of the refractive zone, a transition zone of 2.0 to 3.0 mm was added, making the entire ablation diameter 7.0 to 8.0 mm. More recently, the refractive untreated zone was enlarged to 6.0 mm and the total ablation zone to 9.0 mm.

In hyperopic PRK, the main disadvantages have been regression due to epithelial hyperplasia, annular haze, and central corneal scars (apical scars). These complications seem to be avoided by LASIK; however, the main problem in lamellar surgery for hyperopia has been the development of the flap (safety and being sufficiently large enough to perform the peripheral ablation of stromal tissue).

Typical complications of LASIK, either myopic or hyperopic, are epithelial ingrowth, flap irregularities, and striae. LASIK can be safely performed for low hyperopia (+1.00 to +3.00 D) and good results are still achievable for medium hyperopia (+3.00 to +5.00 D). For high hyperopia (+5.00 to +8.00 D), LASIK is not recommended because of loss of BCVA. In primary hyperopia with astigmatism lower than 1 D and presbyopic patients, our preferred method is treatment with noncontact LTK using the Sunrise Sun 1000 corneal shaping system. In all other cases of hyperopia up to 5 D and hyperopic astigmatism, LASIK is performed. The example in Figures 24C-1a through 24C-1c demonstrate the results of such a patient after hyperopic LASIK. In these figures, treatment of hyperopic astigmatism occurred on the flat meridian at 30°. The laser ablation was performed in plus cylinder treating +1.5 +2.5/120°, OZ = 6.0 mm, peripheral ablation depth of 53 μm. The UCVA increased from 20/63 (0.32) to 20/32 (0.63) in this amblyopic eye, BCVA was preoperatively +3.0 -2.5/20° = 20/32 (0.63), 1 month postoperatively +1.25 -0.75/20° = 20/20- (1.0).

Our current hyperopic LASIK technique includes the use of a microkeratome producing a 9.5 mm flap by a down to upward rotational cut (Hansatome). The excimer ablation is performed with a scanning laser that produces a 200 μm spot and lasers the cornea in a randomized fashion (Keracor 217). In all patients currently treated with this technique, we use a 6.0-mm OZ.

The most important step in hyperopic treatments is the centration of the excimer ablation. Even small decentrations will cause optical problems for the patient, which can be detected by videokeratography. The Keracor 217 has an active eye tracker, which allows a perfectly centered ablation once the tracker is activated. We use the line-of-sight centration technique rather than pupil-based centration. The patient fixates on a red fixation light (while the untreated eye is covered), and the laser is locked in this position. The centration maneuver is done after the lamellar cut has been performed, and the peripheral ablation of corneal tissue is immediately performed. After cleaning the stromal bed and inner side of the flap with BSS, the flap is repositioned. Potential debris is cleaned with a cannula that floods BSS under the replaced flap. The surgeon watches the flap for a 2-minute period to make sure the flap is reattached. During these 2 minutes, the central flap is moistened with BSS

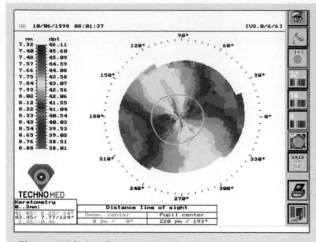

Figure 24C-1a. Preoperative corneal topography map of the right eye showing a mean corneal power of 42.24 D and a corneal astigmatism of 2.42 D (Technomed C-Scan, regular map).

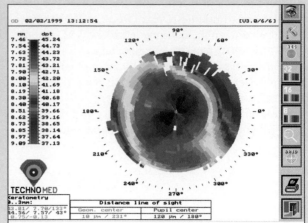

Figure 24C-1b. One-month postoperative corneal topography map of the right eye demonstrating a mean corneal power of 44.19 D and a corneal astigmatism of 0.75 D (Technomed C-Scan, regular map).

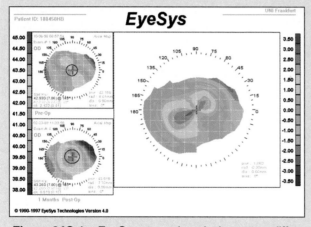

Figure 24C-1c. EyeSys corneal analysis system difference map showing an increase in corneal power of 1.66 D.

and the gutter of the reattached flap is checked with a wet Merocel sponge.

After antibiotic eye drop application the patient rests for approximately 1 hour, and the flap position is rechecked at the slit lamp. Postoperative visits are usually performed in our clinic at 1 day, 1 week, 1, 4, and 12 months postoperatively. Postoperative treatment consists of steroid/antibiotic eyedrops instilled three times a day for the first week. Only if interface problems occur are topical nonsteroids or steroids used for a longer period.

Treating Hyperopia

Luis Antonio Ruiz, MD

We have been using LASIK for hyperopia for 5 years with the Chiron Technolas Keracor 116. Because of the good results we have achieved, we have used it regularly to correct up to 8 D with an optic zone of 4.2 and 4.5 mm and a peripheral ablation of 8.5 to 8.8 mm.

After reviewing 350 operated eyes 1 year after surgery, we have found, on average, the following results:

	Preop	1 month	1 year
VASC	20/60	20/50	20/30
VACC	20/20	20/30	20/25
Sphere	+3.50	-0.30	+0.2

After the first postoperative year, there is remarkable stability with all these parameters. The accuracy and safety will be analyzed with another group of patients.

The characteristics of the Schwind excimer laser with fractal masks have led us to use it routinely for hyperopic corrections.

By reducing the ablation time, we have better and faster recovery. For +10 D correction, the ablation time with the Schwind laser is approximately 34 seconds, or about one-twentieth the time required with other lasers.

Some other important characteristics of this laser are:
- Ablations with large optical zone of 7.0 mm
- Good and reliable eye tracking system
- Astigmatic algorithm with positive or negative cylinders

With these considerations, we have corrected up to +17 D with excellent results (eg, aphakic patients). Following is a summary of the results by groups.

VASC

100 eyes	Preop	1 month	6 months
+0.75 to +4.0	20/80+	20/30+	20/30+
n = 35			
+4.25 to +8.0	20/80	20/40+	20/30
n = 55			
+8.25 to +17	20/400	20/60	20/50
n = 10			

VACC

	Preop	1 month	6 months
+0.75 to +4.0	20/20-	20/25+	20/20-
+4.25 to +8.0	20/25	20/25-	20/25
+8.25 to +17	20/30	20/40-	20/30

Sphere

	Preop	1 month	6 months
+0.75 to +4.0	+2.15	+0.39	+0.48
+4.25 to +8.0	+5.29	+0.75	+0.62
+8.25 to +17	+12.77	+1.22	+1.10

Tables 24D-1 and 24D-2 demonstrate the distribution of postoperative refractive errors. Both groups are similar, but the Schwind group has a much greater safety rate.

In conclusion, it is possible to correct hyperopia with LASIK (even in very high degrees) with safety, accuracy, and fast recovery. Even in patients with very high curvature after surgery we have not encountered problems, because they still have good vision and the contrast sensitivity test is always better postoperatively than preoperatively.

Table 24D-1

SAFETY
Lines of vision (BSCVA)
(postoperative 6 months vs preoperative)

Technolas			Schwind	
52.4%	0.4%	+ 2 o >	0	77%
	1.4%	+ 1	12.2%	
	50.6%	0	64.8%	
	28.6%	- 1	17.6%	
	19%	- 2 o >	5.4%	

Table 24D-2

ACCURACY
(6 months postoperatively)

Technolas		Schwind
11.9%	< -1 D	2.78%
78.6%	± 1 D	75%
9.5%	> +1 D	22.22%

QUALITY OF VISION AFTER LASIK

Michael C. Knorz, MD

All refractive surgical procedures change the optics of the eye. Part of this change, namely the change in overall refractive power, is the actual purpose of the procedure and is therefore welcomed. Another part leads to undesired side effects and should therefore be minimized. When I started to perform LASIK in 1993, a few of us who performed this procedure corrected refractive errors up to -30 diopters (D) in some patients. The more we learned about LASIK in the years to follow, the more we became aware of the importance of a new aspect of refractive surgery: the quality of vision we provide to our patients.

Our patients and staff were excited about an uncorrected vision of 20/25, or 0.8, after we performed a correction of -20 D. However, as time went by, more and more of these patients told us how excited they were, but they reported good vision in bright light, and their next words were "...well, as soon as I am in a room everything gets blurry and foggy. Can you do anything about this?" In the beginning we might not have listened carefully enough, but with increasing experience most of us heard this story over and over again, so we started to look for possible ways to do better. Our interest focused not only on visual acuity and refraction, but we began to investigate the quality of vision after refractive surgery in great detail.

In this chapter, we will consider corneal refractive surgical procedures only. The influence of the lens will therefore be neglected for the purpose of this chapter. This leaves the change in corneal refraction and the diameter of the pupil to be considered. The change in corneal refraction is defined by the diameter of the part of the cornea that was corrected and by the amount of correction (and, to a lesser extent, by the diameter and steepness of the transition zone, if any was used). In addition, the centration of the ablation zone plays a significant role.

For the purpose of this study, we will also initially assume a well-centered zone of correction. The diameter of the zone that received the full amount of correction will only be given. This zone will be called the planned optical zone. It is the part of the cornea that receives full correction by the excimer laser ablation. As the ablation is performed in the stroma and as some epithelial remodeling will occur after treatment, the diameter of the finally achieved optical zone is somewhat smaller than the diameter of the planned optical zone. For the purpose of this chapter, however, we will use the planned optical zone. We will compare different amounts of correction at a given zone size but with varying pupil sizes to estimate the quality of vision under different lighting conditions. Finally, we will look at the effect of decentration on optical quality.

METHODS

We used the Technomed C-Scan corneal topography system. This system offers a software module called "ray tracing analysis." Simplified, this software will, for a given topographic map, trace rays of light through the cornea and pupil and calculate the image on the retina. The effect of the lens will not be included. Any retinal compensation mechanisms (eg, Stilles-Crawford effect) will not be considered either. The software will then create a pictorial that shows the actual topographic map on the lower left, a surface quality map on the upper left, and a kind of a color-coded light intensity graph on the right side (Figure 25-1). On the upper right side, the light intensity is viewed from the side. The narrower the distribution, the better the quality. A broad base, on the other hand, suggests poor image quality due to a lot of light scattering. On the lower right, the same is shown in a two-dimensional display. Blue colors indicate a high light intensity, red colors indicate a low light intensity. Ideally, there should be two distinct small blue spots on the two-dimensional map shown on the lower right. Due to some aberrations inherent to any optical system, an

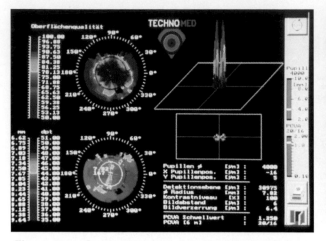

Figure 25-1. Ray-tracing map of the Technomed C-Scan system in an eye after LASIK to correct -3 D.

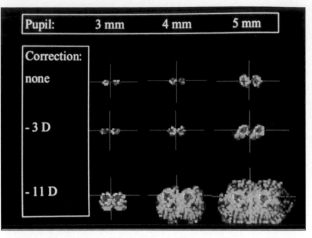

Figure 25-2. Point images in normal eyes and in eyes after LASIK for myopia at different pupil sizes (images calculated using ray tracing by the Technomed C-Scan).

ideal image cannot be expected. Simplified again, this two-dimensional graph can be directly compared to what the patient sees: two well-defined small blue spots indicate excellent quality of vision, while large halos indicate very poor quality of vision. The halo visible in this graph is similar to the halo a patient will experience around light at the given pupil size.

This does not, however, take into consideration the psychophysical mechanisms of compensation we use unconsciously to compensate for the halos. Fortunately, our brain, much like an image-processing computer, filters the unwanted information (the halo), and the halo is not subjectively perceived. This process explains why many of our highly myopic patients who underwent LASIK function reasonably well and do not complain of halos. On the other hand, even if the halos are not perceived, the sheer amount of scattered light will reduce contrast sensitivity and quality of vision in these patients.

Below the two graphs on the right of the c-scan, the pupil size and, among other values, the predicted visual acuity are given. The observer can manually change the pupil size for a given map, and the system will then recalculate the image for this new pupil size. The quality of vision for a given topographic map can therefore be simulated at different pupil sizes.

We will compare a normal cornea to different myopic corrections and one hyperopic correction. All eyes were treated with LASIK using the Keracor 117 C excimer laser and the Automated Corneal Shaper (ACS). The following corrections were included:

- -3 D, 6.0 mm planned optical zone
- -11 D, 5.0 mm planned optical zone
- +5 D, 5.5 mm planned optical zone

We will use the color-coded light intensity maps

only because I feel they provide the best way of understanding the optical effects of corneal refractive surgery.

Myopia Correction

The calculated retinal images of a normal eye, an eye that received a -3 D correction, and an eye that received a -11 D correction were plotted in Figure 25-2. Figure 25-2 clearly demonstrates that the quality of vision decreases with increasing pupil size for a given amount of correction. Part of this decrease is normal and due to increasing optical aberrations with larger pupil sizes, as visible by the increasing blur circles even in a normal eye at large pupil sizes.

Comparing a -3 D correction to a normal eye, we see that results are almost identical, and that a faint halo is visible even at large pupil sizes. This demonstrates a high quality of vision after LASIK in low myopia. Using a 6 mm or larger planned optical zone size, we will therefore provide excellent quality of vision to patients with low myopia.

Results are very different in high myopia. Looking at a -11 D correction with a 5.0 mm planned optical zone, a significant loss of visual quality becomes obvious even at small pupil sizes. The halos are large and confluent, which correlate to a clinically significant loss of visual quality. These findings correlate again with our clinical observation that small optical zones and/or high amounts of correction lead to subjective visual impairment in a certain number of patients.

The results presented in myopia lead, with some simplification, to the following conclusions:

1. Myopia of up to -5 D may be correctable without loss of visual quality
2. Myopia of -5 to -10 D may be correctable with some, probably acceptable, loss of visual quality.

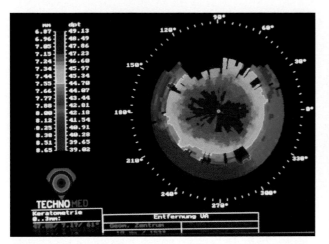

Figure 25-3. Refractive power map after LASIK to correct +5 D (Technomed C-Scan, optical zone 6.0 mm).

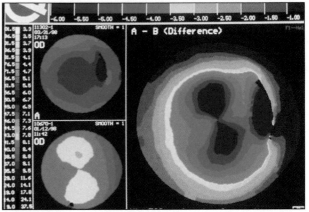

Figure 25-4. Axial power maps and differential map before and after LASIK to correct -5 D of myopia and -2 D of astigmatism (preoperative map, lower left; postoperative map, upper left; differential map, right; Tomey TMS-1).

3. Myopia of more than -10 D is correctable only with significant visual loss.
4. The diameter of the planned optical zone should be as large as possible (at least 6.0 mm).
5. The flap size should be large enough to accommodate the large ablation zones.

In the correction of myopia, we must not only consider the predictability of our treatment but also the quality of vision that can be achieved. We must inform our patients accordingly. We must tell them that quality of vision will be extremely poor in corrections of more than about -10 D, and we should discourage them from undergoing LASIK, as other procedures provide better quality of vision, such as phakic intraocular lenses (IOLs). We must also tell patients that some loss of visual quality will occur in corrections of about - 5 to - 10 D, especially in patients with large pupils. On the other hand, the above results are very encouraging in low myopia. We can inform these patients that LASIK will not alter their quality of vision at all, and that the most recent technologies, such as customized ablation (see Chapter 26), may even improve their quality of vision as compared to the preoperative level.

It was previously stated that the planned optical zone should be at least 6.0 mm in diameter. This requirement by itself limits the amount of correction that can be performed as the amount of corneal tissue that can be safely removed is limited. Today, most surgeons agree that minimal thickness of the stromal bed after the ablation should be 250 μm or even 50% of the total corneal thickness, whichever is larger. We must therefore consider corneal thickness in each individual eye treated. In very thick corneas, we may be able to push the limit toward higher corrections, as more tissue can be safely ablated. In thin corneas, on the other hand, the limit may even be

lower, as there is less tissue to be ablated. It is important we understand these relations and use them both in treatment planning and patient counseling.

Hyperopia Correction

Figure 25-3 shows the topographic map of an eye that underwent LASIK for +5 D of hyperopia. A 6.0 mm planned optical zone was used, and the ablation was well centered, as is clearly visible in the figure. Figure 25-4 shows the pre- and postoperative axial power maps, as well as the differential map of an eye that underwent LASIK for -5 D of myopia and -2 D of with-the-rule astigmatism (right eye). The postoperative refraction of the right eye at 1 year is +0.25 D, and uncorrected visual acuity (UCVA) is 20/16, or 1.25. Halos were not perceived during the day but a faint halo was sometimes visible around light sources at night. It is not disturbing and visible only when willingly paying attention, but its presence shows that the ray-tracing images provide a valid means to evaluate the effect of corneal refractive surgery on the optical or visual quality of the eye.

Figure 25-5 compares the calculated retinal images of these two eyes. Comparing hyperopic and myopic corrections, the halo is larger after hyperopic corrections than after myopic corrections, which indicates a lower quality of vision after hyperopic corrections. These findings are consistent with clinical observations and partially explain why the upper limit of hyperopic corrections is about +5 D, whereas it is about -10 D for myopic corrections.

Decentration

Figure 25-6 shows a -8 D correction (5.5 mm planned optical zone) that is significantly decentered. Looking at the light intensity distribution of the calculated retinal

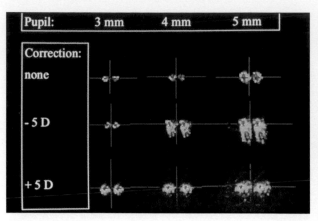

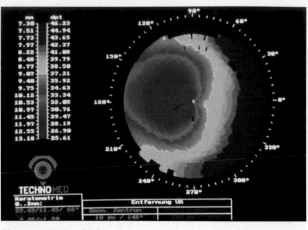

Figure 25-5. Point images in normal eyes and after LASIK for hyperopia and myopia at different pupil sizes (images calculated using ray tracing by the Technomed C-Scan).

Figure 25-6. Refractive power map of a decentered myopic ablation (-8 D, 5.5 mm planned optical zone using the Technomed C-Scan).

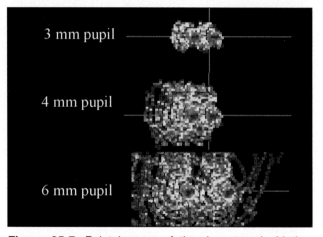

Figure 25-7. Point images of the decentered ablation shown in Figure 25-5 at different pupil sizes (images calculated using ray tracing by the Technomed C-Scan).

image at different pupil sizes (Figure 25-7), the significant loss of visual quality and severe complaints of patients can be clearly appreciated. Even with a small pupil, large and decentered halos are formed. These patients will complain about monocular diplopia in most situations, except in bright sunlight. They will precisely describe the shape and orientation of the second image, and it is quite understandable that they are extremely unhappy with their vision. Treatment is difficult in these patients. Nonsurgical treatment includes the use of miotic drops and rigid gas-permeable contact lenses.

Surgical treatment used to be more an art than a science but became far more predictable following the introduction of customized ablations, so-called topographic-assisted LASIK, based on corneal topography (see Chapter 26). Figure 25-7 stresses that any decentration of the ablation will further decrease visual quality and must be avoided at any cost. The chance of decentration can be minimized by carefully observing a number of variables during surgery. My personal approach is first to ensure that the position of the patient's head under the laser is horizontal and that it remains so during the ablation. Second, I center the treatment on the center of the entrance pupil. Third, I use the active eye tracker of the Keracor 117C or 217 excimer laser, and I visually confirm that the coaxial treatment beam is precisely in the center of the entrance pupil once the eye tracker is locked on target. Finally, I monitor fixation during the ablation, as the eye tracker will shift once the focal plane is changed. Using these precautions, decentration is extremely rare.

CONCLUSION

The purpose of this chapter was to demonstrate the importance of quality of vision when performing refrac-

tive surgery. The described technique of ray-tracing analysis provides an excellent tool to understand the relationship of optical zone size, amount of correction, and pupil size in formation of the retinal image. The key benefit of this understanding is the ability to better advise patients on what to expect. We now know that low myopia can be corrected without loss of quality of vision. We also learned that moderate to high myopia can be corrected only once some loss of quality of vision is accepted, especially in patients with large pupils. We finally came to understand why the amount of correction that can be performed at the cornea is limited, and that extreme myopes as well as high hyperopes will have a poor quality of vision after LASIK. Other techniques, such a phakic IOLs or clear lens extraction, will provide a higher quality of vision in these patients and thus seem to be justified despite lack of long-term follow-up.

CUSTOMIZED ABLATIONS IN LASIK

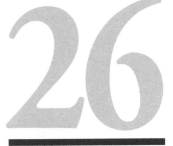

Michael C. Knorz, MD

INTRODUCTION

Current ablation algorithms are either spherical with or without a peripheral transition zone, or elliptical to correct astigmatic errors. They do not allow for customized treatments of corneal irregularities, such as irregular astigmatism. Human corneas, however, are not symmetric or regular; about 40% show some degree of irregularity or asymmetry. These minute irregularities cannot be corrected with spectacles or soft contact lenses, and they will also not be corrected with laser-assisted in situ keratomileusis (LASIK) or photorefractive keratoplasty (PRK) using standard ablation profiles. Surface asymmetries of the cornea may only be corrected with hard contact lenses, which is one of the reasons why hard contact lenses offer a better quality of vision than soft lenses, provided they are tolerated by patients. The use of customized ablation patterns in LASIK is aimed in just the same direction. The ultimate goal is to provide hard contact lens-like vision to our patients, thereby improving their quality of vision beyond that achieved with spectacle correction.

The technology required to perform customized ablations is available. Spot-scanning or flying spot excimer lasers provide the technological platform to perform ablations of any shape. Corneal topography enables us to measure the shape of the cornea with great precision, and elevation-based systems like the Orbscan provide an even better basis for the calculation of the required ablation.

Could we combine corneal topography and scanning lasers to create customized ablations? This question posed quite a challenge when we started to treat our first patients with so-called topography-assisted LASIK a few years ago. The system definitely worked, but a lot of fine tuning was required to establish the algorithms used today. In this chapter, I will describe the long-term

results of our first patients and then the results achieved with the current treatment algorithm. In our first group, we treated patients with severe corneal irregularities following trauma or corneal surgery. Once we had established that the idea worked, we started to treat "normal" eyes, which meant those 40% of eyes that exhibited some degree of asymmetry but we are still classified as within the normal range.

PART I: TREATMENT OF SEVERE CORNEAL IRREGULARITIES

Patients

In our initial prospective study, we evaluated 29 eyes of 27 patients treated between July 1996 and July 1997. Inclusion criteria included irregular corneal astigmatism due to trauma or previous corneal surgery. We considered topography-assisted LASIK their last option prior to performing a corneal graft. Eyes were divided into four groups:

- Group 1 (post-keratoplasty group) consisted of six eyes (five patients) with irregular corneal astigmatism after penetrating keratoplasty. All grafts were performed more than 2 years prior.
- Group 2 (post-trauma group) consisted of six eyes (six patients) with irregular corneal astigmatism after corneal trauma. Trauma dated back more than 2 years in all eyes.
- Group 3 (decentered/small optical zones group) consisted of 11 eyes (10 patients) with irregular corneal astigmatism after PRK (one eye) or LASIK (10 eyes) due to decentered or small optical zones. All patients complained of halos and image distortion even during the day.
- Group 4 (central islands group) consisted of six eyes (six patients) with irregular astigmatism

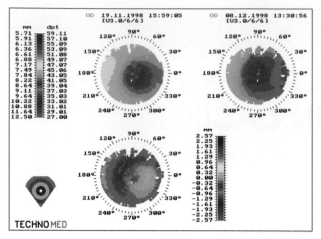

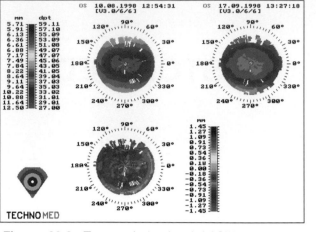

Figure 26-1. Topography-assisted LASIK to treat decentration. The preoperative topographic map (upper left) shows a decentered optical zone following treatment of myopia. The postoperative topographic map (upper right) shows a centered optical zone after treatment with topographically guided LASIK. The differential map (lower left) shows that recentration was achieved by an asymmetrical, customized ablation.

Figure 26-2. Topography-assisted LASIK to enlarge small optical zones. The preoperative topographic map (upper left) shows the small optical zone, the postoperative map (upper right) shows the significantly enlarged optical zone after treatment. The differential map is shown on the lower left.

after PRK (two eyes) or LASIK (four eyes) due to central islands or keyhole patterns. All patients complained of blurred vision or image distortion even during the day.

Procedure

Surgery was performed using topical anesthesia and the Automated Corneal Shaper (8.5-mm flap, 160-µm thickness plate). We used the Keracor 117C excimer laser. This laser uses a 2.0-mm beam, which is scanned across the cornea at a shot frequency of 50 Hz. It was modified by including an aperture that allows the use of both a 1.0-mm beam and a 2.0-mm beam.

Topography in the initial study was performed with the Corneal Analysis System (EyeSys System 2000, Software Version 3.10 and 3.20, EyeSys Premier, Irvine, Calif, USA). The ablation was based on the preoperative corneal topographic map. Once the topography was taken, the true curvature map data (axial radii of curvature) were copied and sent to Bausch & Lomb Surgical Technolas. The axial radii of curvature were converted into true corneal height values using a special software program and algorithm developed by Technolas. We had to provide the desired postoperative corneal refractive power (target k-value in diopters), the maximum ablation depth ,and the manifest refraction. The target k-value was determined as follows: the k-values of the steepest and flattest corneal meridian within the central 4.0-mm zone were taken and the mean value of these two was calculated. Because we were aiming for emmetropia in all eyes, the spherical equivalent of the

manifest refraction was then added to the mean k-value. Based on this data, Technolas calculated a session file that basically contained information for the scanning laser on which ablation pattern to perform. The session file was transferred to us by e-mail and loaded into the Keracor 117C excimer laser just prior to treatment.

Results

Figure 26-1 shows the treatment of a decentered myopic correction using topography-assisted LASIK, and Figure 26-2 shows the treatment of a small optical zone using topography-assisted LASIK. The results of our initial study using the Corneal Analysis System were presented at the American Academy of Ophthalmology Annual Meeting in New Orleans in 1998 and submitted for publication to *Ophthalmology*. The results are shown in part in Table 26-1. In the post-keratoplasty group and in the post-trauma group, corrective cylinder was significantly reduced as compared to the preoperative value. The topographic success rate was defined as either the planned correction fully achieved or the attempted correction partially achieved (decrease of irregularity of more than 1 diopter (D) on the differential map and/or increase of optical zone size by at least 1.0 mm). The success rate was highest in the decentered/small optical zones group (91%), followed by the post-trauma group who had a success rate of 83%. The lowest success rate was observed in the central island group- only 50%. Overall, 14 of the 29 eyes were reoperated (48%) due to regression of effect or undercorrection. The rate of reoperations was lowest in the decentered/small optical

Table 26-1			
REFRACTION, VISUAL ACUITY, AND CORNEAL TOPOGRAPHY 12 MONTHS AFTER TOPOGRAPHY–ASSISTED LASIK			
	Group 1 **post-keratoplasty**	**Group 2** **post-trauma**	**Group 3** **decentered/small**	**Group 4** **central islands**
No of eyes	n = 6	n = 6	n = 11	n = 6
Preop cylinder	5.83 ± 1.25 D (4.00 to 8.00 D)	2.21 ± 1.35 D (1.00 to 5.00 D)	0.73 ± 0.71 D (0 to 2.00 D)	1.42 ± 1.13 D (0 to 3.50 D)
Cylinder at 12 mos	2.96 ± 1.23 D* (1.50 to 4.50 D)	0.50 ± 0.84 D** (0 to 2.5 D)	0.36 ± 1.05 D (0 to 3.5 D)	0.50 ± 0.84 D* (0 to 2.00 D)
Success rate (topography as planned or improved)	66% (n = 4)	83% (n = 5)	91% (n = 10)	50% (n = 3)
Reoperation rate	50% (n = 3)	50% (n = 3)	36% (n = 4)	50% (n = 3)

*$p = 0.01$; **$p = 0.001$

zones group—36% as compared to 50% in all other groups (see Table 26-1).

These results demonstrate that topography-assisted LASIK definitely works. We were able to significantly reduce irregularities in these extremely irregular corneas. On the other hand, our results demonstrated that most eyes were undercorrected, and we had to adjust the algorithm to take care of the undercorrection. Finally, the problem of targeting the right spot on the cornea must be addressed. The results of group 4 (central islands) were poor, which suggests that we may not have hit the right target in these eyes featuring small and circumscribed irregularities. Ideally, the laser should be locked on a topographic map of the cornea prior to treatment, and that is what we are currently working on to improve the results in these rare cases.

PART II: CUSTOMIZED ABLATIONS IN NORMAL EYES

Patients

Based on the very encouraging results in severely irregular corneas, we started another study involving routine treatments in so-called "normal" eyes. We treated one eye of the patients with standard LASIK, and one eye with topography-assisted LASIK. Surgery on the second eye was performed 1 day after the first eye. Preoperative refraction was -7.85 ± 1.4 D in the topography-assisted LASIK eyes, and -7.12 ± 1.6 D in the fellow eyes. Mean preoperative spectacle-corrected visual acuity was 20/22 ± 20/95 in the LASIK-treated eyes and 20/19.8 ± 20/105 in the TA-LASIK treated eyes.

Procedure

The Hansatome microkeratome was used to cut a 9.5-mm hinged flap. The 180-μm thickness plate was used in all eyes. After the cut, suction was released, and the corneal flap was then carefully displaced upward using a blunt spatula. The coaxial Helium-Neon (He-Ne) laser of the Keracor 117C excimer laser was centered over the middle of the entrance pupil, and the eye tracker was engaged. Active eye tracking was used in all eyes as it seems to be essential to guarantee reproducible centration. After the ablation, the back of the flap and the stromal bed were irrigated, and the flap was replaced. Topical treatment with gentamicin and dexamethasone eyedrops was started and continued for 5 days (one drop three times daily).

Topography was performed using the C-Scan topography system and the Orbscan system. The ablation was based on the preoperative corneal topographic map. Three maps were taken, and data were copied and sent to Bausch & Lomb Surgical Technolas. We had to provide the desired postoperative corneal refractive power (target K-value in diopters) and the manifest refraction, as previously explained. Technolas calculated a session file, which was again transferred to us by e-mail and loaded into the Keracor 117C excimer laser just prior to treatment. We also received a pictorial (Figure 26-3), depicting the patient and treatment data (upper left), the preoperative corneal topographic map (lower left), the calculated ablation (as a color-coded map, upper right), and the predicted postoperative corneal topography map (lower right). When commercially available, the software to customize ablations will be installed on the topography system to avoid the need for file transfers via e-mail.

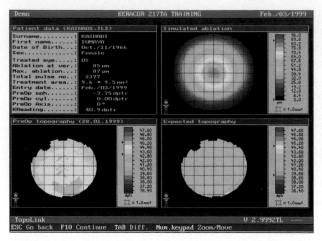

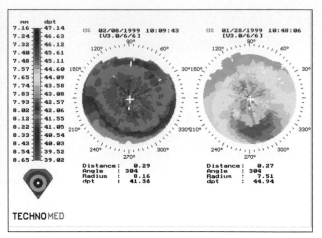

Figure 26-3. Pictorial of the calculated treatment of an eye with slightly asymmetric with-the-rule astigmatism. Shown are the patient and treatment data (upper left), the preoperative corneal topographic map (lower left), the calculated ablation (as a color-coded map, upper right), and the predicted postoperative corneal topography map (lower right)(courtesy of Maria Arbelaez, MD).

Figure 26-4. Side-by-side comparison of the pre- and postoperative corneal topographic maps of the eye corresponding to the treatment plan shown in Figure 26-3. The preoperative map (right) shows with-the-rule astigmatism, which is slightly asymmetric, the lower half meridian being steeper than the upper half meridian. The postoperative map (left) shows a centered and symmetrical ablation zone, demonstrating the benefits of customized ablations based on corneal topography (courtesy of Maria Arbelaez, MD).

Results

Figure 26-4 shows one of the eyes treated with topography-assisted LASIK. The preoperative map (right) shows with-the-rule astigmatism, which is slightly asymmetric, with the lower half meridian being steeper than the upper half meridian. The postoperative map (left) shows a centered and symmetrical ablation zone, demonstrating the benefits of customized ablations based on corneal topography. Preoperative refraction was -3 sphere -0.5 cyl axis 180°, spectacle-corrected acuity was 20/20. Postoperative refraction was plano, and uncorrected visual acuity was 20/10.

Postoperatively, uncorrected acuity was 20/26 ± 20/111 and spectacle-corrected acuity was 20/25 ± 20/143 in the LASIK group, and 20/25 ± 20/133 and 20/23 ± 20/117, respectively, in the topography-assisted LASIK group. Mean spherical equivalent was +0.46 D ± 0.42 D in the LASIK group and +0.14 D ± 0.21 D in the topography-assisted LASIK group. Two eyes in the LASIK group showed a residual astigmatism of -0.5 D and -0.75 D, respectively, while none of the eyes in the topography-assisted LASIK group showed residual astigmatism.

These early results indicate that topography-assisted LASIK works at least as well as a standard LASIK treatment in so-called "normal" eyes and may well be superior in the treatment of astigmatism. To date, the number of eyes treated is still too low for final conclusions. Nevertheless, topography-assisted LASIK seems likely to replace the standard symmetrical ablation pattern used today, enabling us to customize our treatments to the individual needs of our patients.

The work presented here is not based on one individual but on the support of many of my colleagues and friends all over the world. Those who contributed significantly include Dr. Maria Clara Arbelaez, Dr. Jorge Alió, Dr. Stephen G. Slade, Dr. Michiel Kritzinger, and Dr. Thomas Neuhann. All of us were supported by a dedicated team from Bausch & Lomb Technolas in Munich that included Dr. Kristian Hohla, Dr. Gerhard Yousseffi, Martina Sohr, and many others not mentioned by name. I am pleased for the opportunity to thank all of them for their dedication and support.

LASIK CORRECTION OF IRREGULAR ASTIGMATISM

Jorge L. Alió, MD, PhD
Fernando Rodríguez-Mier, MD

27

INTRODUCTION

Benefits of lamellar refractive surgery using laser-assisted in situ keratomileusis (LASIK) include a larger range of refractive errors to be treated more effectively, a relatively shorter visual rehabilitation period postoperatively, a relatively pain-free experience for patients, and a desired minimal healing response as compared to other refractive surgeries. But, as in all kinds of refractive surgery, complications exist that affect visual acuity. One of the most serious is irregular astigmatism.[1]

Precise apposition of wound surfaces after LASIK is essential to normal corneal wound healing, and a wide variety of circumstances can lead to a failure in the healing process. It is important that the clinician is able to identify the intraoperative and postoperative LASIK complications. Recognized complications are microkeratome-related complications and photoablation-related complications. Difficulties with microkeratomes, which may result in flap irregularities, are not uncommon. Photoablation following the creation of the flap has complications similar to those seen in photorefractive keratectomy (PRK). Overhydration or dehydration of the corneal stromal bed may contribute to irregular ablation with resulting astigmatism or unprecise refractive outcome. Photoablation decentration may cause irregular postoperative astigmatism. Following photoablation, the corneal flap must be replaced as closely as possible to its original position. Preplaced marks facilitate correct flap repositioning. Flap wrinkling and torsion, although minimally noticeable under the operating microscope, may nevertheless cause postoperative irregular astigmatism. Epithelial ingrowth causes interface irregularity and visual aberration, often necessitating debridement. Postoperative astigmatism in these instances may also be irregular. Finally, irregular astigmatism may be induced by other previous refractive procedures such as RK, LTK, PRK, and ALK. Among others, penetrating keratoplasty, corneal trauma, and previous keratitis are also potential sources of irregular astigmatism.

Three different corneal refractive procedures have been developed and used by us for the correction of irregular astigmatism: The first procedure, developed by our group, was named selective zonal ablations (SELZA). It is performed using a broadbeam excimer laser. The second procedure also developed by our group, named excimer laser assisted by sodium hyaluronate (ELASHY). It is performed using a flying spot Plano C-Scan excimer laser. An international group under a study protocol has used the third procedure, named topographic-linked excimer laser ablation (topolink). It is performed using a flying spot Plano C-Scan. The procedures were selected according to the irregular astigmatism plane of location and the corneal topographic pattern.

In this chapter we will comment on our experience with a significant number of patients using these techniques.

CLINICAL CLASSIFICATION OF IRREGULAR ASTIGMATISM

In corneal refractive surgery using LASIK, the surgeon uses an automated or manual microkeratome for the creation of the corneal flap and stromal bed. Once the flap is made, the excimer laser is used to ablate tissue from the bed for the planned correction, depending on the capabilities of the laser. Irregular astigmatism may be caused by flap irregularities (Figure 27-1a), stromal bed irregularities (Figure 27-1b), or both (Figure 27-1c), inducing a corneal surface irregularity. First, we must decide where the irregularity is: at the flap, the stromal bed, or in both. Then we must understand the corneal surface topography pattern. We have used the EyeSys 2000 (Holladay Diagnostic Summary, Houston, Texas,

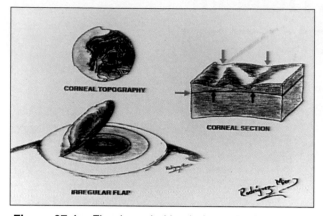

Figure 27-1a. Flap irregularities induced by folds, wrinkles, irregular thin flap, flap dislocation, epithelial ingrowth, free cap, lost cap, etc.

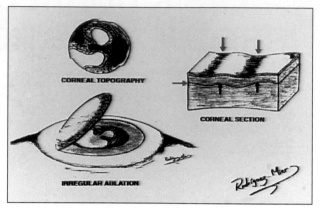

Figure 27-1b. Stromal bed irregularities induced by irregular photoablation, decentered photoablation, irregular cut, etc.

USA) corneal topographer and the C-Scan color ellipsoid topography unit (Technomed Technology, Gmb-H, Germany). For treatment purposes, we have found two corneal topographic patterns: irregular astigmatism with defined pattern and irregular astigmatism with undefined pattern.

CORNEAL TOPOGRAPHY PATTERNS OF IRREGULAR ASTIGMATISM

Irregular Astigmatism With Defined Pattern

Irregular astigmatism with defined pattern is defined as those cases in which the corneal topography map shows a steep area of at least 2.0 mm diameter at the 6.0 mm optical zone area. The corneal topographic irregularity in the central 3.0 mm of the corneal center was classified into five groups:

1. Decentered ablation: shows a corneal topographic pattern with decentered myopic ablation more than 1.5 mm in relation to the center of the cornea. The flattened area is not centered in the cornea; the optical zone of the cornea has one flat and one steep area (Figure 27-2a).
2. Decentered steep: shows a corneal hyperopic treatment decentered more than 1.5 mm in relation to the center of the cornea (Figure 27-2b).
3. Central island: shows an image with an increase in the central power of the ablation zone for myopic treatment ablation at least 3.00 diopters (D) in height and 1.5 mm in diameter, surrounded by areas of lesser curvature (Figure 27-2c).
4. Central irregularity: shows an irregular pattern

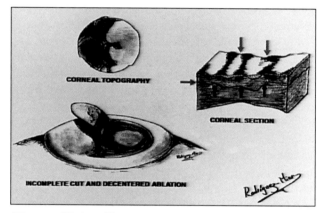

Figure 27-1c. Flap and stromal bed irregularities induced by the LASIK cut.

with more than one area no larger than 1.0 mm and no more than 1.50 D in relation to the flattest radius, located in the area of the myopic ablation treatment (Figure 27-2d).

5. Peripheral irregularity: shows a corneal topographic pattern similar to the central island extending to the periphery. The myopic ablation is not homogeneous. There is a central zone measuring 1.5 mm in diameter and 3.00 D in height that is connected with the periphery of the ablation zone in one meridian (Figure 27-2e).

Irregular Astigmatism With Undefined Pattern

Irregular astigmatism with undefined pattern is defined as a surface with multiple irregularities (big and small, steep and flat areas) with more than one area measuring over 3.0 mm in diameter included in the central area of 6.0 mm (Figure 27-3). The difference between flat and steep areas is not possible to calculate in the profile map. Delta k (keratometry) appears as a

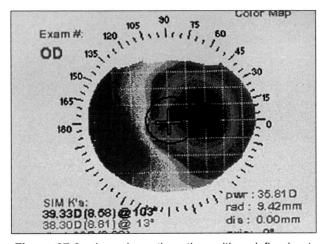

Figure 27-2a. Irregular astigmatism with a defined pattern: decentered ablation.

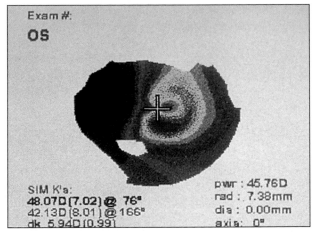

Figure 27-2b. Irregular astigmatism with a defined pattern: decentered steep.

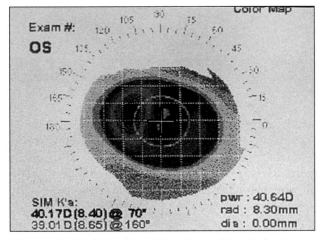

Figure 27-2c. Irregular astigmatism with a defined pattern: central island.

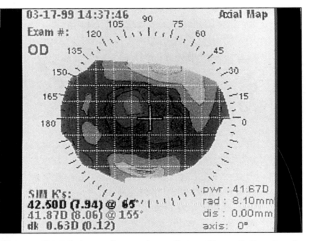

Figure 27-2d. Irregular astigmatism with a defined pattern: central irregularity.

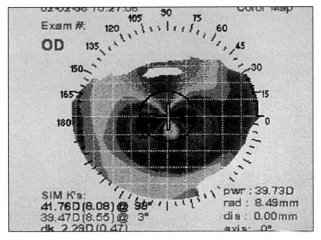

Figure 27-2e. Irregular astigmatism with a defined pattern: peripheral irregularity.

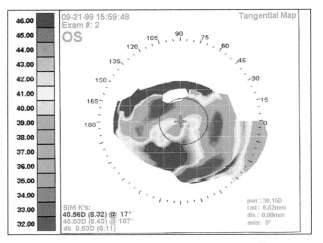

Figure 27-3. Irregular astigmatism with undefined pattern.

plane line or irregularly irregular line. Normally, delta k is the difference between the steep k and the flat k given in diopters at the cross of the profile map.[2] This corneal topography classification is useful to define terms and concepts, to understand the postoperative visual symptoms, and to create a topographic basis for a new treatment.

PREOPERATIVE EVALUATION

A complete preoperative ocular examination was performed, including ocular history, keratometry, ultrasonic pachymetry (Ophthasonic Pachymeter Teknar Inc, St. Louis, Mo, USA), and computerized corneal topography. Preoperative uncorrected and best-corrected visual acuity was recorded using a neutral Boston rigid gas-permeable contact lens. During the preoperative and postoperative period, corneal quality was studied using data offered by the Holladay Diagnostic Summary (corneal uniformity index [CUI], predicted corneal acuity [PCA] and corneal topographic maps).

SURGICAL PROCEDURES WITH THE EXCIMER LASER

We have used three different methods for the surgical correction of irregular astigmatism. At the present time, we use three surgical procedures with the excimer:

1. Selective zonal ablation (SELZA). This is a quantitative method useful for improving irregular astigmatism with defined pattern (Figures 27-2a through 27-2c).[2]
2. Excimer laser assisted by sodium hyaluronate (ELASHY). This is a qualitative method useful for improving irregular astigmatism with undefined pattern (Figure 27-3).[3]
3. Topographic-linked excimer laser ablation (topolink). This is both quantitative and qualitative, and useful for improving irregular astigmatism with defined pattern achieving a refractive programming outcome in the same procedure.

In all cases, we used the topical anaesthesia oxibupacaine 0.2% drops; no patient required sedation. Postoperative treatment consisted of instillation of topical tobramycin 0.3%, nonpreserved artificial tears, and diclofenac sodium 0.1% four times a day. When the excimer laser procedure was performed on the corneal surface, we used a soft contact lens, and after complete re-epithelization of the cornea, topical steroid therapy of fluorometholone acetate 0.1% drops was initiated and continued for three months.

Statistical Analysis

Statistical analysis was performed with the SPSS/Pc+4.0 for Windows (SPSS Inc, Madrid, Spain). Measurements were typically reported as the mean ± 1 standard deviation (using $[n - 1]^{1/2}$ in the denominator of the definition for standard deviation, in which n is the number of observations for each measurement) and as the range of all measurements at each follow-up visit. Statistically significant differences between data sample means were determined by the Student's t test; P values less than 0.05 were considered significant. Additionally, the Mann Whitney U test was applied in the group that underwent ELASHY.

Analysis of the data concerning predictability, safety, and efficacy of the procedure was performed in each series using previously published criteria.[4]

1. SELZA

In this study, we reported the results of a prospective clinically controlled study performed on 23 eyes of 18 patients with irregular astigmatism induced by refractive surgery. All cases were treated with SELZA using an excimer laser of broad circular beam (VISX 20/20, 4.02, VISX Inc, Sunnyvale, Calif, USA). Surgical planning was applied using the Munnerlyn formula,[5] modified by Buzard,[6] to calculate the depth of the ablation depending on the amount of correction desired and the ablation zone. In this formula, the resection depth is equal to the dioptric correction, divided by three, and multiplied by the ablation zone (mm) squared. We used an empirical correction factor of 1.5, to avoid under-corrections:

$$\text{Ablation depth} = \frac{(\text{dioptric correction}) \times 1.5 \times (\text{ablation zone})^2}{3}$$

How to Perform SELZA

Usually we use ablation zones of 2.0 to 3.0 mm, depending on the steep area of the corneal topography to be modified. The ablation zone is determined by observing the color map. This form of videokeratoscopy provides additional information about the irregular zones, and the profile map gives the values for performed ablation. In all cases, treatment was performed on the center of the steeper area of irregularity. When the patient had previous LASIK, we lift the flap or make a new LASIK cut and then perform excimer laser ablation using phototherapeutic keratectomy (PTK) mode.

The technique is based on subtraction of tissue to eliminate the induced irregular astigmatism and to achieve a uniform corneal surface using the excimer laser.

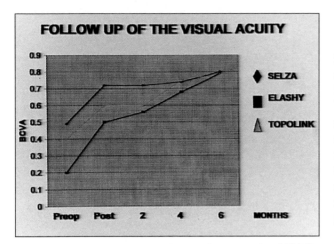

Figure 27-4. Follow-up of visual acuity in SELZA, ELASHY, and topolink.

Results

Visual acuity improved significantly, attaining (in many instances) near best-corrected visual acuity (BCVA) before the initial refractive procedure. The difference between BCVA before and after the therapeutic procedure proved to be highly statistically significant (p < 0.005). The BCVA at 1 month after surgery was 0.6 ± 0.1 (range: 0.6 to 1.0). After 2 months it was 0.8 ± 0.1 (range: 0.7 to 1.0). After 3 months, it was 0.8 ± 0.1 (range: 0.7 to 1.0). These were as good as the initial BCVA of 0.7 ± 0.1 (range: 0.7 to 1.0). The visual acuity pre selective ablation improved from 0.4 ± 0.1 (range: 0.3 to 0.9) to 0.8 ± 0.1 (range: 0.7 to 1.0) (Figure 27-4). We had no patients with one or more lost lines of BCVA.

The *corneal uniformity index* pre- versus post-selective zonal ablation with excimer laser improved from 58 ± 0.3% (range: 30 to 90) to 87 ± 0.8% (range: 70 to 100), a change that was also statistically significant (p < 0.005). The safety of the procedure was 96% (22 eyes). The *safety index* was equal to 1.5, which is the ratio of mean postoperative BCVA over mean preoperative BCVA; this is most easily calculated by converting the values of geometric mean acuities to decimal values. The *efficacy* of the procedure in the percent of uncorrected visual acuity (UCVA) 20/40 was 85%.

The *predictability* (astigmatic correction) using the corneal uniformity index (CUI) was expressed as a percentage. Various relationships between the preoperative CUI and the surgically induced postoperative CUI provided information about the magnitude of irregular astigmatism correction and corneal surface uniformity. The correction index, which is the ratio of mean postoperative CUI of 87 ± 0.8% (range: 70 to 100) over mean preoperative CUI of 58 ± 0.3% (range: 30 to 90) was equal to 1.5.

Discussion

The selective zonal ablation technique under the indicated conditions and parameters, showed satisfactory results for the correction of irregular astigmatism induced by refractive surgery (Figures 27-5a and 27-5b). Visual acuity improved in the postoperative period, achieving values near initial BCVA prior to the initial surgical procedure. The CUI evaluating the 3.0 mm central diameter showed improvement in the early postoperative period and stabilization after 3 months, just as visual acuity (p < 0.005). Normally, this refractive procedure requires a stable corneal topography and adequate interpretation.[7]

2. ELASHY

We reported the results of a prospective clinically controlled study performed on 20 eyes of 20 patients with irregular astigmatism induced by LASIK. All cases were treated with ELASHY using a Plano C-Scan excimer laser in PTK mode with the Technolas 217 C-LASIK. Ablation was assisted by a mask of sodium hyaluronate 0.25% dyed with fluorescein. All patients had irregular astigmatism with undefined pattern.

How to Perform ELASHY

In cases in which the irregular astigmatism was induced by a flap irregularity (superficial irregular astigmatism), the ablation was performed on the corneal surface. The epithelium was removed using the excimer laser assisted by viscous masking. When the irregularity was in the stroma below the flap, we lifted the flap wherever possible and then performed stromal ablation. After the procedure, the flap was repositioned. We centered the action of the laser on the corneal center and used eye tracking. After this, one drop of 0.25% sodium hyaluronate dyed with fluorescein was applied to the cornea. The physical characteristics of sodium hyaluronate confer important dispersive and cohesive rheological properties.[8] The photoablation rate was similar to that of corneal tissue, forming a stable and uniform coating on the surfaces of the eye, filling depressions on the cornea, and effectively masking tissues to be protected against ablation by the laser pulses. This contributes to a smoother surface of the cornea after the procedure and most probably a reduction of haze formation and less scarring when the procedure was performed on corneal surface.[9] With the use of one drop of fluorescein, together with the masking solution, it is possible to observe the spot and the effect of the laser.[9] Because fluorescent light is emitted during ablation of corneal tissue, cessation of

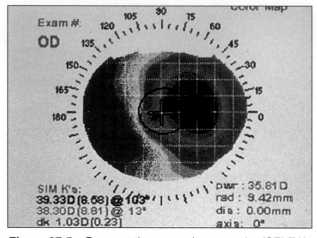

Figure 27-5a. Preoperative corneal topography (SELZA).

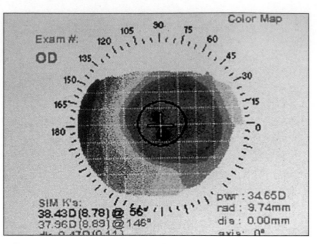

Figure 27-5b. Postoperative corneal topography (SELZA).

the fluorescence signifies complete removal of the viscous mask and tissue.

Results

Following surgery, visual acuity improved significantly and attained values superior to the BCVA before the refractive procedure. The difference from the BCVA before the therapeutic procedure proved to be statistically significant (p < 0.01, Student t test). The previous visual acuity was 20/200 (range 20/90 to 20/200), and at 3 months after surgery it was 20/30 (range: 20/30 to 20/50), remaining stable. We did not have any patients with one or more lines of lost BCVA (Figure 27-4). Visual recovery was slow, usually achieved at 2 to 3 months postoperatively. There was no difference between surface and stromal treatment.

The CUI pre versus post therapeutic procedure was improved from 35 ± 0.5% (range: 10 to 60) to 98 ± 0.5% (range: 70 to 100). Corneal optical quality was good. These results proved to also be statistically significant (p < 0.01, student t test). As with BCVA, the CUI was stable between 2 and 3 months postoperatively. It correlated with the predicted corneal acuity (PC acuity).

The procedure was highly safe, with a safety index equal to 6, which is the ratio of mean postoperative BCVA (20/30) over mean preoperative BCVA (20/200) expressed as a decimal (Figure 27-6). The efficacy index of the procedure in the percent of BCVA 20/40 postoperatively was 87%. The astigmatic correction was evaluated in its ability to improve the corneal surface. We used the distortion map (EyeSys 2000) for this and the corneal surface quality (C-Scan).

The average ablation depth was 65 microns (range: 45 to 75 microns). The corneal ablation was equal to three-fifths (60%) for 100 mm entered in the software of

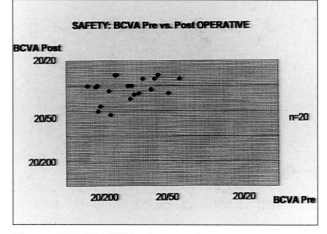

Figure 27-6. ELASHY safety results.

the excimer laser. When the laser ablation was performed on the corneal surface, we increased by 50 microns, which was necessary for the epithelial and Bowman's layer ablation. The epithelium was ablated if the preoperative corneal topography showed an irregular flap. In Figure 27-7, we observe that in a normal procedure with excimer laser, the programmed ablation is theoretically similar to the achieved corneal ablation (straight line), while with viscous masking solution, the line had an exponential increase determined by the substance used (curve line).

We obtained a significant improvement in irregular astigmatism using excimer laser assisted by sodium hyaluronate 0.25%. In all patients, the irregular astigmatism was decreased with slight modification of refractive error. Concerning the retractive result, we obtained overcorrections in 55% and undercorrections in 45%.

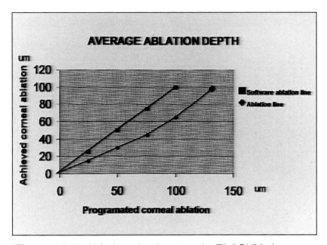

Figure 27-7. Ablation depth curve in ELASHY; the average ablation depth was 65 mm.

Discussion

Using a viscous masking solution (sodium hyaluronate 0.25%) together with fluorescein is very useful to observe the excimer laser action and corneal ablation. The excimer laser was programmed in PTK mode for ablation amounts of 25 microns while observing the corneal surface until a maximum of 100 microns was delivered. The corneal ablation was three-fifths (60%) for each 100 microns programmed in the software of the excimer laser. When the laser ablation was performed on the corneal surface, we increased the ablation by 75 microns, which was necessary for the epithelium ablation under the viscous mask. The patients included in our study had a minimal corneal thickness of 420 microns in their thinner portion; we also made sure corneal ablation did not leave the cornea with a value less than 390 microns (Figure 27-8).

3. TOPOLINK

Following early studies, the exquisite precision with which the excimer laser ablation, when assisted by corneal topography, could improve the irregular astigmatism was shown. The aim of this study was to create a regular corneal surface in 29 eyes of 29 patients with irregular astigmatism induced by LASIK. All cases were treated with the Plano C-Scan excimer laser with the Technolas 217 C-LASIK assisted by the C-Scan ellipsoid topography.

How to Perform Topolink

We performed several corneal topographies from the same eye. The automated corneal topographer software selected the four most nearly equal. These corneal maps, the refractive error, the pachymetry value, and desired k-

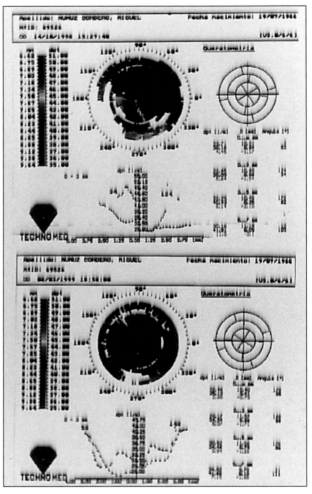

Figure 27-8. Preoperative (above) and postoperative (below) corneal topography (ELASHY).

readings calculated on the basis of the aforementioned data for each patient were sent to Technolas by modem. The information was analyzed and a special software program for each patient was created, loading it in the Technolas 217 C-LASIK excimer laser by system modem.

The basis for the topography-assisted procedure was the preoperative topography.[11] This data was transferred into true height data, and the treatment for correcting the refractive values in sphere and astigmatism, taking into account the corneal irregularities, was calculated. After that, a postoperative topography was simulated. With this technique, real customized treatment becomes a reality, not only treating the refractive error but also improving the patient's visual acuity and achieving a programmed refractive outcome.

Results

After 3 months post-surgery, the mean preoperative

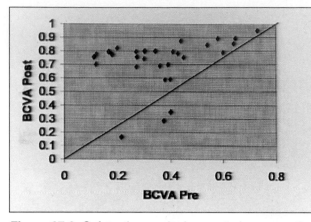

Figure 27-9. Safety: the results in our study were satisfactory in topolink.

UCVA improved from 20/80 ± 0.25 (range: 20/400 to 20/60) to 20/40 ± 0.54 (range: 20/100 to 20/30); mean preoperative BSCVA improved from 20/60 ± 0.20 (range: 20/200 to 20/30) to 20/40 ± 0.15 (range: 20/60 to 20/30) (see Figure 27-4). This proved to be statistically significant (p<0.001).

Even though emmetropia was our goal, it was considered more important to achieve a regular corneal surface. The spherical equivalent of the individual refraction was taken into account in determining the corneal k-value. Preoperatively, mean sphere was 0.75 ± 4.50 D (range: -5.75 to +3.70 D) and mean cylinder was -2.05 ± 3.08 D (range: -6.00 to +2.56 D). Three months after surgery, the mean sphere was 0.75 ± 1.25 D (range: -1.75 to +1.50 D) and the mean cylinder was 0.75 ± 1.00 D (range: -1.78 to +2.00).

Corneal topography improved significantly, and the mean corneal surface quality was improved from 45% (range: 60% to 35%) to 86.6% (range: 96.43% to 60.06%). The corneal surface was left smooth and ray-tracing was improved, showing improvement in peak distortion, coinciding with the improvement of the visual acuity. In 74.23% of patients, visual aberrations disappeared.

The safety of the procedure was 79.31% (23 eyes). After surgery, three eyes (10.34%) were unimproved (Figure 27-9). In these patients, UCVA, BSCVA, and corneal topography was exactly equal to preoperative values. In three eyes (10.34%) regression was observed 2 months after surgery. The efficacy of the procedure in percent of UCVA 20/40 was 69.68%. The predictability was 76.56%.

Regarding patient satisfaction, 23 patients said their vision was better, three patients noticed no change, and three patients initially said their vision was improved but 2 months later felt it was worse.

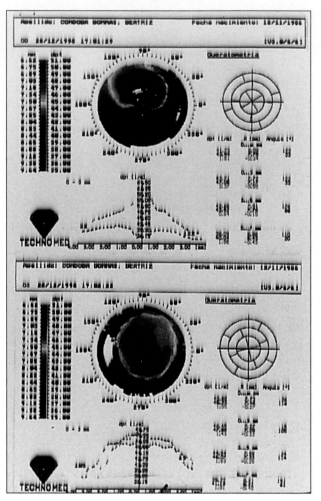

Figure 27-10. Preoperative (above) and postoperative (below) corneal topography (topolink).

Discussion

Using the corneal topographic map as a guide, excimer laser ablation can be used to create a more regular surface with improved visual acuity. In a program consisting of a combination of phototherapeutic and photorefractive ablation patterns, the amount of tissue to be removed is calculated on the basis of the diameter and height of the irregular areas of the corneal surface (Figure 27-10).

With this procedure some irregular astigmatism cannot be corrected. Twelve patients could not be selected as candidates using the corneal topographer software, because some of the following criteria were present:

1. Difference between steep and flat meridians was more than 10 D at the 6.0 mm treatment area
2. Corneal pachymetry was not sufficient (< 400 microns)
3. Diameter of the corneal topography more than 5.0 mm

4. Corneal topographies there are different

5. Corneal topography showed an extremely undefined pattern

This study showed that topographic-assisted LASIK (topolink) may be useful for irregular astigmatic correction, but we observed a percentage of undercorrection and regression. Future studies with more patients should provide further advances in topography-linked excimer laser ablation.

SUMMARY

Although videokeratography provides a great deal of qualitative information about a patient's corneal topography through pattern recognition and color scale, this information alone is not suitable for evaluating clinical trial data collected from a large group of patients with irregular astigmatism. The statistical analysis of topographic data essential for a scientific study can be obtained from numerical indices derived from raw topographic data. In turn, these indices provide quantitative and qualitative points to guide and assess the effects of therapy.[12]

Irregular astigmatism has a variety of appearances on videokeratography. Generally, every deviation from a pure ellipsoidal shape is called irregular astigmatism. Induced irregular astigmatism from refractive surgery can be devastating to vision when it occurs centrally within the pupillary area. It can be present even on a surface that clinically appears relatively smooth.[13] Functionally, irregular astigmatism is that component of astigmatism that cannot be corrected with spectacles. LASIK can induce irregular astigmatism in the flap, in the stromal bed, or in both; the corneal topographic map may demonstrate both defined pattern and undefined pattern.

We have performed three different corneal refractive treatments using the excimer laser for the correction of irregular astigmatism, taking into account the irregular astigmatism pattern, with variable results:

Decentered ablation was improved in 89.65% of eyes using SELZA and in 93% eyes using topolink. Decentered steep was improved in 63.43% of eyes using SELZA, in 26.45% of eyes using ELASHY, and in 86.23% of eyes using topolink. Central island was improved 92.3% of eyes using SELZA, in 47.56% of eyes using ELASHY, and in 89.24% of eyes using topolink. Central irregularity was improved in 72.56% of eyes using SELZA, in 85.65% of eyes using ELASHY,

and in 84.12% of eyes using topolink. Peripheral irregularity was improved in 88.95% of eyes using SELZA, in 64.62% of eyes using ELASHY, and in 72.69% of eyes using topolink. Undefined pattern was improved in 15.12% of eyes using SELZA and in 93.23% of eyes using ELASHY. Topolink was effective in those cases that fit the selection criteria now present for this technique.

REFERENCES

1. Trokel SL, Srinivasan R, Braren B. Excimer laser surgery of the cornea. *Am J Ophthalmol.* 1983;96:705-710.

2. Alió JL, Rodríguez-Mier FA, Artola A. Selective zonal ablations with excimer laser for correction of irregular astigmatism induced by refractive surgery. *Ophthalmology.* Accepted for publication June 1999.

3. Alió JL, Rodríguez-Mier FA. Excimer Laser assisted by sodium hyaluronate for correction of irregular astigmatism. *Journal of Refractive Surgery.* Submitted for publication July 1999.

4. Koch DD, Kohnen T, Obstbaum SA, Rosen ES. Format for reporting refractive surgical data (letter). *J Cataract Refract Surg.* 1998;24:285-287.

5. Munnerlyn C, Koons S, Marshall J. Photorefractive keratectomy: A technique for laser refractive surgery. *J Cataract Refract Surg.* 1988;14:46-52.

6. Buzard K, Fundingsland B. Treatment of irregular astigmatism with a broad beam excimer laser. *Journal of Refractive Surgery.* 1997;13:624-636.

7. Seitz B, Behrens A, Langenbucher A. Corneal topography. *Current Opinion in Ophthalmology.* 1997,8;IV:8-24.

8. Kornmehl EW, Steiner RF, Puliafito CA. A comparative study of masking fluids for excimer laser phototherapeutic keratectomy. *Arch Ophthalmol.* 1991;109:860-863.

9. Kornmehl EW, Steinert RF, Puliafito CA, Reidy W. Morphology of an irregular corneal surface following 193 nm ArF excimer laser large area ablation with 0.3% hydroxypropyl methylcellulose 2910 and 0.1% dextran 70.1% carboxy-methylcellulose sodium or 0.9% saline (ARVO abstracts). *Invest Ophthalmol Vis Sci.* 1990;31:245.

10. Kreuger RR, Trokel SL. Quantification of corneal ablation by ultraviolet light. *Arch Ophthalmol.* 1986;103:1741-1742.

11. Wiesinger-Jendritza B, Knorz M, Hugger P, Liermann A. Laser in situ keratomileusis assisted by corneal topography. *J Cataract Refract Surg.* 1998;24:166-174.

12. Klyce SD, Smolek MK. Corneal topography of excimer laser photorefractive keratectomy. *J Cataract Refract Surg.* 1993;19:122-130.

13. Gibralter R, Trokel S. Correction of irregular astigmatism with the excimer laser. *Ophthalmology.* 1994; 101:1.310-1.315.

POSTERIOR CHAMBER PHAKIC IOL IMPLANTATION AND BIOPTICS FOR EXTREME REFRACTIVE ERRORS

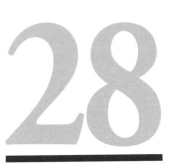

Roberto Zaldivar, MD, Jonathan M. Davidorf, MD,
and Susana Oscherow, MD

BACKGROUND

In the 1950s, after witnessing the early successes of intraocular lenses (IOLs) for correction of aphakia, Strampelli designed a minus power IOL for phakic patients with extreme myopia.[1] Barraquer was the first to report a long-term study of these one piece, polymethylmethacrylate (PMMA), plate anterior chamber angle fixated phakic IOLs. Without the benefit of the operating microscope, nylon sutures, viscoelastics, refined IOL manufacturing, and knowledge of corneal endothelial function, approximately 60% of the lenses had to be removed because of corneal edema or the uveitis-glaucoma-hyphema syndrome.[2]

Phakic IOL surgery was abandoned until renewed interest began with Fechner's modification of the Worst iris claw lens and Baikoff's modification of the Kelman multiflex anterior chamber IOL in the mid 1980s.[3-5] Both of these anterior chamber phakic IOLs have undergone a series of design improvements and have demonstrated reasonable performance regarding efficacy, predictability, and stability of the refractive result for high myopia. Earlier models produced endothelial cell loss; later models showed minimal loss.[6-10]

We began implanting the Baikoff lens (first the ZB model, then the ZBMF model) in 1989. Although we also obtained reasonable efficacy and predictability of the refractive result over a 6-year period, concerns about the small optic zone size (4.0 mm), which created patients' complaints of halos and glare, progressive iris retraction with oval pupils and a large incision size of 6.0 mm lead us to search for a lens with a better design for myopia and one that could also treat hyperopia.

In December 1993, we began implanting the Staar plate posterior chamber phakic IOL (trade named the Implantable Contact Lens [ICL], Staar Surgical AG, Nidau, Switzerland). The ICL is implanted into the posterior chamber of the phakic eye behind the iris and in front of the anterior capsule of the crystalline lens (Figure 28-1). Fyodorov originated this lens style in 1986, using a one-piece silicone collar button phakic IOL with a 500 to 600 nm Teflon coat.[11] Problems with cataract formation and uveitis lead to refinements in lens design, including the incorporation of collagen into the lens material to improve biocompatibility.[12] As the Fyodorov lens evolved through approximately six design changes, investigators achieved encouraging initial results, with 89% of eyes achieving uncorrected visual acuity equal to the preoperative level of best spectacle corrected visual acuity.[11,13]

The current Staar Surgical-AG IOL (ICL) is made of a porcine collagen/hydroxyethylmethacrylate copolymer (trade named Collamer) with a refractive index of 1.450 at 35°C. This Collamer material absorbs ultraviolet radiation and has a light transmittance in the visible region of the spectrum of approximately 90% + 5%. The plate haptic design is quite similar to the existing plate-haptic technology in Staar's model AA-4203V lens for aphakia/cataract surgery. One difference is that the ICL incorporates a forward vault to minimize IOL-crystalline lens contact (see Figure 28-1). It is a foldable lens that may be implanted through a 3.2 mm or smaller corneal incision, at times under topical anesthesia. The central concave/convex optic comes in sizes ranging from 4.65 to 5.50 mm in diameter, depending on the lens power. Available powers are, for myopic lenses, -3.0 to -20.0 diopters (D) and, for hyperopic lenses, +3 to +20 D. Other lens powers are sometimes available. Five lens lengths are manufactured, ranging from 11 to 13 mm, to accommodate different eye sizes.

Phakic IOL surgery offers some distinct advantages over current corneal refractive techniques. While both photorefractive keratectomy (PRK) and laser in situ keratomileusis (LASIK) have demonstrated encouraging results for the treatment of low to moderate myopia,

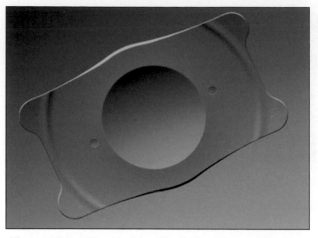

Figure 28-1a. The Implantable Contact Lens (ICL). Two partial thickness positioning dimples can be seen outside the border of the optic portion of the lens (courtesy of Staar Surgical).

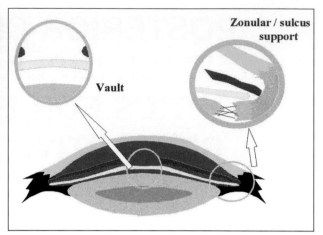

Figure 28-1b. The Staar Collamer posterior chamber phakic intraocular lens. The drawing illustrates phakic IOL vaulting and zonular/ciliary sulcus support of the haptics.

hyperopia, and astigmatism, the large ablation depths, smaller ablation zones, increased optical aberrations, and poorer predictability have raised doubts that the cornea is the appropriate site for correction of extreme refractive errors.[14-30]

Phakic IOL surgery obviates the need to violate the corneal visual axis. In the case of posterior chamber phakic IOL surgery, potential corneal scarring is limited to a peripheral, astigmatically neutral, clear cornea incision. In addition, the effective optical zone size is larger than the size achieved with PRK or LASIK. With excimer laser ablation, the ablation diameter is normally decreased in order to prevent the need for excessive ablation depths. For example, with the VISX Star excimer laser, the ablation diameter is typically reduced from 6.0 mm to 5.5 mm for myopia greater than -6 D. The effective optical zone created by an ablation diameter of 5.5 mm is likely smaller than 5.5 mm, even in the setting of perfect ablation centration. In the case of the ICL, the full 4.65 to 5.50 mm of the lens optic is available for refracting light rays. Moreover, a 5.50 mm optical zone at the level of the crystalline lens receives more light rays than a 5.50 mm optical zone at the level of the cornea (Figure 28-2).

Phakic IOL implantation does not preclude the use of keratorefractive procedures following phakic IOL implantation for the correction of residual myopia and/or astigmatism. Performing these secondary procedures allows for fine tuning of the refractive result. Currently, we prefer to treat eyes with preoperative myopia of approximately -18 D or greater with a two-step procedure we have named "bioptics."[31] In these eyes, the posterior chamber phakic IOL is implanted to

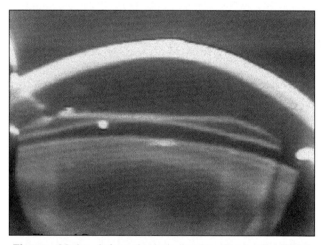

Figure 28-1c. Infrared photograph, slit mode (Nidek EAS-1000 anterior segment analyzer) demonstrating IOL vault over crystalline lens.

achieve a target postoperative residual refraction of -1.5 to -12 D spherical equivalent refraction (with or without astigmatism). The residual myopia (and astigmatism, when present) is corrected with LASIK no sooner than 1 month after phakic IOL implantation.

The ICL received the European Community Mark of Approval in May 1997, which allowed unrestricted marketing distribution of the ICL throughout all European Union countries. In the United States, the ICL is being studied under an Food and Drug Administration (FDA)-approved Investigational Device Exemption (IDE) by a limited number of investigators. The ICL clinical trial was granted expansion to Phase 3 in October of 1998, final FDA approval is pending.

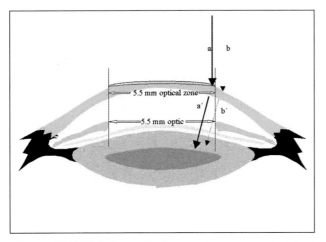

Figure 28-2. Relative optical zone size in corneal versus intraocular surgery. Incident light rays at the edge of a 5.5 mm optical zone (a) on the surface of the cornea are refracted toward the visual axis (a') and traverse the iris plane (i) well within a 5.5 mm pupil. Incident light rays peripheral to a 5.5 mm optical zone on the surface of the cornea (b) are refracted toward the visual axis (b') and may still traverse the 5.5 mm optic of a posterior chamber phakic IOL.

PREOPERATIVE EVALUATION

Patient Selection

We prefer to use LASIK for eyes with up to -10 or -12 D of myopia and up to +4 D of hyperopia. Patients with refractive errors outside this range are considered for ICL implantation. Patients with co-existing astigmatism, or with myopia or hyperopia outside the range in which the ICL could be expected to correct the entire refractive error, are still candidates for ICL implantation. The residual astigmatism (and myopia or hyperopia, when present) is treated with LASIK following ICL implantation (bioptics). Refractions should be stable, as they should be prior to any refractive procedure. In the US FDA study, patients with myopia of -7 D or greater or with hyperopia of +3 D or greater are potential ICL candidates. The guidelines for enrolling patients in the FDA study require that patients have no more than 2.5 D of refractive cylinder. Eyes may undergo astigmatic keratotomy prior to receiving an ICL, but secondary refractive procedures following ICL implantation are not permitted in the FDA study.

Exclusion criteria include previous intraocular surgery, corneal pathology (eg, keratoconus, infectious keratitis, dry eye syndrome, corneal degeneration), visually significant cataract, glaucoma, proliferative diabetic retinopathy, and retinal breaks. Patients with advanced systemic disease are also excluded. Because the ICL takes up space within the anterior segment, it is advised

that prospective patients have anterior chamber depths of at least 3.0 mm. Because the spectrum of hyperopia includes nanophthalmos, particular attention should be paid to anterior chamber depth when considering ICL implantation into hyperopic eyes.

Preoperative Examination

Patients are instructed to discontinue wearing hard contact lenses and rigid gas-permeable contact lenses for at least 2 weeks before preoperative measurements are taken and surgery is performed. Preoperative examinations should include measurement of uncorrected visual acuity, best spectacle-corrected visual acuity with manifest and cycloplegic refractions, keratometry, corneal topography (axial and tangential maps) and diameters (EyeSys corneal topographer), pachymetry, specular microscopy (Konan Noncon Robo, H-iogo, Japan), A-scan ultrasonography, slit lamp biomicroscopy, applanation tonometry, anterior segment infrared photography (Nidek EAS 1000), and dilated funduscopy. If necessary, gonioscopy and B-scan ultrasonography are also performed. Because potential patients tend to have high refractive errors and because ICL power calculations are performed assuming a vertex distance of 12.5 mm, attention to vertex distance is perhaps even more important in phakic IOL surgery than in other areas of refractive surgery. We measure corneal diameter with the computerized calipers on the videokeratographer (white-to-white). It is important to perform a detailed dilated funduscopic examination for predisposing retinal breaks in patients at high risk for spontaneous retinal detachment, such as those with extreme myopia.

ICL Power Calculation and Sizing

ICL power calculations are performed with formulas developed by Olsen and modified by Zaldivar. The independent variables in the formula are preoperative spherical equivalent refraction, vertex distance, average keratometry, corneal thickness, and actual anterior chamber depth. The power of the implanted ICL does not match the patient's spherical equivalent refraction. For example, an eye with -18 D of myopia will likely require an ICL of -20 D. In addition, because the ICL is not manufactured in powers greater than -20 D, a secondary refractive procedure is needed to fully correct eyes with over -18 D of myopia at the spectacle plane (bioptics). Lens power selection is less critical when bioptics is planned, because with bioptics, residual refractive errors are corrected with LASIK. The target spherical equivalent refraction following myopic ICL implantation for bioptics eyes is between -1 to -12 D. The length of the implanted ICL is determined by the patient's horizontal corneal diameter (white-to-white), which is verified in

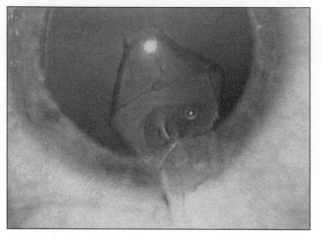

Figure 28-3a. ICL implantation: injecting the lens. The injector tip is placed within the corneal wound as the ICL is delivered.

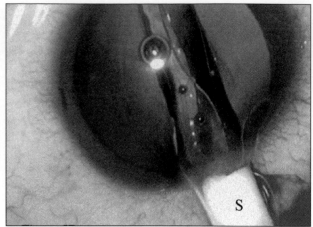

Figure 28-3b. The ICL continues to unfold within the anterior chamber. The injector barrel and Merocel sponge (S) do not enter the eye.

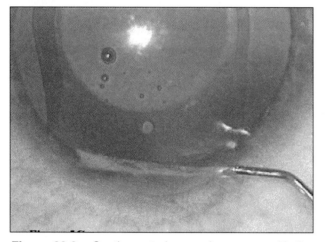

Figure 28-3c. Gentle posterior nasal pressure with the Zaldivar ICL manipulator is used to position one of the temporal footplates. Each of the four footplates is positioned independently.

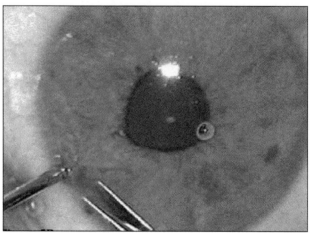

Figure 28-3d. The Zaldivar iridectomy forceps help create a patent surgical iridectomy.

surgery with calipers. For myopic eyes, the size of the ICL is chosen to be the horizontal corneal diameter plus 0.5 mm, rounded to the nearest 0.5 mm increment. For hyperopic eyes, the ICL is matched to the actual horizontal corneal diameter. The goal is to achieve proper anterior IOL vaulting and secure fixation.

SURGICAL TECHNIQUE

Laser Iridotomies

In order to decrease the incidence of postoperative pupillary block, we began placing peripheral laser iridotomies at least 4 days preoperatively. Patients initially received a single superior iridotomy; subsequently, we began placing two superior iridotomies positioned

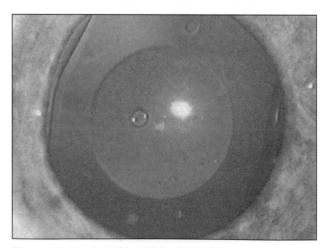

Figure 28-3e. A well-positioned ICL prior to instillation of a miotic agent.

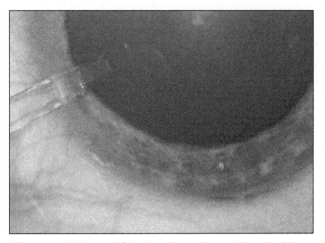

Figure 28-4a. ICL implantation: the incision. Paracentesis fashioned with the Zaldivar Anterior Procedure (ZAP) diamond knife.

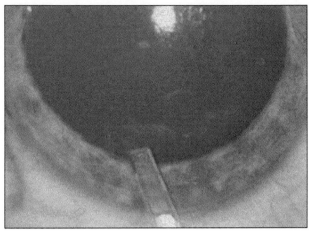

Figure 28-4b. ICL implantation: the incision. ZAP knife used for constructing a shelved 3.0 mm temporal clear cornea incision.

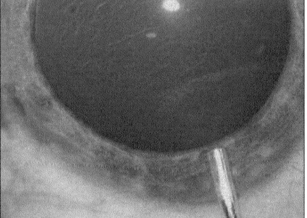

Figure 28-4c. ICL implantation: the incision. A cohesive viscoelastic is injected into the anterior chamber through the temporal incision.

between 60 to 90 degrees apart in order to decrease the likelihood of iridotomy occlusion by the phakic IOL haptics. Iridotomies should be 250 to 500 mm in diameter and located superiorly (covered by the upper eyelid) in the peripheral iris. At first, we only used the Nd: YAG laser (single burst, 3 to 10 mJ). We now recommend using the argon green laser prior to applying the Nd: YAG spots in order to decrease iris bleeding and pigment deposition on the phakic IOL (argon settings: 50 micron spot size, 650 to 1000 mW power, and 0.2 to 0.5 second duration). In hyperopic eyes, myopic eyes with dark irides, and eyes with possible nonpatent laser iridotomies, surgical iridectomies should be performed. The Zaldivar iridectomy forceps (ASICO, Westmont, Ill) facilitates this maneuver (Figures 28-3a through 28-3c).

Preoperative Medications and Anesthesia

Patients are counseled immediately before surgery in order to decrease the need for sedation. Oral alprazolam was administered as needed. One hour before surgery, tropicamide 1%, phenylephrine 2.5%, diclofenac, and gentamicin (a fluoroquinolone may be substituted) are applied serially. Patients are then taken to the preoperative holding area where they are fitted with a hair net and their eyes and lids are cleaned and scrubbed with an iodine eye scrub. A gauze pad is placed over the temporal periorbital region to absorb fluid drainage during the procedure.

Anesthesia is achieved with either peribulbar or topical lidocaine. If topical anesthesia is to be used, nonpreserved lidocaine (1%) is given beginning 20 minutes prior to surgery. ICL patients seem to have a more difficult time tolerating topical anesthesia than typical cataract patients, perhaps because they are often younger in age (no cataract, more widely dilating pupils). We, therefore, often prefer peribulbar anesthesia (lidocaine 2%, duracaine 0.5%, and hyaluronidase). When optimal dilation and anesthesia are obtained, the patient is taken to the operating room, the eyelids are prepared with povidone-iodine, the head is draped with a sterile field, and a lid speculum is placed.

ICL Implantation

A 2.8 mm temporal clear corneal incision and superior paracentesis are performed with the ZAP diamond knife (Figures 28-4a through 28-4c). For cases in which topical anesthesia is used, a supplement of preservative-free intraocular lidocaine is instilled into the anterior

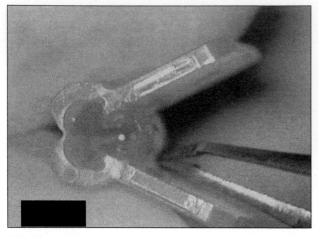

Figure 28-5a. ICL implantation: folding the lens. Nontoothed forceps are used to ensure that the ICL is completely within the loading area prior to folding the cartridge.

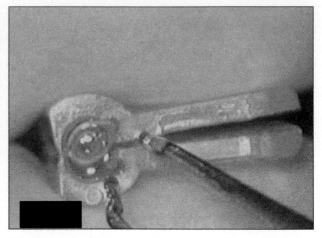

Figure 28-5b. Once loaded, gently feed the ICL into the cartridge barrel.

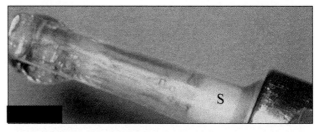

Figure 28-5c. The injector is properly loaded with the ICL. The 5.0 mm piece of Merocel sponge (S) can be seen at the proximal end of the cartridge barrel.

chamber. Hydroxypropyl-methylcellulose is then injected into the anterior chamber (OcuCoat, Storz). The viscoelastic should have good cohesive properties and be of low viscosity to facilitate easy removal following ICL implantation. Corneal endothelium protection by the viscoelastic is of less concern than in cataract surgery, because the crystalline lens is not being phacoemulsified.

The ICL should be kept well hydrated in a sterile container of balanced salt solution (BSS) until loading. Under direct visualization with the operating microscope, the ICL is positioned in the lens insertion cartridge (MicroStaar, Staar Surgical) (Figures 28-5a through 28-5c). A forceps insertion is not recommended because of the increased possibility of inadvertently damaging the crystalline lens. Within the lens injector cartridge, the ICL should be oriented so that its long axis is aligned with the center of the cartridge and both sides of the ICL must be completely within the loading area. Viscoelastic will facilitate these manipulations. A 1.0 mm diameter wedge of Merocel microsurgical sponge is cut and placed behind the cartridge within the lens injector to protect the ICL from the injector arm.

The injector tip is then placed within the wound (but not into the anterior chamber) and the lens is slowly injected into the anterior chamber, anterior to the iris plane, ensuring proper orientation (see Figure 28-3). During insertion, the ICL tends to rotate upside down. Current ICL models are angulated so that proper orientation is essential. The ICL has two dimples on the anterior surface that serve as positioning holes. One hole is located next to the distal footplate, and the second is located next to the proximal footplate. An upside-down lens would show inversion of these positioning holes. Often, it is difficult to assess ICL orientation while the

lens is inside the injector. Rotating the injector while inserting the ICL, which maintains proper lens position throughout the procedure, facilitates proper orientation. In the case of an inverted ICL, the lens should not be repositioned inside the eye. Instead, the ICL should be removed with forceps and re-injected in its proper orientation, minimizing the risk of cataractogenesis.[31,32]

After proper insertion, the ICL should rest anterior to the iris with the footplates reaching just beyond the pupil margin. Each ICL footplate is positioned independently. Gentle posterior pressure with the Zaldivar ICL manipulator is used to place the temporal haptic beneath the iris (see Figure 28-3c). The nasal haptic is then positioned in a similar fashion. Do not attempt to lift the iris. A rotational technique ("dialing-in" the temporal haptic) was abandoned early on because it produced increased postoperative pigment dispersion and posed an increased risk to the crystalline lens.

In order to ensure the ICL is not captured by the iris, the ICL is not blocking the iridotomies, and aqueous is flowing freely through the iridotomies, acetylcholine is injected into the anterior chamber to induce miosis. Diluted Miostat or Carbachol is preferred, as Miochol (CIBA Vision, Duluth, Ga) often elicits only a brief

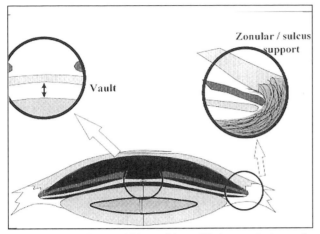

Figure 28-6. Proper ICL vaulting. Slit lamp photograph shows ICL vaulting over the anterior lens capsule. Note the clarity of the crystalline lens of this eye 2 years after ICL implantation.

response. Remaining viscoelastic is removed with gentle irrigation and aspiration using the phacoemulsification system (AMO Prestige, Allergan, Irvine, Calif, USA). It is important to remove all remaining viscoelastic in order to guard against pupillary block, since the viscoelastic may precipitate and block an otherwise patent iridotomy postoperatively.[33]

While the surgical maneuvers are identical in myopic and hyperopic eyes, the shallower anterior chambers of the hyperopic eyes require extra care during phakic IOL insertion in order to avoid corneal endothelium contact.

Topical tobramycin-dexamethasone, gentamicin, and 500 mg of oral acetazolamide are given at the conclusion of the surgery. Only eyes that receive peribulbar anesthesia are patched. Eyes that receive topical anesthesia are given protective eye shields for bedtime use only. Postoperative medications include 0.3% dibekacin qid for 1 week, 1% prednisolone qid for 1 month, and a Betablocker (eg, 0.5% timolol) bid for 1 month. In the FDA protocol, ofloxacin bid for 1 week and a regimen of tobramycin dexamethasone tapered over 16 days is advised.

Secondary Refractive Procedures— Bioptics

Most commonly, we perform LASIK no sooner than 4 weeks following ICL implantation. We call this two-staged procedure bioptics, and it has some advantages over a single-staged ICL implantation.[31] First, as mentioned above, it allows the surgeon to treat eyes that are outside the range of current ICL models and enables one to surgically correct co-existing astigmatism. In addition, with bioptics the refractive result can be fine tuned. Especially in patients with a high level of preoperative

myopia, the ICL power calculation may be somewhat inexact. Limitations in predictability are partly related to choosing phakic IOL powers based on spectacle refractions, and an imprecise refraction endpoint directly translates into ICL power miscalculations. After significantly reducing the level of myopia by ICL implantation, the patient's endpoint of refraction should be more precise with the new lower level of myopia. LASIK for low to moderate myopia and myopic astigmatism is quite effective and should yield predictable results.[15,17,20-22]

After we described this technique, other colleagues have suggested similar procedures combining other phakic IOL implants with automated lamellar keratoplasty (ALK) prior to the intraocular procedure.[34] Excimer laser ablation is then performed 1 month after IOL implantation. The majority of these cases have been performed with anterior chamber IOLs, such as the NuVita MA20 (Bausch & Lomb Surgical/Chiron Vision, Irvine, Calif, USA) or Iris-Claw lens (Ophtec, Groningen, Netherlands).

Performing ALK prior to LASIK is mandatory when using anterior chamber IOLs due to the potential risk of endothelial damage during the flap dissection. Flattening of the central cornea, both due to the suction ring and passage of the microkeratome head during LASIK, can induce cornea-IOL contact. With a posterior chamber phakic IOL, however, the position of the IOL minimizes the risk of corneal endothelial injury during LASIK.

An inconvenience of performing the flap dissection prior to phakic IOL implantation is that patients are then subjected to a higher incidence of epithelial ingrowth due to lifting the flap 1 month later. Bioptics performed with a foldable posterior chamber phakic IOL enables the surgeon to elevate the flap only once, minimizing the incidence of epithelial ingrowth.

Second (Fellow) Eye Surgery

Because of the high level of refractive error in ICL patients, long delays in second eye surgery is often poorly tolerated due to the burden of postoperative anisometropia. We wait a minimum of 2 days between eyes before implanting an ICL in the fellow eye. In the FDA clinical trial, patients are required to wait a minimum of 6 months before receiving an ICL in the fellow eye.

POSTOPERATIVE EXAMINATIONS

ICL patients must be examined the day of surgery, 3 to 5 hours postoperatively. The examining physician must ensure that no iris capture or pupillary block has occurred and the anterior vaulting of the ICL is adequate prior to releasing the patient (Figure 28-6). The intraocular pressure should be checked and the iridotomies examined to verify patency. Dilated or swollen iris tissue may temporarily occlude iridotomy sites, which may lead to pupillary block.

Routine postoperative examinations are scheduled at 1 day, 1 month, 3 to 6 months, 12 months, 18 to 24 months, then every year after surgery. Subjective complaints should be detailed. Uncorrected visual acuity, best spectacle-corrected visual acuity, automated keratometry, applanation tonometry, and slit lamp biomicroscopy, endothelial cell count, and infrared photography of the anterior segment are performed at each examination. ICL vaulting, pigment dispersion, and crystalline lens clarity should be particularly observed. Lens clarity and pigment on the ICL surface is graded from 0 to 4+ by direct visualization at the slit lamp. Gonioscopy and dilated funduscopy are performed as needed. If improper IOL vaulting or excessive pigment dispersion is identified, removal of the ICL is indicated and the surgeon may consider exchanging the ICL for one of different length, keeping in mind that the greater the ICL length, the more pronounced the vault.

RESULTS

The refractive and visual results following ICL implantation are characterized by a large reduction in the preoperative level of myopia or hyperopia and by substantial gains in best spectacle-corrected visual acuity, particularly in myopic eyes.

In a recent study of 124 highly myopic eyes that underwent ICL implantation (mean preoperative spherical equivalent refraction -13.38 + 2.23 D, range -8.50 to -18.63 D), we found that 69% (86 eyes) achieved a postoperative spherical equivalent refraction within 1 D of emmetropia.[31] A tendency toward undercorrection was encountered, partly because ICL powers are selected based on spectacle refractions. In their study of 15 myopic eyes receiving Staar's posterior chamber phakic IOL, Assetto, et al achieved a postoperative spherical equivalent refraction within 1 D of emmetropia in 31% of eyes.[35] With the benefit of refined ICL power calculation formulas and in setting lower overall preoperative myopia (mean -7.75 D, range -7.25 to -9.375 D), all of the initial 10 eyes (100%) enrolled in the FDA clinical trial achieved a postoperative spherical equivalent refraction within 1.125 D of emmetropia.[36]

We encountered somewhat better predictability of the ICL procedure for the correction of high hyperopia compared to our high myopia results.[37] Of 24 eyes that received an ICL for the correction of hyperopia (mean preoperative spherical equivalent refraction +6.51 + 2.08

D, range +3.75 to +10.50 D), we achieved a postoperative spherical equivalent refraction of + 1.00 D in 79% (19 eyes). The lower absolute value of the spherical equivalent refraction in the hyperopic group may have contributed to the better predictability. In addition, the preoperative manifest refraction (which is the major determinant in phakic IOL power calculations) in hyperopic eyes may be more reliable than in myopic eyes because of the spectacle-induced magnification in preoperative hyperopes. In contrast, myopic eyes may experience a more poorly defined preoperative refractive endpoint because of spectacle-induced minification.[38,39] The baseline refraction and refractive outcome of the initial 10 hyperopic eyes enrolled in the FDA study were similar to ours. The mean baseline spherical equivalent refraction was +6.63 D (range +2.50 to +10.88 D), and all 10 eyes (100%) achieved a postoperative spherical equivalent refraction within 1 D of emmetropia.[40]

The most dramatic results have been demonstrated with the bioptics procedure for the correction of extreme myopia, despite a much higher level of preoperative myopia. Of 67 eyes with a mean preoperative spherical equivalent refraction of -23.00 + 3.60 D, 85% achieved a postoperative spherical equivalent refraction within 1 D of emmetropia.[31]

Because of a reduction in preoperative spectacle-induced minification in myopic eyes, 76% of bioptics eyes and 36% of ICL-only eyes experienced a gain of two or more lines of vision.[31,32] Gains in best spectacle-corrected visual acuity in hyperopic eyes were less frequent than in myopic eyes, probably because the hyperopic eyes experienced spectacle-induced magnification preoperatively. Despite this, 8% (two eyes) of hyperopic eyes in our study and 20% (two eyes) of the initial eyes in the FDA study experienced a gain of two or more lines of best spectacle-corrected visual acuity.[37,40] An examination of best contact lens-corrected visual acuity (as opposed to best spectacle-corrected visual acuity) may offset some of the discrepancy in visual acuity gains between the myopic and hyperopic populations. Affording patients improved spectacle-corrected visual acuity has inherent merits of its own, however as patients become able to achieve functional vision in spectacles, giving them a reasonable vision correcting alternative to contact lenses.

The incidence of best spectacle-corrected visual acuity loss of two or more lines was 1% (two eyes) in our initial 148 eyes that received ICLs for the correction of myopia or hyperopia.[37,37] Of our initial 67 eyes that underwent bioptics for extreme myopia, no eyes lost more than one line of best spectacle-corrected visual acuity. The most important potential pitfall of bioptics is that patients are exposed to the known and unknown risks of two refractive procedures. In our recent report on the bioptics procedure, all eyes tolerated increased intraocular pressure during the microkeratome pass and there were no flap complications produced by the recent sutureless temporal clear corneal incision.[31] This has implications for patients who have experienced a "refractive surprise" following conventional cataract surgery-we can offer these patients LASIK to correct their residual refractive error once refractive stability has been attained.

Iatrogenic cataractogenesis is the major theoretical concern of posterior chamber phakic IOL implants such as the Staar ICL. Following ICL implantation, insufficient vaulting may lead to cataract formation either by

1. Mechanical irritation of the anterior lens capsule
2. Obstruction of aqueous circulation to the anterior crystalline lens

Poor vaulting may result from the implantation of an ICL with too small of a horizontal diameter. In contrast, excessive vaulting may occur if an ICL with too large a horizontal diameter is implanted, which may lead to iris chaffing and pigment loss. Vaulting is also influenced by the model of ICL used. Certain ICL models have a smaller posterior radius of curvature, which allows for more space between the posterior face of the ICL and the anterior face of the crystalline lens. Trindade and colleagues recently demonstrated peripheral ICL-crystalline lens touch by ultrasound biomicroscopy in nine eyes that received a Staar Collamer posterior chamber phakic IOL.[41] Only one eye, however, demonstrated possible central IOL-crystalline lens touch. The authors noted that unequivocal touch of the ICL and the crystalline lens could not be demonstrated because of limitations in the resolution of the ultrasound biomicroscope. Assetto, et al performed postoperative axial densitometry on 12 eyes that received the Collamer IOL and found no opacities of the crystalline lens.[35] In our original series of myopic eyes that underwent primary phakic IOL implantation, one eye (0.9%) developed an anterior subcapsular cataract as a result of preoperative laser iridotomy.[32] No phakic IOL-induced lenticular changes were noted in that series. However, in our bioptics series, one eye developed an anterior subcapsular cataract because of inadequate ICL vaulting over the crystalline lens. Trindade and Pereira recently reported a case of cataract formation 6 months after uneventful implantation of a myopic Staar ICL. Visual recovery was achieved after removing the phakic IOL and performing phacoemulsification with implantation of a foldable IOL through the same unenlarged self-sealing corneal incision.[42] Forthcoming reports with longer follow-up will help determine the incidence of cataractogenesis following posterior chamber phakic IOL implantation. No visually significant intraoperative or postoperative complications occurred in the initial 20 eyes that received ICLs in the FDA clinical trial.[36,40]

CONCLUSION

Refinements in lens design, power calculation formulas, and surgical technique have made posterior chamber phakic IOL implantation a promising technique for the correction of high myopia and hyperopia. By performing LASIK following ICL implantation to correct planned residual refractive errors (the two-staged bioptics procedure) more extreme levels of myopia, hyperopia, and eyes with significant co-existing astigmatism may be safely corrected. With appropriate patient selection, careful surgical manipulations, and close patient follow-up, excellent outcomes may be anticipated.

REFERENCES

1. Strampelli B, Sopportabilits' di lenti aciliche in camera anteriore nella afachia e nei vizi di refrazicne. *Ann Ottalmol Clin Ocul.* 1954;80:75-82.
2. Barraquer J. Anterior chamber plastic lenses. Results and conclusions from five years' experience. *Trans Ophthal Soc UK.* 1959;79:393-424.
3. Baikoff G, Joly P. Comparison of minus power anterior chamber intraocular lenses and myopic epikeratoplasty in phakic eyes. *J Refract Corneal Surg.* 1990;6:252-260.
4. Praeger DL, Momose A, Muroff LL. Thirty-six month follow-up of a contemporary phakic intraocular lens for the surgical correction of myopia. *Annals of Ophthalmology.* 1991;23:6-10.
5. Fechner PU, Strobel J, Wicchmann W. Correction of myopia by implantation of a concave Worst iris-claw lens into phakic eyes. *J Refract Corneal Surg.* 1991;7:286-298.
6. Baikoff G, Colin J. Intraocular lenses in phakic patients. *Ophthalmol Clin North Am.* 1992;5:789-795.
7. Perez-Santonja JJ, Iradier MT, Sanz-Iglesias L, Serrano JM, Zato MA. Endothelial changes in phakic eyes with anterior chamber intraocular lenses to correct high myopia. *J Cataract Refract Surg.* 1996;22:1017-1022.
8. Landesz M, Worst JGF, Siertsema JV, van Rij G. Correction of high myopia with the Worst myopia claw intraocular lens. *Journal of Refractive Surgery.* 1995;11:16-25.
9. Krumeich JH, Daniel J, Bast R. Closed-system technique for implantation of iris-supported negative-power intraocular lens. *Journal of Refractive Surgery.* 1996;12:334-340.
10. Baikoff G, Arne JL, Bokobza Y, et al. Angle fixated anterior chamber phakic IOL for myopia of -7 to -19 D. *Journal of Refractive Surgery.* 1999;14:282-293.
11. Fyodorov SN, Zuev VK, Aznabayev BM. Intraocular correction of high myopia with negative posterior chamber lens. *Ophthalmosurgery.* 1991:3:57-58.

12. Neumann AC. Update on three IOLs for myopia. In: Schonfeld AR. *Ocular Surgery News*. Dec 1, 1993. Presented at the ESCRS Annual Symposium, Innsbruck, Austria, September 1993; Fechner PU. Phakic PCL is promising for high myopia. In: Schonfeld AR, *Ocular Surgery News International Edition*. 1993;4:12. Presented at the ESCRS Annual Symposium, Innsbruck, Austria, September 1993.

13. Fyodorov SN, Zuyev VK, Tumanyan NR, Suheil AJ. Clinical and functional follow-up of minus IOL implantation in high-grade myopia. *Ophthalmosurgery*. 1993;2:12-17.

14. Aron-Rosa DS, Colin J, Aron B, et al. Clinical results of excimer laser photorefractive keratectomy: a multicenter study of 265 eyes. *J Cataract Refract Surg*. 1995;21:644-652.

15. Machat JJ. *Excimer Laser Refractive Surgery: Practice and Principles*. Thorofare, NJ, SLACK Incorporated; 1996.

16. Waring GO, Lindstrom KK. Published results of refractive keratotomy. In: Waring GO. *Refractive Keratotomy for Myopia and Astigmatism*. St. Louis, Mo: Mosby;1992.

17. Guell JL, Muller A. Laser in situ keratomileusis (LASIK) for myopia from -7 to -18 diopters. *Journal of Refractive Surgery*. 1996;12:222-228.

18. Menezo JL, Martinez-Costa R, Cisneros A, et al. Excimer laser photorefractive keratectomy for high myopia. *J Cataract Refract Surg*. 1995; 21:393-397.

19. Pop M, Aras M. Multizone/multipass photorefractive keratectomy: six month results. *J Cataract Refract Surg*. 1995;21:633-643.

20. Salah T, Waring GO, El Maghraby A, Moadel K, Grimm SB. Excimer laser in situ keratomileusis under a corneal flap for myopia of 2 to 20 diopters. *Am J Ophthalmol*. 1996;121:143-155.

21. Zaldivar R, Davidorf JM, Oscherow S. Laser in situ keratomileusis for myopia from -5.50 to -11.00 diopters with astigmatism. *Journal of Refractive Surgery*. 1998; 14(1):614-619.

22. Zaldivar R, Davidorf JM, Shultz MC, Oscherow S. LASIK for low myopia and astigmatism with a scanning spot excimer laser. *Journal of Refractive Surgery*. 1997;13(7).

23. Buratto L, Ferrari M, Genisi C. Myopic keratomileusis with the excimer laser: 1-year follow-up. *J Refract Corneal Surg*. 1993;9:12-19.

24. Helmy DA, Dalay A, Badawy TT, Sidky AN. Photorefractive keratectomy and laser in situ keratomileusis for myopia between 6.00 and 10.00 diopters. *Journal of Refractive Surgery*. 1996;12:417-421.

25. Salz JJ, Salz JM, Salz M, Jones D. Ten years experience with a conservative approach to radial keratotomy. *J Refract Corneal Surg*. 1991;7:12-22.

26. Kim WJ, Lee JH. Long-term results of myopic epikeratoplasty. *J Cataract Refract Surg*. 1993;19:352-355.

27. Goosey JD, Prager TC, Goosey CB, Allison ME, Marvelli TL. Stability of refraction during two years after myopic epikeratoplasty. *J Refract Corneal Surg*. 1990;6:4-8.

28. Lohmann CP, Gartry DS, Kerr Muir M, et al. Haze in photorefractive keratectomy: its origins and consequences. *Lasers Light Ophthalmol*. 1991;4:15-34.

29. Seiler T, Wollensak J. Results of a prospective evaluation of photorefractive keratectomy at 1 year after surgery. *German Journal of Ophthalmology*. 1993;2:135-142.

30. Chan WK, Heng WJ, Tseng P, et al. Photorefractive keratectomy for myopia of 6 to 12 D. *Journal of Refractive Surgery*. 1995;11:S286-S292.

31. Zaldivar R, Davidorf JM, Oscherow S, Ricur G, Piezzi V. Combined posterior chamber phakic intraocular lens and laser in situ keratomileusis: bioptics for extreme myopia. *Journal of Refractive Surgery*. In press.

32. Zaldivar R, Davidorf JM, Oscherow S. Posterior chamber phakic intraocular lens implantation for extreme myopia. *Journal of Refractive Surgery*. 1998;14:294-305.

33. Deitz MR. Human implants of implantable contact lenses. Proceedings from the sixth annual Ocular Surgery News Symposium. New York, NY. September 1997.

34. Guell J. The adjustable refractive surgery concept (ARS). *Journal of Refractive Surgery*. 1998;14:271.

35. Assetto V, Benedetti S, Pesando P. Collamer intraocular contact lens to correct high myopia. *J Cataract Refract Surg*. 1996;22:551-556.

36. Sanders DR, Brown DC, Martin RG, Shepherd J, Deitz MR, DeLuca M. Implantable contact lens for moderate to high myopia: phase 1 FDA clinical study with 6 month follow-up. *J Cataract Refract Surg*. 1998;5:607-11.

37. Davidorf JM, Zaldivar R, Oscherow S. Posterior chamber phakic intraocular lens implantation for high hyperopia. *Journal of Refractive Surgery*. 1998;14:306-311.

38. Applegate RA, Howland HC. Magnification and visual acuity in refractive surgery. *Arch Ophthalmol*. 1993;111:1335-1342.

39. van der Heijde GL. Some optical aspects of implantation of an IOL in a myopic eye. *European Journal of Implant and Refractive Surgery*. 1989;1:245-248.

40. Brown D, Deitz M, Martin R, Shepherd J. Implantable contact lens for hyperopia: US FDA study. Presented at the American Academy of Ophthalmology Annual Meeting, San Francisco, 1997.

41. Trindade F, Pereira F, Cronemberger S. Ultrasound biomicroscopic imaging of posterior chamber phakic intraocular lens. *J Cataract Refract Surg*. 1998(5):497-503.

42. Trindade F, Pereira F. Cataract formation after posterior chamber phakic intraocular lens implantation. *Journal of Refractive Surgery*. 1998(12):1661-1663.

Combined LASIK Surgeries

José Güell, MD, PhD and Mercedes Vázquez, MD

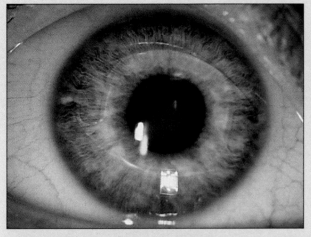

Figure 28A-1. ARS (adjustable refractive surgery) concept: 6.0 mm Artisan phakic IOL plus LASIK for the correction of a –19 D young myopic patient

Combined procedures have been performed in order to get an additive effect on refractive efficacy and predictability, as well as postoperative visual quality, when correcting high myopia and/or astigmatism.[1]

The goal of these combined techniques is to reduce myopia and/or astigmatism with the first procedure: Artisan lens implantation[2] or arcuate keratotomy,[3] correcting the residual sphere and/or cylinder with LASIK as a second procedure, and maintaining the largest possible optical zone in both.

In high myopic candidates for this two-stage procedure, it is possible to perform the lamellar cut at the time of the first surgery, with the phakic IOL implantation, avoiding the possible risks associated with the microkeratome once the IOL is inside the eye.

After all the sutures have been removed and the residual cylinder has been stable for at least a 6-week period, the final refraction is adjusted with LASIK by lifting the flap and performing the ablation with the excimer laser, as with our standard LASIK enhancement. This approach is what we termed ARS: adjustable refractive surgery.[4]

The ARS concept[5] has different advantages in different surgical situations. When an anterior chamber phakic or aphakic IOL is present, we avoid IOL-endothelial touch. When a posterior chamber phakic IOL is present, we avoid the possible luxation of the IOL in the anterior chamber. When we have a high myopic pseudophakic

eye, an elongated eye with the natural lens, we avoid the possible peripheral retinal damage associated with the suction pressure developed during LASIK.

AK is an effective procedure to correct astigmatism, but its results are more accurate when correcting lower degrees of astigmatism. Astigmatic myopic LASIK is also less predictable with astigmatism higher than 3 D, and the tendency is to undercorrect, especially if we plan to correct the sphere at the same time a large amount of tissue removal is necessary. This is why we have assessed the additive effect of both procedures together in patients with astigmatism higher than 3 D. The patients undergo arcuate keratotomy, and once the residual cylinder is stable for at least a 6-week period, LASIK is performed. We have achieved good results with a mean astigmatism reduction of 85%, and with a better quality of vision than using LASIK alone.

Using a 4.0 to 5.5 mm optical zone when implanting a phakic IOL alone or when performing arcuate keratotomy, it is possible to correct high degrees of myopia or astigmatism, but because of the possibility of glare, halos, and contrast sensitivity loss, we do not recommend this option. With these combined techniques it is possible to maintain a 6.5 mm optical clear zone due to the additive effect of both procedures, drastically reducing the possibility of glare, night halos, and reduced quantity and quality of vision at night.

The most important aspect of these combined techniques is its safety both from the clinical and visual quality aspects. Also, the fact that performing LASIK as a second procedure to correct residual ametropia allows us to increase the predictability of the technique.

REFERENCES

1. Güell JL, Gris O, Muller A, Corcóstegui B. LASIK for the correction of residual refractive errors from previous surgical procedures. *Ophthalmic Surgery and Lasers.* 1999;30:5341-349.
2. Güell JL, Vazquez M, Gris O, Muller A, Manero F. Combined Artisan lens and laser in situ keratomileusis to correct high myopia. *Journal of Refractive Surgery.* In press.
3. Güell JL, Vazquez M. The correction of high astigmatism with astigmatic keratotomy combined with LASIK. *J Cataract Refract Surg.* Pending publication.
4. Güell JL. The adjustable refractive surgery concept (ARS). *Journal of Refractive Surgery.* 1998;14:271.
5. Güell JL. The adjustable refractive surgery concept: phakic IOL plus LASIK. *Eye World.* 1998;3(12):15-16.

MYOPIC AND HYPEROPIC LASIK ENHANCEMENTS

Louis E. Probst, V, MD
Jeffery J. Machat, MD

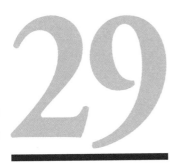

INTRODUCTION

The dramatic results that patients experience following LASIK are not completely stable during the first few postoperative months. As the degree of myopia increases, so does the amount of regression from the initial myopic correction, thus the subsequent need for enhancement procedures. The maximal regression typically occurs between 2 to 4 weeks postoperatively, after which relative refractive stability is achieved. A smaller amount of regression is generally noted from 1 to 3 months postoperatively.

For high myopia, we treat the majority of the myopia in the first procedure and the residual myopia during the enhancement procedure. A golfing analogy is useful when describing this concept to patients: the first procedure will get them onto the "green" and the second procedure will "putt" them into the "hole."

The enhancement procedure is associated with a lower surgical risk and greater predictability, as the flap can be lifted rather than cut if the enhancement is performed before 6 months postoperatively and a much smaller, more precise excimer laser ablation is required. This two-step method is also very effective in avoiding hyperopic overcorrections. At The Laser Center (TLC), during the preoperative counseling process, we inform all patients who have greater than 10 diopters (D) of myopia that they will require an enhancement procedure. By preparing each patient for the need for enhancements, we have found that they are very accepting of the second procedure, although the majority of patients will not require further surgery.

LASIK enhancement procedures are mainly performed with the lamellar technique of lifting the original flap or performing a second pass with the microkeratome. Photorefractive keratectomy (PRK) should not be used for LASIK enhancements, as the surface ablation will thin the corneal flap and has been associated with significant postoperative confluent haze in 4 of the 6 cases attempted by two TLC centers.

PRINCIPLES OF MYOPIC AND HYPEROPIC LASIK ENHANCEMENTS

All excimer laser refractive procedures modify the refracting power of the cornea by altering the anterior corneal curvature by the process of photoablation. The correction of myopia involves increased relative flattening of the central cornea compared to the peripheral cornea, which reduces the anterior corneal curvature and hence reduces the refractive power of the treated area. Because the maximal corneal stromal tissue will be photoablated from the central cornea, the thickness of the central cornea becomes important when LASIK is performed for high refractive errors with large ablation depths.

The average central cornea thickness is approximately 550 ± 100 microns. Since flap thickness during the LASIK procedure is generally 160 microns, the average cornea will have 390 microns of posterior stromal tissue left for ablation. When the multi-multizone ablation technique is used with the ablation pattern distributed between 3.6 and 6.2 mm, the average stromal ablation per diopter will be approximately 10 microns.

It has been recommended that at least 250 microns of posterior stromal tissue be left after the myopic LASIK procedure to avoid a loss of corneal integrity and subsequent development of corneal ectasia. Since we have observed iatrogenic keratoconus after automated lamellar keratoplasty (ALK) with 200 microns of remaining posterior stromal tissue, we generally elect to leave at least 250 microns of posterior stromal tissue. Therefore, the maximal myopic correction that should be performed on a patient with a 550 microns cornea using a full multizone technique is generally less than 14 D ([550 μm - 160 μm - 250 μm]/10 μm per D = 14 D).

A simpler and less mathematically complex way of calculating the safe maximal myopic correction is to always leave at least 400 microns of total stromal tissue following LASIK.[2] With an average flap thickness of 160 microns, approximately 240 microns of posterior corneal stromal would be left to maintain corneal integrity. For the average 550-micron cornea, this would allow a maximal myopic correction of 15 D ([550 μm - 400 μm]/10 μm per D = 15 D). With a single zone LASIK technique, the ablation per diopter would be increased to 15 microns and would allow the maximal correction of 10 D ([550 μm - 400 μm]/15 μm per D = 10 D). Modified multizone LASIK algorithms with increased zone depths of 30 microns result in an ablation of 12.5 microns per diopter and would allow a maximal correction of 12 D ([550 μm - 400 μm]/12.5 μm per D = 12 D).

Some surgeons have recommend that the depth of the stromal ablation not exceed more than 50% of the preoperative pachymetry value. Using this method, the average 550-micron cornea with a 160-micron flap would have 115 microns available for ablation (550 μm/2 - 160 μm = 115 μm) for a correction of 11.5 D (115 μm/10 μm per diopter) and 275 microns of posterior stromal tissue.

Regardless of the calculation method, a minimum of 200 microns of central posterior stromal tissue should be preserved for myopic LASIK, and ideally 240 to 250 microns. It should be noted that the distribution of the central stromal thinning is different following ALK and LASIK. With ALK, a 4.2-mm lamellar disc is removed from the center of the visual axis, creating uniform thinning over the entire area where the tissue was removed. With LASIK, however, excimer ablation using either the single zone or the multizone techniques, results in a gradient of thinning maximal only in the very central region of the ablation zone, with the remaining posterior stromal tissue maintaining substantially more thickness. Therefore, corneal integrity should be better preserved following LASIK compared to ALK.

While these calculations are crucial for preoperative planning and patient counseling prior to the original LASIK procedure, they are no less important during the myopic LASIK enhancement procedure. All patients must have preoperative pachymetry prior to the enhancement procedure to determine whether an adequate amount of posterior stromal tissue remains to allow for an enhancement procedure to be performed.

During a myopic enhancement procedure, we always leave at least 200 microns of posterior stromal tissue, and ideally 240 microns. Since enhancement ablations are generally performed at the 6.2 mm ablation zone, approximately 20 microns of stromal tissue is ablated per diopter of correction. Therefore, a post-LASIK patient with pre-enhancement pachymetry readings of 440 microns would have the absolute maximal amount of tissue to allow a 2.0 D correction if the flap thickness was 160 microns ([440 μm - 160 μm - 240 μm]/ 20 μm per D = 2.0 D). If, however, the flap needs to be recut (as we recommend 6 months post-LASIK and perform at 200 microns), there would be no further posterior stromal tissue available for safe ablation (440 μm - 200 μm - 240 μm = 0 D) without risking the corneal integrity and potential postoperative corneal ectasia. In general, we do not recommend enhancing eyes with less than 400 microns of total remaining corneal tissue.

The maximum correction for hyperopic LASIK (H-LASIK) is not governed by the depth of the ablation but rather the limitations on the amount of steepening that can be successfully performed on the cornea. H-LASIK removes tissue at approximately 15 microns per diopter of hyperopic correction, however much more corneal tissue is removed since the ablation is performed over the peripheral cornea. The peripheral cornea is generally thicker than the central cornea, so corrections of more than +6.0 D are technically possible with a scanning excimer laser. However, clinical experience has shown that H-LASIK should generally not be performed for over +4.0 to +5.0 D due to increased risk of regression, decentrations, and loss of best-corrected visual acuity (BCVA). These principles are critical when considering an H-LASIK enhancement.

PREOPERATIVE EVALUATION

Potential candidates for a LASIK retreatment should have an evaluation at 1 to 3 months following the original LASIK procedure, as most of the regression will have occurred by this point and the LASIK flap can still be easily lifted. Most of the regression occurs by 1 month and stability is achieved by 3 months, so the enhancement procedure can be planned at 1 month for 3 months postoperatively. The lower the degree of pre-LASIK myopia, the earlier the enhancement can potentially be performed: a -3.00 D myope could be safely enhanced at 1 month while a -12 D myope should wait the full 3 to 4 months prior to enhancement (Table 29-1). Full preoperative evaluation should include a review of the original procedure to identify any unusual surgical difficulties and the refractive history. Preoperative testing should include refraction, pachymetry, computerized

	Table 29-1	
	LASIK ENHANCEMENTS	
Error	**Comment**	**Treatment**
Hyperopia		
	Normal cornea	Hyperopic LASIK at 4 months
	Thin cornea	LTK at 6 months
Myopia		
	1 to 3 D preop	Myopic LASIK at 1 month
	3 to 6 D preop	Myopic LASIK at 2 months
	Greater than 6 D	Myopic LASIK at 3 to 4 months
Regression	Wait for stability	Myopic LASIK
Astigmatism	Wait for stability	LASIK at 3 to 4 months

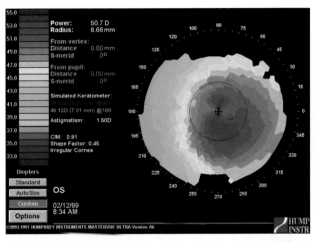

Figure 29-1. Decentered ablation following a +6.0 D hyperopic LASIK correction.

videokeratography, and corneal examination to identify any additional concerns such as epithelial ingrowth, flap striae, or a flap melt.

The preoperative refraction allows the identification of residual or regressive myopia and astigmatism. There should be no more than 0.25 to 0.50 D change in the refractive error over the last 2 postoperative months in order to allow reasonable predictability for the enhancement procedure. Often, uncorrected visual acuity (UCVA) is better than the myopia measured post-LASIK would suggest. For example, a -2.25 D regressive myopia post-LASIK may have a visual acuity of 20/60, which is the UCVA generally observed for -1.25 D primary myopia (the UCVA of a primary myope can be estimated by moving up one Snellen line from 20/20 for each 0.25 D of myopia, so a -1.25 D myope would be expected to have a UCVA of 1.25/0.25 = five lines up from the 20/20 Snellen visual acuity line, or 20/60). If such a discrepancy exists, we perform a more conservative enhancement to account for the better UCVA. This often

results in a retreatment for 60% to 70% of the refractive error. Any remarkable discrepancy between the uncorrected visual acuity and the post-LASIK refractive error suggests that a central island or decentered ablation may be present on computerized videokeratography. The enhancement procedure strategy is to always be conservative in order to avoid postoperative hyperopia.

Preoperative pachymetry must be performed for all post-LASIK patients to identify the amount of residual posterior stroma available for ablation. This measurement should be correlated to the preoperative refraction and UCVA in order to determine the most efficacious and safe correction that can be performed. Corneal videokeratography will also identify central islands, decentered ablations, and epithelial ingrowth, which can alter the method of treatment.

LASIK enhancements following primary H-LASIK should be approached with caution. Large H-LASIK corrections of over +4.0 D will often be associated with considerable regression. While these eyes can be technically retreated, this will induce tremendous central corneal steepening. This keratoconus-like configuration of the cornea can produce dry eye-like symptoms due to poor wetting of the central steep cornea. Other concerns after excessive H-LASIK include fluctuations in vision and a loss of BCVA. Preoperative topography is essential for the identification of decentered ablations following H-LASIK (Figure 29-1).

LASIK enhancements can also be preformed following other refractive corneal procedures such as radial keratotomy, photorefractive keratectomy, and penetrating keratoplasty (Tables 29-2 to 29-4). Each of these situations are unique with their own indications, techniques, and risks. Patients should be fully informed of both the benefits and additional risks of LASIK after previous corneal surgery.

Table 29-2

LASIK AFTER RK

Indications
- Stable refraction
- Residual myopia or hyperopia
- Regular astigmatism
- Eight or less radial incision
- Optical zone of 3.0 mm or greater

Risks
- Unstable postoperative refraction
- Decreased postoperative refractive predictability
- Flap fragmentation
- Epithelial ingrowth
- Persistent starburst and night glare
- Persistent diurnal variation
- Potential increase in corneal anatomical instability

Preoperative
- Refractive stability
- Early morning refraction
- Eight or less radial incisions
- Optical zone at least 3.0 mm
- Radial incisions well healed
- No epithelial cysts
- No reduction in BCVA

Procedure
- 200-micron depth plate with ACS
- Target slight myopia
- Monocular treatment
- Extreme care with flap manipulation
- Alignment of flap and radial incisions

Postoperative
- Expect greater refractive fluctuations initially
- Watch for epithelial ingrowth
- Do not lift flap after LASIK with RK
- Recut at 6 months for enhancements

SURGICAL TECHNIQUES

There are two main methods of performing an enhancement following LASIK: lifting the original flap and recutting another flap.[2] During the first 6 months following the original LASIK procedure, we recommend that patients have the flap lifted and the ablation performed in the original plane. The flap is quite easy to lift up to 6 months postoperatively. While we have lifted flaps up to 14 months following LASIK, this technique becomes progressively more difficult after the 6-month period. Although patients can experience 24 hours of discomfort following this procedure due to the epithelial defects that often occur along the edge of the flap, this technique is much safer, as it has none of the risks associated with another pass of the microkeratome.

After 6 postoperative months, we recommend the

Table 29-3

LASIK AFTER PRK

Indications
- Stable refraction
- Residual myopia or hyperopia
- Regular astigmatism
- Adequate corneal thickness

Risks
- Persistence of superficial corneal haze
- Epithelial defects
- Epithelial ingrowth
- Reduction in corneal anatomic integrity

Preoperative
- Refractive stability
- Adequate corneal thickness
- No corneal haze
- No history of recurrent erosion after PRK
- Well-centered ablation on topography
- No loss of BCVA

Procedure
- 200 microns depth plate with ACS
- Minimal topical anesthetic
- Lubrication to protect epithelium

Postoperative
- Watch for epithelial ingrowth

Table 29-4

LASIK AFTER PK

Indications
- Stable refraction
- Residual myopia or hyperopia
- Regular astigmatism
- Adequate corneal thickness
- Sutures out for at least 1 year
- Reasonable BCVA

Risks
- Unstable postoperative refraction
- Decreased postoperative refractive predictability
- Epithelial ingrowth
- Dehiscence along graft edge
- Induction of graft rejection
- Greater enhancement rate

Preoperative
- Wait 12 months after sutures are out
- Stable refraction
- Ensure regular astigmatism on topography

Procedure
- Center suction ring on graft
- Minimize suction time
- Wait 2 weeks before performing ablation (?)

Postoperative
- Topical steroids for 1 to 2 weeks to prevent rejection
- Watch for ingrowth
- Wait 4 months for enhancement
- Lift flap for enhancement

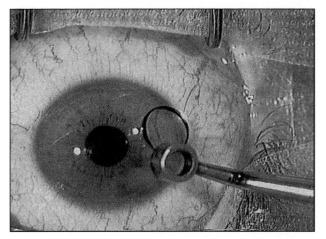

Figure 29-2. Lifting the corneal flap: the marking circles are placed to assist with flap realignment at the end of the procedure (photos reprinted with permission from Machat JJ, Slade SG, Probst LE. *The Art of LASIK, Second Edition.* Thorofare, NJ: SLACK Incorporated; 1999).

flap be recut. This technique offers the advantage of a comfortable eye postoperatively without epithelial defects and a rapid rehabilitation of vision, usually by the next postoperative day. However, recutting the flap is associated with all the risks of the original lamellar procedure, including corneal perforation, flap configuration problems, free flaps, and lost flaps There are also added risks associated with recutting a cornea that has already had a lamellar cut and is centrally flattened because of the original LASIK stromal ablation, including a higher risk of a centrally thin or perforated flap and the potential to generate a free corneal wedge of tissue where the two flaps intersect if the original flap has not adequately healed.

Lifting the Original Flap

Preparation of the eye should include avoidance of the liberal use of topical anesthetic, as is commonly done for PRK. Topical anesthetics are toxic to the corneal epithelium, which is preserved with LASIK. Irrigation of the fornices with balanced salt solution (BSS) removes debris from the tear film. Preoperative antibiotics and Voltaren are instilled routinely and 2 to 3 mg of lorazepam is given sublingually 10 to 15 minutes prior to the procedure.

The patient is taken to the slit lamp biomicroscope and the edge of the flap is marked with a sharp instrument, such as fine forceps like the Suarez or the Machat spreader. This initial step, which was developed at TLC, is essential, as it allows simple, rapid reopening of the flap with minimal epithelial trauma and maximal postoperative comfort. It is not necessary to create an epithelial defect that can cause the patient discomfort following the

procedure, but only to indent the epithelium sufficiently to allow detection of the mark under the excimer laser operating microscope. If the flap edge is not marked at the slit lamp biomicroscope, it may be impossible to discern the flap edge under the surgical microscope because of lack of tangential illumination.

The patient is then aligned underneath the surgical microscope and the eye is thoroughly anesthetized in the fornices prior to the insertion of the eyelid speculum. As with the original LASIK procedure, it is useful to use a drape or tape the eyelashes underneath the speculum to ensure that they do not interfere with the flap. The Probst tape tucker provides a convenient and painless method of tucking the eyelid tape or surgical drape into the conjunctival fornices so that the eyelashes are completely separated from the operative area. The adjustable titanium Liebermann eyelid speculum offers excellent exposure, and the locking mechanism ensures that patient eyelid squeezing is minimized.

A bladed lid speculum can also be used for LASIK enhancements, which provide some advantages over draping the lids. The bladed speculum provides adequate exposure particularly when an extra strong variety is used, such as the Probst LASIK enhancement power speculum (Storz). The bladed speculum cannot be used for primary LASIK, as the suction ring will not fit into the central opening, however this is not an issue for LASIK enhancements. Lid draping is not required, as the blades will isolate the lashes from the eye. Finally, patients often find the bladed speculum more comfortable, as less localized pressure is placed on the lids.

The cornea is then marked temporally with one or two 3.75-mm optical zone markers that have been covered with gentian violet (Figure 29-2). In the primary LASIK procedure, two optical zones markers of different sizes (3.25 mm and 3.75 mm) for four-point alignment are used so that the flap can be correctly oriented using the disparate circle sizes should a free flap occur. When performing an enhancement procedure by lifting the flap with an intact hinge, the risk of a free flap is minimal, therefore two different sized optical zone markers are not necessary. These corneal marks are placed in a straddling position over the flap edge so that both the flap and the peripheral cornea are marked. It is helpful to place one of the markers over the indented epithelial mark as well, as this will further facilitate finding the lamellar plane of the original LASIK incision. Correct repositioning of the flap following the enhancement procedure is indicated by the proper realignment of these corneal marks.

A spreader is then inserted at the interface indicated by the demarcated flap edge (Figure 29-3). Marking allows precise placement of the spreader and therefore

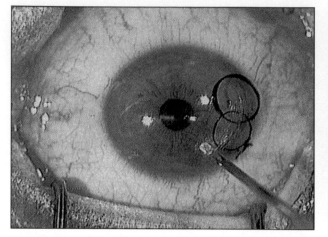

Figure 29-3. Lifting the corneal flap: the Machat spreader is inserted under the corneal flap and the temporal edge of the flap is gently opened.

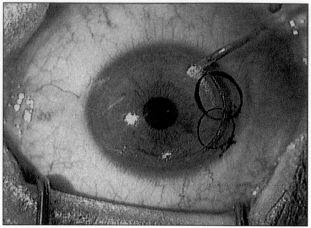

Figure 29-4. Lifting the corneal flap: the Machat spreader has been moved circumferentially in order to open the temporal aspect of the flap.

minimizes unnecessary trauma to the surrounding tissue. Gentle down and inward pressure is usually sufficient to place the spreader within the lamellar plane of the LASIK flap. This step can also be performed at the slit lamp, creating a 1 to 2 o'clock pocket to insert the spreader. The spreader is passed along the healed cut edge peripherally (Figure 29-4). Typically, the flap adhesion is along the cut edge of Bowman's layer for approximately 0.5 to 1.0 mm. The spreader should be moved and oriented so that the lamellar dissection is only along the flap edge. The tendency to further insert the spreader beneath the flap should be avoided, as this may introduce epithelial cells underneath the flap and contribute to postoperative epithelial ingrowth. Once the flap edge has been sufficiently dissected, the flap is gently grasped with nontoothed forceps and with slow and steady nasal traction it can be reflected back onto the conjunctiva (Figure 29-5). During this step, it is important to not reposition or regrasp the flap, as this can result in epithelial displacement. The main concern when lifting the flap should be preservation of epithelium. Any extra disruption of the epithelium will increase postoperative discomfort and the risk of epithelial ingrowth. If a LASIK enhancement by lifting the flap is done well, there will be not greater discomfort or risk of epithelial ingrowth as compared to the primary LASIK procedure.

Once the peripheral healed edge along Bowman's layer has been opened, the strength of the stromal adhesion is extremely variable. While the most consistent factor associated with strong stromal adhesion is increased postoperative time, patients with aggressive wound-healing characteristics and with flap problems, such as stromal melt or haze, may also have increased stromal adherence.[2] Epithelial ingrowth within the interface tends to prevent adhesion of the flap to the stromal bed, allowing

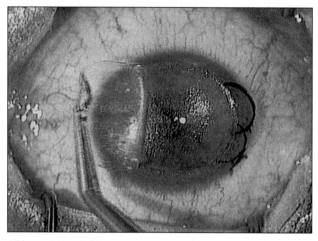

Figure 29-5. Lifting the corneal flap: nontoothed forceps are used to reflect the flap nasally.

the flap to be lifted more easily in this region. If a strong adhesion is encountered, a blunt instrument such as the cyclodialysis spatula found on the other end of the Machat spreader is inserted beneath the flap and a gentle lamellar dissection is performed. Some surgeons have advocated using filtered BSS to dissect the interface, however this will alter the stromal hydration and can therefore affect efficacy of the enhancement excimer ablation.[2]

Once the flap has been reflected back, the interface is inspected under high magnification for any evidence of epithelium or debris that has been introduced underneath the flap. Any epithelium that is hanging over the peripheral edge of interface bed, present on the stromal interface, or present on the reflected flap surface must be removed by gently scraping those affected areas with a sharp surgical blade (Figure 29-6) that is regularly

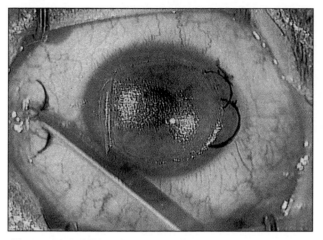

Figure 29-6. Lifting the corneal flap: the stromal bed and undersurface of the corneal flap are gently scraped to remove debris or epithelium.

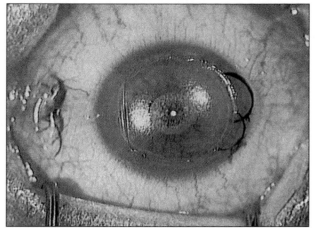

Figure 29-7. Lifting the corneal flap: the excimer laser ablation is performed centered on the center of the pupil. The pretreatment protocol has been performed using the Chiron Technolas Keracor 116 excimer laser at 3.0 mm.

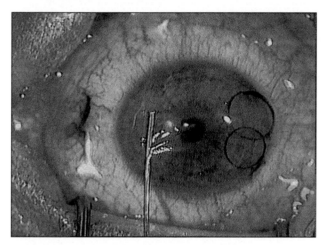

Figure 29-8. Lifting the corneal flap: after the flap has been replaced, a cannula is placed beneath the flap and it is refloated into its original position as indicated by realignment of the corneal markings.

inspected and cleaned of the epithelial debris that accumulates on its surface. If this process is carefully and meticulously performed, risk of epithelial ingrowth is similar or less than the risk of epithelial ingrowth associated with recutting the corneal flap, and the complications associated with recutting are avoided.

The ablation is then performed according to the preoperative calculations (Figure 29-7). Since the patient has free movement of the eye during the enhancement procedure, constant verbal encouragement must be to fixate on the fixation light and to resist squeezing the eyes, which can cause Bell's phenomena. The pneumatic suction ring without the actual application of suction can be used to stabilize the eyes of patients unable to maintain their eye position or patients with nystagmus. The central corneal stroma can be dried with filtered air, a surgical spear, or wiped with a spatula in order to avoid central accumulations of fluid and central island formation.[2] Scanning excimer laser systems such as the Chiron Technolas 217 or broadbeam excimer laser systems equipped with a pretreatment nomogram, as developed by Machat, such as the VISX Star do not require central island compensation techniques.

Following the ablation, the reflected flap and stromal bed along the hinge are hydrated with several drops of BSS. An instrument such as the blunt forceps or a cyclodialysis spatula is inserted under the nasal hinge of the reflected flap and the flap is gently replaced with one smooth motion temporally. The interface is then thoroughly irrigated with filtered BSS injected through a flat cannula such as a hydrodissection needle or a flattened blunt-tipped 25-gauge cannula that has been inserted along the lamellar plane underneath the flap (Figure 29-8). Irrigation can be used for up to 10 seconds to remove debris, fibers, and small air bubbles that are often noted on close inspection of the flap interface. Excessive fluid irrigation should be avoided, as it can result in the corneal flap swelling, poor flap adhesion, and incorrect flap alignment. After interface irrigation, the cannula is gently withdrawn to allow the flap to "float" into its correct position. Wet surgical spears are then lightly wiped from nasal to temporal flap positions to remove the remaining interface fluid. Generally, perfect flap alignment is observed at this point, however if the corneal markings indicate misalignment, the flap should be refloated and wiped again so positioning can be reassessed.

The patient is instructed to maintain fixation on the fixation light for about 2 minutes, to allow for adequate adhesion to form between the flap and the stromal bed.

Filtered compressed air can be used to promote flap adhesion, however this should be used conservatively as it often results in flap shrinkage along the flap edge.[2] Surgeons should resist the temptation to poke and prod the flap and the flap edge during this waiting period, as this invariably results in a disturbance in the flap alignment and does not speed the process of flap adhesion. If little BSS was used, the flap will generally seal in 1 minute, however, when an excessive amount of BSS irrigation is used, flap adhesion can take as long as 5 minutes. The majority of flaps will form adequate adhesion in 2 to 3 minutes.

A final check of the corneal flap involves the assessment of two factors: flap alignment and flap adhesion. Proper flap alignment is confirmed not only by realignment of the circular corneal markings but also by the edge gape test, the Probst surface test, and the retroillumination test. The edge gape test involves a quick circumferential check of the flap edge to ensure that excessive gape is not present in one location, indicating that the flap may be displaced in the opposite direction (Figure 29-9). The Probst surface test involves inspection of the reflection of the light reflex off the dry surface of the cornea. Any ripples or lines identified when the microscope illumination light reflects off the dried corneal surface may indicate that corneal striae and/or flap misalignment are present. The retroillumination test also allows the identification of subtle flap striae by projecting the fixation beam directing through the center of the pupil with the surgical microscope illumination light turned off. If any problems are identified with the corneal flap it should be refloated.

Tests of the flap adherence include the striae test and the blink test. The Slade striae test involves gently pressing along the cut corneal edge peripheral to the flap with the blunt forceps to ensure that the striae are transmitted through to the flap indicating that it is well adhered to the stromal bed (see Figure 29-9). The side of blunt forceps can then be wiped peripherally along the flap edge to confirm the flap adherence, smooth the flap edges, or realign the flap edges. The blink test is performed after the lid speculum has been carefully removed from the eye so that the arms of the speculum do not touch the flap edges. The patient is asked to blink several times, the eyelids are opened, and the flap edges are examined once again. Occasionally, slight displacement of the superior edge of the flap with a few associated striae will be noted. If the flap is displaced, it must be refloated, and if the flap is not demonstrating adequate adherence, it must be left to stabilize with the eyelid speculum in place for 1 or 2 more minutes and then retested.[2] If flap striae are present only in the superior position, they can be elimi-

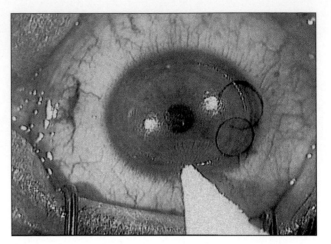

Figure 29-9. Lifting the corneal flap: the gutter test involves examining the small gap between the peripheral flap and the cornea. Asymmetry found on the gutter test indicates that the flap may not be accurately placed. The Slade striae test is performed by gently pressing on the corneal edge peripheral to the flap to ensure that the striae are transmitted through to the flap, indicating good flap adherence.

nated by instructing the patient to look down, smoothing the striae with the side of the blunt forceps or a Merocel sponge, and then waiting another minute for readhesion.

Recutting the Original Flap

Six months after the original LASIK procedure the corneal flap becomes very adherent, making the process of lifting the flap more difficult and time consuming. This also invariably results in more epithelial defects and some degree of flap distortion. For these reasons, we recommend recutting the flap after this postoperative period. Many high-volume LASIK surgeons routinely recut a new flap for retreatment at 3 months or earlier, however, the risks and benefits of this technique must be considered. At TLC, we use the Chiron Vision Automated Corneal Shaper (ACS) microkeratome for our LASIK procedures.

The advantages to performing a second microkeratome pass are that the basic dynamics of the original LASIK procedure are unchanged, the nomogram for the excimer ablation is still applicable, and excessive flap and flap edge manipulation are avoided, so postoperative pain and discomfort are minimized.[2] Additionally, since there is less displacement of epithelial cells around the rim of the flap, theoretically the incidence of epithelial ingrowth is expected to be less than after the original flap is manually relifted. This, however, has not been found to be clinically significant, since we began scraping and cleaning the undersurface of the flap and the stromal bed during LASIK enhancements performed by lifting the flap.

The disadvantages of performing the second microkeratome pass are three-fold. The eye is once again subjected to the risks of the previous microkeratome pass, which include ocular perforation, thin flap, short flap, free flap, or an irregular flap. Additionally, the corneal contour has now been altered so that the central cornea is significantly flattened often to less than 40 D, as measured by computerized videokeratography. While clinically this does not seem to cause a problem with flap creation because the peripheral edge of the cornea where the microkeratome engages is still its original steepness, this does increase the risk of free, perforated, and thin flaps. Finally, performing a second microkeratome pass requires an additional lamellar cut be made in the cornea. Most surgeons will perform the second lamellar cut at the same depth as the original cut, however this can result in a loose lamellar wedge of stromal tissue if the postoperative period has been too short and adequate healing of the original lamellar cut has not occurred.[2] We prefer to wait at least 6 months, with a minimum of 3 months, before the second lamellar cut to ensure that a firm bond has occurred between the original flap and the stromal bed. We generally perform the second microkeratome pass at 200 microns to compensate for the flatter cornea and to minimize the risk of creating a free wedge of cornea.

The technique used to perform the second microkeratome pass is identical to the original LASIK procedure.[1] The microkeratome is religiously and systematically checked prior to each procedure using the "look, listen, and feel" tests. The microkeratome is examined under the microscope to ensure that blade quality is excellent, the stopper is in place, the plate number is correct and fully inserted, and blade oscillation is consistent. The microkeratome is run through the pneumatic suction ring to ensure smooth passage. A change in the pitch of the microkeratome motor as it advances and reverses can provide clues about improperly assembled equipment or a weak motor. The head of the microkeratome and the plate screw are felt to ensure they are firmly attached.

After the eye has been appropriately prepared and anesthetized and the lid speculum has been placed as previously described, the cornea is peripherally marked using the Machat marking technique with two optical zone markers of different sizes so that a free flap could be appropriately replaced and reoriented if necessary. The pneumatic suction ring is placed on the eye and displaced 0.5 to 1.0 mm nasally on the cornea to displace the hinge of the corneal flap more medially, away from the area of ablation. The suction ring can also be displaced slightly inferiorly to avoid cutting through excessive superior corneal neovascularization.

The authors utilize the following technique for small orbits and deep-set eyes when it is often difficult to get adequate suction; this technique can be used successfully for all eyes. Downward pressure on the eyelid speculum will cause the eye to proptose, increase the tautness of the conjunctiva, and cause the palpebral opening to slightly increase, allowing placement of the pneumatic suction ring with firm downward pressure for 1 to 2 seconds to create a firm seal before the suction is activated. The suction is then applied and the level verified by the meter on the base unit to ensure adequate suction has been achieved.

Once suction is achieved, the pneumatic suction ring is lightly supported. Downward pressure on the suction ring can result in prolapsing conjunctiva and elevation of the eyelid speculum above the plane of the microkeratome, which makes smooth passage of the microkeratome extremely difficult. The suction ring should not be torqued, as this may result in loss of suction. The intraocular pressure is then checked with the Barraquer applanation tonometer to confirm a level greater than 65 mm Hg.

The experienced LASIK surgeon does not need to check the size of the LASIK flap when using the fixed LASIK suction ring, as the size of the flap can be predicted by the preoperative curvature and diameter. The corneal surface is wetted with several drops of proparacaine in order to ensure smooth passage of the microkeratome and minimize epithelial defects. The dovetail of the microkeratome is then gently rotated into the track of the pneumatic suction ring and advanced. If the microkeratome gears do not engage, the foot pedal is briefly depressed first to engage the gears of the microkeratome into the track of the pneumatic suction ring and next to perform the second microkeratome cut. Once the microkeratome has been fully advanced nasally, it is fully reversed and gently removed from the track of the pneumatic suction ring.

The suction ring may be left in place to stabilize the eye, however, the suction itself is released so the period of high pressure with its associated retardation of the ocular perfusion is minimized. The corneal flap is then reflected nasally onto the edge of the pneumatic suction ring and the excimer ablation is performed. When the ablation process is complete, the stromal bed as well as the reflected corneal flap is generously wetted to ensure that there is no adhesion of the epithelial surface of the corneal flap to the suction ring. The flap is then gently replaced in the same manner previously described and the suction ring is removed from the eye after the patient has been instructed to maintain eye in its primary position. The flap is floated and then alignment and positioning are checked in the same manner as previously described.

If the microkeratome cut is thin, perforated, asymmetrical, or short, some surgeons advocate performing PRK 1 week after with a transepithelial approach, however this approach can yield postoperative corneal haze and irregular astigmatism. The best management of an intraoperative flap complication is to close the flap and realign the flap edges as closely as possible, then recut a new flap with a 180-micron or a 200-micron depth plate 3 months later.

POSTOPERATIVE CARE

The postoperative regimen is identical for the two lamellar procedures. Two days of rest are recommended. At TLC, our postoperative protocol following LASIK involves the use prednisolone acetate 1.0% and ofloxacin 0.3% four times a day for 4 days. The prednisolone drops are increased one drop every hour on the second day to address any subclinical cases of LASIK interface keratitis. Patients are instructed to avoid rubbing or squeezing the eyes, particularly during the first postoperative day and extending through the first postoperative week. By 24 to 48 hours postoperatively, visual recovery is usually complete and the flap and cornea are clear.

If epithelial defects are bothersome, a contact lens with a topical nonsteroidal anti-inflammatory drug (NSAID) drop, such as Voltaren, and corticosteroid-antibiotic combination drop, such as Tobradex, for the first 24 to 48 hours will provide increased postoperative comfort.

RESULTS OF MYOPIC LASIK ENHANCEMENTS

The results of LASIK enhancements performed at TLC, The Windsor Laser Center were retrospectively reviewed for a total of 209 cases with follow-up ranging from 1 to 12 months. The average preoperative spherical equivalent (SE) refractive error was -1.95 + 0.78 D SE (range: -4.5 to -0.38 D SE). Follow-up data were not available for each interval in some cases. The total number of cases recorded for follow-up was 159 cases at 1 month, 122 cases at 3 months, 51 cases at 6 months, and nine cases at 1 year.

This retrospective review found that many post-LASIK enhancement patients do not return for follow-up. Those that do return have generally not achieved 20/20 uncorrected visual acuity (UCVA) and are therefore seeking further treatment. Therefore, there is a negative bias in the data, as the most successful patients are not represented.

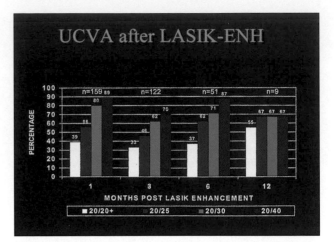

Figure 29-10. The results of LASIK enhancements for 209 eyes with the follow-up data for 1, 3, 6, and 12 months. At 6 months follow-up in 51 eyes, 87% of cases achieved at least 20/40 uncorrected visual acuity.

The efficacy of the procedure was evaluated by determining the percentage of eyes that achieved each level of acuity (Figure 29-10). At 3 months follow-up, 31.1% of eyes achieved at least 20/20 visual acuity, and 71.3% of eyes achieved at least 20/40. At 6 months follow-up, 37.3% of eyes achieved at least 20/20 visual acuity, and 88.2% of eyes achieved at least 20/40. At 12 months follow-up, 44.4% of eyes achieved at least 20/20 visual acuity, and 66.7% of eyes (six of nine eyes) achieved at least 20/40. Since these results are for enhancements, procedures alone, they add to the postoperative LASIK eyes that achieved 20/40 or better UCVA from the primary procedure. Because many highly myopic eyes have reduced best-corrected visual acuity (BCVA) prior to surgery, these UCVA results tend to underestimate the success of the procedure. We have adjusted our excimer ablation nomograms so that now virtually all patients achieve at least 20/30 UCVA.

Predictability of the enhancement procedure was also evaluated (Figure 29-11). At 3 months follow-up, 51.6% of eyes were within + 0.5 D of emmetropia, and 76.2% were within + 1.0 D of emmetropia. At 6 months follow-up, 58.8% of eyes were within + 0.5 D of emmetropia, and 86.3% were within + 1.0 D of emmetropia. At 12 months follow-up, 77.8% of eyes were within + 0.5 D of emmetropia, and 77.8% were within + 1.0 D of emmetropia. The scattergram of the attempted and achieved refractive results illustrates that only one eye was significantly overcorrected and the majority of the eyes outside + 1.0 D of emmetropia were undercorrected (Figure 29-12).

The average SE refractive error was found to be -0.33 + 0.84 D at 1 month, -0.63 + 0.92 D at 3 months, -0.69 +

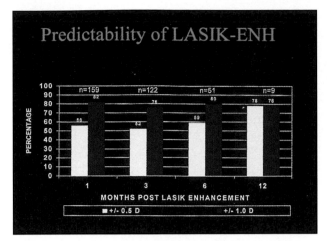

Figure 29-11. The predictability of LASIK enhancements at 1, 3, 6, and 12 months postoperatively.

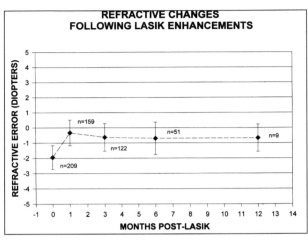

Figure 29-12. The scattergram demonstrates the predictability of LASIK enhancements at 6 months follow-up of 51 eyes. Only one eye was significantly overcorrected, while the remaining eyes not within 1.0 D of emmetropia were undercorrected.

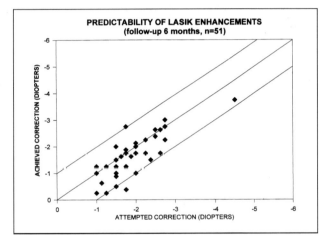

Figure 29-13. The postoperative refractive change after LASIK enhancements for the 1, 3, 6, and 12 months follow-up data. While there was a significant myopic regression in myopia between the first and the third postoperative month, after this point refractive stability was achieved with no significant change in the average spherical equivalent refractive error.

1.1 D at 6 months, and -0.67 + 0.9 D at 12 months (Figure 29-13). ANOVA (analysis of variance) indicated a significant difference in refractive change over time, however further analysis with the Tukey-Kramer multiple comparisons test indicated that only the refractive change from the 1 to the 3 months was significant; there was not significant change in the average SE refractive error from 3 to 6 or 12 months. Therefore, while significant regression was initially noted following the enhancement procedure, stability of the refractive result was achieved about 3 months following the enhancement procedure.

Safety of the LASIK enhancement procedure was reviewed for a change in the postoperative BCVA (Figure 28-14). At 3 months post-LASIK, 14% of eyes lost one line of Snellen acuity, and 1.6% lost two lines. No patient had a greater visual loss. Conversely, a gain of one Snellen line was achieved in 8% of eyes, two Snellen lines in 3% of eyes, and three Snellen lines in 0.8% of eyes. At 6 months post-LASIK, 14% of eyes lost one line of Snellen acuity, 1.9% lost two lines, and no patient had a greater visual loss, while a gain of one Snellen line was achieved in 15% of eyes. At 12 months post-LASIK, 11% of eyes lost one line of Snellen acuity, while a gain of one Snellen line was achieved in 22% of eyes with no eyes gaining or losing greater amounts of BCVA. These results indicate that LASIK is a relatively safe procedure with few eyes experiencing a significant loss in BCVA.

Epithelial ingrowth that required removal occurred in two eyes, and flap striae was treated in one eye. Both these complications were treated without a loss in BCVA or a significant change in refractive outcome. One eye lost two lines of BCVA at the 1-month follow-up visit because of moderate haze that had developed at the flap interface. One patient had a dislodged flap that was eventually removed, but UCVA recovered to 20/25 after phototherapeutic keratectomy (PTK).

This study found that no eyes lost more than two lines of BCVA and between 1.6 to 1.9% of eyes lost two lines of BCVA after the LASIK enhancement procedure. The US Food and Drug Administration (FDA) phase III PRK excimer laser trials found 1% of eyes treated with the VISX laser, and 3% of eyes treated with the Summit laser lost a similar amount of BCVA. Lindstrom noted that for PRK to be considered approvable by the FDA, less than or equal to 5% of eyes could lose two lines of Snellen acuity, and less than or equal to 0.2% of eyes could lose five lines of Snellen acuity (serious adverse reaction). Therefore, loss in BCVA found in this study of LASIK enhancements is comparable the results of the FDA PRK trials and significantly less than what would be considered approvable by the FDA.

CONCLUSIONS

Initial undercorrections and regression result in a significant number of post-LASIK eyes with residual refractive error. This refractive error is effectively treated with a LASIK enhancement procedure that can achieve excellent visual acuity and good stability. The uncommon complications of corneal flap striae, epithelial ingrowth, and even dislodged/lost flaps can be effectively managed without comprise of BCVA. H-LASIK enhancements should be approached with caution due to the limitations of central corneal steepening. LASIK enhancements allow the refractive surgeon to further improve the results of the original LASIK procedure in an efficacious, safe, and predictable manner.

REFERENCES

1. Machat JJ. LASIK procedure. In: Machat JJ, ed. *Excimer Laser Refractive Surgery.* Thorofare, NJ: SLACK Incorporated; 1996.
2. Machat JJ. LASIK retreatment technique and results. In: Machat JJ, ed. *Excimer Laser Refractive Surgery.* Thorofare, NJ: SLACK Incorporated; 1996.
3. McDonald MB, Talamo JH. Myopic photorefractive kerate-ctomy: The experience in the United States with the VISX excimer laser. In: Salz JJ, ed. *Corneal Laser Surgery.* St. Louis, Mo: Mosby-Year Book; 1995.
4. Thompson KP, Steinert RF, Daniel J, Stulting D. Photorefractive keratectomy with the Summit excimer laser: The phase III US results. In: Salz JJ, ed. *Corneal Laser Surgery.* St. Louis, Mo: Mosby-Year Book; 1995.
5. Machat JJ. Preoperative PRK patient evaluation. In: Machat JJ, ed. *Excimer Laser Refractive Surgery.* Thorofare, NJ: SLACK Incorporated; 1996.

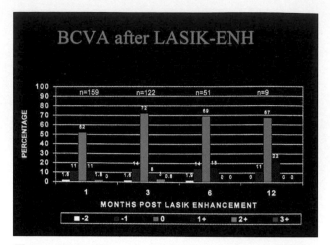

Figure 29-14. Changes in BCVA following the LASIK enhancement found that most eyes experienced no overall gain or loss of BCVA at each of the follow-up visits. At 6 months follow-up in 51 eyes, 14% of eyes lost one line, and 1.9% of eyes lost two lines of Snellen acuity, while 15% of eyes actually gained one line of Snellen acuity. No greater loss or gain of BCVA acuity was found.

LASIK Retreatment by Flap Elevation

Arun Brahma, MB, FRCOphth and Charles McGhee, MB, FRCOphth, PhD

Table 29A-1	
CALCULATING THE AMOUNT OF CORRECTION NEEDED FOR REGRESSION AFTER PRIMARY LASIK	
Refractive error prior to primary treatment	-10.00 D sphere/-1.00 D cyl 180
Spherical equivalent (SEQ 1)	-10.50 D
Refractive error after treatment (RET)	-1.50 D
Percentage regression = (RET/SEQ 1) x 100	(-1.50/-10.50) x 100 = 14.3%
Treatment correction for retreatment	-1.50 + (-1.50 x 14.3%)= -1.72 D

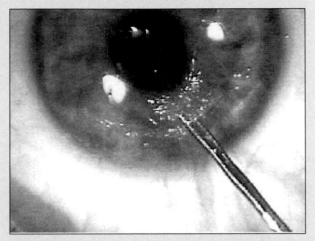

Figure 29A-1. Breaking peripheral LASIK flap adhesions to create entry into the interface superiorly with a blunt instrument.

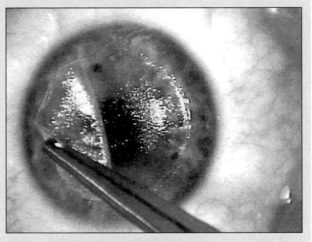

Figure 29A-2. Reflecting the LASIK flap with nontoothed forceps after all peripheral flap adhesions have been broken.

LASIK is a relatively predictable treatment for myopia, but a significant proportion of eyes require enhancement to reduce undercorrection or regression.

According to reports, the flap can be lifted up to 1 year after the primary treatment for further ablation of the underlying stromal bed, but in our experience this is best done within 3 months. This prevents trauma to the flap when excessive force may be required to enter the interface due to the healing process. The procedure can be divided into five basic steps:

Calculate the amount of retreatment required. This amount takes into account the percentage of regression compared to the primary refractive error. This is added to the manifest correction. This is illustrated in Table 29A-1.

Mark the flap edge. This is best achieved at the slit lamp just prior to treatment, as slit lamp optics and light sources are superior to most excimer laser microscopes. The epithelium overlying the flap edge at the 12 o'clock position can be marked with a variety of instruments or a hypodermic needle.

Lift the flap. This is often the most difficult part of the procedure. A blunt fine instrument, such as a cyclodialysis spatula, is gently introduced into the interface superiorly (Figure 29A-1). Once in the interface, the spatula is swept along the periphery of the flap in a fashion similar to opening an envelope. If the flap cannot be separated without excessive force, the procedure should be aborted. Creating epithelial tags and introducing them into the interface must be carefully avoided, since this may give rise to an epithelial ingrowth later. The temptation to use a sharp instrument to separate the interface should be avoided, as accidental perforation of the flap

may occur. Once separated along the edge, the flap is grasped with a nontoothed forceps opposite to the hinge and slowly lifted from the bed (Figure 29A-2).

After the flap is elevated, the ablation is performed as in primary LASIK (Figure 29A-3).

Flap replacement. Per the primary procedure, the flap is floated onto the stromal bed. Loose tags of epithelium must be kept out of the interface to avoid ingrowth, which is more common after retreatment. The flap may be wiped with three to four strokes of a wet microsponge to achieve a wrinkle-free edge approximation (Figure 29A-4).

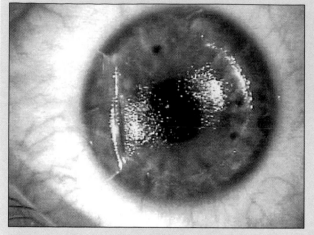

Figure 29A-3. Ablation of the stromal bed with the LASIK flap resting nasally.

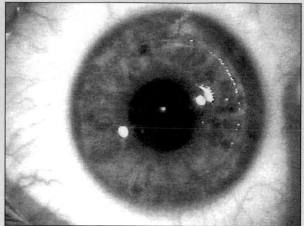

Figure 29A-4. Appearance of the LASIK flap following completion of the enhancement procedure.

Treating Overcorrection

Klaus Ditzen, MD

PURPOSE

In refractive procedures such as PRK or LASIK, most overcorrections occur in correcting myopic refractive errors; only rarely do they occur in hyperopic and astigmatic treatment.

The average thickness in caucasian myopic eyes is between 520 and 580 microns. The average energy to treat myopic eyes lies between 250 and 300 mJ, the average hertz frequency is between 20 Hz (full area ablation system, broad beam and small slit scanning system) and 30 to 100 Hz (flying spot scanning system with 1.0 to 2.0 mm top-hat or gaussian spotmode).

Depending on the age of the patient, the corneal thickness, the beam and energy mode, or the ablation time, there will be overcorrections in attempting to achieve emmetropia after the primary refractive ablation.

How it is possible to treat the overcorrection?

METHOD

Overcorrected PRK Procedures

Six months after primary PRK we start with the new treatment.

a. We have the best results after transepithelial excimer ablation with a two-thirds correction of the overcorrected diopters from the remaining superficial stromal haze. We have done it with a broadbeam slit scanning laser system (MEL 60), but other laser systems are just as useful.

b. A secondary LASIK procedure can be performed in overcorrected eyes up to +3 D. Six months after the first PRK, we will use the microkeratome (either automated or nonautomated) with a 130-micron plate to produce a temporal nasal or down-up flap. For the following excimer laser ablation we use the same technique as described above.

c. With more than +3 D overcorrection in myopic PRK, we will use HO-YAG-LTK (laser thermokeratoplasty). It is possible to use a contact or noncontact system (Technomed or Sunrise). We coagulate the stromed tissue with eight spots (D = 1.0 mm) on a 7.0 mm circle around the pupillary center. The depth of coagulation should be 80% of the corneal tissue; the time of coagulation 1 to 2 seconds.

Overcorrected LASIK Procedures

a. The earliest time to correct overcorrections is 3 months postoperatively. With a Buratto or Slade hook, we lift the flap from the superior side (in cases with a temporal-nasal cut) or from the temporal side (in cases with a down-up cut). With this technique, we avoid a rupture or flap hole and disruption of the epithelium. With the same hook, we open the flap to the hinge. The following excimer laser technique is the same as previously described.

In postoperative overcorrections up to +3 D of more than 1½ years, we perform a new LASIK procedure with a thicker plate (180 microns) to achieve a clean stromal surface. Microkeratome and excimer laser technique will be the same as before. After the laser ablation, we wash out the inner side of the hinge and ablated stromal side with BSS. We then replace the flap, remove the fluid from the interface with a suction tube, and dry the cornea for 2 minutes.

c. After 3 months postoperatively, overcorrections more than +3 D we will use the transepithelial HO-YAG-LTK technique as previously described.

RESULTS

With PRK after PRK, LASIK after PRK, and LTK after PRK, we have seen a short recovery time, especially in LASIK after PRK. The predictability and stability are good. In safety (BSCVA) and efficacy (UCVA), we gained an average of one to two lines.

In LTK after PRK, we lost two lines in two of 20 eyes (10%) from an irregular astigmatism.

In reopening the flap and LASIK after LASIK, we lost no lines. On the average, we gained one line in safety (BSCVA) and efficacy (UCVA). Stability (refraction) and predictability were good. In LTK after LASIK, we lost two lines in two from 20 eyes (10%) from an irregular astigmatism. However, the recovery time was quicker and the regression slower, as with LTK after PRK.

CONCLUSIONS

To treat overcorrections in myopia it is necessary to wait 6 months after primary PRK and 3 months after primary LASIK. PRK after PRK, LASIK after PRK, and reopening the LASIK flap can be done between 3 and 6 months postoperatively. LASIK after LASIK can be done after 1 ½ years postoperatively. In all cases, a two-thirds ablation of the residual diopters will be enough in all cases up to +3 D overcorrection. Stability (refraction), predictability, safety (BSCVA), and efficacy (UCVA) will be good.

In overcorrections more than +3 D, it is better to perform an HO-YAG-LTK treatment. Here, however, there is a danger of loss of lines from producing an irregular astigmatism! Overcorrected astigmatism is accompanied by an arcuate cut to flatten the steep meridian. Overcorrected hyperopic eyes cannot be treated in the case of regression.

Enhancements

Andreu Coret Moreno, MD

INTRODUCTION

Even though the LASIK technique and the predictability and UCVA that we obtain are better every day, the patients' expectations of vision make enhancements a frequent occurence. Essentially, there are two ways to do it: lifting the original flap or cutting a second flap.

PRINCIPLES OF LASIK ENHANCEMENTS

1. We consider the possibility of enhancement when the difference between the UCVA and BCVA is two or more lines on the Snellen scale, except in monovision cases.

   Another less frequent option is to perform a radial keratotomy when we have a low residual refraction and there is not enough remaining corneal tissue. PRK must not be used for a LASIK enhancement because it is associated with a high incidence of haze.

2. Most regression appears during the first postoperative month and stability is achieved usually around the third month, which is why enhancements can be scheduled between the first and the third month. The lower the pre-LASIK corrected refraction, the sooner the enhancement can be performed because stability will be achieved sooner. In myopias higher than 10 D and especially in patients with presbyopia, it is advisable to perform a two-step treatment to obtain a better final result and also to avoid overcorrections.

3. One of the most important preoperative tests for any patient that is going to be operated on is pachymetry; however, in enhancements, pachymetry is even more important to identify the amount of residual posterior stroma that can be ablated. The amount of stroma to be removed basically depends on the residual refraction, the

chosen optical zone, and the excimer laser to be used.

It is recommended to leave at least 200 to 250 microns of residual posterior stroma after a LASIK or enhancement surgery to avoid future development of corneal ectasia. An easy method to calculate this is to leave at least a whole corneal thickness between 380 to 400 microns after LASIK or enhancement surgery. If we calculate a flap thickness of 160 microns, we will have 220 to 240 microns of stromal posterior thickness left.

In patients with borderline pachymetries, there are different points to consider:

3.1 It is always best to undercorrect or decide on another intraocular technique than to excessively reduce the optical zone because that will decrease the visual quality in mesopic conditions.

3.2 The patient must be warned that there is a possibility of a posterior stroma shortage, making enhancement impossible.

3.3 For hyperopic patients or in enhancement surgeries for overcorrection, pachymetry is not important because the ablation takes place peripherally and not centrally.

4. Corneal topography is useful to detect central islands or decentrations, but also to identify corneal curvature, because this must be maintained between 33 D to 49 D after enhancement if we do not want to really increase the risk of losing BCVA.

SURGICAL TECHNIQUE

There are two surgical techniques: lifting the original flap or cutting a second flap.

Lifting the Flap

During the first year after LASIK surgery, we always recommend lifting the original flap. It is relatively easy and usually much safer because it avoids all the risks associated with the microkeratome (free caps, irregular cuts, etc). Microkeratome-related risks increase in enhancements because of a second cut on a flattened (myopia) or curved (hyperopia) cornea in its central zone, which is still poorly adhered. Although time is the biggest factor in flap adherence, patients with aggressive healing (keloid formers) or with flap irregularities, slim flaps or peripheral hemorrhage (small cornea, superior pannus, or use of a large suction ring in relation to the cornea) can also enhance stromal adhesion. In these cases, enhancement must take place within 6 months after the primary surgery. However, epithelial ingrowth tends to prevent flap adhesion to the stromal bed, making it easier to lift the flap in that area.

The surgical technique begins with marking the temporal area with the Machat marker. In most cases it is not necessary to examine the patient under the slit lamp to determine the edge of the initial flap, even though in some cases it can be useful. If the cornea is dry, pressing on the limbal area will clearly show the edge by the striae that will appear. To get into the interface, press down and inward with a satin crescent knife. The rest of the flap is then desiccated with a cyclodialysis spatula, beginning with the edges of the hinge. Once the flap is lifted, it is as important to clean the interface as the underside of the flap to remove epithelial debris. After the laser ablation, the flap is hydrated with BSS and repositioned with the cyclodialysis spatula. Afterward, the interface is irrigated with BSS filtered through a flat hydrodissection cannula. With a wet Merocel sponge, the excess BSS is removed from the interface. If little BSS is used, it is enough to wait 1 minute for the flap to be perfectly adhered.

Cutting a Second Flap

One year after LASIK, it is better to cut a new flap because in most cases, the original flap is very well adhered and makes surgery more difficult and long, creating more epithelial defects, flap distortions, and interface epithelial ingrowth.

The surgical technique to make a second cut is exactly the same as for primary LASIK. The only difference is to use a 180 to 200-micron depth plate and larger suction ring to avoid cutting on the same plane as the primary cut.

LASIK AFTER PREVIOUS CORNEAL SURGERY

Jorge L. Alió, MD, PhD,
Walid H. Attia, MD

Laser-assisted in situ keratomileusis (LASIK) is gaining acceptance as a versatile refractive surgical procedure. LASIK is gaining popularity due to quick visual rehabilitation, minimal postoperative discomfort, and the ability to correct variable forms and high degrees of refractive errors with minimal postoperative complications. LASIK efficacy has been reported in several studies for the correction of primary refractive errors such as myopia, hyperopia, and astigmatism. However, there have been very few studies reporting the use of LASIK in treating patients with residual refractive errors following other corneal or nonrefractive refractive procedures. LASIK is an evolving surgical technique with both therapeutic and refractive indications, especially in cases where refractive defects or irregular astigmatism have been induced by previous refractive surgery, trauma, or penetrating keratoplasty. This chapter is dedicated to study the use of LASIK in treating the following residual refractive problems after different corneal surgical procedures:

1. Radial keratotomy (RK)
2. Astigmatic keratotomy (AK)
3. Photorefractive keratectomy (PRK)
4. Laser thermokeratoplasty (LTK)
5. Penetrating keratoplasty (PKP)
6. Automated lamellar keratoplasty (ALK)
7. Epikeratophakia
8. Corneal trauma

LASIK AFTER RK

RK was a widely used surgical technique to correct myopia. It flattens the central cornea indirectly through peripheral radial incisions, however the amount of central flattening that can be achieved is limited.[1,2] The most common side effect of this procedure is overcorrection or undercorrection. Waring, et al in 1994 reported the result of a multicenter prospective evaluation of an RK study in which 43% of patients had a hyperopic shift of 1 diopter (D) or more by 10 years after treatment.[3] Treatment of hyperopia after RK has been a complicated problem. To avoid this problem, most radial keratotomy surgeons prefer to perform conservative initial surgery as a safeguard against the development of hyperopic shift, with intentionally undercorrected postoperative results, thus increasing the incidence of patients with significant undercorrection. Eventually, this group will need additional treatment. Myopic regression is a common finding following RK and is more evident in young patients; again this group of patients will need additional treatment.

Residual Myopia After RK

Unexpected or intentional residual myopia after RK may be due to a large optical zone, few incisions, or shallow incisions. Each patient's corneal reaction to the procedure differs.[4] A number of patients with residual myopia after RK exist and need additional treatment. Correcting residual myopia can be done by spectacles, contact lenses, or reoperations either by redeepening, or extending the RK incisions, or performing additional RK incisions. However, although there are many nomograms for performing radial keratotomy,[5,6] nomograms for enhancing refractive procedures do not exist. Reoperations cannot be based on the same calculations used in the initial surgery because the predictable effect of adding incisions and reducing optical zones is lower than in primary nomograms.[7] An increase in the incidence of microperforations is observed with RK enhancement procedures.[8] Overcorrection is another serious complication that has been reported in several studies using RK as an enhancement procedure.[5,9] While young patients may be able to accommodate to compensate for an overcorrection now, in time the patient will be complaining of severe and early presbyopia.

Photorefractive keratectomy is another form of treat-

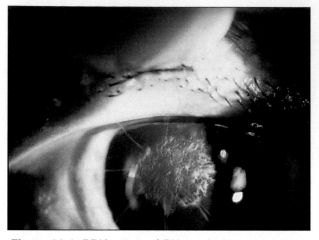

Figure 30-1. PRK on top of RK, producing severe haze with marked surface irregularity.

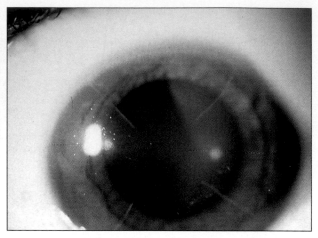

Figure 30-2. LASIK on top of RK, minimal haze can be seen 1 month after LASIK.

ment, but today there is a major concern about using it after RK. Several complications have been reported, including different degrees of haze and regression due to keratocyte activation, dehiscence of the RK incisions during scraping of the epithelium, and significant decrease in best spectacle-corrected visual acuity (BSCVA) due to surface irregularity and subepithelial scarring[10-11] (Figure 30-1). Azar, et al in 1998 advised against using PRK to correct residual myopia after RK in patients with high amounts of pre-RK and residual post-RK myopia.[4]

LASIK is more likely to provide an accurate result with early and long-term stability without the risk of haze.

Hyperopia After RK

Progressive hyperopia is a common complication following RK. It may result from lack of preoperative cycloplegic refraction, extending the radial incisions to the limbus, multiple RK enhancement procedures, redeepening procedures, extended contact lens wearing after RK, and possibly postoperative ocular rubbing.[12]

Treatment of hyperopia after RK is a complicated problem.13 Hexagonal keratotomy was used, but the results were not predictable. Grene lasso sutures are more predictable but still not highly efficient. Thermal keratoplasty shows variable degrees of regression; thus, it is not reliable in treating hyperopic shift after RK. Hyperopic PRK has a high incidence of postoperative haze and disappointing results.

Hyperopic LASIK is a promising technique in the management of these cases, especially with new reliable software for treating hyperopia.

The Cornea After RK

RK incisions can be seen for a long time after sur-

gery. These incisions never completely heal. Epithelial ingrowth may be found in the RK incisions. Patients wearing contact lenses may have deep vascularization especially in deep incisions. Flat corneas are more common in patients with overcorrections.

LASIK After RK

LASIK seems to be an attractive alternative to correct residual myopia and hyperopic shift after RK. However, due to the fact that the cornea underwent previous RK surgery, it requires special handling both preoperatively and postoperatively to get the best results, to avoid any refractive surprise, and to decrease the possibility of developing haze (Figure 30-2).

Preoperative Considerations

LASIK should only be attempted after 1 year post-RK, with a stable refraction for at least the last 6 months, and a corneal topographic pattern stable for two consecutive examinations in a 1-month interval. Timing is very important, especially with patients showing regression after RK. Overactive healing is responsible for this regression, and its effect may continue after LASIK if it is performed too early.

Patients wearing contact lenses should discontinue use for at least 15 days before evaluation. Soft contact lenses should be discontinued for 15 days before LASIK, and both hard and gas-permeable contact lenses should be discontinued for at least 1 month before LASIK. In patients with blood vessels in the incisions, more time is needed to allow for blood vessel regression.

If the patient has irregular astigmatism, or if the astigmatic value is larger than the spherical value, topographic linked excimer laser ablation (topolink) is preferred. A classic LASIK procedure will produce unpredictable results.

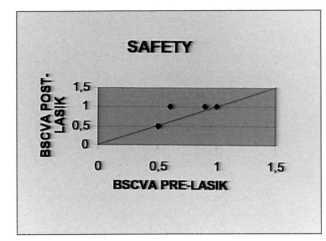

Figure 30-3. BSCVA pre- and post-LASIK in the undercorrected group of LASIK after RK.

Contraindications

Post-RK corneas are unstable corneas that may cause unpredictable results, thus great care is needed while dealing with these corneas. LASIK should not be performed if one or more of the following items exist.

- Epithelial ingrowth: epithelial inclusions in the RK incisions is a serious problem and LASIK should be avoided in these cases, as the epithelium may pass under the flap, causing flap melting.
- Macroperforation: LASIK should not be attempted in any case with prior macroperforations.
- Deep vascularization: may be found in the deep incisions and is more common in patients who wear contact lenses.
- Flat cornea: LASIK on flat corneas may cause a free cap, which will make it difficult to achieve good results, as the diameter of the cut will not be large enough to perform hyperopic ablation.
- Unstable refraction: this should be excluded before any attempt to perform LASIK; the patient may end up with an unpredictable and untreatable refractive condition.

Intraoperative Considerations

In post-RK corneas, we are cutting across RK incisions, and it is well-documented that these incisions never completely heal. Our main concern is to prevent opening of the incisions while creating the flap. As long as the RK incisions are well-healed without epithelial ingrowth at the time of surgery, a safe regular cut can be performed with a 160 μm blade; however, it is better to use a thicker depth blade. A 180 μm or 200 μm blade is safer, but the corneal thickness and amount of ablation determine this. It is important to always keep the corneal epithelium wet during the cut, this will serve as a lubricant and facilitate the pass of the microkeratome.

Lifting the flap should be done very carefully with a wide spatula, while avoiding forceps to grab the edge of the flap. This will protect the incisions from splitting apart. Perfect fixation is needed. If it is not maintained, eccentric correction and unpredictable astigmatism could result. When replacing the flap, good apposition is mandatory; this will prevent migration of the epithelium, especially if an incision in the flap is opened. During the procedure, avoid traumatizing the epithelium to avoid any epithelial scraping, which may cause keratocyte activation and increase in corneal haze.

Applying a contact lens after surgery is not necessary unless there is opening in one or more of the RK incisions in the flap.

If we are treating hyperopic shift, we attempt to obtain a large flap at least 9.5 mm, by using a large suction ring to avoid hinge syndrome. Fixation is usually more difficult with these patients. For better results, we give the patient extra training in fixation.

Results (Pilot Study)

Ten myopic patients had previous RK. After 1 year, six patients had significant undercorrection, and the other four patients developed overcorrection. LASIK was done to correct the residual refractive defects in the 10 patients.

Patients with undercorrection showed the following results 3 months after LASIK: the mean spherical equivalent changed from -2.50 D ± 2.47 (-6.25 to -0.50) to 0.12 D ± 0.26 (-0.25 to +0.50). Mean BSCVA improved from 0.75 ± 0.24 (0.5 to 1.0) to 0.83 ± 0.25 (0.5 to 1.0) (Figure 30-3), and mean uncorrected visual acuity (UCVA) significantly improved from 0.33 ± 0.22 (0.1 to 1.0) to 0.80 ± 0.24 (0.5 to 1.0).

Patients with overcorrection showed the following results 3 months after LASIK: the mean spherical equivalent changed from 1.87 D ± 0.66 (1.00 to 2.50) to -0.25 D ± 0.50 (-0.50 to 0.50). Mean BSCVA improved from 0.72 (0.6 to 0.8) to 0.80 (0.7 to 0.9) (Figure 30-4), and mean UCVA improved from 0.52 (0.4 to 0.6) to 0.70 (0.6 to 0.8). Treating both undercorrection and overcorrection with LASIK following RK is almost equally safe, effective, and highly predictable (Figures 30-5a and 30-5b). There were no major intraoperative or postoperative complications.

Conclusions

Although LASIK for the correction of residual refractive errors after RK seems to be a promising and safe procedure, great care should be taken with the flap during the entire procedure to avoid possible complications.

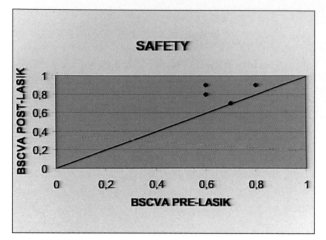

Figure 30-4. Mean BSCVA pre- and post-LASIK in the overcorrected group of LASIK after RK.

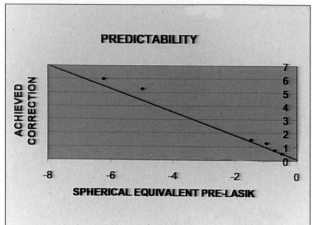

Figure 30-5a. Predictability in the undercorrected group.

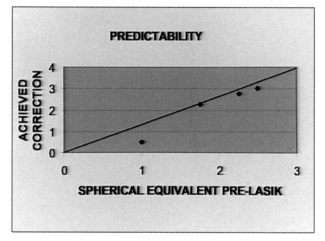

Figure 30-5b. Predictability in the overcorrected group.

LASIK AFTER AK

As the treatment of spherical refractive errors, myopia, and hyperopia evolved, treatment of astigmatism has lagged behind. The incidence of clinically significant astigmatism varies between 7.5% to 75%.[14] However, an astigmatic refractive error of more than 2.0 D is less common, between 3% and 15%.[15] Astigmatism corrected by spectacles may cause distortion due to the meridional magnification.[16] Contact lenses may alleviate this problem, but not all patients can tolerate them. Here, the discussion is limited to the surgical correction of naturally occurring mixed astigmatism more than -3.0 D.

The general goal of incisional or ablative astigmatic surgery is to reduce the magnitude of astigmatism by flattening the cornea at its steepest meridian, steepening the cornea at its flattest meridian, or a combination. Any corneal incision flattens the cornea adjacent to it and at

the meridian perpendicular to the cut. AK is a common method to correct astigmatism and is a very powerful tool in reducing astigmatism. It flattens the steep cylinder axis and, at the same time, steepens the flat axis, a process known as coupling.[17] The coupling ratio (flattening/steepening ratio) depends on the location, length, and depth of the incision. In patients with large amounts of astigmatism, AK can be used to significantly lessen the astigmatism, however it is important to consider the patient's refractive error and how astigmatism-reducing surgery will affect the spherical equivalent.

The benefits of AK are greater in patients with myopic astigmatism. Transverse incisions in the cornea cause flattening in the meridian of the incision and steepening of the meridian 90° away. Arcuate or curvilinear incisions have been reported as more effective than straight transverse incisions.[18,19] The distance between the AK and the center of the pupil is an important factor as well. The smaller the distance, the smaller the optical zone, with a higher incidence of irregular astigmatism near the pupil resulting in a poor visual quality, especially in low-light conditions.

McDonnell and colleagues were the first to report the success of toric sculpting of the cornea with an excimer laser to correct regular corneal astigmatism.[20] This initial success encouraged refractive surgeons to use the same principle to correct astigmatism. The current approach to correct astigmatism by excimer laser, involves a nonradially symmetrical ablation of the corneal tissue, with greater ablation in the steep axis and minimal or no ablation in the flat axis.[21] Recently, the Technolas, LaserSight, Autonomous, and Nidek lasers have been used to correct astigmatic errors in which the scanning beam moves along the axis of astigmatism and differentially ablates the cornea.

The Cornea After AK

Following uncomplicated AK, the anatomical structure of the cornea does not show significant alteration, both in the superficial layers and the deep stroma. Scars from the previous arcuate keratotomy are usually seen at a 7.0 mm optic zone. There is no need to avoid cutting through them with the microkeratome. A LASIK procedure can be carried out without special intraoperative precautions.

Performing LASIK After AK

The predictability of AK is of great concern for refractive surgeons, undercorrection, overcorrection, and change in the axis are complications that must be dealt with and corrected. Undercorrection is more common and better tolerated than overcorrection. In spite of several medical and surgical options used to manage these conditions, results are not predictable, but with LASIK we are getting more predictable and stable results.

Coupling effect and hyperopic shift in the spherical equivalent are commonly seen after AK. For small amounts of myopia in association with astigmatism, the astigmatic surgery may be all the patient needs. However, astigmatism associated with high myopic or hyperopic spherical error will need a second approach in an attempt to achieve emmetropia. Radial keratotomy, photorefractive keratotomy, or LASIK can treat coupling and residual refractive defects. LASIK has proved itself as the most predictable and reliable procedure in dealing with most refractive errors.

Preoperative Considerations

Allowing the refraction to stabilize is just as important in astigmatic surgery as in any other form of refractive surgery. We wait about 3 months after AK to perform LASIK; this period suffices in achieving a stable refraction. Usually in astigmatic correction with or without spherical error, treatment is based on the manifest refraction for axis correction; however, if the refractive axis differs from the topographic axis by more than 10°, we prefer to use the topographic axis. Patients who wear contact lenses should stop use of soft for 3 days and hard contact lenses for 2 weeks before getting manifest refraction results. Patients with binocular spectacle-corrected astigmatism are showing adaptation to the meridional magnification induced by their spectacles. Surgical correction of their astigmatism may result in torsional diplopia, and re-adaptation may take months. We discuss this problem with astigmatic patients before any surgery to correct astigmatic errors is attempted.

With irregular astigmatism, normal LASIK treatment is contraindicated. It may worsen the condition, and it is advisable to treat these cases with the topography-assisted lasers.

Intraoperative Considerations

In cases of previous AK, LASIK can be carried out as normal. The procedure has proven to be very safe following AK. All LASIK steps can be carried out as usual, as long as the procedure does not take place before 3 months following AK. Centration should be very precise and accurate to avoid decentration, which is usually more common with astigmatic treatment. Corneal topography should be our guide to achieve the best possible centration.

Results (Pilot Study)

Ten patients with mixed astigmatism underwent AK. The mean spherical equivalent after AK was +0.57 D ± 2.8 (-1.5 to +6.0). The mean astigmatic value after AK was -1.50 D ± 0.60 (-0.5 to -2.5). Mean BSCVA was 0.76 ± 0.15 (0.4 to 0.9), and mean UCVA was 0.51 ± 0.16 (0.3 to 0.8). All patients underwent LASIK surgery in an attempt to correct the residual refractive error. In all cases, the procedure was carried out at least 3 months after AK. One month after LASIK, mean spherical equivalent was +0.87 D ± 0.5 (0.0 to +2), mean BSCVA was 0.76 ± 0.16 (0.4 to 1.0), and mean UCVA significantly improved to 0.73 ± 0.14 (0.4 to 0.9). Three months after LASIK, mean spherical equivalent became +0.60 D ± 0.31 (0.25 to 1.25), mean BSCVA improved to 0.79 ± 0.17 (0.4 to 1.0) (Figure 30-6), and mean UCVA was 0.74 ± 0.18 (0.4 to 1.0). The cylinder's vector-corrected change was 1.61 D ± 0.71. LASIK after AK proved to be safe, highly efficient (Figure 30-7), and predictable. There were no adverse events during LASIK and no major complications were reported during or after the procedure.

Conclusions

Patients with a residual refractive defect after AK can benefit from LASIK. For the best results, LASIK should be done 3 months after AK. There were no problems with the cut, and with handling the flap. Surgeons are advised to treat the cornea as a virgin one.

LASIK AFTER PRK

Since the introduction of excimer laser PRK,[22] there has been a steady increase in the number of PRK procedures performed worldwide.[23] The most frequent complications after PRK are regression, haze, central islands, decentered ablations, as well as other less frequently seen complications.[24] An estimated 10% to 20% of patients require a repeat PRK procedure for significant

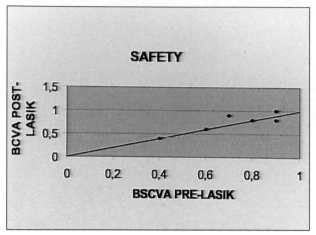

Figure 30-6. BSCVA before and after LASIK.

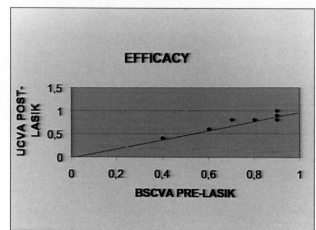

Figure 30-7. BSCVA before LASIK against UCVA after LASIK. The procedure proved to be highly efficient.

regression. Regression is caused by the corneal wound healing response, which may differ from one patient to another and results in various refractive outcomes and incidence of complications.

The Cornea After PRK

It is now well documented that the cornea demonstrates specific acute and delayed responses to excimer laser ablation. Epithelial wounds usually heal over a period of months following PRK. The epithelium first slides to cover the defect initially it is thinner than normal, but later hyperplasia takes place, and the number of cells becomes greater than normal. Epithelial hyperplasia may be responsible for postoperative regression. The basement membrane, which is removed during PRK, usually regenerates with focal discontinuities and duplication. Normal epithelial attachment complexes are regenerated within weeks to months after surgery.[25] Stromal changes continue for months or even years after PRK. After closure of the epithelial defect, keratocytes begin transformation into activated fibroblasts and migrate into the treated region, so that the subepithelial 10 to 15 microns become hypercellular. These activated keratocytes synthesize new collagen and extracellular matrix, which may contribute to corneal haze that is observed postoperatively. The new collagen lacks the organized lamellar arrangement characteristics of corneal stromal collagen fibers.[26] Proteoglycans, including keratan sulfate and hyaluronic acid, are produced in response to the injury. The produced hyaluronic acid may change the water balance and thus create disruptions in the lamellar arrangement.[26] Depending on the depth of ablation, Bowman´s layer may be partially or completely excised during the procedure.[25]

Performing LASIK After PRK

PRK retreatment for significant regression will significantly reduce residual myopia. However, the risk of further regression, haze and loss of visual acuity exists.[27] In addition, treating residual myopia by PRK is less successful than primary PRK.[30] LASIK has been used primarily to treat moderate to high myopia because of its superiority over PRK for this range of refractive error.[28] Many surgeons are now advocating the use of LASIK rather than PRK for lower levels of myopia, because LASIK preserves Bowman's layer, decreases the amount of disruption of keratocytes and anterior stromal collagen, and avoids the large epithelial defect seen with surface PRK.[29] Because LASIK causes less regression and haze, we studied the results of LASIK in treating residual myopia after primary PRK.

Preoperative Considerations

It is clear that regression and haze are the most common complications after PRK. These complications will determine, to a great extent, the outcome of treating these patients with LASIK.

- Regression: the amount of regression after PRK is related to the amount of myopic correction attempted. The deeper the ablation, the more frequently regression occurs. Regression may continue over months, thus a stable refraction is important to prevent further regression after LASIK. An interval of 1 year is usually enough to achieve a stable refraction. This should be documented by repeated refraction and corneal topography at least twice within 1 month before any attempt to perform LASIK.
- Haze: the grade of haze present after PRK can affect the outcome of LASIK. The incidence of

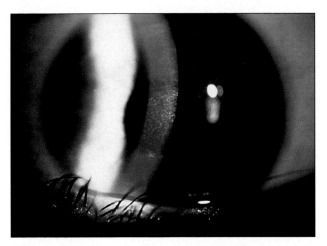

Figure 30-8. Haze in the early post-LASIK period, 1 week after LASIK.

regression after LASIK is higher in corneas with grade 2 haze or more. In patients with grade 2 or more corneal haze, our target should be overcorrection to compensate for expected postoperative regression. In patients with minimal to no corneal haze, our target is emmetropia, as regression is less likely to occur. For example, in a patient with manifest refraction of -4.0 D with corneal haze grade 2, the LASIK surgical plan should be -5.0 D. The immediate postoperative overcorrection will be compensated by the expected regression.

Intraoperative Considerations

The cut is a critical step in performing LASIK after PRK. The flap should be as thick as possible—not less than 160 μm—the thicker the better. With a thin flap, we may encounter two problems:

- First, the microkeratome blade will pass through a peripherally normal clear cornea, and then through a more tough area due to the previous PRK treatment. This will affect the smoothness of the cut in the corneal stroma, resulting in an irregular surface. With a thicker blade, we can avoid this problem by passing beneath the previous PRK treatment area.
- Second, after PRK, Bowman's membrane may be partially or completely removed, thus the flap will be more liable to wrinkles due to lack of Bowman's membrane support. This can be compensated by creating a thicker flap. Patients with a keratometric value less than 40 D are more likely to have a free cap and require care in creating the flap.

Postoperative Treatment

Patients who undergo LASIK after PRK should be managed with the same regimen used after PRK, using extensive steroids for a long period. Although after a regular LASIK procedure prolonged steroid therapy is not necessary, we found it very effective in decreasing the amount and incidence of haze in LASIK after PRK (Figure 30-8).

Results (Pilot Study)

Thirty patients with regression after PRK were treated by LASIK. The procedure was performed at least 12 months after PRK. The mean pre-LASIK spherical equivalent was -3.65 ± 1.9 (-1.75 to -6.0), mean pre-LASIK BSCVA was 0.7 ± 0.23 (0.4 to 1.0), and mean UCVA was 0.24 ±0 .41 (0.1 to 0.6).

Results after LASIK

Mean UCVA significantly improved to 0.4 ± 0.29 (0.2 to 0.8) at 1 month, 0.6 ± 0.26 (0.2 to 0.9) at 3 months, and 0.6 ± 0.18 (0.2 to 1.0) at 6 months (Figure 30-9). One month after LASIK, BSCVA was 0.5 ± 0.31 (0.2 to 0.9); at 3 months, BSCVA was 0.7 ± 0.22 (0.2 to 1.0); and at 6 months, BSCVA was 0.7 ± 0.17 (0.4 to 0.1) (see Figure 30-9). In 78% and 85% of eyes, UCVA was better than 0.5 at 3 and 6 months respectively. Only one eye lost more than two lines of BSCVA after LASIK; this was related to severe haze that developed following an intraoperative flap complication in which the flap was cut into two halves. At the end of follow-up, 98% of the patients where within ± 1.0 D of intended refraction and 77% were within ± 0.5 D.

Conclusions

LASIK seems to be a good alternative to correct post-PRK regression; the procedure is safe, effective, and highly predictable. The curve of visual improvement after LASIK seems to follow that of PRK (decrease in immediate postoperative visual acuity, followed by an improvement after the first month). This could be related to the significant amount of haze observed in this group of patients immediately after LASIK, therefore aggressive and prolonged use of topical corticosteroids is necessary. The microkeratome cut is more difficult after PRK than with virgin corneas. The flap has to be as thick as possible to avoid the increased risk of developing wrinkles and an irregular surface.

LASIK AFTER LTK

When hyperopic errors are corrected by corneal refractive surgery, the goal is to steepen the central cornea in an amount proportional to the hyperopic error to be corrected.

With recent advances in laser technology, LTK was

studied for the correction of hyperopia. Erbium, CO_2, and holmium (Ho): YAG lasers were investigated as potential candidates for this procedure. The CO_2 (10.6 mm) LTK was studied by Peyman, et al, and resulted in superficial retraction of the corneal collagen, as well as early regression of the refractive effect.[31] Yr-erbium-glass laser spots (1.54 mm) resulted in extensive penetration and tissue necrosis.[32]

Ho: YAG laser (2.06 microns) LTK was then used for the correction of hyperopia. Ho: YAG LTK changes the anterior corneal curvature by using the infrared laser energy heat generated in the cornea to change the anterior corneal curvature.[33] The corneal collagen shrinks by 30% to 45% of its original length at temperatures ranging from 58°C to 60°C. Higher temperatures cause tissue necrosis and relaxation.[34] Stromal haze at the treatment site extends from 50% to 70% of the corneal thickness.[35]

LTK flattens the periphery and thus steepens the central area. The results from Koch[36] indicate that this could be a promising technology to correct low to moderate hyperopic refractive error. Alió, et al[37] recommend that algorithms to improve final results should include an initial calculated overcorrection adjusted to variables that influence regression, such as age and corneal thickness. However, in spite of all these refinements, regression of effect has been a major limitation to the potential refractive outcome of LTK. Regression is variable and may even be total. It was found to be mainly a biophysical mechanism,[38] which proved difficult or impossible in most cases to be solved with LTK retreatment.

The Cornea After LTK

After LTK, the opacities in each treatment spot (average diameter is 0.7 mm) decrease with time. After 2 months, they can be observed only under the slit lamp. Although the degree of opacity decreases over time, it is usually present for a long period after LTK. The density and depth of haze are related to the pulse energy. Up to 1 year after LTK, the mean central corneal thickness was slightly thinner than the preoperative value. However, after 2 years, the mean central corneal thickness was almost identical to the preoperative value. From our observations, it seems that the cornea remains unstable for a long time after LTK treatment, especially with unsuccessful treatment. The corneas in these patients tend to return to their original preoperative topographic status, with a multifocal irregular corneal surface.

Performing LASIK After LTK

Many patients previously treated with LTK are seeking an alternative surgical treatment for the correction of their residual refractive error. LASIK may offer a good alternative for these corrections. With LASIK, it is possi-

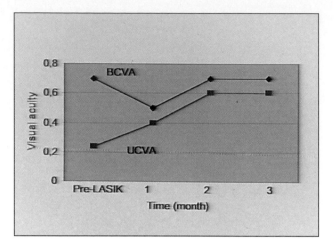

Figure 30-9. Change in the mean BCVA and UCVA over time pre-LASIK, 1, 2, and 3 months after LASIK.

ble to ablate the corneal periphery by stromal photorefractive ablation and prevent strong epithelial regression with the overlying flap.[39] With virgin hyperopic corneas, LASIK proved to be very efficient, safe, and predictable. However, laser energy is expected to have its own effect at the level of the previous LTK spots, and this may significantly influence its effect on the correction achieved, stability of the refractive results, and corneal wound healing. Thus, performing LASIK on corneas with previous LTK treatment requires special care in both preoperative evaluation and intraoperative precautions to achieve the best possible results.

The only contraindication for this procedure is the presence of a dense corneal opacity that interferes with vision; but even in cases developing irregular astigmatism, topography-linked excimer laser ablation can be used.

Preoperative Considerations

As regression is the main complication after LTK and may continue over a variable duration, LASIK should be postponed until regression has stopped. This might take up to 1 year or even more.

Factors affecting regression:

- Age. Greater regression is seen in young adults with relatively elastic stromal tissue and Bowman's membrane, thus complete refractive stability is essential before LASIK.
- High pre-LTK hyperopia invites greater and prolonged regression. We need to have at least three consecutive stable corneal topographies over 3 months before performing LASIK.

It is important to distinguish between undercorrection and regression; undercorrection is present in the immediate postoperative period, while regression occurs

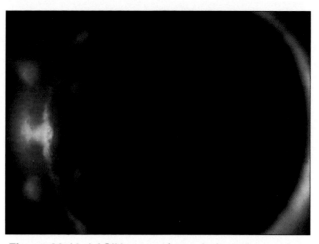

Figure 30-10. LASIK cut performed along the previous LTK spots, producing a characteristic ring-shaped haze.

during the course of healing. However, a longer interval between the two operations allows us to perform more accurate surgery and avoid future complications. With our patients, we wait at least 1 year after LTK to perform LASIK. Patients with pre-LTK high degrees of hyperopia should wait up to 18 to 24 months, as they usually show more regression. In general, no LASIK attempt should be considered unless we have a stable refraction and corneal topography for 2 consecutive months. Corneal topography is important to assess the size and shape of the optic zone and to plan the new surgery.

Biomicroscopic examination is important in assessing the sites, degree, and extension of stromal scars, usually seen at the LTK treatment sites, to plan the LASIK cut.

Intraoperative Considerations

Centration is always essential. Decentration is more common in hyperopic patients and will be more accurate and easier if corneal topography is used to assess centration.

The LASIK cut should be performed away from the LTK corneal spots, otherwise the cornea will show dense ring-shaped haze (Figure 30-10).[40] Although this does not influence the immediate visual result, the long term stability of the achieved refractive results are still unknown.

A large flap is always preferable to allow perfect peripheral corneal ablation; the flap should be 8.5 mm or more.

Results (Pilot Study)

Twenty-three eyes with significant regression following noncontact LTK treatment underwent LASIK in an attempt to correct their refractive error. LASIK was performed at least 18 months after the LTK treatment. The pre-LASIK mean spherical equivalent changed from +3.14 D ± 1.82 (+0.50 to +6.50) to +0.52 D ± 1.71 (-2.75 to +3.75) 6 months after LASIK. There was a significant change in refraction between the preoperative and postoperative spherical equivalent values at 1, 3, and 6 months (p < 0.05). There was a minor insignificant change between the pre-LASIK mean BSCVA (0.74 ± 0.15, range: 0.4 to 1.0) and the post-LASIK mean BSCVA at 6 months (0.74 ± 0.18, range: 0.4 to 1.0). Three patients lost one line of BSCVA, and two patients lost more than one line of BSCVA. Six months after LASIK, UCVA significantly improved from a mean value of 0.36 ± 0.16 (0.1 to 0.7) to 0.61 ± 0.25 (0.2 to 1.0). Although the procedure seems to be safe (Figure 30-11), it was not as effective. Six patients (26%) showed no change in preoperative BSCVA from the postoperative UCVA. Three patients (13%) gained one or more Snellen lines, five patients (21%) lost one Snellen line, and nine patients (39%) lost two or more Snellen lines (Figure 30-12). Seventeen patients (73%) were within ±1 D of intended hyperopic correction. Four patients (27%) had regression during the period of 6 months after LASIK. Regression ranged from 0.75 D to 3.75 D; we believe this regression was a continuation of the regression taking place after LTK.

Conclusions

Hyperopic LASIK is a good alternative for the correction of residual refractive error after holmium LTK. Efficacy and predictability are inferior to that of virgin hyperopic corneas that undergo LASIK, but the procedure seems to be equally safe. We should keep in mind that these corneas are unstable, and a completely stable corneal topographic map is very important to decrease the incidence of further regression after LASIK. To avoid the development of severe haze after LASIK, we perform the LASIK cut away from the previous LTK spots.

LASIK AFTER PKP

PKP is a procedure frequently performed worldwide, with more than 34,000 yearly in the United States.[40] Most of these cases are left with refractive errors both spherically and cylindrically that may cause variable degrees of anisometropia. Irregular astigmatism is frequently found after PKP, leading to significant limitation in visual performance.

The visual result after PKP is influenced by biological and refractive factors. The biological quality of the donor tissue and episodes of graft rejection affect the transparency of the graft.

Despite the corneal graft being optically clear, a high

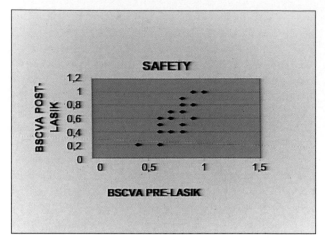

Figure 30-11. BSCVA before LASIK and at 6 months after LASIK.

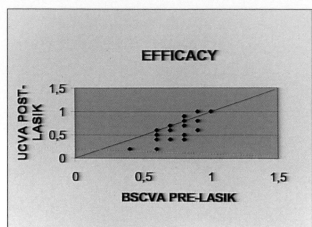

Figure 30-12. BSCVA before LASIK against UCVA at 6 months after LASIK.

astigmatism average of 4 to 6 D,[42] and irregular astigmatism associated with the spherical error explains why these patients are unable to reach BCVA with spectacles or contact lenses.

In summary, the main aspects involved in the optical and refractive outcome of this surgical procedure include the following:

Biological factors:
- Quality of the donor cornea
- Difference in thickness between the donor and recipient corneas
- Wound healing
- Underlying corneal disease

Surgical factors:
- Graft-recipient disparity
- Wound dehiscence
- Wound configuration
- Eccentric trephination of donor or host cornea
- Previous astigmatism of donor cornea
- Previous anterior segment surgery (PKP, phacoemulsification, RK)
- Time of suture removal and suturing technique are the most important of all. The double-running 10-0 nylon sutures or the combined interrupted and continuous sutures can minimize irregular post-keratoplasty astigmatism when compared with interrupted sutures.[43,44]

In addition to the wound healing process, there are different responses according to the age of the patient. The younger the patient, the stronger and faster the wound healing. Wound integrity is determined by the amount of whitening and scarring at the PKP wound, especially if associated with vascular invasion.[45]

The authors would like to acknowledge Dr. Valerio De Iorio for his assistance in the production of this section.

Corneal Refractive Surgery

Several techniques are available to correct refractive errors after PKP:

- Incisional surgery: effective but unpredictable due to the different quality of the donor cornea, wound healing, and tensional forces of the cornea generated by the wound healing structure.
- PRK: produces problems due to laser interaction with wound healing, increasing the risk of haze. Moreover, this can lead to a major risk of graft rejection due to the removal of the epithelium and Bowman's membrane.
- LASIK: may be the best alternative treatment, especially with the help of topography-linked excimer laser ablation (topolink). With LASIK, we are able to offer an improvement in visual acuity with fast visual recovery and less pain.

Performing Excimer Laser After PKP

Surgical correction of the refractive error following PKP depends on corneal regularity.

For spherical defects associated with regular astigmatism, we perform:

- Standard LASIK treatment with or without previous AK. In cases of astigmatism more than 4 D, we usually perform AK followed by LASIK.

For irregular astigmatism, we perform:

- Topolink
- Excimer laser ablation assisted by sodium hyaluronate (ELASIIY)
- Selective excimer laser zonal ablation (SELZA)

(These procedures are explained in Chapter 27.)

Preoperative Considerations

Preoperative ophthalmologic evaluation:

- Medical history: it is essential to investigate the causes that led to PKP, with special attention to herpetic keratitis, previous graft rejection, and keratoconus, which may induce severe astigmatic effect, especially after suture removal. Systemic diseases affecting the healing process, as collagen vascular diseases, must be excluded. This might affect the outcome of LASIK.
- UCVA and BCVA (with spectacles and rigid/gas-permeable contact lenses).
- Refraction should be stable for the last two months before LASIK treatment.
- Pinhole visual acuity is a rapid method to diagnose the presence of irregular astigmatism.

Details concerning the graft:

- Date of surgery, date of suture removal, diameter of corneal button, signs of wound integrity, healing, site and depth of neovascularization.
- Corneal topography. we must have a series of two stable consecutive corneal topographies with a 2-month interval to assure a low activity of wound healing and corneal remodeling.[45] Recently, the Orbscan elevation maps, the corneal uniformity index (EyeSys), and potential corneal visual acuity (Technomed) give quantitative estimation of corneal regularity not only at the anterior surface but also at the posterior surface of the cornea.
- Slit lamp biomicroscopy: to plan the cut, it is important to study the presence and extension of corneal neovascularization, the amount of wound scarring, the presence of ectatic areas at the level of previous stitches or dehiscence that could limit or render the LASIK procedure more dangerous.
- Endothelial microscopy: although LASIK is not dangerous to the corneal endothelium,[46] it is always advisable to ascertain the endothelial condition before surgery, considering that the cornea after PKP has continuous cell loss.[47] A LASIK procedure should not be considered if the corneal endothelium is severely decreased or at high risk of decompensation.
- Peripheral and central corneal pachymetry: it is important to measure 8 to 16 corneal points, using the topographic map as a guide, especially at the wound level and at the sites where the cornea seems thinner upon slit lamp examination to avoid perforation of undetected ectasia.

LASIK Indications

- Significant spherical and/or astigmatic errors induced by PKP, especially if not correctable with spectacles or contact lenses.
- Anisokonia due to postoperative refractive defect.

High Risk Cases and LASIK Contra-indications

- Herpetic keratitis represents a well-known contraindication to excimer laser treatment.[48,49] In corneas with post-herpetic PKP, we must consider the possibility not only of keratitis recurrence, but also the risk of allograft rejection due to the reactivation of latent herpes simplex virus present in the corneal nerve and in the keratocytes[50] under the effect of the excimer laser and mechanical trauma.
- Diffuse corneal neovascularization could represent a considerable problem during surgery.
- Corneal inflammation is a contraindication—it increases the risk of rejection.
- High residual astigmatism can render LASIK unuseful even with topolink. Alternative procedures should be considered to treat irregular astigmatism.
- The presence of sutures is a relative contraindication. In fact, an average of 8.8 D of astigmatism has been reported after suture removal,[13] so it is mandatory to postpone the operation.
- Bad optical quality of the donor button.
- Corneal ectasia.

Preoperative Medications

We can divide post-PKP patients into four main groups suitable for prophylactic therapy before undergoing LASIK:

1. Patients with no history of graft rejection or herpetic keratitis. To prevent an eventual rejection we should use topical steroids, dexamethasone 0.1%, or prednisolone 1%, one drop four times a day for 15 days before surgery and for 1 month after surgery.
2. Patients with previous rejection episodes. Topical treatment includes dexamethasone 0.1% or prednisolone 1%, one drop four times a day for 15 days before surgery and 1 month after surgery. Systemic treatment: 1 mg/kg per day of prednisolone, 5 days before and after surgery, and then tapered.
3. Patients with previous herpetic keratitis. In order to avoid recurrence and/or rejection: systemic acyclovir 800 mg per day for 15 days before surgery and 1 month after surgery.
4. Patients with history of herpetic keratitis and rejection. Systemic acyclovir 800 mg per day for

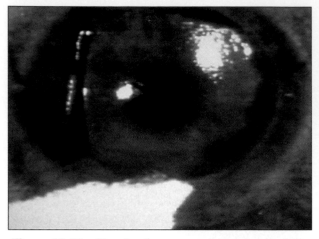

Figure 30-13a. Bleeding from neovessels after performing the microkeratome cut. A sponge wetted with phenylephrin was used to control bleeding (this patient underwent PKP 4 years before LASIK).

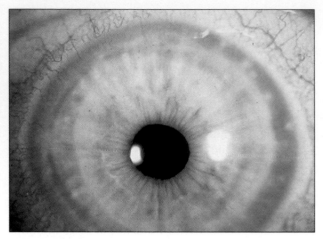

Figure 30-13b. The same eye 1 week after LASIK, with perfect flap adhesion.

15 days before surgery and 1 month after surgery. Systemic low grade steroids: 15 mg per day for 15 days before surgery and 1 month after surgery.

When to Operate

An interval of 18 to 24 months after PKP is enough for the graft to form a stable union with the host's peripheral cornea.[45,51]

The corneal topography should be stable for 2 months after removing the stitches.

There are particular circumstances in which it is recommended to perform LASIK treatment earlier, as in young patients intolerant to contact lenses who require fast recovery of their binocular vision.[45]

Kritzinger performs laser ablation 2 weeks after the microkeratome cut, allowing the cornea to achieve its new refractive configuration after releasing the tensional forces of the fibrotic wound.[52]

Patients should be informed of the possibility of undergoing more than one procedure to reach the best refractive results.

Intraoperative Considerations

Flap diameter: The flap diameter should be as small as possible to avoid bleeding from the injured corneal neovascularization, which could affect the quality of ablation, clarity of the interface, and increase the risk of rejection. If this happens, the surgeon has to clean the interface. If bleeding is severe, we apply to the peripheral limbus a sponge soaked with phenylephrine to induce vasoconstriction in the feeder vessels before ablation (Figures 30-13a and 30-13b).

Hinge position: To avoid hinge syndrome, we do not perform the cut opposite the astigmatic axis by using lateral, oblique, or down-up position. The thickness of the flap should not be less then 160 µm.

Figures 30-14a through 30-14c show the sequence of changes in the corneal topography before and after customized ablation (topolink) in a patient with previous PKP.

Conclusions

There are few published reports concerning LASIK after PKP[45,51,52] and the long-term refractive stability after suture removal.[43] It is very difficult to achieve predictable refractive results after LASIK performed on eyes with previous PKP surgery. If we can not guarantee emmetropia to these patients, at least we can offer them benefits by reducing the astigmatism of this "unstable biological tissue."

In summary. the main aspects involved and to be remembered in LASIK after PKP are:
- Corneal stability
- Corneal regularity
- First reduce the astigmatism with AK if necessary
- Size of the flap
- Hinge position
- Corneal vessels
- Prophylactic therapy against rejection and herpetic keratitis

LASIK AFTER ALK

ALK is a lamellar refractive surgery technique used to change the anterior surface of the cornea by removing a portion of the corneal stroma. In ALK, a three-piece suction ring is used to create the flap. The suction ring also enables us to determine and perform the second

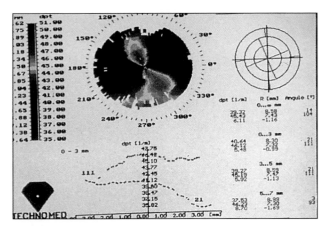

Figure 30-14a. Corneal topography after PKP and before LASIK.

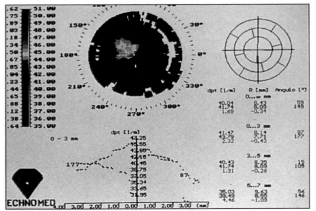

Figure 30-14b. The same eye on the first postoperative day after LASIK.

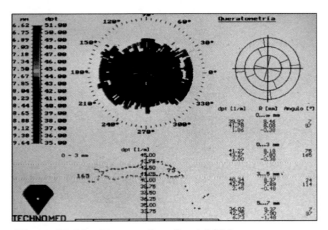

Figure 30-14c. Two months after LASIK.

refractive cut. Myopic treatment depends on removing a portion of the central corneal stroma. Hyperopic treatment uses a transverse circular cut of corneal lamellae at 70% depth of the corneal thickness and 6.0 mm diameter. Predictability is the main problem we faced in the past with this type of surgery, resulting in a high incidence of over or undercorrection. Now, these patients are requiring a second surgery to correct residual refractive error. Here we report the outcome of LASIK in treating these patients.

The Cornea After ALK

The following features may be found in the cornea after ALK: nonadherent or lost cap, epithelial growth in the interface, and regular or irregular astigmatism. Concerning visual outcome, it is true that this technique is relatively efficient in the correction of myopia. However, it is also true that any minimal decentration between the two corneal cuts could produce distortion of the central optical zone, leading to irregular astigmatism and subjective visual alterations such as glare, diplopia,

and decrease in the contrast sensitivity. In myopic treatment, ALK will produce a small central depression corresponding with the central corneal cut. In hyperopic treatment, we may find induced keratoconus due to central corneal ectasia.

Performing LASIK After ALK

LASIK may be an efficient tool in treating residual refractive error after ALK, but as it uses a lamellar cut, additional technical and intraoperative problems may arise, which might render this technique very difficult and unsafe in some cases. Thus, careful patient selection is mandatory to improve the outcome of this procedure.

Preoperative Considerations

After ALK, time is the most important factor to assure good corneal healing. Albino Parisi reported a case of an involuntarily dissected and elevated ALK flap during a LASIK attempt 6 months after ALK.[11] A period of 2 years is essential to achieve a stable corneal condition and to decrease the possibility of such a major complication. The refractive state of the cornea should be stable to improve the predictability of the treatment. We carefully study the corneal topography of these patients to exclude the possibility of induced keratoconus (central corneal ectasia) after hyperopic ALK treatment, which is a contraindication for LASIK.

Intraoperative Considerations

The LASIK cut is the most critical step; it should be performed superficial to the previous cut, which is difficult to judge. The cut may pass parallel to or intersect with the previous ALK cut, inducing irregular astigmatism or increasing the already present astigmatism. In cases of undiagnosed induced keratoconus, the LASIK cut will be too deep, the cornea will be thinner and more ectasia will develop, inducing major complications and a

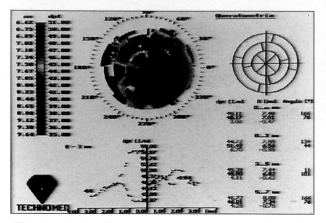

Figure 30-15a. Severe irregular astigmatism following LASIK 26 months after a previous hyperopic treatment by ALK.

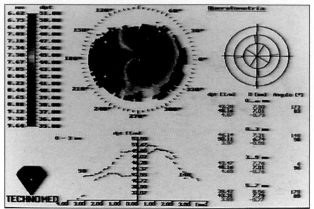

Figure 30-15b. The same patient showing a significant improvement 2 weeks after excimer laser ablation assisted by sodium hyaluronate.

significant decrease in the visual acuity. It is advisable to abort the procedure as soon as any difficulty is encountered in performing the cut to avoid further complications. We experienced some problems with the LASIK cut as it intersected with the previous ALK keratectomy, producing an irregular surface (Figures 30-15a and 30-15b).

Conclusions

LASIK is not a highly predictable procedure in treating a residual refractive defect after ALK. Careful patient selection and a 2-year interval between surgeries should be enough to improve the efficacy and predictability of the procedure. Other techniques to treat irregular astigmatism (Chapter 27) should be considered in treating these patients.

LASIK AFTER EPIKERATOPHAKIA

Epikeratophakia was used to treat adult aphakia, pediatric aphakia, and severe myopia. This technique is obsolete due to the high incidence of complications, including lack of predictability, poor optical results, almost constant irregular astigmatism, chronic epithelial defects with scarring, tissue melting, long period of time to recover BSCVA due to lack of corneal transparency, undercorrection, overcorrection, glare, diplopia, and reduced contrast sensitivity. Also, the procedure is not totally reversible, as it was previously thought to be.

Before LASIK treatment, it is important to assess corneal transparency and measure the button diameter. During LASIK, the cut should be done within the lamellar button by creating the smallest possible flap to avoid

peripheral lamellar dissection. We have limited experience with these cases and further studies are needed to evaluate the long-term refractive outcome.

LASIK AFTER CORNEAL TRAUMA

Several types of trauma, such as penetrating corneal wounds, chemical burns, and radiant energy, could affect the cornea. It is very important before performing a LASIK treatment to check the presence of corneal opacity, neovascularization, and irregular astigmatism. In the presence of a corneal scar, we avoid cutting through it, especially if it is close to the limbus, to avoid bleeding from the new vessels. The possibility of cutting through corneal ectasia should be excluded by evaluating the pachymetric value of the suspected zone. The quality of laser ablation and its rate differ according to the density of the corneal scar, thus the patient should be advised that he or she might need more than one procedure to correct the refractive defect. Topography-linked excimer laser ablation (topolink) should be useful in most cases.

FUTURE OF LASIK AFTER OTHER CORNEAL SURGERIES

Regression, undercorrection, and overcorrection are possible complications following various refractive surgical procedures. LASIK has proved to be a safe method in treating these refractive defects in most cases. However, these corneas are usually unstable. With careful patient selection, preoperative evaluation and intraoperative management, we can usually improve the efficacy and predictability of this procedure.

REFERENCES

1. Villaseñor RA, Cox KO. Radial keratotomy: reoperations. *Journal of Refractive Surgery.* 1985;1:34-37.

2. Salz JJ. Radial keratotomy. In: Thompson FB, ed. *Myopia Surgery: Anterior and Posterior Segments.* New York, NY: Macmillan; 1990.

3. Waring GO III, Lynn MJ, McDonnel PJ. PERK study group. Results of the prospective evaluation of radial keratotomy (PERK) study 10 years after surgery. *Arch Ophthalmol.* 1994;112:1298-1308.

4. Azar DT, Benson RA, Hardten DR. The PRK after RK study group. Photorefractive keratectomy for residual myopia after radial keratotomy. *J Cataract Refract Surg.* 1998;24:303-311.

5. Salz JJ, Salz JM, Salz M, Jones D. Ten years experience with a conservative approach to radial keratotomy. *J Refract Corneal Surg.* 1991;7:12-22.

6. Werblin TP, Stafford GM. The Casebeer system for predictable keratorefractive surgery: 1-year evaluation of 205 consecutive eyes. *Ophthalmology.* 1993;100:1095-1102.

7. Sawelson H, Marks RG. Two-year results of reoperations for radial keratotomy. *Arch Ophthalmol.* 1988;106:497-501.

8. Gayton JL, Van Der Karr M, Sanders V. Radial keratotomy enhancements for residual myopia. *Journal of Refractive Surgery.* 1997;13:374-381.

9. Werblin TP, Stafford GM. Radial keratotomy predictability (letter). *Ophthalmology.* 1994;101:416.

10. Hahn TW, Kim JH, Lee YC. Excimer laser photorefractive keratotomy to correct residual myopia after radial keratotomy. *J Refract Corneal Surg.* 1993;9(suppl):S25-S29.

11. Durrie DS, Schumer DJ, Cavanaugh TB. Photorefractive keratectomy for residual myopia after previous refractive keratectomy. *J Refract Corneal Surg.* 1994;10:S235-S238.

12. Salz JJ, Assil KK, Colin J. Radial keratotomy. In: Serdarevic O, ed. *Refractive Surgery: Current Techniques and Management.* New York: Igaku-Shoin Medical Publishers. 1997;27-36.

13. Deitz MR, Sanders DR. Progressive hyperopia with long-term follow-up of a radial keratotomy. *Arch Ophthalmol.* 1985;103:782-784.

14. Duke-Elder SS, Abrams D. Ophthalmic optics and refraction. In: *System of Ophthalmology. Vol 5.* St.Louis, Mo: CV Mosby; 1970.

15. Buzard K, Shearing S, Relyea R. Incidence of astigmatism in a cataract practice. *Journal of Refractive Surgery.* 1988;4:173.

16. Guyton DL. Prescribing cylinders: the problem of distortion. *Surv Ophthalmol.* 1977;22:177-188.

17. Thompson V. Astigmatic keratotomy. In: Serdarevic O, ed. *Refractive Surgery: Current Techniques and Management.* New York: Igaku-Shoin Medical Publishers. 1997.

18. Duffey RJ, Jain VN, Tachah H, et al. Paired arcuate keratotomy. A surgical approach to mixed and myopic astigmatism. *Arch Ophthalmol.* 1988;106:1130-1135.

19. Merlin U. Curved keratotomy procedures for congenital astigmatism. *Journal of Refractive Surgery.* 1987;3:92-97.

20. McDonnell PJ, Moreira H, Terrance N, et al. Photorefractive keratectomy for astigmatism-initial clinical results. *Arch Ophthalmol.* 1991;109:1370-1373.

21. Vajpayee RB, Taylor HR. Photorefractive keratectomy for astigmatism. In: Serdarevic O, ed. *Refractive Surgery: Current Techniques and Management.* New York: Igaku-Shoin Medical Publishers. 1997; 207-216.

22. Munnerlyn CR, Koons SJ, Marshall J. Photorefractive keratectomy: a technique for laser refractive surgery. *J Cataract Refract Surg.* 1988;14:46-52.

23. Seiler T, McDonnell PJ. Excimer laser photorefractive keratectomy. *Surv Ophthalmol.* 1995;40:89-118.

24. Kim JH, Sah WJ, Kim MS, et al. Three-year results of photorefractive keratectomy for myopia. *Journal of Refractive Surgery.* 1995;11(3suppl):418-20.

25. Wu WCS, Stark WJ, Green WR. Corneal wound healing after 193-nm excimer laser keratectomy. *Arch Ophthalmol.* 1991;109:1426-1432.

26. Tuft SJ, Zabel RW, Marshall J. Corneal repair following keratectomy: a comparison between conventional surgery and laser photoablation. *Invest Ophthalmol Vis Sci.* 1989;30:1769-1777.

27. Chayet AS, Assil KK, Montes M, Espinosa-Lagana M, Castellanos A, Tsioulias G. *J Refract Corneal Surg.* 1990;6:335-339.

28. Pallikaris IG, Papatzanaki ME, Stathi E. Laser in situ keratomileusis. *Lasers Surg Med.* 1990;10:463-468.

29. Fiander DC, Tayfour F. Excimer laser in situ keratomileusis in 124 myopic eyes. *Journal of Refractive Surgery.* 1995;11(3suppl):S234-8.

30. Sutton G, Kalski RS, Lawless MA, Rogers C. Excimer retreatment for scarring and regression after photorefractive keratectomy for myopia. *Br J Ophthalmol.* 1995;79:756-759.

31. Andrews AH. Modification of rabbit corneal curvature with the use of carbon dioxide laser burns. *Ophthalmic Surg.* 1980;11:325-329.

32. Kanoda AN, Sorokin AS. Corneal curvature change using energy of laser radiation. In: Fydorov SN, ed. *Microsurgery of the Eye.* Moscow:Mir Publishers; 1987:147-154.

33. Koch DD, Berry MJ, Vassiliadias AJ, et al. Noncontact holmium: Yag laser thermal keratoplasty. In: Salz JJ, ed. *Corneal Laser Surgery.* St. Louis, Mo: Mosby-Year Book, Inc; 1995.

34. Moreira H, Campos M, Sawush MR, et al. Holmium laser thermokeratoplasty. *Ophthalmology.* 1993;100:752-761.

35. Koch DD, Abarca A, Villarreal R, et al. Hyperopia correction by noncontact holmium: yag laser thermal keratoplasty: clinical study with 2-year follow-up. *Ophthalmology.* 1996;103:731-740.

36. Koch D, Aborca A. Laser thermal keratoplasty. *Ophthalmology.* 1996;103:1525-1536.

37. Alió JL, Ismail M, Sanchez-Pego JL. Correction of hyperopia with noncontact Ho: yag laser thermal keratoplasty. *Journal of Refractive Surgery.* 1997;113:17-22.

38. Ismail MM, Perez Santonja JJ, Alió JL. Correction of hyperopia and hyperopic astigmatism by laser. In: Serdarevic O, ed. *Refractive Surgery: Current Techniques and Management.* New York: Igaku-Shoin Medical Publishers. 1997.

39. Ditzin K, Huschka H, Pieger S. Laser in situ keratomileusis for hyperopia. *J Cataract Refract Surg.* 1998;24:42-47.

40. Attia WH, Alí0 JL, Perez Santonja JJ. LASIK following LTK regression in hyperopic patients. *Journal of Refractive Surgery.* Submitted for publication April 1999.

41. Eye Bank Association of America. *1996 Eye Banking Statistical Report.* Eye Bank Association of America, Washington, DC; 1996.

42. Vail A, Gore SM, Bradley BA, et al. Corneal graft survival and visual outcome. A multicenter study. *Ophthalmology.* 1994;101:120-7.

43. Hoppenreijs VP, Van Rij G, et al. Causes of astigmatism after penetrating keratoplasty. *Doc Ophthalmol.* 1993;85:21-34.

44. Busin M, Monk T, Al Nawaiseh I. Different suturing techniques variously affect the regularity of postkeratoplasty astigmatism. *Ophthalmology.* 1998;105:1200-1205.

45. Lam DS, Leung AT,Wu JT, Tham CC, Fan DS. How long should one wait to perform LASIK after PKP? *J Cataract Refract Surg.* 1998;24:6-7.

46. Perez-Santonja JJ, Sakla HF, Alió JA. Evaluation of endothelial cell changes 1 year after excimer laser in situ keratomileusis. *Arch Ophthalmol.* 1997;115:841-846.

47. Bourne WM, Hodge DO, Nelson LR. Corneal endothelium 5 years after transplantation. *Am J Ophthalmol.* 1994;118:185-196.

48. Pepose JS, Laycock KA, Miller JK, et al. Reactivation of latent herpes virus by excimer laser photokeratectomy. *Am J Ophthalmol.* 1992;144:45-50.

49. Vrabec MP, Durrie DS, Chase DS. Recurrence of herpes simplex after excimer laser keratectomy. *Am J Ophthalmol.* 1992;116:101-102.

50. Xie LX, Dong XG, Kaufman HE. Investigation of herpes simplex virus type-1 latency in corneas. *Chin Med J Engl.* 1993;106(4):288-91.

51. Parisi A, Salchow DL, et al. Laser in situ keratomileusis after automated lamellar keratoplasty and penetrating keratoplasty. *J Cataract Refract Surg.* 1997;23:1114-1118.

52. Kritzinger MS. Corneal transplant patients far better with LASIK than PRK. *Ocular Surgery News.* 1998,16:34.

LASIK After PKP

Michiel S. Kritzinger, MD

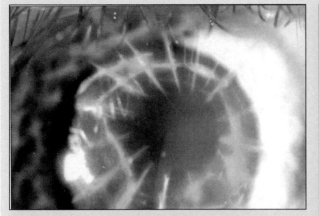

Figure 30A-1. Futile RK attempts at crossing the fibrotic ring.

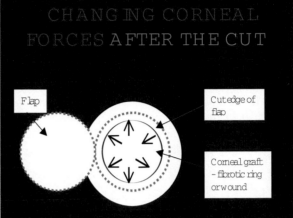

Figure 30A-2. Cutting the fibrotic PKP wound ring creates new forces into the button, which changes the spherical and cylindrical powers, as well as the axis of the astigmatism.

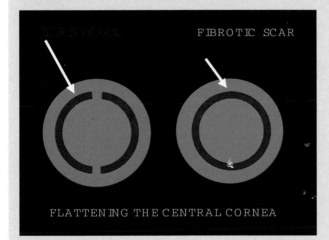

Figure 30A-3. With LASIK PKP surgery, the UCVA postoperatively is the same as the BCVA preoperatively. LASIK will play a major role in the visual rehabilitation of the ametropic eye following PKP.

There is rarely an ideal refractive error outcome after PKP surgery. Usually there is moderate to high myopia or hyperopia and astigmatism. In the past, incisional refractive surgery was attempted but was usually met with frustrating visual results. In the new excimer laser era, PRK is also not the refractive surgery of choice because it induces severe haze and fibrosis, which rarely clears.

LASIK is the ideal final refractive treatment for PKP refractive errors but with a different approach and technique:

1. All corneal sutures must be removed before planning LASIK surgery.
2. Wait 4 months after the last suture is removed so the cornea can stabilize.
3. First do the microkeratome cut without lifting the flap or irrigating the interface, then wait another 4 weeks before applying the new refractive error treatment.

The refraction changes the most with a full-thickness 160-micron flap, which includes the PKP fibrotic ring. It changes the least with a small thin flap, which consist of only the PKP button.

4. The fibrotic PKP wound ring has an intrastromal corneal ring segment (ICRS) effect when doing LASIK treatment with a resultant hyperopic shift, or contra wise less myopic regression postoperatively.
5. The incidence of enhancement surgery is higher than in normal LASIK surgery due to severe refractive errors.
6. More buttonholes are cut in the flaps due to steep corneas of different K values for the button and peripheral cornea.
7. It is more difficult to lift the flap in enhancement surgery due to the PKP wound scar.
8. More regression postoperatively is seen when using infant and elderly donor material being.
9. You may spring a leak from the corneal bed because you are treating, especially in hyperopia, the corneal wound as well.
10. Too many enhancements result in fluctuating vision due to a cornea that is too thin.

LASIK After PKP

Antonio Marinho, MD

INTRODUCTION

Penetrating keratoplasty (PKP) is usually associated with large residual refractive errors. On many occasions, a clear cornea and a perfect surgery seem a failure for the patient because of residual ametropia. Myopia and astigmatism (sometimes very high) are the most common refractive errors found after PKP. Different techniques of trephining and suturing, as well as the intraoperative use of several devices to avoid astigmatism, have not in many instances solved this problem.

HOW TO CORRECT AMETROPIA AFTER PKP

Ametropia after PKP has been treated surgically in several ways. Incisional surgery (arcuate incisions) has been used in astigmatism with different results (corrections from 40% to 100% were reported) but is almost always associated with significant regression. PRK has also been applied to post-PKP cases with good refractive results. However, significant haze was observed in many cases, sometimes as late haze (even 2 years after PRK) and very resistant to treatment (Figure 30B-1). LASIK, on the other hand, can be performed without complications from a primary case.

WHEN TO PERFORM LASIK

LASIK should be performed in all cases after PKP when the ametropia is not easily corrected with glasses or contact lenses. An important point is the timing of surgery. LASIK can only be performed 2 years after PKP and not before.

HOW TO PERFORM LASIK AFTER PKP

When performing LASIK after PKP, we must create a flap as large as possible. In every case, the diameter of the flap must be larger than the diameter of the graft. A thick flap (180 microns) is also advisable.

After PKP, the cornea is sometimes not stable even 2 years after surgery and this is probably the cause of some unpredictable results reported after LASIK.

To avoid this problem, the following surgical method is advised:

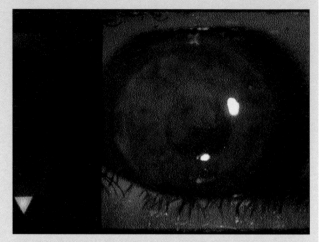

Figure 30B-1. Late haze after PRK.

1. Create the flap.
2. Check the refraction and topography weekly until it is stable.
3. Lift the flap and perform the laser ablation only when refraction and topography are stable (usually 3 weeks after creating the flap).

RESULTS

Refractive results of LASIK are not as accurate (corneal instability) as in primary cases. In most cases a residual astigmatism is observed. We must also consider that in most cases, we are not aiming for emmetropia but only trying to make the use of glasses or contact lenses acceptable.

CONCLUSIONS

LASIK is a useful and safe method to reduce significant ametropias induced by PKP. LASIK is not associated with more complications than in primary cases. The following guidelines are important to maximize results.

1. Perform LASIK only 2 years after PKP.
2. Create a flap larger than the graft.
3. Do not perform the ablation immediately; wait (at least 3 weeks) until the topography and refraction are stable.

LASIK is the only refractive procedure safe and effective enough to use after PKP.

LASIK in PKP

Claudio Genisi, MD

INTRODUCTION

PKP, because of the current donor selection criteria by eye banks, mechanized instruments, and standardized surgical techniques, has reached a very high level of anatomical success; in eyes with keratoconus, the pathology that most frequently necessitates this operation, the success rate is about 95%. However, perfect corneal transparency alone cannot be considered an index of functional success because postoperative refractive errors often prevent satisfactory visual recovery. The correction of postoperative refractive errors in patients after PKP was often a problem due to the abnormal response of the transplanted cornea, since it exhibited different characteristics from those of the normal cornea.

The outcome of incisional techniques used inside and outside the transplanted button is difficult to predict. With time, there is a tendency for ectasia of the wound margin and on occasion there is rejection. In a large number of cases, excimer laser PRK will provoke late onset, very dense haze. This usually requires the surgeon to perform a repeat PKP (T. Tervo, *Cornea*, January 1996).

The LASIK technique has specific advantages and produces results that are unquestionably superior to previous techniques.

PATIENT SELECTION

Patient selection is very important. The amount and type of refractive error must be clearly determined. Myopic patients are evaluated with the same criteria used for normal corneas. Pachymetry, corneal curvature, and pupillometry are measured. Under normal conditions, there are usually no problems with correction of up to 10 to 11 D.

The biggest problem is with astigmatism, which ideally must be regular, and preferably with symmetrical bowtie topography. Eyes with irregular astigmatism and those with ectasia of the wound margin of the corneal transplant should not undergo LASIK because ectasia is often associated with a weak wound, which may perforate under the high IOP necessary for the LASIK procedure.

The following should also be excluded because of the risk of a free cap: patients with a corneal curvature of less than 39 D and astigmatism greater than 8 D with the flattest axis parallel to the microkeratome's path.

Biomicroscopy must be very accurate. The surgeon must evaluate the wound and the degree of scar formation very carefully. The LASIK technique should not be performed before 3 years after PKP and at least 6 months after suture removal.

In the event of sectorial epithelial fibrosis, the possibility of retreatment must be considered. Fibrosis is often the real reason for the development of astigmatism.

SURGICAL TECHNIQUE

The surgical technique is basically the same as the classical technique. However, there are some variations. The advised cut thickness is 160 to 180 microns. A depth less than this may create a risk of damage from the blade pass relative to the wound.

The diameter of the flap cut should ideally be greater than the diameter of the PKP flap, so that the lamellar cut can eliminate the astigmatism induced by scarring and allow hyperopic treatments to be performed with a large bed.

In my experience, the results from excimer laser ablation (Chiron Technolas 117C PlanoScan) appear to be slightly poorer, probably because of the different hydration of the PKP flap. As a result, the refractive correction must be increased by 10%.

With significant subepithelial fibrosis limited to a single corneal sector, the procedure should be performed in two steps. First, the lamellar cut should be performed with the microkeratome without the refractive treatment. Four to 5 days later, after further evaluation of the refraction and topography, the flap is raised and the refractive procedure is performed. In this way, overcorrection of the astigmatism induced by scar traction forces of the fibrosis is avoided.

CONCLUSIONS

In 1 year, I performed 25 LASIK operations in patients who had prior PKP. In terms of precision, complications, and outcome, the results appeared to be identical to those performed on normal corneas.

In comparison to incisional techniques and PRK, the LASIK technique would appear to be far superior in terms of results and safety.

LASIK After RK

Laurence Lesueur, MD and Jean-Louis Arné, MD

Secondary ametropia resulting from RK is relatively frequent. This may now be corrected with LASIK.

SURGICAL PROCEDURES TO CORRECT AMETROPIA AFTER RK

Residual myopia, stable and progressive hyperopia, and astigmatism may be encountered after RK. In cases of residual myopia, redeepening of the same incisions is possible, but this is only efficient for residual myopia less than 1.5 D. In cases of astigmatism after RK, radial and transverse incisions could cross and lead to a healing problem. Hexagonal incisions cannot correct residual hyperopia. PRK could be performed in these situations, but the risk of developing haze and regression would be much greater than after a primary procedure. Thus, in these indications of secondary ametropia after RK, LASIK appears to be the most accepted surgical procedure.

The advantage of performing LASIK after RK is its ability to correct secondary myopia, hyperopia, and astigmatism without risk of developing pathological haze and regression of the refractive effect.

Preoperative Evaluation

- Uncorrected visual acuity and best-corrected spectacle visual acuity
- Refraction under cycloplegia
- Corneal topography is essential to eliminate keratoconus or corneal ectasia with irregular astigmatism
- Corneal thickness by pachymetry
- Slit lamp examination of the corneal incisions
- Surgical Procedure of LASIK after RK

In comparison with a primary LASIK procedure, some differences are encountered with LASIK after RK. It is better to use a microkeratome capable of cutting a large flap (diameter > 8 mm) with a thickness of 160 μm. Particular care must be taken in cutting the corneal flap with the microkeratome.

The major risk is that incisions may reopen when manipulating the flap. It is sometimes difficult to preoperatively evaluate the degree of incision healing. This complication increases the rate of epithelial ingrowth.

A flat cornea is frequent after RK and also runs the risk of a free flap.

INDICATIONS FOR LASIK AFTER RK

- Stability of the refraction greater than 1 year
- No ongoing consecutive hyperopia
- Wait at least 4 years after the last RK procedure
- No more than eight radial incisions without transverse incisions
- Good healing of the incisions
- Absence of epithelial cysts
- Absence of fibrosis
- Absence of corneal ectasia (corneal topography)
- Pachymetry greater than 500 μm
- Surgeon's experience with LASIK

TREATMENT OF PREOPERATIVE COMPLICATIONS

If the incisions reopen during suction, the procedure must be stopped. In cases of widely gaping incisions or a free cap, a suture must be placed after the procedure.

The rate of epithelial ingrowth is lower when the stromal interface is very carefully irrigated after repositioning the corneal flap.

CONCLUSION

Few series of LASIK after RK have been published to date; however, there is a general consensus that LASIK is the best surgical technique for correction of secondary ametropia after RK. Eyes with corneal complications after RK must be excluded for this treatment. After RK, the LASIK procedure is technically more difficult than the primary LASIK procedure.

LASIK ENHANCEMENT FOLLOWING OTHER INTRAOCULAR PROCEDURES

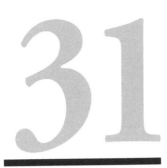

José L. Güell, MD, PhD
Mercedes Vázquez, MD

INTRODUCTION

Refractive surgical techniques have undergone major improvements over the last 15 years. Cataract surgery, including phacoemulsification with intraocular lens (IOL) implantation, penetrating keratoplasty, refractive corneal surgery (such as radial keratotomy [RK] and photorefractive keratectomy [PRK]), reconstructive surgery following ocular trauma, and more recently, the increasing use of both anterior or posterior chamber phakic IOLs to correct refractive errors, have continued to improve in quality and predictability. At the same time, more exacting demands from the surgeon, as well as increased patient expectations from ophthalmic surgery, are creating a demand for more predictability, with a goal in most cases of emmetropia and good uncorrected vision.

While keratoplasty with good anatomic results has become achievable, and good extracapsular cataract extraction or phacoemulsification with a lens implant is no longer considered technically difficult, the goal for both the surgeon and the patient is to increasingly approach emmetropia without the need for additional optical corrections. This has been achieved in cataract surgery by improvement in biometry and lens calculation formulas, and in keratoplasty with selective suture removal, topographic control of suture removal, and running suture adjustment in the early postoperative period. Refractive accuracy in both RK and PRK continue to be important goals, which are being achieved.

In an attempt to meet patient expectations, refinements in previous ocular surgery have been attempted to obtain the best possible uncorrected vision. Examples include arcuate keratotomy, relaxing incisions following keratoplasty, or cataract surgery in an attempt to reduce residual astigmatism. RK has been used to enhance the refractive results of PRK, and the reverse situation is also

true. Laser-assisted in situ keratomileusis (LASIK), as a means to enhance the refractive result of previous ocular surgery, is gaining widespread acceptance. Our experience with this technique will be further described in this chapter.

Cryolathe myopic keratomileusis was first described by Barraquer.[1-5] To avoid corneal damage due to freezing,[6] Swinger, et al[7] developed the nonfreeze keratomileusis technique. Numerous studies comparing[8,9] and reviewing[10-14] both procedures have been carried out since then. Ruiz[15] introduced keratomileusis in situ with an automated microkeratome. Buratto described the use of the excimer laser for the refractive or second cut, both on the cap and in situ, in the late 1980s. Shortly after, Pallikaris described the flap technique.[16-19] LASIK combines the advantages of laser ablation[20] (high accuracy and flexibility on corneal tissue ablation) with the advantages of intrastromal or lamellar surgery, preventing complications common in photorefractive techniques, such as haze or refractive instability secondary to ablation on the epithelial-Bowman's membrane complex. Numerous studies have now been carried out that show LASIK efficacy in correcting low, medium, and high myopia with excellent predictability and stability, although most of these studies lack long-term follow-up.

During the last 4 years, we have been using LASIK to correct myopia and astigmatism from -0.50 up to -14 diopters (D). We have found LASIK to be effective in correcting residual refractive errors following previous refractive procedures. The techniques and results are described below.

SURGICAL TECHNIQUE

Between March 1994 and August 1996, LASIK was performed to correct residual myopia and astigmatism in 87 eyes of 62 patients who were previously operated on with other refractive surgical techniques. Twenty-six of the eyes had previously undergone phacoemulsification with IOL implantation, 20 eyes had undergone penetrating keratoplasty (PK), 22 eyes had undergone RK, 10 eyes had undergone PRK, four eyes had undergone penetrating ocular trauma requiring corneal suturing with and without additional intraocular surgery, and five eyes were following phakic IOL implantation.

Spherical refractive errors between -0.50 and -9.75 D and astigmatic cylindrical errors between -0.75 and -6.00 D were corrected.

As with our normal LASIK cases, calculations were based on manifest refraction, although slight modifications based on the cycloplegic refraction were sometimes taken into account if there was a great difference between the two.

The period between the first surgery and the LASIK enhancement procedure was 11 ± 8.2 (3 to 20) months, although this period varied between different operations. For example, after cataract or phakic IOLs, surgery was normally 3 months after and with PK, it was 16 months. In those cases where sutures were still present, all sutures had been removed at least 8 weeks prior to the LASIK procedure.

A mild tranquilizer (5 mg of diazepam) is given 30 minutes before the operation. Ultrasonic central pachymetry (five measurements immediately after performing the last videokeratography) is then performed. Topical anesthesia (oxybuprocaine and tetracaine HCL) is given, one drop every 5 minutes for 15 minutes prior to the procedure, administering the last drop once the patient is already positioned on the operating table. The procedure is performed under the coaxial microscope of our Keracor 117 (Chiron Technolas) with indirect illumination. The ablation profile has been previously programmed in the laser, and the microkeratome and laser performance have been thoroughly checked. Laser fluence is checked in the routine manner with the Mylar plate to verify that between 63 and 65 pulses remove 99% of the film.

The surgical area is prepared in the same manner as with any other anterior segment surgery, and the Barraquer lid speculum is placed. The microkeratome suction ring (Automated Corneal Shaper, Chiron Vision ALK-E series nr 256) is centered over the pupil. This usually places it centered on the limbus, except in those very special cases with a clearly eccentric pupil. A 160-micron plate is normally used to attempt a 160-micron flap. For a smooth lenticle resection, it is most important to wet the corneal surface with Ringer's lactate, as well as the suction ring track prior to the microkeratome cut. A new, sterile blade is used for each procedure.

After the flap is made, the microkeratome and suc-

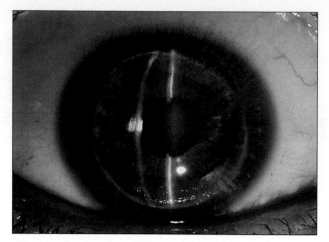

Figure 31-1. LASIK after keratoplasty.

tion ring are removed just as in those eyes in which primary LASIK is performed. Our laser system works with an active eye tracker system. The eye tracker is a system that detects eye movements through an infrared camera following the movements of the eye without interrupting the flow, thus maintaining centration during photoablation. Of course, you can adjust the maximum permitted area of movement where the laser will not stop. Prior to lifting the lenticle, the eye tracker is turned on. In order to be perfectly sure of the patient's fixation point on the cornea and its relationship with the pupil area, we prefer to verify it with the lenticle in its original position because sometimes this requires additional time, and it is preferable not to alter the stromal hydration. Once the eye tracker is centered, the lenticle is reflected using our spatula, and approximately 15 seconds later, the ablation is initiated using the 50 Hz scanning method (Keracor 117 CT). In some cases, we noticed the eye tracker does not work well, specifically at the end of the photoablation; that means the eye tracker is not correctly reading the pupil because of an excess of reflections over the ablated stroma. If this happens, it is recommended to switch off the eye tracker and continue centration in the standard way.

Once the ablation is completed, the interface is washed with balanced salt solution (BSS) and softly rubbing with our soft silicone cannula. When we observe a completely clean interface, the lenticle is repositioned, always over a wet bed. For the next 2 minutes, Merocel sponges are used to dry the resection border. A striae test is performed, the lid speculum is carefully removed, and gentamicin and diclofenac or ketorolac drops are instilled.

After the procedure, the eye is not patched except in unusual situations in which trauma to the eye is a risk (unusually nervous patients). Oral analgesic medication

Table 31-1						
LASIK RESULTS FOLLOWING VARIOUS INTRAOPERATIVE TECHNIQUES						
Primary surgery	**# eyes**	**±1 D SE predictability (%)**	**±1 D Ast predictability (%)**	**UCVA ≥ 20/40 efficacy lines (%)**	**Loss 2+ BSCVA safety (%)**	**±0.5 D SE stability (6 mos) (%)**
Phaco	26	96	91	85	0	98
PK	20	70	53	62	0	61
RK	22	75	61	89	0	85
PRK	10	90	96	55	0	97
Trauma	4	95	92	96	0	100
Phakic IOL	5	88	92	80	0	100
Total	87	77.0	70.11	70.11	0	94.3

SE = spherical equivalent; Ast = astigmatism; UCVA = uncorrected visual acuity; BSCVA = best spectacle-corrected visual acuity; Phaco = phacoemulsification; PK = penetrating keratoplasty; RK = radial keratotomy; PRK = photorefractive keratectomy; IOL = intraocular lens.

or topical diclofenac is used as needed. Broad spectrum topical antibiotics are used during the first week, with artificial tears continued for the first 6 weeks. Patients are instructed to not rub their eyes for 8 weeks.

In those patients who have previously undergone penetrating keratoplasty, we empirically used topical steroids for 8 weeks postoperatively, three times daily for the first 2 weeks, tapering to twice daily for the next 2 weeks and once daily for the remainder. All patients are examined at 1 day, 1 week, 1, 3, 6, and 12 months following surgery. A complete ophthalmologic exam is carried out, except at postoperative day 1, when only uncorrected visual acuity and slit lamp biomicroscopy is performed.

RESULTS

Refraction

Mean refractive spherical equivalent at 6 months was -0.70 D (standard deviation: 0.65). Refractive accuracy at the 6-month period was 95.7% ± 6.10. Seventy-seven percent of the eyes were within ± 1.0 D and 57.4% within 0.5 D of emmetropia. This is similar to our LASIK results on virgin eyes. For more details on refractive results see Table 31-1, in which the results obtained with LASIK following different previous procedures are detailed.

Stability up to 6 months is ± 0.50 D in 94.3% of patients in every group. An important exception was a patient with 2.00 D of induced astigmatism who originally had penetrating keratoplasty. In any case, in those LASIK after PK patients, we expect to have refractive changes throughout a 2-year period.

Visual Acuity

Preoperatively, best spectacle-corrected acuity (BSCVA) was 5/10 or better (20/40 or better) in 78 of 87 eyes (89.65%). Six months postoperatively and including all eyes in the same grouping, 83 of 87 eyes (95.40%) were 5/10 or better. This slight improvement in BSCVA results is fundamentally due to the cylinder reduction in post-PK eyes. Some post-keratoplasty residual astigmatism was extremely high (> 4.00 D), and as this was corrected in the cornea, a better corrected vision was obtained. At 6 months, uncorrected visual acuity (UCVA) was 5/10 or better in 61 of 87 eyes (70.11%)

Astigmatism

No postoperative irregular astigmatism in any case was observed, once again correlating with results that we obtained with LASIK on normal eyes when there were no intraoperative or postoperative flap complications.

Sixty-one of 87 eyes had no residual refractive astigmatism, 16 of 87 eyes had reduced astigmatism, maintaining the original axis, with most of these eyes having undergone previous penetrating keratoplasty. Ten of 87 eyes had less astigmatism than preoperatively, though on a different axis.

INDICATIONS

LASIK is a good option to correct the residual myopia and/or astigmatism after a first procedure, refractive or not. It is well recognized that predictability is good when treating low to moderate myopia, but decreases in high myopia.[21]

LASIK enhancement is recommended in cases of undercorrection or residual astigmatism after intraocular surgery, especially after lens surgery with IOL implantation, penetrating keratoplasty, radial or astigmatic keratotomy, photorefractive keratectomy, corneal suturing after trauma, or phakic IOL implantation. Nevertheless, some considerations must be taken into account depending on the patient or the first procedure already performed.

In patients nearing presbyopia, we always consider the option of monovision. It is extremely important to discuss this point with the patient to avoid unrealistic expectations.

When the first procedure was penetrating keratoplasty, it is important to obtain a large flap, because in most cases, we are dealing with high astigmatism and we will work with large ablation zones. In those cases in which the residual astigmatism is higher than -4.0 D, it is our recommendation to first do an arcuate keratotomy, and once refraction is stable, perform LASIK. We have improved our predictability with this combined technique.[22] Some other points to be considered in performing LASIK after PK are:

1. It might be a better approach to first do the lamellar cut and wait for refractive stabilization, because spherical and cylindrical changes seem to appear after this alone.
2. Before proceeding with LASIK surgery, it is extremely important to explore the donor-recipient interface to avoid a lamellar cut across an extremely thin cornea.
3. Remember that with very young donor tissue we must expect to have larger refractive regression (this might be more common in keratoconus patients).

Another point to be considered, especially in those patients who have suffered from trauma, is irregular astigmatism, because a better solution may be contact lenses.

One concern with anterior chamber phakic IOLs is the possibility of endothelial-IOL touch during the microkeratome cut, even though we have not noticed differences between endothelial cell counts after LASIK in our Artisan Iris Claw phakic IOL patients.[23,24] With posterior chamber phakic IOLs, the fear is luxation of the IOL to the anterior chamber during suction. That is why in high myopic and hyperopic candidates for clear lens extraction with IOL implantation or those with phakic IOL implantation in which bioptics is expected, we recommend performing the lamellar cut at the time of the first surgery. This concept is what we have called adjustable refractive surgery (ARS).[25]

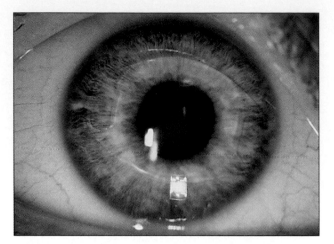

Figure 31-2. LASIK after Artisan phakic IOL implantation.

COMPLICATIONS

LASIK enhancement procedures present similar complications as those observed with LASIK on virgin eyes.

No microkeratome-related complications were observed in this group of patients. This is probably related to the many precautions used in this particular group. In the first case of reoperation for undercorrected LASIK, following undercorrected eight-incision radial keratotomy, an important complication occurred. During the standard enhancement flap dissection with our spatula, the old RK incisions came apart. The operation was completed successfully; however, the patient presented with recurrent corneal erosion symptoms for 3 months following the procedure. This was controlled using topical hyperosmotic agents. From this, we concluded that LASIK reoperations on patients originally treated by incisional surgical procedures should always be carried out with a new cut and not by means of flap lifting, as we ordinarily do. In fact, we recommend the same for a LASIK enhancement after LASIK in a PK patient.

Epithelial ingrowth was not clinically significant in this group of patients, although in some cases the presence of small epithelial islands at the edge of the flap (no larger than 1.0 mm) were seen. The incidence of epithelial ingrowth was higher in those overcorrected RK patients treated with LASIK, although the results are not included in this series. Contrary to our LASIK experience on virgin eyes, night vision was not a particular problem in this patient group (subjective analysis). We did notice a slight daytime visual fluctuation (a new complication from our previous LASIK experience) in those patients who previously underwent RK and, in particular, on those cases in which there was a high residual undercorrection. This was probably related to the aggressiveness of the previous incisional surgery.

The main complication was a slight undercorrection, just as we have seen in our normal LASIK series.

Reoperations for undercorrection were performed on five of 26 previous phacoemulsification cases (19.23%), nine of 20 (45%) previous penetrating keratoplasty cases, four of 22 (18.8%) previous keratotomy cases, and one of 10 (10%) previous PRK cases. No cases of LASIK over previous penetrating ocular trauma or phakic IOLs for high myopia required reoperation. This resulted in a 21.83% incidence of reoperations secondary to undercorrection. There were no reoperations due to interface problems.

SUMMARY

Presently, we are using LASIK to correct myopia with or without astigmatism, from -0.50 to -12.00 D, either as a primary treatment or as an enhancement treatment to correct residual refractive errors following previous ocular surgery.

LASIK combines the advantages of intrastromal or lamellar surgery in avoiding epithelial-stromal interaction with the advantages of laser ablation (ie, high precision and flexibility and the ability to carry out spherical and cylindrical stromal ablation). The main advantages of LASIK, as compared to PRK[26-29] include faster useful visual acuity recovery, elimination of pain in the immediate postoperative period, lack of haze or scarring secondary to epithelial-stromal interaction (probably the main cause of anterior corneal opacity and refractive instability following PRK), the ability to correct a wider range of myopia with or without associated astigmatism, and an extremely lower incidence of rejection episodes after PK.

LASIK advantages as compared to RK[16,30] (within the myopic range in which both procedures are applicable) include refractive stability over a longer time period (noting that we only have a 4-year follow-up period with LASIK), and a greater resistance to ocular trauma with LASIK as compared to RK. In addition, enhancement procedures are simpler following LASIK than following RK. Generally speaking, LASIK is easier to carry out than nonfreeze myopic keratomileusis[8,10-12,14] or standard in situ keratomileusis.[15,31]

More refractive surgeons feel that RK enhancement after primary RK should only be considered if the residual myopia is less than 1.50 D,[32,33] and in most cases, should be avoided completely.[34] In the last few years,

there has been an increased interest in dealing with undercorrected RK by means of PRK, with good results obtained by a large number of researchers,[27,29,35-39] even proposing a two-stage treatment for high myopia.[40]

Some groups, however, have noticed a clear tendency toward hyperopia,[41] while others have noticed a lower predictability and higher incidence of haze[42] than the one seen following PRK on a virgin eye. Phakic IOL and ALK have also been suggested for undercorrected RK.[43,44]

Despite the intra- and postoperative methods for reducing residual cylinder with suture manipulation and/or removal, astigmatism is still the most common complication after penetrating keratoplasty.

Techniques such as wedge resection[45,46] or relaxing incisions in their various forms[47-49] are useful, though with low predictability. Other researchers have used not only incisional surgery but also lamellar surgery[50] to correct myopic spherical residual errors, though predictability was poor and astigmatism could not be addressed. In some cases, PRK provided very good results to correct both spherical as well as cylindrical defects,[35,51-53] however, severe complications have been published, such as significant regression and haze as compared to virgin eyes,[54,55] as well as a higher frequency of graft rejection episodes.[56,57]

Despite improvement in IOL calculation formulas for cataract surgery, it is not infrequent to find residual refractive defects, especially in highly myopic and hyperopic eyes. The use of corneal refractive surgery to correct smaller defects has been used, as well as IOL exchange or the insertion of a piggyback IOL in those cases where the refractive defect was significant. Both RK[58] and PRK can also be useful, taking into account the previously discussed advantages and disadvantages of each procedure.

Until recently, most surgeons treated PRK undercorrection with additional RK, although RK has also been used. Most feel, however, that a repeat PRK with transepithelial laser ablation is preferable. We prefer to use LASIK for undercorrection after lens surgery and PRK.

There is little literature regarding refractive defects after anterior segment ocular trauma. Most descriptions are related to calculation of IOL power and the need for rigid contact lenses and/or potential penetrating keratoplasty. Fundamentally, these techniques try to correct high refractive errors as opposed to small residual defects. In these cases, we have also successfully used LASIK.

A refractive surgical technique now becoming popular and having potential advantages is the use of phakic refractive IOLs. Despite the fact that it is a technique with a high degree of predictability and also has the possibility to exchange powers, small residual refractive spherical defects may result, and the issue of astigmatism has not been completely addressed.

On the other hand, in high myopia with spherical equivalents higher than -12.00 D, it is extremely important to have a minimal 6.0 or 6.5 mm optical zone, both for corneal ablation procedures and for intraocular lenses into a phakic eye, but it is usually impossible to work with so large optical zones when we are dealing with high myopia (to reduce ablation corneal depth or peripheral IOL thickness in these high minus powers, we need to reduce the optical zone in both procedures). That is why we implemented the combination of a 6.0 mm optical zone Artisan Iris Claw IOL and LASIK with 6.0 mm optical ablation zone in the correction of high myopia. Moreover, performing LASIK as the second procedure for correcting the residual ametropia permitted us to finally have a very highly predictable procedure.[23,24] Finally, we implemented the term ARS (adjustable refractive surgery) in all those cases in which we were planning to combine intraocular and corneal refractive surgery. The rationale in doing the lamellar cut during the intraocular surgery was to avoid any possibility of contact between the endothelium and the IOL during suction in LASIK or any other possible complication related to suction in an eye with an IOL.[25]

From our LASIK experience (October 1993 to present), we feel that LASIK is a safe procedure to obtain good corrected and uncorrected visual acuity, lack of endothelial trauma, and is also easy to enhance. Up to 12 D of correction, with or without additional astigmatism, is highly predictable. LASIK is our technique of choice to correct myopic/astigmatic refractive defects, both on virgin eyes and on eyes that have undergone previous surgical procedures.

CONCLUSIONS

It is important to stress in our experience the high safety and predictability in the correction of up to 12 D of spherical myopia and up to 4 D of astigmatism, both in virgin eyes and in eyes that have undergone previous surgical procedures. It is also important to note the very low complication rate we have seen in this range and on the procedure's high stability. It is our treatment of choice to correct most residual refractive errors following penetrating keratoplasty (where it has become extremely important in advancing the rehabilitation of visual function) and after cataract surgery with intraocu-

lar implant, particularly in those highly myopic and hyperopic patients in which biometric techniques still present predictability problems.

LASIK also provides an excellent method to correct the residual refractive defects following phakic IOL implantation, especially in correcting high myopia and hyperopia.

In the phakic IOL patient, LASIK enhancement avoids the risk of repeat intraocular surgery (IOL exchange) and allows correction of residual astigmatism rather than perhaps inducing more astigmatism with another intraocular procedure.

Finally, even though LASIK is an excellent way to correct refractive defects, it is not perfect and continues to evolve. New technical advances in the technique will undoubtedly improve the procedure in the near future. Small laser beam scanning technology is improving ablation quality. There is no doubt that tracking technology is also improving centration with higher quality and safety, and in the near future, solid state lasers may be used for corneal ablation. On the other hand, technological improvements in microkeratomes will also help in obtaining better visual quality results.

From the surgeon's viewpoint, it is a great advantage to be able to use the same procedure to correct different refractive defects in different clinical situations. As with other surgical techniques, the more the technique can be used, the more proficient the surgeon can become.

REFERENCES

1. Barraquer JI. Queratomileusis para la corrección de la miopia. *Arch Soc Amer Oftal Optom.* 1964;5:27-48.
2. Swinger CA, Barraquer JI. Keratophakia and keratomileusis: clinical results. *Ophthalmology.* 1981;88:709-715.
3. Barrraquer J, Viteri E. Results of myopic keratomileusis. *Journal of Refractive Surgery.* 1987;3:98-101.
4. Swinger CA, Barker BA. Prospective evaluation of myopic keratomileusis. *Ophthalmology.* 1984;91:785-792.
5. Barrraquer C, Gutierrez AM, Espinosa A. Myopic keratomileusis short-term results. *J Refract Corneal Surg.* 1989;5:307-313.
6. Baumgartner SD, Binder PS. Refractive keratoplasty histopathology of clinical specimens. *Ophthalmology.* 1985;92:606-1615.
7. Swinger CA, Krumeich J, Cassiday D. Planar lamellar keratoplasty. *Journal of Refractive Surgery.* 1986;2:17-24.
8. Couderc JI,, Lozano Moury F, De Charance B. Resultats compares des keratomileusis myopiques avec et sans congelation. *Ophthalmologie.* 1988;2:293-296.
9. Zavala KY, Krumeich J, Binder PS. Laboratory evaluation of freeze vs. nonfreeze lamellar refractive keratoplasty. *Arch Ophthalmol.* 1987;105:1125-1128.

10. Saragoussi JJ, Hanna K, Jobin D, De la messeliere S, Besson J, Pouliquen V. Resultats du keratomileusis myopique. Etude retrospective a propos de 40 cas. *J Fr Ophthalmol.* 1988;11:311-316.

11. Saragoussi JJ, Abenhaim A, Hanna K. Le keratomileusis myopique. *Bull Belge Ophthalmol.* 1989;233:67-94.

12. Keratomileusis: visual and corneal evolution. *European Journal of Implant and Refractive Surgery.* 1989;1:179-170.

13. Zavala KY, Krumeich J, Binder PS. Clinical pathology of nonfreeze lamellar refractive keratoplasty. *Cornea.* 198;7:223-230.

14. Laroche L, Gauthier L, Thenot JC, et al. Nonfreeze myopic keratomileusis for myopia in 158 eyes. *J Refract Corneal Surg.* 1994;10:400-412.

15. Ruiz LA. *Keratomileusis in situ.* American Academy of Ophthalmology; 1986.

16. Pallikaris IG, Papatzanaki ME, Siganos DS, Tsilimbaris MK. A corneal flap technique for laser in situ keratomileusis human studies. *Arch Ophthalmol.* 1991;109:1699-1702.

17. Pallikaris I, Papatsanaki M, Stathi E, Frenschock O, Georgiadis A. Laser in situ keratomileusis. *Lasers Surg Med.* 1990;10:463-468.

18. Pallikaris IG, Siganos DS. Excimer laser in situ keratomileusis (LASIK) versus photorefractive keratectomy for the correction of high myopia. *J Refract Corneal Surg.* 1994;10:498-510.

19. Pallikaris I. Tecnica de colgajo corneal para la queratomileusis in situ mediada por laser: estudios en humanos. *Arch Ophthalmol (Spanish).* 1992;3:127-130.

20. Gomes M. Keratomileusis in situ using manual dissection of corneal flap for high myopia. *J Refract Corneal Surg.* 1994;10(2suppl):225-257.

21. Güell JL, Muller A. Laser in situ keratomileusis (LASIK) for myopia from -7 to -18 diopters. *Journal of Refractive Surgery.* 1996;22:222-228.

22. Güell JL, Vázquez M. Combined surgery to correct high astigmatism: arquate keratotomy and laser in situ keratomileusis (LASIK). *J Cataract Refract Surg.* In press.

23. Güell JL, Vázquez M. Combined surgery to correct high myopia: Worst Iris Claw phakic intraocular lens (IOL) and laser in situ keratomileusis (LASIK). *Journal of Refractive Surgery.* In press.

24. Vázquez M, Güell JL, Gris O, et al. Combined surgery to correct high myopia: Worst Iris Claw phakic intraocular lens (IOL) and laser in situ keratomileusis (LASIK). *Ophthalmic Research.* 1998;30(S1):138.

25. Güell JL. The adjustable refractive surgery concept (ARS) (Letter). *Journal of Refractive Surgery.* 1998;14:271.

26. Seiler T, Wollensak J. Myopic photorefractive keratectomy with the excimer laser. One-year follow-up. *Ophthalmology.* 1991;98:1156-1163.

27. Machat JJ, Tayfour F. Photorefractive keratectomy for myopia: preliminary results in 147 eyes. *J Refract Corneal Surg.* 1993;9(suppl):16-19.

28. Kim JH, Tae WH, Young CL, Cheon KL, Woo JS. Photorefractive keratectomy in 202 myopic eyes: 1-year results. *J Refract Corneal Surg.* 1993;9(suppl):11-16.

29. Epstein D, Fagerholm P, Hamberg-Nystrom H, Tengrowth. Twenty-four month follow-up of excimer laser photorefractive keratectomy for myopia. *Ophthalmology.* 1994;101:1558-1563.

30. Salz JJ, Salz JN, Salz M, Jones D. Ten year's experience with a conservative approach to radial keratotomy. *J Refract Corneal Surg.* 1991;7:12-22.

31. Arenas-Archilla E, Sanchez-Thorin J, Naranzo-Uribe J, Hernandez-Lozano A. Myopic keratomileusis in situ: a preliminary report. *J Cataract Refract Surg.* 1991;17:424-35.

32. Coulon P, Poirier L, Williamson W, Verin P, Roques JC. Results of reoperation for undercorrection of radial keratotomies: apropos of 25 cases. *J Fr Ophtahlmol.* 1993;16(2):95-102.

33. Montard.M, Piquot X, Bosc JM, Posposil A. Reoperation after radial keratotomy. When is it indicated? *J Fr Ophthalmol.* 1991;14(3):177-80.

34. Poirier L, Coulon P, Williamson W, Barac'h D, Mortemousque B, Verin P. Effect of peripheral deepening of radial keratotomy incisions. *J Refract Corneal Surg.* 1994;10(6):621-4.

35. Nagy ZZ, Suveges I, Nemeth J, Fust A. The role of excimer laser photorefractive keratectomy in treatment of residual myopia followed by radial keratotomy. *Acta Chir Hung.* 1995-96;35(1-2):13-19.

36. Ko ML, Gow JK, Bellavance F, Woo G. Excimer photorefractive keratectomy after undercorrected radial keratotomy. *Journal of Refractive Surgery.* 1995;11(3suppl):S280 83.

37. Durrie DS, Schumer DJ, Cavanaugh TB. Photorefractive keratectomy for residual myopia after previous refractive keratotomy. *J Refract Corneal Surg.* 1994;10(2suppl):S235-8.

38. Gallinaro C, Cochener B, Mimouni F, Colin J. Treatment by refractive photokeratectomy of undercorrections after radial keratotomy. *J Fr Ophthalmol.* 1994;17(12):746-9.

39. Seiler T, Jean B. Photorefractive keratectomy as a second attempt to correct myopia after radial keratotomy. *J Refract Corneal Surg.* 1992;8(3):211-4.

40. Lee YC, Park CK, Sah WJ, Hahn TW, Kim MS, Kim JH. Photorefractive keratectomy for undercorrected myopia after radial keratotomy: 2 years follow-up. *Journal of Refractive Surgery.* 1995:11(3suppl):S274-79.

41. Meza J, Perez-Santonja JJ, Moreno E, Zato MA. Photorefractive keratectomy after radial keratotomy. *J Cataract Refract Surg.* 1994;20(5):485-9.

42. Ribeiro JC, McDonald MB, Lemos MN, Salz JJ, Dello-Russo JV, Aquavella JV, et al. Excimer laser photorefractive keratectomy after radial keratotomy. *Journal of Refractive Surgery.* 1995;11(3):165-9.

43. Lyle WA, Jin GJ. Initial results of automated lamellar keratoplasty for correction of myopia: 1-year follow up. *J Cataract Refract Surg.* 1996;22(1):31-43.

44. Buratto L, Ferrari M, Genisi C. Myopic keratomileusis with the excimer laser: 1-year follow-up. *J Refract Corneal Surg.* 1993;9:12-19.

45. Frucht-Pery J. Wedge resection for postkeratoplasty astigmatism. *Ophthalmic Surg.* 1993;24(8):516-8.

46. Lugo M, Donnenfeld EO, Arentsen JJ. Corneal wedge resection for high astigmatism following penetrating keratoplasty. *Ophthalmic Surg.* 1987;18:650-653.

47. Seitz B, Naumann GO. Limbus parallel keratotomies and compression sutures in excessive astigmatism after penetrating keratoplasty. *Ger J Ophthalmol.* 1993;2(1):42-50.

48. Kirkness CM, Ficker LA, Steele AD, Rice NS. Refractive surgery for graft-induced astigmatism after penetrating keratoplasty for keratoconus. *Ophthalmology.* 1991;98:1786-92.

49. Jacobi PC, Hartmann C, Severin M, Bartz SK. Relaxing incisions with compression sutures for control of astigmatism after penetrating keratoplasty. *Graefes Arch Clin Exp Ophthalmol.* 1994;232:527-32.

50. Roholt PC. Automated lamellar keratoplasty after penetrating keratoplasty. Symposium of cataract IOL and refractive surgery. *American Society of Cataract and Refractive Surgeons.* San Diego, Calif; April 1995.

51. Hordan LT, Binder PS, Kansar BS, Hetzmann J. Photorefractive keratectomy to treat myopic and astigmatism after radial keratotomy and penetrating keratoplasty. *J Cataract Refract Surg.* 1995;21:268-273.

52. Dunker GW, Shhröder E. Excimer laser correction of high astigmatism after keratoplasty. *J Cataract Refract Surg.* 1996;22:313-317.

53. Lampos M, Hertzog L, Gardus J, et al. Photorefractive keratectomy for severe post-keratoplasty astigmatism. *Am J Ophthalmol.* 1992;114:429-436.

54. John ME, Martines E, Cvintal T, Mellor-Filho A, Soter F, Barbosa de Sousa MC,et al. Photorefractive keratectomy following penetrating keratoplasty. *J Refract Corneal Surg.* 1994;10(2suppl):S206-S10.

55. Tuunanen TH, Ruusuvaara PJ, Uusitalo RJ, Tervo TM. Photoastigmatism keratectomy for correction of astigmatism in corneal grafts. *Cornea.* 1997;16(1):48-53.

56. Hersh PS, Jordan AJ, Mayers M. Corneal graft rejection episode after excimer laser phototherapeutic keratectomy. *Arch Ophthalmol.* 1993;111:735-736.

57. Epstein RJ, Robin J. Corneal graft rejection episode after excimer laser phototerapeutic keratectomy. *Arch Ophthalmol.* 1994;112:157.

58. Au YK, Lucius RW, Granger B. Radial keratotomy in an elderly patient after ECCE/IOL. *J Cataract Refract Surg.* 1993;19(3):415-6.

SUGGESTED READING

Buratto L, Ferrari M. Excimer laser intrastromal keratomileusis case reports. *J Cataract Refract Surg.* 1992;18(1):3741.

Choyce DP. Residual myopia after radial keratotomy successfully treated with Baikoff ZB5M IOLs (letter). *J Refract Corneal Surg.* 1993;9(6):475.

TREATMENT OF EPITHELIAL INGROWTH

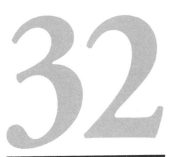

Heriberto Marotta, MD

Epithelial ingrowth is a laser-assisted in situ keratomileusis (LASIK) postoperative complication that occurs when certain factors associated with the creation and handling of the corneal flap take place during surgery. For this reason, we must pay special attention to technical details in order to avoid it.

When this complication is detected, it is necessary to accurately diagnose it early on. Its evolution must be followed and adequate treatment must be provided so that normal corneal transparency can be restored, avoiding changes from irreversible consequences such as corneal melting.

Epithelial ingrowth develops in the interface, slowly in the beginning and for one to several weeks following LASIK. We have precociously observed areas of less corneal transparency, which turn into a whitish or milky acumulus in the interface. They may present as various shapes, such as an extended peninsula or small epithelial cysts or nests, or as epithelial pearls. This is one of the most frequent complications after LASIK. An early diagnosis allows us to follow its evolution and treat it in case it should progress centrally, produce alterations of the corneal flap, or alter the patient's visual acuity. When epithelial ingrowth remains stable and shows no signs of progression, it should be checked periodically. It has rarely been known to regress spontaneously.

The most common clinical sign of epithelial ingrowth is the loss of local transparency, but symptoms can also include interface lucency, an area of brightness or luminosity, and an epithelial cyst or pearl.

The incidence of epithelial ingrowth is directly related to the surgeon's experience with the LASIK procedure. Between 2% and 10% of surgeons new to the technique have reported this complication, whereas the percentage drops dramatically to between 1% and 2% in more experienced surgeons.

The incidence of epithelial ingrowth also increases after enhancements. When we dissect or lift the edge of the flap, we generate epithelial defects or irregularities called "tags" on the margins of the flap, which allow epithelial migration toward the stromal interface. Also, it is more frequent in hyperopic LASIK patients as, employing ablation zones of larger diameter, we may ablate the edge of the cut bed. To prevent this, protect the edges with a sponge and spatula. Patients of advanced age with a history of recurrent corneal erosion, and those who during the immediate postoperative period have edema or inflammation of the edges of the flap and excessively decentered ones, present a greater risk of experiencing this complication.

In cases of LASIK after previous radial keratotomy, an ingrowth of epithelial plugs may occur, and in case the incision of the flap edge is reopened, the epithelial defect created there may lead to the beginning of epithelial invasion. Most cases of epithelial ingrowth are asymptomatic, but some patients complain of a foreign-body sensation due to epithelial irregularity of the flap edge, a drop in the best-corrected visual acuity (BCVA), a decrease in contrast sensitivity, pain, photophobia, and irregular astigmatism.

Should there be a foreign body sensation during the immediate postoperative period, we should instill a drop of fluorescein and observe the flap edge, to see if it spreads into the interface. This indicates that there is a connection to the outside due to poor adherence of the flap to the stromal bed, and through this, epithelial migration may develop. The principal causes are:

- Poor adherence of the flap
- Epithelial ablation of the flap/bed margin
- Dislocated or decentered flap
- Buttonholes in the flap
- Striae and folds of the flap
- Epithelial alterations of the flap edge, such as epithelial tags in enhancements

The pathology is observed better at the slit lamp with direct tangential focal illumination and appears as white

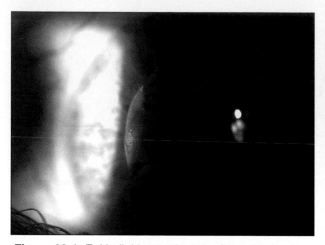

Figure 32-1. Epithelial ingrowth at the flap edge.

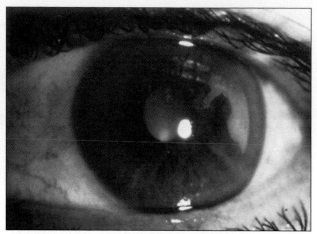

Figure 32-2. Epithelial nests or epithelial cysts.

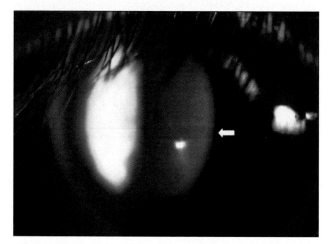

Figure 32-3. Epithelial cyst related to a fold or incomplete flap.

to greyish white color, with fluorescein retention areas at the flap edge. Surface irregularities may be seen corneal topography as irregular astigmatism. In order to determine whether it affects the visual axis or reaches the pupillary area and to establish its limits and relation to striae and folds, retroillumination with pupillary dilatation is useful.

The most common form of epithelial ingrowth is the 2.0 mm thin, white line at the edge of the flap, which generally is of very slow progression (Figure 32-1). Other more aggressive forms progress and require treatment. Most of the time, they appear in the shape of epithelial nests or cysts (Figure 32-2), or related to folds or incomplete flaps (Figure 32-3). If they do not progress, they still may cause melting in the epithelial ingrowth area.

The most aggressive forms can progress, affecting the pupillary area in a 2-week period. These require early treatment, as they run the risk of corneal melting due to the persistence of epithelium in the interface.

Melting is related to the liberation of collagenase or other substances from the hypoxic epithelial cells retained in the interface under the corneal flap. Should the epithelial ingrowth cause haze and opacity extending to the pupillary area and affecting the visual axis, glare is produced, as well as ghosting and halos.

Peripheral flap melting causes distortion on the corneal surface, with localized break-up of the lacrimal film, increasing dry-eye problems after LASIK.

In some cases, there may be pain due to irritation of the corneal nerves in the interface, apart from corneal irregularity, which can produce epithelial erosions of the flap edge with irritation and pain.

Epithelial ingrowth is not caused by the implantation of epithelial cells during surgery as was previously believed, but is due to an epithelial defect created during the procedure. In theory, epithelial ingrowth is produced by the following mechanisms:

- Cells of the epithelial surface grow in the interface from the flap edge
- The microkeratome blade introduces the epithelial cells during keratectomy
- Irrigation of the stromal bed after ablation carries the epithelial cells to the interface

There is a theory that microkeratome cuts, with an incidence of 26°, have less probability of creating epithelial ingrowth than those with an incidence of 0°. Another factor to consider would be excessive use of topical anaesthesia, which could weaken the epithelium and retard healing.

Incidence of epithelial ingrowth may be increased by a malfunction of the microkeratome, creating flaps of irregular thickness. These may be vertical alterations, as in gear problems, due to intermittent advancement, or horizontally, due to blade alterations or irregularities in the cut, and thinner caps. In other cases, thicker, vertical alterations are due to poor suction, a badly aligned free cap, or free caps with excessive manipulation, which result in local edema and epithelial alterations of the edge. There is no doubt that complicated flap cases with perforations or incomplete flaps have a greater incidence of epithelial ingrowth.

Many agree that epithelial ingrowth is a complication related to the patient's epithelial adherence. Patients who develop strong, bond-like complexes of basal membrane, which firmly adhere to the overlying epithelium do not develop epithelial cysts.

It is also accepted that epithelial ingrowth is more frequent in thinner flaps. These are more difficult to handle and increase the probability of creating alterations of the flap edge, such as folds, striae, and dislocations, especially for beginning surgeons.

When the epithelial ingrowth is larger it may be progressive and create melting of the flap edge, which looks as though it lost its integrity and becomes thinner, giving the area an eroded appearance.

Stromal melting is a progressive keratolysis, which can turn into irregular astigmatism and loss of best-corrected visual acuity with photophobia and ciliary injection. Its pathogenesis is not completely clear, but it is believed that the interaction between the epithelium and the stroma produces proteases, which are responsible. In approximately 5% of cases, it has developed with epithelial ingrowth area 6 months after its detection.

Different theories exist regarding corneal melting. These include the nutritional theory, the inflammatory theory, and the mixed theory.

The nutritional theory: explains the necrotic phenomena because it affects the passage of glucose from the aqueous humor to more superficial epithelial layers, acting as a barrier, blocking the passage of nutritional sources.

The inflammatory theory: an inflammatory reaction produces cytokines, such as the interleukin -1a; interleukin 6, and tumor necrosis factor (TNF-a). These cytokines could alter the production of plasminogen, collagenase, and proteases, and cause flap lysis.

The mixed theory: nutritional and metabolic mechanisms act together.

Epithelial ingrowth cysts may be classified according to development, location, effect on the visual axis, whether they are asymptomatic or symptomatic, single or multiple, diffuse or localized, and according to their behavior. Cysts more than 2.0 mm from the edge should be treated.

Machat classifies epithelial ingrowth in terms of severity by Grades 1, 2, and 3.

Grade 1: does not require treatment, does not reach 2.0 mm from the edge, is transparent, delimited, nonprogressive, not associated with changes in the flap, and difficult to observe at the slit lamp.

Grade 2: slightly thicker, nest shaped, less than 2.0 mm from the edge, easily visible at the slit lamp, not neatly delimited, greyish white in color, slowly progressive, and should be treated within 2 or 3 weeks.

Grade 3: pronounced in growth, very thick, more than 2.0 mm from the flap edge, easily visible, opaque areas, grey in color, not well delimited, with necrotic areas or loss of transparency, progressive, with melting areas of necrotic epithelium, and must be treated immediately.

Classifications are isolated or associated with other pathologies, such as folds, striae, particles, under- or overcorrections, incomplete or irregular flaps, and holes.

The most important concern for those performing LASIK is to prevent complications. Here, prevention is achieved by means of a neat, refined technique, taking particular care not to produce epithelial damage at the flap edge during the keratectomy, or during edge drying. The flap must also be handled with extreme care, especially where it is everted on the conjunctiva or on a drop of viscoelastic. This helps to prevent the formation of folds. In this manner, we create perfect repositioning and a firm adherence between the flap edge and the stromal bed.

As another means of prevention, we recommend the use of the wet-wet technique, and proper irrigation of the interface to ensure no cellular particles or detritus remain in it. We recommend drying the edge of the flap with a Merocel sponge which leaves no particles. The superior hinge also provides another means of prevention. The flap must be protected during the photoablation, especially in hyperopia cases.

To obtain excellent results, we must recognize epithelial ingrowth, follow its evolution carefully, and treat it when necessary. Epithelial cysts must be treated when they are progressive or when we detect irregular astigmatism within the first 3 months. This helps avoid stromal melting which, if it advances toward the visual axis, may produce permanent halos, ghosting, and glare.

There is a consensus among different authors who attest to the urgency of treating epithelial ingrowth within 2 to 4 weeks to avoid sequelae. Most also agree it is important to treat cases in which the growth extends beyond 2.0 mm from the edge of the flap. Those that advance and grow are associated with flap melting or altered visual acuity.

Precise differential diagnosis is required for:
- A foreign body in the interface, such as mucus on

the ocular surface, dragged there by excessive washing, or talc due to the use of gloves

- Stromal inflammatory reaction
- Infection

Results are generally satisfactory when epithelial ingrowth is removed early, thus preserving the integrity of the flap. After melting occurs, treatment is difficult, as in this state the stromal scar is irreversible. There are also technical difficulties because the flap is firmly adhered to the stroma in that area. Lifting it is very difficult and the risk of damaging the flap increases.

Once epithelial ingrowth is diagnosed and while we monitor the case, we recommend topical therapy with steroids to decrease the inflammatory reaction, which may develop into melting. An infection, on occasions, begins with very similar signs and symptoms. Therefore, topical antibiotics should be administered. We can discontinue this medication when we are sure it is only an inflammatory process.

We must remember that flap melting destroys the epithelial surface. This is associated with alterations of the lacrimal film increasing dry-eye problems that usually appear after LASIK. Lubricants or artificial tears should be routinely used.

Once we decide to treat the complication, we must select proper treatment. Accepted proposed treatments include:

1. Total or partial lifting of the flap
2. Flap lifting associated with PTK
3. Flap lifting associated with the application of alcohol
4. Incision and expression of the cyst
5. Removal by laser photodisruption with Nd: YAG laser
6. Casebeer technique

Removal with a YAG laser has been proposed by Guillermo Avalos and by other authors using picosecond intrastromal laser (ISL). The YAG laser has been successfully employed in the treatment of islands of peripheral epithelial nests using 1.2 to 2.0 mJ of power, focusing slightly behind the cyst or epithelial nest. Once applied, we observe bubbles forming in the inside, which disappear together with the cyst in a few hours. Generally, 30 to 40 shots are enough. If the residue persists, it can be removed approximately 2 weeks later. Treatment with the YAG laser must be done very carefully as it may leave permanent scars. These cysts in the theoretical model could be treated perfectly with the picosecond laser.

Incision and expression is a simple procedure for peripheral islands. The epithelial nest is incised directly through the flap with a gauged, calibrated diamond knife

for radial keratectomy, at no more than 250 microns, then the cyst's epithelial cells are expressed. It is easy to perform but presents two problems: a. it leaves scars, and b. it requires a very high percentage of enhancements. For these reasons, we do not recommend this technique.

Casebeer technique: Casebeer has designed a needle in order to avoid lifting the flap completely. It is a 27-gauge bent needle that is inserted through the flap edge. This technique employs two 90° bent needles in such a way that the liquid draining hole is forward in one and backward in the other. The bevel edges of the needles are smooth so as not to produce any damage in the faces of the flap and bed. When we enter the interface in search of the epithelial nest, we do so with the front irrigation cannula, which dissects the tract until reaching the virtual space where the cyst is. Here we wash it. Then we change to back irrigation to drag cellular debris from the area and remove it from the interface. If cleaning has been insufficient, the operation should not be repeated in the same tunnel; it is better at 45° to 90° from the original entrance. On some occasions, we can use smooth forceps to remove epithelial remnants.

Flap lifting: when performing this technique, we must take various factors into account. First, we must diagram the location of the epithelial ingrowth, taken from its observation at the slit lamp with tangential illumination. This is particularly important because the surgical microscope lacks this kind of light, rendering it very difficult to determine the exact position of the cyst or epithelial ingrowth.

Second, we must remember we could generate a refractive change. In most cases, we are treating a slight irregular astigmatism and it would be better, as Probst advises, not to combine this cleaning of cysts with enhancements of residual ametropia.

Third, we should only treat clinically significant cysts, as treatment in itself is a potential producer of epithelial ingrowth. Basically, the treatment consists of lifting the flap and removing the epithelium with a combination of scraping and irrigation. This technique should be carefully performed by an expert, as it creates the following potential complications:

1. Damage to the corneal flap.
2. Dislocation of the flap and/or folds when replaced.
3. Incomplete removal or recurrence of the cyst.

On some occasions, there may remain irregular, over-elevated areas in addition to the resulting astigmatism. Some authors recommend prior identification of the flap edge at the slit lamp under topical anaesthesia. If we depress the cornea under high magnification, we can clearly see the edge of the flap and can create continuity

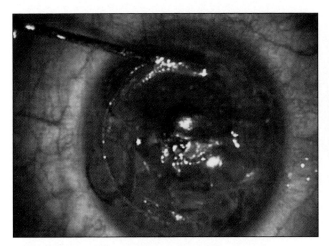

Figure 32-4. Lifting the flap edge with a spatula.

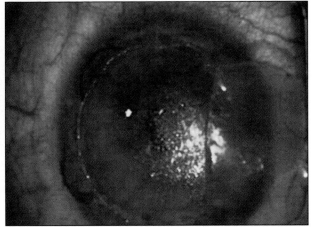

Figure 32-5. The flap is pulled back nasally with non-toothed forceps.

with a cyclodialysis spatula or a Sinskey hook, in order to make it more visible under the surgical microscope.

The cornea should be premarked as usual, so the flap may be replaced in its original position. We penetrate under the flap with a Fukasaku, Machat, or Paton spatula, or any other specially designed for enhancements. Once we have penetrated the interface with the spatula, we advise against advancing any further than 1.5 mm. trying to separate the flap edge with delicate manipulation. This will help avoid epithelial damage or epithelial tags, which can produce postoperative problems such as pain due to erosions, discomfort, or epithelial ingrowth recurrences (Figure 32-4).

Once the debridement is done and the epithelial edge is separated, we carefully grasp it with a Kelman-type smooth forceps temporally and lift it nasally with a slow but steady movement, taking care to use enough strength with the forceps to hold the flap firmly without damaging it (Figure 32-5).

Treatment continues with the removal of the epithelium from the interface with a simple maneuver. If we detect membranes, we perform a peeling of these membranes with thin, smooth forceps. Working in this way, we remove remnants with only slight stromal trauma.

Next, we use a 64 Beaver blade to scrape the stromal faces of the flap and stromal bed. This maneuver has to be done with extreme care, placing the cutting edge of the blade at a 45° angle, advancing opposite to this angle's vertex (Figures 32-6a through 32-6c) with the object of minimizing the possibility of damage to either the flap or the bed. This can be achieved by always moving from center to periphery so as not to implant cells in the central area, and checking and cleaning the blade after every pass. The stromal face of the flap is more difficult to clean. We ask the patient to fixate temporally to expose its surface more directly. It is here that the previ-

ous drawing assumes special importance, as it is very difficult to center the effected area again through the microscope.

Another way of cleaning the interface is a Merocel sponge, which must be discarded after each pass so as not to drag peripheral cells toward the center. We prefer these sponges because they do not shed particles. We then wash the surface with a microfiltered balanced saline solution. We use a 27-gauge tip-angled silicone cannula, replace the flap as we do in LASIK, and finally irrigate the interface abundantly in order to eliminate any epithelial remnants or debris that might have accidentally been left (Figure 32-7).

Flap alignment must be carefully performed, lining up previous marks. We then carefully dry the flap edge using a Merocel sponge. Afterward, we perform a striae test to check adherence. Lastly, the speculum is carefully removed and we check the flap again with a blink test.

We prefer to occlude these cases for at least 6 to 8 hours. Some authors propose partially lifting the flap. We do not agree with this technique, as it can favor the appearance of folds or striae postoperatively. Complete flap lifting gives a much more regular surface.

We treat these patients with tobramycin and dexamethasone ointment every 3 to 5 hours, applying ocular lubricants as well. Follow-up is daily until the epithelium heals completely. Visual rehabilitation occurs within 3 to 5 days, and the best results are obtained in cases in which the epithelium is not damaged.

Probst found a 10% recurrence between week 1 and week 4 after the operation. Personally, I have never had recurrences using this technique, and I recommend it as a treatment of choice for cysts accompanied by folds or striae, and in cases of long duration. For this reason, it is important to treat acutely and recurrences are rare.

Flap lifting associated with PTK: indicated in recur-

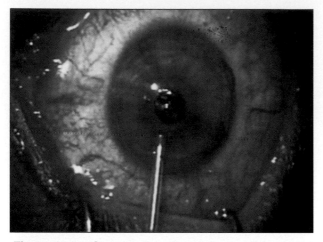

Figure 32-6a. Scraping the stromal face of the stromal bed with a sharp blade.

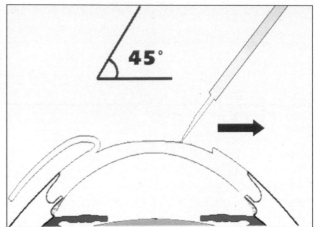

Figure 32-6b. Scraping the stromal face of the flap with a sharp blade.

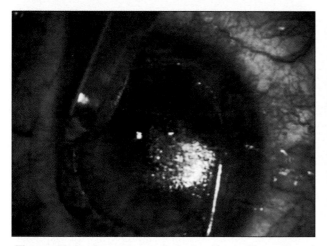

Figure 32-6c. Proper way of placing the cutting edge of the blade to scrape the stroma.

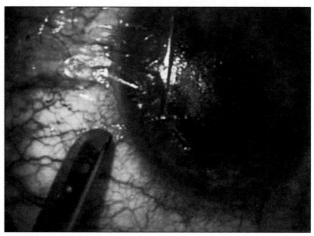

Figure 32-7. The stromal bed is irrigated to remove epithelial remnants or debris.

rences or primarily in severe cases. Once scraping and washing are complete, a PTK is planned with a 6.5 mm optical zone. The surface is carefully dried and the shots are applied on the stromal face of the flap and on the bed, knowing that residual epithelial nests will be ablated and will produce necrosis of isolated epithelial cells upon the stromal faces. Two shots should be enough to destroy these remnants.

In order to ablate the flap stromal face and to make the beams take a perpendicular incidence, lift the flap with a spatula. Once it is perpendicular to the laser beam, the shots are fired. We can use a spatula specially designed for this, such as the Wilson LASIK spoon, with a diameter approximately the same as that of the flap.

During the postoperative period, the cornea appears clear. Irregular astigmatism is not induced with this technique. Other authors, such as Alfredo Castillo and collaborators, recommend this technique in cases of

enhancement to eliminate the interface epithelial cells, with an application of 10 laser pulses upon the stromal bed of the flap.

After lifting the flap and removing the epithelium, others, such as Roger Onnis, recommend topical applications of alcohol on the stroma, with a sponge to loosen the epithelium in this area. This is based on the principle that alcohol destroys epithelial cells. After this, the procedure continues as described.

In cases in which epithelial ingrowth develops into severe corneal melting, there are techniques for its treatment. If the melt turns into a significant distortion of the corneal surface associated with visual alteration of the lacrimal film with dry-eye syndrome, and it extends toward the visual axis producing glare, ghosting, and halos with visual distortion and a decrease of the BCVA, this is probably caused by a lacrimal alteration that produces poor oxygenation of the epithelial surface. It is more frequent in those patients with a history of dry-eye filamentous keratoconjunctivitis or lagophtalmos. These cases are to be treated aggressively to prevent them from growing into ulcers or infections of the flap.

According to Pérez Santoja and coworkers' statistics, peripheral flap melting that does not affect visual acuity, is found in 10.9% of treated eyes with a 12-month follow-up.

First, the flap has to be lifted, then cleaned and replaced. In most of these cases it is difficult because they are thin, irregular flaps. If tissue necrosis advances, the necrotic tissue must be removed, as it might grow deeper or become infected. In this case we must try to lift the flap and cut the hinge to create a free flap. This free flap is carved and rotated, so as to allow the transparent part of the same to remain over the visual axis, leaving part of the stroma uncovered, re-epithealizing in a second phase. In most of these cases sutures are unnecessary. A lamellar corneal graft would be the technique of choice in these cases to restore corneal transparency in the visual axis.

Epithelial ingrowth is a relatively frequent complication. Although techniques to treat it are constantly being developed, prevention is fundamental to avoid its appearance. The success of treatments is based upon the implementation of a refined technique.

BIBLIOGRAPHY

Bas AM, Onnis R. Excimer laser in situ keratomileusis for myopia. *Journal of Refractive Surgery.* 1995;11(3suppl): S229-233.

Buratto L, Brint S. *LASIK: Principles and Techniques.* Thorofare, NJ: SLACK Incorporated; 1998; 124-127.

Castillo A, Diaz VD, Gutierrez A, Tolendo N, Romero F. Peripheral melt of flap after LASIK. *Journal of Refractive Surgery.* 1998;14:61-63.

Davidorf J, Zaldivar R, Oscherow S. Results and complications of laser in situ keratomileusis by experienced surgeons. *Journal of Refractive Surgery.* 1998;14:114-122.

Farah S, Azard D, Gurdal C, Wong J. Laser in situ keratomileusis: literature review of a developing technique. *Journal of Refractive Surgery.* 1998;24:989-1006.

Gimbel H, Anderson Penno E. *LASIK Complications: Prevention and Management.* Thorofare, NJ: SLACK Incorporated; 1999.

Helena MC, Meisler D, Wilson SE. Epithelial growth within the lamellar interface after laser in situ keratomileusis (LASIK). *Cornea.* 1997;16:300-305.

Machat JJ. LASIk Complications and Their Management. In: Machat JJ, ed. *Excimer Laser Refractive Surgery.* Thorofare, NJ: SLACK, Incorporated; 1996.

Machat JJ, Slade SG, Probst L. *The Art of LASIK, Second Edition.* Thorofare, NJ: SLACK Incorporated; 1996; 427-440.

Pallikaris IG, Siganos DS. Excimer laser in situ keratomileusis and photorefractive keratectomy for correction of high myopia. *J Refract Corneal Surg.* 1994;10:498-510.

Perez Santoja JJ, Ayala M, Sakla H, Ruiz Moreno J, Alió JL. Retreatment after LASIK. American Academy of Ophthalmology. *Ophthalmology.* 1999;106.21-28.

Slaha T, Waring GO III, El-Maghraby A, Moadel K, Grimm S. Excimer laser in situ keratomileusis under a corneal flap for myopia of 2 to 20 diopters. *Am J Ophthalmol.* 1996;121:143-155.

Epithelial Ingrowth After LASIK

Charles McGhee, MB, FRCOphth, PhD and Arun Brahma, MB, FRCOphth

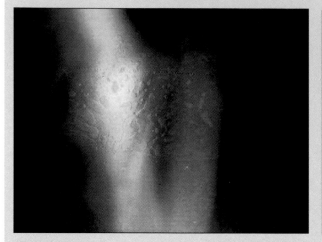

Figure 32A-1. Epithelial ingrowth with microcysts.

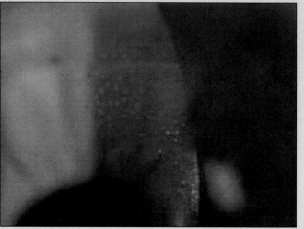

Figure 32A-2. Epithelial ingrowth (1.3 mm).

Epithelial ingrowth is much more common than many beginning LASIK surgeons imagine. It is also much less serious, in the majority of cases, than these surgeons fear. Introduction of individual cells, or small isolated groups of cells, during the LASIK procedure will not normally produce an epithelial ingrowth. For an ingrowth to develop and continue, there must be a continuous connection between the limbal stem cells and the epithelial cells introduced into the interface. Epithelial cells are more commonly introduced when an epithelial abrasion has occurred, when epithelium is disturbed at the flap edge during irrigation or manipulation, when a very thin flap is created and, most importantly, following flap elevation in retreatment cases. The authors have generally noted the most rapidly advancing ingrowths when epithelial defects or widespread prolonged (24 hours) epithelial toxicity is encountered. Meticulous attention to loose epithelium at the time of LASIK minimizes epithelial ingrowth.

Recorded estimates for epithelial ingrowth vary considerably; however, minor epithelial ingrowth (ie, less than 0.75 mm from the flap edge and less than one clock hour of flap periphery) is fairly common on close scrutiny. These minor, nonvision- threatening ingrowths are commonly seen near the flap hinge, do not progress after 6 weeks, and tend to fade, leaving a trace peripheral haze. These may occur in up to 10% to 12% of primary LASIK cases.

A more aggressive epithelial ingrowth, usually associated with epithelial loss or epithelial tags at the time of surgery, may appear within 3 to 5 days and is associated with interface microcysts. These ingrowths usually

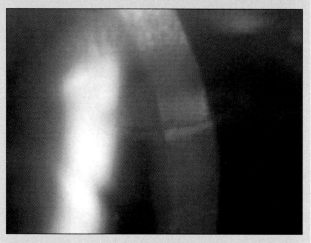

Figure 32A-3. Same eye as in Figure 32A-2 at 6 weeks post-LASIK enhancement with focal, self-limiting flap melt in the region overlying peripheral epithelial ingrowth.

involve at least 2 to 3 clock hours of the peripheral flap and may advance rapidly in the first 6 weeks postoperatively (Figure 32A-1). Fortunately, the majority of these cases are self-limiting at 6 to 8 weeks and should merely be monitored by measuring and documenting the width of the epithelial base and distance of the apex of the ingrowth in relation to the flap edge.

Some epithelial ingrowths (Figure 32A-2), although self-limiting in regard to interface progression, may be associated with minor flap melts 6 weeks to 6 months post-LASIK. These cases must be monitored closely, although intervention is usually not required (Figure 32A-3).

Since flap elevation and removal of the epithelium from the stroma and rear of the flap has variable success, surgical management of epithelial ingrowth should only be undertaken if there is risk to vision. Therefore, in prospective studies, the authors have generally observed these larger epithelial ingrowths by monthly review with the following criteria for intervention:

- Induced topographic astigmatism.
- Epithelium in or very near the pupillary zone.
- Progressive flap melt.
- Compromised visual acuity or visual symptoms that can be related to progression of the ingrowth.

Currently, with this conservative approach, less than 1% of LASIK cases have required treatment for epithelial ingrowth and no eyes with persisting ingrowth have exhibited loss of two lines of BSCVA.

TREATMENT OF FLAP FOLDS AND STRIAE FOLLOWING LASIK

Angela M. Gutierrez, MD

INTRODUCTION

One of the complications of LASIK surgery is the formation of flap folds or striae. These occur more frequently during the surgeon's learning curve and account for approximately 1% of all complications.[1] Clinically, they appear during the postoperative period as loss of best-corrected visual acuity and irregular astigmatism. In some instances, they may alter the corneal surface so severely that conventional treatments are ineffective, requiring lamellar keratoplasty in order to restore the refractive properties of the cornea (Figures 33-1 and 33-2).

There are three linear-shaped alterations of the flap after LASIK: folds, striae, and wrinkles. Folds are continuous usually straight, grayish, and sometimes elevated, lines that can have any orientation depending on hinge location (Figure 33-3). Striae are multiple small, continuous, slightly sinuous lines with a grayish edge and an unelevated darker core (Figure 33-4). Multiple, very small and discontinuous meshlike lines are described as wrinkles (Figure 33-5).

PATHOPHYSIOLOGY

Flap folds were first observed with the technique of in situ keratomileusis,[2] for three reasons:

1. The thickness of the flap in the in-situ technique (130 to 160 microns) was much thinner than that created for the freeze keratomileusis procedure (average 280 microns).[3,4]
2. Running antitorque sutures, which would distribute tension evenly, were substituted for three or four radial stitches changing the total disc cut for an incomplete nasally hinged flap[5] to the peripheral cornea allowed rotational displacement.
3. Folds are usually observed in cases of dislocation. Predisposing factors include exophthalmos, lagophthalmos, excess irrigation and/or excessive stromal hydration and poor flap adherence.[1,6] Patients typically complain of severe photophobia, pain, red eyes, profuse tearing, and poor vision. The displacement of a 1.0 to 2.0 mm shift usually occurs within the first 12 to 24 hours, rarely being complete; one side looks with the shadow while the opposite side looks superimposed on the resection border (Figures 33-6 and 33-7).

From a mechanical standpoint, folds are the result of uneven forces acting on the disc, inducing malposition. We had an opportunity to do the histological study of a flap with folds and found undulations in Bowman's membrane, which created V-shaped troughs in the stroma with a deep obtuse vertex; these troughs were filled by an increased number of squamous corneal epithelial cells. It is important to note that the stromal thickness was reduced by one-half under the vertices of the troughs; this thinning was compensated by the epithelium, keeping the disc thickness uniform[7] (Figure 33-8). No loss of the collagen lamellae was found, but they were compressed under the V-shaped undulations (Figures 33-9 and 33-10). Flap striae are produced by the change in the usual lid-to-corneal curvature relationship, caused by the change in the corneal base curve in high corrections.

Etiology

Folds and wrinkles form during surgery or the early postoperative period when the flap is poorly positioned on the corneal bed or it is displaced by external pressure (rubbing, eye squeezing). The most common cause of wrinkles is excessive dryness.

Striae are more commonly seen with a thin disc covering a larger ablation[8] (see Figures 33-3 through 33-5). Listed below are multiple factors that may contribute to this complication.

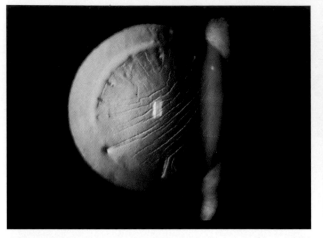

Figure 33-1. Postoperative flap folds in a myopic LASIK patient; a lamellar graft had to be performed.

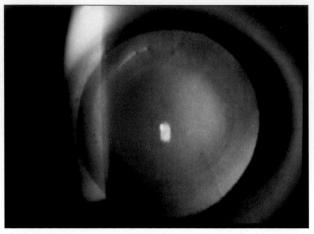

Figure 33-2. Result of the lamellar graft 4 years postoperatively. Note the smooth surface.

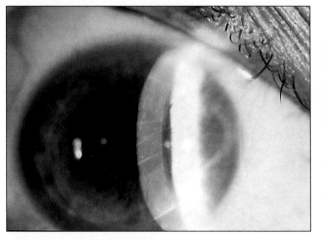

Figure 33-3. Horizontal oblique folds in a nasal hinge flap.

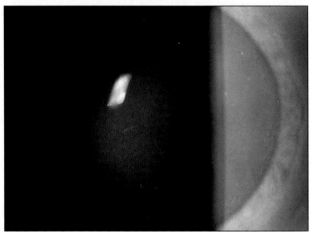

Figure 33-4. Striae in a large ablation for a 14 D myopic patient.

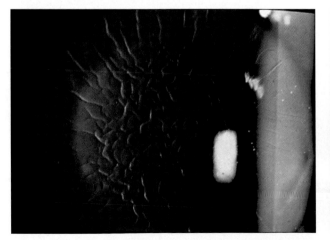

Figure 33-5. Wrinkled flap.

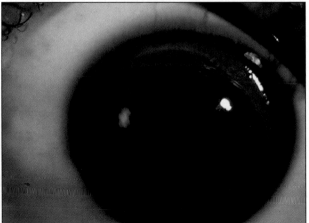

Figure 33-6. Displacement of a nasal hinge flap.

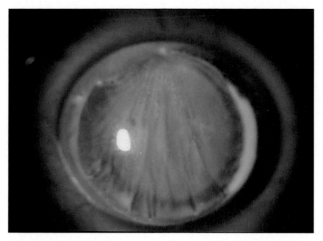

Figure 33-7. Displacement of a superior hinge flap with vertical folds.

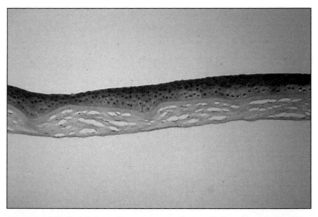

Figure 33-8. Light microscopy plate of the corneal wrinkles in Figure 33-1. Hematoxylin and Eosin x 40 preparation. Corneal flap with folds in Bowman's membrane complicated by an increased number of epithelial layers and reduced stromal thickness. The posterior stromal cut is regular.

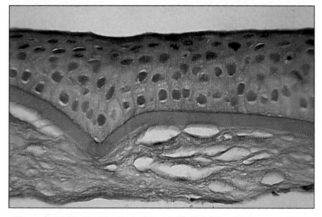

Figure 33-9. Periodic acid schiff (PAS) x 160 procedure. The undulations in Bowman's membrane create V-shaped troughs in the stroma.

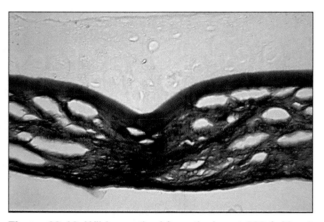

Figure 33-10. Wilder method for reticulum x 160 (without counterstain) corneal lamellae are compressed in some areas of the stroma.

Intraoperative

Folds may be induced during surgery in the following circumstances:

- When the lifted corneal flap is rotated improperly during stromal ablation.
- Incorrect repositioning of the corneal flap; this can be avoided by making adequate apposition of the reference marks.
- In corneas with a previous radial keratotomy, microfolds may occur in front of the incisions in the optic zone. This is due to slight misalignment of the incisions, which creates tension along the flap secondary to the relaxing keratotomy combined with the lamellar cut (Figures 33-11 and 33-12).
- Folds may form due to disc displacement caused by careless removal of the lid speculum or from the patient squeezing the lids too tightly following the procedure. If the patient's lids are not properly closed, friction between the cornea and gauze may create folds.

Wrinkles may result from excessive drying; this may occur when the disc edge is sponge dried, or allowed to dry too much. They may be induced when direct pressure is applied during sponge drying of the disc edge or with the excessive use of air.[9,10]

Striae are usually seen in the optical zone during the later postoperative period.

When large ablations have been performed to correct high myopia, a transient pseudochamber is formed at the ablation center, delaying healing of the central corneal layers and inducing striae.

- In large steep hyperopic ablations, peripheral and circular striae may also be seen.[11]

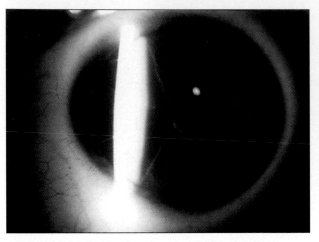

Figure 33-11. Folds after myopic LASIK after RK.

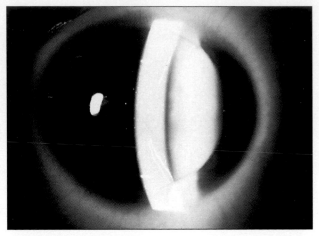

Figure 33-12. Folds after myopic LASIK after RK.

- The combination of a thin disc and a large ablation may contribute to striae.[8]
- Large diameter discs in myopic ablations make adaptation to the new bed more difficult and can induce striae.[3,4,11]

Postoperative

- During the immediate postoperative period, fold formation and disc displacement may be induced as a result of lid squeezing.
- If the patient rubs the eyes or fails to use night shields, folds may result. It is important to remember that although there may be corneal sensitivity in the periphery, there is central hypoesthesia or anesthesia because corneal nerves are severed by the keratectomy, which requires at least 1 month to recover.[12]

CLINICAL FINDINGS

Folds may be detected at slit lamp examination on the day of surgery or at 1-day postoperatively. Retroillumination with maximum pupil dilatation is the best technique. Folds will exhibit specific characteristics in terms of shape, color, and orientation relative to hinge characteristics and location. Horizontal or oblique linear white-grayish folds are seen centrally or in the periphery with a horizontal nasal hinge when the flap is slightly rotated. They are also found if the disc is displaced when removing the speculum (see Figures 33-1 and 33-3).

Vertical or oblique folds are more characteristic of superior hinge discs. They are thinner, more centrally located and have less effect on visual acuity than horizontal ones. Lid pressure on the superior hinge disc[6] aids its reposition; if there is pendular movement, it seldom produces significant folds; these folds have a minor

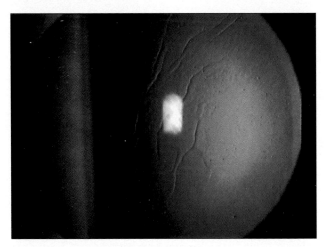

Figure 33-13. Vertical oblique folds in a superior hinge flap.

effect on visual acuity and are easier to reposition and smooth. Folds are commonly associated with inadequate flap positions during replacement or as a result of slippage during the postoperative period (Figure 33-13).

Striae are small continuous, but slightly wavy, lines with a grayish edge and dark core seen in the optic zone of well-repositioned discs (Figures 33-14 and 33-15) with large amounts of corneal flattening; they usually do not affect the visual acuity. Circular striae[11] are sometimes detected by retroillumination under maximum dilatation in the area of maximum peripheral ablation in hyperopic procedures. This phenomenon is caused by the same mechanism giving rise to striae in large central ablations for myopic corrections, resulting in large base curve changes.

When complete flap eversion with the nasal hinge occurs, the greatest complications are interface epithelialization and flap edema, rather than folds or striae (Figure 33-16). With superior hinges, there may be a

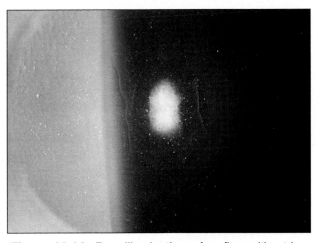

Figure 33-14. Retroillumination of a flap with striae. Notice the small continuous, but slightly wavy, lines with a grayish edge and dark core.

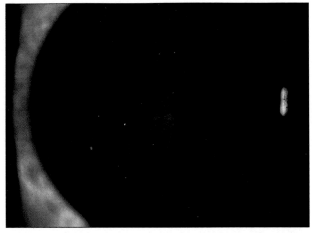

Figure 33-15. Frontal view of a flap with striae. Notice the small continuous, but slightly wavy, lines with a grayish edge and dark core.

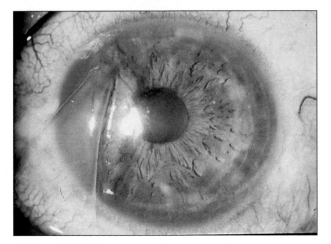

Figure 33-16. Displacement and complete eversion of a horizontal hinge flap.

pendular displacement, but a complete disc eversion is almost impossible. We had no reports of everted discs using the superior hinge technique. When there is a large displacement, arcuate-shaped folds are formed close to the hinge in the upper flap periphery.

Abundant lines with an almost mesh-like pattern on the disc are classified as wrinkles and are seldom seen (see Figure 33-5).

HOW CAN FOLDS AND STRIAE BE AVOIDED?

Potential causes of fold formation during surgery must be considered and the patient must be carefully instructed regarding postoperative care. If postoperative management guidelines are followed, a large number of complications will be eliminated.

It is advisable to plan for a flap thickness equal to or greater than 160 microns for diameters not greater than 8.50 mm in myopic ablations and for aspheric ablations requiring a relatively large correction. Drying the remaining central fluid and edges must be accomplished with great care during surgery, always working from the center to the periphery. In large ablations, it is our recommendation to dry and carefully remove central fluid in order to obtain good apposition of the anterior layers.

In order to avoid excessive disc manipulation, Vidaurri[13] has designed a double U-shaped cannula to irrigate the interface and epithelium at the same time, while replacing the disc on its bed. No sponge drying is required, and he waits 1 minute before removing the speculum. According to this author, the incidence of folds and disc displacement is very low. Flap adherence to the interface must be checked before removing the speculum by applying light pressure peripheral to the disc edge, noting that it should not move and very subtle folds or peripheral striae should radiate across the gutter. This is called the striae test.[1]

After speculum removal, the flap should be rechecked to confirm that no folds have been inadvertently created. The patient is asked to blink in order to determine that there is no movement and that the disc is firmly adhered.[1] We recommend closing the patient's eye with adhesive tape and placing gauze on top to create a tight seal; this is replaced with a protective shield at the conclusion of my surgical session. Some surgeons use only a protective shield and no gauze.

Others favor the temporary use of a bandage contact lens[9,6,14] with the argument that it prevents fold formation because it adheres to the cornea; although some consider the lens to be a source of irritation and folds. We believe that the lens may favor infection, as described by

Barraquer.[3,4] When the epithelium is intact, as is the case of LASIK, the disc itself acts as a contact lens.

Management

Early diagnosis is crucial. Slit lamp examination before discharging the patient allows for early diagnosis and treatment. There are varying opinions concerning treatment, but it is generally agreed that primary treatment is always directed to rehydrate the disc. This can be accompanied by other options, such as mechanical stretching, sutures, de-epithelialization, and bandage contact lenses. The sooner folds are treated, the greater the possibility of their disappearance. Once they have been allowed to remain for several weeks, it is more difficult to correct and eliminate all traces of them, as the cornea has a kind of "memory" in this regard due to changes in Bowman's membrane and the superficial stroma.

Hydration

As soon as folds are detected during the postoperative period, the disc should be hydrated again on the interface and under the flap. Castillo, et al[15,16] suggest using distilled sterile water; Hatsis[8] proposes the use of hypotonic buffered saline solution (80% balanced salt solution [BBS] in distilled water), which induces disc edema and stretches out flap wrinkles, folds, and striae through a hydrodynamic action. Advocates of overhydration with distilled water,[15,16] first rehydrate the disc, then express out the fluid. At that point, folds must have disappeared or, if they have not, they will be readily observed. There are others who propose hydration using donor cornea preserving solutions such as Optisol.[17]

Hatsis states[8] that striae rarely completely disappear, but best-corrected visual acuity improves after hydration.

Our experience in the treatment of folds, wrinkles, and striae is with hydration to provoke transient corneal edema with subsequent corneal stretching and disappearance of the flap irregularities.

Sutures

According to our experience, two stitches can be placed perpendicular to the folds. However, they must be placed under low tension in order to avoid new folds; it is advisable to remove them the next day; this approach is applicable mainly with late postoperative detection. Compression sutures[18] may also be anchored outside the disc, as suggested by Guimaraes[19] and Buratto.[6]

De-epithelialization

This method is used for the treatment of old folds and is done after hydrating the disc.[15,16] Old folds that have been displaced for several days persist even after hydration. Many times, this is due to the fact that there is a larger number of epithelial cell layers over Bowman's

membrane that, when removed, allow for normal re-epithelialization over the smoothed membrane.

Contact Lenses

Some surgeons propose contact lens insertion instead of sutures after rehydrating the disc.[6,9] Others support de-epithelialization with placement of a contact lens.

Finally, the most important method to prevent fold formation is excellent surgical technique. Gentle disc treatment with minimal manipulation of corneal tissue, combined with precise patient instructions regarding postoperative care (with the aim of avoiding ocular trauma at all cost) will provide the greatest success.

REFERENCES

1. Slade SG. LASIK complications and their management. In: Machat JJ, ed. *Excimer Laser Refractive Surgery*. Thorofare, NJ: SLACK Incorporated; 1996.
2. Casebeer JC, Ruiz LA, Slade S. *Lamellar Refractive Surgery*. Thorofare, NJ: SLACK Incorporated; 1996; 88-89.
3. Barraquer JI. *Queratomileusis y Queratofaquia*. Bogotá: Editorial Arco;1980; 23-24.
4. Barraquer JI. *Cirugía Refractiva de la Córnea*. Bogotá: Instituto Barraquer de América; 1989.
5. Pallikaris IG, Papatzanaki ME, Siganos DS, Tsilimbaris MK. A corneal flap technique for in situ keratomileusis. *Arch Ophthalmol.* 1991;145:1699-1702.
6. Buratto L, Brint SF, Ferrari M. Complications. In: Buratto L, Brint SF, eds. *LASIK: Principles and Techniques*. Thorofare, NJ: SLACK Incorporated; 1998; 121-122,126.
7. Barraquer F. Personal comunication; 1999).
8. Hatsis A. Modified technique successfully removes flap wrinkles, reduces striae. *Ocular Surgery News*. 1999;8:34-35.
9. Suárez E, Cardenas JJ. Intraoperative complications of LASIK. In: Buratto L, Brint SF, eds. *LASIK: Principles and Techniques*. Thorofare, NJ: SLACK Incorporated; 1998.
10. Torres F. Personal comunication; 1999.
11. Barraquer C. Personal comunication; 1997.
12. Tervo T, Barraquer C, Latvala T. Corneal wound healing and nerve morphology after excimer laser in situ keratomileusis (LASIK) in human eyes. *Journal of Refractive Surgery*. 1996;6:677.
13. Vidaurri Leal Jesús. Personal comunication.
14. Pallikaris IG, Siganos DS. *LASIK*. Thorofare, NJ: SLACK Incorporated;1998; 134,161.
15. Castillo A, Diaz D, Garcia J, Hernández JI, et al. Poster. American Society of Cataract and Refractive Surgery Meeting. San Diego, Calif; 1998.
16. Hernández JL. Personal comunication; 1999.
17. Hoyos J. Personal comunication; 1996.
18. Rama P, Chamon W, et al. Excimer laser intrastromal keratomileusis (LASIK). In: Azar DT, ed. *Refractive Surgery*. Stamford, Conn: Appleton & Lange; 1997; 463-464.
19. Guimaraes RQ, Rowsey JI, Reis-Guimaraes MF, et al. Suturing in lamellar surgery: bra technique. *J Refract Corneal Surg*. 1992;8:84-87.

Intraoperative and Postoperative Flap Striae

Roger F. Steinert, MD

INTRAOPERATIVE STRIAE

Current approaches to smoothing the flap and avoiding striae at the end of the procedure vary widely, as presented in earlier chapters. No matter which technique is employed, however, the surgeon must carefully examine the eye for the presence of striae once the flap is repositioned. Coaxial and oblique illumination should be used at the operating microscope. Checking the patient at the slit lamp 15 to 30 minutes postoperatively is important to detect immediate flap slippage as well. If present, striae should be immediately corrected by refloating and stroking the flap smooth. A protective plastic shield for the first 24 hours is advisable to discourage touching of the eyelids and inadvertent disruption of the flap.

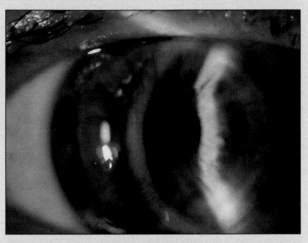

Figure 33A-1. Macrostriae from edge slippage.

POSTOPERATIVE STRIAE

Macrostriae represent full thickness, undulating stromal folds (Figure 33A-1). These invariably occur due to initial malposition or postoperative flap slippage. Careful examination should disclose a wider gutter on the side where the folds are most prominent. This situation should be rectified as soon as it is recognized, as the folds rapidly become fixed. Under the operating microscope or at the slit lamp, a lid speculum is placed; the flap is lifted; copious irrigation is used in the interface; and the flap is stroked repeatedly until the striae resolve. Hypotonic saline or sterile distilled water as the irrigating solution will swell the flap and may reduce the striae, but swelling reduces flap diameter, which widens the gutter, and delays flap adhesion due to prolonged endothelial dehydration time. A bandage soft contact lens should always be employed for at least 24 hours to stabilize the flap until full re-epithelialization occurs. In severe cases of intractable macrostriae, a tight 360° anti-torque running suture may be placed, but irregular astigmatism may be present after suture removal.

Microstriae are fine, hair-like optical irregularities best seen on red reflex illumination or light reflected off the iris. Microstriae are fine folds in Bowman's layer. This anterior location accounts for the disruption of best-corrected visual acuity that microstriae may cause. Computer topography does not usually show these fine irregularities. A few striae may not be visually significant. Mild loss of acuity or other optical symptoms such as ghost images usually improve over time as the epithelial thickness adjusts to the folds and restores a more regular anterior tear film.

Optically significant striae should be addressed, however. Microstriae will only resolve with hydration of Bowman's layer. While this will eventually occur with prolonged stroking of the epithelial surface with a moistened surgical spear sponge or irrigating cannula, microstriae usually disappear within minutes of deliberate de-epithelialization of the area over the microstriae. Several drops of sterile distilled water speed the disappearance of microstriae. If the striae persist, the flap should be lifted and the interface irrigated. A bandage soft contact lens is then applied with an antibiotic and mild steroid until re-epithelialization is established.

Striae of the Flap

Gordon Balazsi, MD

Striae are the most common flap-related cause of loss of best-corrected visual acuity after LASIK. Microstriae are very fine and best observed on retro- or oblique illumination, and their effect on optical quality varies from insignificant to severe. Macrostriae are very significant wrinkles of the full flap thickness that result in a serious loss of visual acuity.

Striae most commonly appear in the immediate postoperative period (< 24 hours) as a result of flap displacement. Approximately 1% of eyes present with microstriae on the first day after surgery. Fortunately, the vast majority of these are clinically insignificant. Very rarely (3/10,000 eyes), microstriae can be induced by ablation of a significant depth of tissue resulting in a flap-to-bed mismatch (high myopic astigmatism) or an asymmetric corneal scar, and attempts to stretch the flap flat are not always successful. Macrostriae are also very rare (3/10,000 eyes).

Risk factors for postoperative flap displacement include squeezing by the patient, thin flap (associated with dull blades, inadequate suction, very large corneas), flap edema (excessive hydration/manipulation). Preventive measures include giving all patients oral diazepam and a lot of "vocal local." Dr. Mullie and I inspect all blades preoperatively on a diamond blade scope; we use a 200-micron depth plate for large corneas greater than 12.5 mm; we have evolved a dry surgical technique with minimal flap manipulation. Immediately postoperatively, the eyes are inspected at the slit lamp, covered with clear plastic shields, and most importantly, the patients are instructed to keep their eyes closed for at least 4 hours. All patients are re-examined early the following morning.

Clinically insignificant microstriae not associated with a gape of the flap edge should be left alone. All other striae should be treated as early as possible. Incipient epithelial ingrowth through a wound gape is best detected with fluorescein.

Smoothing techniques can be best observed with oblique illumination from the operating microscope or a muscle light. We do not recommend retroillumination of a dilated pupil, as it causes photophobia.

If striae are detected within 24 hours, it is usually sufficient to relift the flap, float it with several drops of BSS, and stroke its epithelial surface with a standard bent-tip 27-gauge cannula (a wet sponge does not provide sufficient drag) perpendicular to the orientation of the folds. Smoothing may take several minutes and may be incomplete. At the end, the flap is refloated and stroked from the hinge to the opposite side of the optical zone. Excessive pressure past this point will compress the flap back toward the hinge and worsen the folds.

After 24 hours, the folds can be more rigid and require more vigorous stretching than is possible with this epithelial approach alone. It then becomes important to attack the inner surface of the flap as well. This is best achieved by asking the patient to look in the direction opposite the hinge and folding the flap back on the exposed conjunctiva. We prefer to use direct pressure from the heel of a cyclodialysis spatula to vigorously stroke the folds. This may require several minutes, and the patient aware of pressure on the globe. The flap is then repositioned, and the procedure completed with the epithelial approach previously described. Even though the flap can usually be successfully smoothed out with this method, it usually takes several days for the ridges of differential stromal edema to resolve.

Before removal of the speculum, the flap is allowed to re-adhere for 3 minutes while the epithelial surface is kept moist. The eye is re-examined 30 minutes later, before the patient is discharged. The patient must keep the lids closed for 4 hours. Only rarely is a bandage lens or lid taping necessary.

LASIK DECENTRATION AND CENTRAL ISLANDS

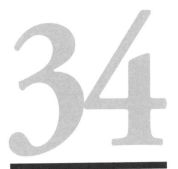

Steven E. Wilson, MD, Mark Walker, MD,
Stephen D. Klyce, PhD

Optimal visual performance following laser-assisted in situ keratomileusis (LASIK) is directly related to the quality of the corneal contour and the geometric relationship of the change in corneal contour to the entrance pupil, and, therefore, the overall alignment with other components of the ocular system. There are numerous anomalies of corneal topography that may occur following LASIK that represent irregular astigmatism and contribute to a less than optimal clinical outcome. Two of the most common complications are decentration and central islands. These can produce a patient's perception of poor visual quality. This chapter delineates the causes of decentration and central islands following LASIK and provides recommendations regarding treatment.

DECENTRATION OF THE LASIK PROCEDURE

Decentration of LASIK can be divided into decentration of the flap created with the microkeratome and decentration of the excimer laser ablation. Each of these may cause serious degradation of uncorrected and best-spectacle corrected visual acuity due to irregular astigmatism and may lead to annoying or disabling visual disturbances such as multiple images, starbursting, and glare.

Decentration of the Flap

Decentration of the flap is common following LASIK and is attributable to improper positioning of the suction ring when preparing to cut the flap. Typically, flap decentration is easily avoided by monitoring the position of the suction ring relative to the limbus as suction is applied. The suction ring often has a tendency to migrate when suction is applied. This may trigger a decentration. This effect can be minimized by firm posterior pressure on the microkeratome ring by the surgeon

as suction is initiated. If decentration is detected prior to making the cut, the vacuum should be released and the suction ring repositioned. However, even a few seconds of suction tend to produce a compression gutter that will guide the suction ring back to the original decentered position. If this occurs, it may be necessary to wait a few minutes until the compression gutter disappears to establish a new centration of the suction ring. Sometimes overcompensating the placement of the ring in the direction opposite the decentration prior to initiating suction is helpful in obtaining a centered suction.

The smaller the intended flap, the more critical the centration. Microkeratomes such as the Automated Corneal Shaper (ACS) that produce flaps averaging around 8.0 to 8.5 mm are more prone to symptomatic decentration. These smaller flaps should be centered relative to the entrance pupil consistent with optimal visual performance.[1] Such centration will also minimize flap edge effects under darker lighting conditions, when dilation is more likely to include the scarred periphery of the flap within the edge of the entrance pupil. Proximity of the flap edge to the pupil may result in deflection of rays to produce multiple images, ghosting, or starbursting. One of the advantages of microkeratomes such as the Hansatome is the 9.5 to 10.5 mm flaps created with larger size rings. These are far less likely to be of clinical significance in the event of a small decentration. The optical benefits of this far outweigh the limbal bleeding that may occur in some eyes with larger flaps. Bleeding is easily managed with a topical vasoconstrictor, Merocel sponges, and placement of the flap back into its original position.

If a decentered flap has already been cut, the surgeon must evaluate whether the degree of decentration is likely to produce optical symptoms. It is important to consider the size of the pupil under scotopic conditions for the individual eye. This may be approximated through the operating microscope by reducing the illumination and dimming the lights in the operating room. One rule of thumb, derived from clinical observation of patients with decentered flaps, is to consider aborting the LASIK procedure if the edge of the laser ablation (typically 6.0 mm in diameter) will fall closer than 0.5 mm from the edge of the flap. For example, for a normally centered 10 mm flap with a 6.0 mm ablation, there will be approximately 2.0 mm of clearance between the edge of the ablation and flap edge. If the flap is decentered such that the ablation would end only 0.3 mm from the edge of the flap, one should abort the procedure.

As noted above, decentration resulting in the edge of the ablation infringing within 0.5 mm of the edge of the flap is likely to be symptomatic. Also, the higher the level of attempted correction, the more likely a decentration will be symptomatic since power transitions are higher in the periphery of ablations with greater corrections.

Often, the hinge of the flap will be within the intended ablation zone despite a flap that is otherwise sufficiently centered. In these cases, it is important to protect the flap so that a double ablation of the bed near the hinge and the flap itself do not occur. Such a double ablation will produce localized flattening of corneal contour and may induce irregular astigmatism.[2] The edge of the flap can be protected during laser ablation with a contact lens cut in half, a metal blade edge, or other suitable instrument.

Anomalies of corneal topography consistent with visual distortions (Figure 34-1) are commonly noted in eyes with the ablation falling adjacent to the flap edge. Typically, there is a postoperative steepening of the corneal topography just outside the edge of the flap where the ablation is too near the edge. This is likely due to the effect of the edge of the flap creating an abrupt transition of power resulting in steepening of surface contour at that position on the cornea. If this abrupt steepening lies within the zone overlying the entrance pupil, visual distortions are likely.

If the surgeon decides the subsequent ablation is likely to fall near or overlap the edge of the flap, then the best course of action is to replace the flap without excimer laser ablation. In such cases, the flap can typically be recut approximately 3 months after the original procedure.

Symptoms of patients with decentered flaps that were ablated with the excimer laser may be very difficult to treat. Attempts to eliminate corneal topographic irregularities that result are usually a failure and may worsen symptoms since intentionally decentered balancing ablations will overlap the edge of the flap. A rigid gas-permeable contact lens can be used to cover such irregular-

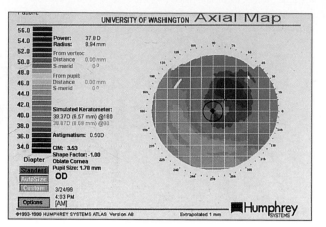

Figure 34-1. A decentered flap. The edge of the ablation that was centered on the pupil fell within 0.5 mm of the edge of the flap that was decentered in the superior direction. Note the corneal contour appears steep just outside the ablation zone in the inferior cornea. This apparent inferior steepening was not present prior to LASIK and is likely related to the edge of the flap being within the pupillary zone since the central corneal thickness was 0.5 mm after the procedure. The patient had a one-line decrease in best spectacle-corrected visual acuity and complained of a double image and glare that was increased under scotopic conditions.

ities if a fitting is possible. In some cases, a corneal transplant may be needed to eliminate disabling visual symptoms. Custom surface ablations with scanning lasers may be used in the future to try to regularize topography overlying the entrance pupil. This possible treatment is discussed later in this chapter.

Decentration of the Excimer Laser Ablation

Decentration of the ablation has become less frequent as lasers have included better systems for monitoring the entrance pupil. As with all refractive surgical procedures, the ablation should be centered on the entrance pupil to optimize visual performance. The key to avoiding problems with decentered ablations is prevention. The surgeon should strive to monitor the treatment and temporarily halt and recenter the ablation if a drift of fixation is noted. Constant encouragement of the patient to fixate on the fixation target is helpful. Tracking systems may further decrease the incidence of ablation decentration in LASIK. Even lasers with tracking systems may, however, yield a decentered ablation, as it is the surgeon who achieves the centering rather than the laser system.

Little is known about the degree of ablation decentration that must be present to induce symptoms. It is not uncommon to encounter completely asymptomatic patients with decentrations greater than 1.0 mm relative to the entrance pupil. What can be stated is that the

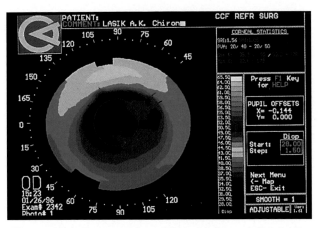

Figure 34-2. Decentration of the ablation relative to the entrance pupil. The ablation was decentered inferiorly. The pupil is indicated by the black circle. The patient complained of a ghost image seen with this eye, despite 20/20 uncorrected vision.

chance of encountering loss of best spectacle-corrected vision, multiple images, glare, starbursting, or other abnormalities increases as the level of decentration increases. Many patients with such a decentration will only experience difficulty at night when the pupil is dilated.

Treatment of patients with decentrations should begin with medical attempts to decrease symptoms since modalities currently available to surgically treat them are suboptimal. Constriction of the pupil with dilute pilocarpine will often improve symptoms. This is especially useful in older patients with diminished accommodation, but can be attempted regardless of age. One-half percent pilocarpine is the typical starting concentration, but further decrease in concentration can be attempted using custom solutions. Patients have been noted anecdotally in whom .10% pilocarpine is effective in constricting the pupil and decreasing symptoms attributed to decentration. The lower the concentration, the less the effect on accommodation. One might predict that a topical adrenergic antagonist that triggers pupil constriction without affecting accommodation would be useful for treating these eyes. Unfortunately, such a medication is not currently available.

Eyes with decentration of the LASIK ablation frequently have astigmatism induced by the displacement between the pupil and the ablation. Correction of astigmatism with astigmatic keratectomy or spectacles, based on the refractive cylinder, may be helpful in alleviating some symptoms.

Again, a rigid gas permeable contact lens can effectively eliminate symptoms of decentration if an appropriate fit can be obtained. The higher the original correction, the more difficult this is likely to be. It is, however, important to exclude this as a possibility prior to pro-

ceeding with an attempt at surgical correction.

Currently, any attempt at surgical correction of symptomatic LASIK decentration must be customized and is certainly more art than science. One method that has been used to reduce symptoms is to attempt to produce an ablation with equal decentration in the opposite direction. Typically, this involves lifting the flap and protecting a portion of the initial ablation with 2% methylcellulose solution or some other masking agent (Figure 34-2) while attempting to extend the inadequate ablation in the opposite direction. An approximation of the amount of decentration can be obtained from the corneal topography. Then, with the flap lifted, methylcellulose is applied to protect a portion of the bed from further ablation beginning approximately 1.0 mm away from the central pupil toward the direction of the original decentration (see Figure 34-1). It is wise to attempt this manipulation in a stepwise fashion, with each treatment being restricted to less than 2 diopters (D). An advantage of LASIK is that such retreatments can be performed several times at 1- to 2-week intervals with reduced risk of significant haze.

Linkage of corneal topography to excimer ablation will likely become the treatment of choice for decentration of ablations in LASIK. One could envision that a subtraction between the decentered topography and an ideal correction topography being entered into a small beam scanning laser to direct a correcting ablation. At present, the accuracy of corneal topographic measurements is such that these attempts may need refinement. Since there is currently no technique for monitoring topography during the ablation, topographically linked ablations must be confined to "snap shot" treatments in which only the preoperative corneal topography is utilized. Because of this, sophisticated techniques must be employed to carefully align the eye using 4 degrees of freedom—X, Y, Z—and rotation. Treatment of decentrations will likely provide optimal cases for testing the efficacy of topographically linked excimer laser ablations.

CENTRAL ISLANDS

Central islands are irregular elevations of corneal contour that occur within the bounds of the ablation zone following LASIK (Figure 34-3a). Many clinicians and scientists identify a central island as significant if it measures more than 1.5 mm in diameter and 3 D in elevation on topographic analysis, but all such definitions are arbitrary.[3] Smaller central islands that do not fulfill these definitions may cause symptoms and interfere with an optimal outcome following surgery.

Symptom-producing elevations of corneal topography within the ablated zone are not always central and frequently are not islands. Other shapes, such as peninsulas are also frequently noted. Each of these produces irregular astigmatism and interference with optimal visual function. For the sake of clarity in discussion, however, we will refer to each of these elevations in corneal contour within the ablated zone as central islands.

Symptoms attributable to central islands include decreased uncorrected visual acuity due to undercorrection and best spectacle-corrected visual acuity due to irregular astigmatism. Other frequently noted symptoms include image distortion, multiple images, starbursting, and glare.

Little has been published regarding the occurrence of central islands following LASIK. In the authors' experience, they are more common with some brands of excimer lasers than with others. For example, in one series the incidence of central islands following LASIK with the Summit Apex laser was approximately 5% prior to the presently incorporated central island software, while the incidence with the VISX Star S2 was less than 0.5% (SE Wilson, unpublished data, 1999). Central islands also vary in incidence with the level of attempted correction, with the incidence increasing with higher treatment levels.

In order to understand the principles of limiting central islands and other topographic elevations in LASIK, it is important to understand the etiologies. Several potential mechanisms have been suggested.

Degradation of optics by the excimer laser and a resulting cold spot in the center of the ablation is likely to be one source of central islands. Such degradation of the optics occurs with all excimer lasers. Sudden failure of optical components may occur in some cases with a clustering of severe central islands. Central islands caused by this mechanism should show a correlation between their magnitude (diameter and power) and the amount of attempted correction.

A plume of debris is ejected from the corneal surface during excimer laser ablation. Several authors have suggested that a vortex may occur sporadically over the ablation and deposit debris selectively within the center of the treated zone.[4,5] Subsequent excimer laser pulses would be blocked by the plume vortex itself or deposited debris. Central islands that are generated by this mechanism should be confined to broad beam excimer lasers and eliminated by scanning lasers. A recent study of scanning laser photorefractive keratectomy (PRK) for myopia showed the complete absence of central islands.[6] Additionally, a sporadic vortex would be expected to produce a random incidence of central islands as has been reported.[7]

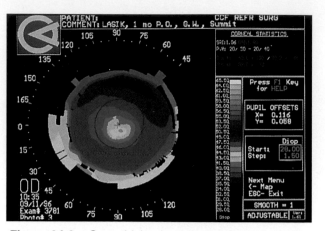

Figure 34-3a. Central islands and peninsulas. A central island is present 1 month following LASIK. Best spectacle-corrected visual acuity was reduced by two lines.

Nonuniform fluid distribution within the ablated zone is another potential cause of central islands.[8] A shiny area may develop during LASIK in the center of the ablated zone, indicating an accumulation of fluid from the stroma. This concentration of fluid absorbs and reflects subsequent excimer laser pulses owing to the fact that high energy ultraviolet (UV) light can induce substantial changes in the refractive index of water. Shockwaves generated by excimer laser pulses may concentrate this fluid that emerges from the bare stroma in the center of the ablation. Additionally, the process of epithelial debridement has been found to produce an anterior stromal edema that could contribute to surface fluid appearance.[9]

What preventative measures can be taken to limit the development of central islands following LASIK? First, the performance of the excimer laser must be monitored carefully. This can be done with available paper and plastic schemes that provide a good indication of beam homogeneity. Although time consuming, some users check the power of an ablation made in plastic with a lensometer every few ablations, or in some cases after every ablation. A regular schedule of preventative maintenance is helpful. It is important to heed clues to optical damage, such as rapid changes in indicators of laser performance within only a few treatments following a gas fill. Treatment should be suspended and the laser serviced prior to proceeding when there is a sudden change in the performance of the laser. Utilization of evacuation nozzles with excimer lasers such as the VISX Star S2 may limit vortex formation and central deposition of plume debris, but care must be taken in the design of such systems since they may actually contribute to vortex formation in some cases.

Some surgeons utilize central island pretreatments in which an initial central ablation is performed prior to the

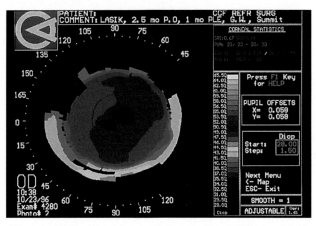

Figure 34-3b. Treatment of the cornea in Figure 34-3a was performed 2 months after primary LASIK. Retreatment was performed with the Summit Apex laser using 45 bursts of patient training A. At 1 month after retreatment, the central island was reduced and best spectacle-corrected visual acuity returned to the preoperative level.

broad ablation for optical correction. For example, the authors found that pretreatment with 40 bursts of the patient training A was effective in reducing central islands during LASIK performed with the Summit Apex laser. This was a crude and empirical measure that was, however, effective. Some lasers now incorporate additional central treatment designed to limit central islands into the ablation algorithm. The VISX Star S2 and Summit Apex Plus incorporate this type of automated pretreatment. This appears to be effective since the incidence of central islands is now markedly reduced.

Finally, it is important that the surgeon monitor the center of the ablation during excimer laser treatment with LASIK. The ablation should be interrupted and the stroma wiped with a lint-free sponge if fluid accumulation is detected in the center of the ablation.

Use of a scanning laser may limit the incidence of central islands that are attributable to vortex with central debris deposition. Scanning ablation may or may not eliminate central islands that are attributable to nonuniform fluid distribution. Any fluid accumulation in the center of the ablated zone would still be absorbed by a scanning laser and could create a central island. If shock waves from a broad beam laser are an important component in the central accumulation of fluid, then scanning lasers would tend to reduce the incidence of fluid-derived central islands.

What treatment can be performed once a central island is generated following LASIK? The authors' experience is that central islands that occur with LASIK are much less likely to recede spontaneously than with PRK. We have observed central islands for more than 1 year following LASIK and have seen little tendency for

change beyond 3 to 4 months following surgery. We recommend following the central island with refraction and corneal topography at 1 to 2-month intervals. If no changes are noted over this 3- to 4-month interval and the patient remains symptomatic, retreatment will likely be needed.

It may be necessary to distinguish central islands from kerectasia (a steepening of the cornea following refractive surgery), which has been reported in a limited number of case reports. Kerectasia should certainly be considered if progression of a central island is noted with corneal topography over time. More suspicion is warranted with corneas that have received high levels of correction or the thickness of the bed has been decreased to less than 250 μm. Careful preoperative screening with topography is also essential to reduce risks to keratoconus cases.[10] Recent studies have suggested that scanning slit topography technology might be useful in detecting kerectasia. However, the accuracy of these measurements have not been verified and may, in fact, represent artifact (see comment in referenced article).[11]

Treatment of a central island is often more art than science. Corneal topography can provide guidance regarding appropriate planning for re-ablation. Thus, the topographic map can be used to obtain an estimate of the elevation and diameter of the central island. Some investigators have relied heavily upon these measurements.[12] However, keep in mind that these measurements, especially of power or elevation, may not be accurate. We prefer a conservative approach even though additional treatment may be required. The actual excimer laser ablation may vary between clinicians. Some prefer to use the excimer laser in phototherapeutic mode, in some cases with varying diameters of minimal treatment. Thus, if the diameter of the central island is measured to be 2.0 mm and 3 D in power, then 25 bursts could be given at 2.0 mm, 25 bursts at 1.7 mm, and 25 bursts at 1.5 mm beneath the flap with the laser in phototherapeutic keratectomy (PTK) mode (Figure 34-3b). If the central island is not directly in the center of the initial ablation, an attempt can be made to decenter the retreatment according to the corneal topographic analysis of decentration. Retreated corneas are then analyzed with corneal topography 1 to 2 weeks after surgery and additional treatment given if a residual, symptomatic, central island remains. Other more empirical strategies are used by some clinicians: some might utilize 40 to 50 bursts of the Summit patient training A algorithm to provide treatment of an island 1.5 to 2.0 mm in diameter. Again, the residual island, if any, would need to be analyzed a few weeks after surgery and consideration given to additional treatment.

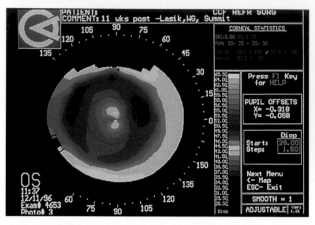

Figure 34-3c. A central island is present at 11 weeks after LASIK.

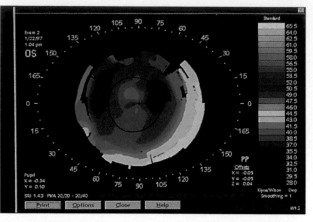

Figure 34-3d. Retreatment with 45 bursts of patient training A resulted in a decrease, but not elimination, of the central island. The patient noted an improvement in visual acuity.

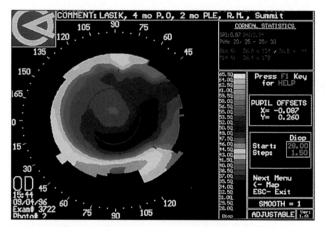

Figure 34-3e. A cornea with a peninsula present following LASIK. There was a one- to two-line decrease in best spectacle-corrected visual acuity in this case.

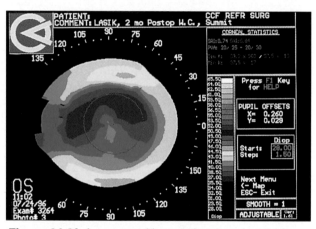

Figure 34-3f. A cornea with a peninsula present following LASIK. There was a one- to two-line decrease in best spectacle-corrected visual acuity in this case.

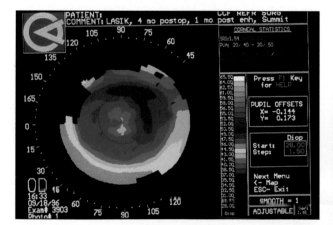

Figure 34-3g. A cornea with a peninsula present following LASIK. There was a one- to two-line decrease in best spectacle-corrected visual acuity in this case.

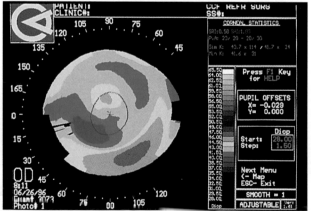

Figure 34-3h. A cornea with a decentered ablation relative to the entrance pupil along with a decentered central island.

Peninsulas and other irregular elevations are much more difficult to treat. Treatment of the central component of the elevation can be attempted with broad beam lasers, but the peripheral elevation will not be treated. Scanning/tracking lasers offer the promise of correction of these irregular shapes; however, such treatment will itself be dependent upon the accuracy of the topographic analysis and the ability to properly align the cornea under the laser prior to treatment. Future investigation will determine the utility of this linkage between corneal topography and excimer ablation for correction of irregular surfaces.

Supported in part by National Eye Institute grants EY10056 and EY03311.

Dr. Klyce has been a paid consultant to Tomey Corporation, Waltham, Mass, USA. The other authors have no commercial or proprietary interests in any of the products discussed in this chapter.

REFERENCES

1. Uozato H, Guyton DL. Centering corneal surgical procedures. *Am J Ophthalmol.* 1987;103:264-70.
2. Wilson SE. LASIK: management of common complications. *Cornea.* 1998;17:459-67.
3. Kampmeier J, Tanzer DJ, Er H, Schallhorn SC, LaBree L, McDonnell PJ. Significance of corneal topography in predicting patient complaints after photorefractive keratectomy. *J Cataract Refract Surg.* 1999;25:492-9.
4. Lin DTC. Corneal topographic analysis after excimer photorefractive keratectomy. *Ophthalmology.* 1994;101:1432-1439.
5. Noack J, Tonnies R, Hohla K, Birngruber R, Vogel A. Influence of ablation plume dynamics on the formation of central islands in excimer laser photorefractive keratectomy. *Ophthalmology.* 1997;104:823-30.
6. Coorpender SJ, Klyce, SD, McDonald, MB, et al. Small beam tracking excimer laser PRK topography. *J Cataract Refract Surg.* In press.
7. Klyce SD, McDonald MB. Computerized corneal topography of surface ablations with the Tomey TMS-1. In: Salz JJ, McDonnell PJ, McDonald MB, eds. *Corneal Laser Surgery.* St Louis, Mo: Mosby; 1995, 93-108.
8. Oshika T, Klyce SD, Smolek MK, McDonald MB. Corneal hydration and central islands after excimer laser photorefractive keratectomy. *Journal of Refractive Surgery.* 1998;24:1575-80.
9. Klyce SD, Karon MD, Ruberti JW, Smolek MK, Goto T. Epithelial debridement initiates acute anterior stromal edema. *Invest Ophthalmol Vis Sci.* 1999;40:S193.
10. Kalin NS, Maeda N, Klyce SD, Hargrave S, Wilson SE. Automated topographic screening for keratoconus in refractive surgery candidates. *CLAO J.* 22:164-167, 1996.
11. Wang Z, Chen J, Yang B. Posterior corneal surface topographic changes after laser in situ keratomileusis are related to residual corneal bed thickness. *Ophthalmology.* 1999;106:406-9.
12. Manche EE, Maloney RK, Smith RJ. Treatment of topographic central islands following refractive surgery. *J Cataract Refract Surg.* 1998,24:464-70.

Treating a Decentered Ablation

Melania Cigales, MD

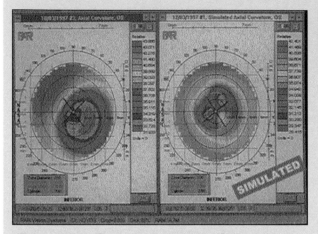

Figure 34A-1. Case of decentered LASIK and its simulated topography treatment.

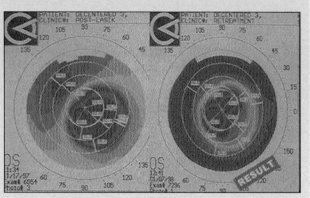

Figure 34A-2. Decentered LASIK and its result after treatment guided by simulated topography.

Decentered ablations can lead to irregular astigmatism and cause symptoms of glare, night vision problems, ghosting, and diplopia. Irregular astigmatism induced by decentration is difficult to correct with glasses or conventional surgery because there are not two axes 90° apart, but rather two hemicorneas—one steep and the other flat.

We treat decentered ablations by performing a new ablation on the opposite side under topographic simulation guidance. Elevation topography is required for this purpose. We use the PAR Vision System topographer (New Hartford, NY, USA). The surgery is a two-step procedure consisting of centering the ablation first and then treating the residual refractive error.

SIMULATION TECHNIQUE

We first identify for the center of the flattened area in the topography. In this point the elevation map shows a depression in microns off of the perfect sphere. Then we determine the opposite point ("mirror point") and its elevation in microns. The mirror point will be the center of the new ablation and the depth will be the sum of the depression plus the elevation. After that we need to determine the optical zone representing the best simulation.

Using this data (mirror point + depth + optical zone) we perform the simulation in the topography unit to obtain the simulated topography. Figure 34A-1 shows a case of decentered LASIK and its simulated topography, where the flattest area has is recentered.

SURGICAL TECHNIQUE

In cases of decentered LASIK, the flap is lifted using the technique normally employed in retreatments. In cases of decentered PRK, a flap is created using the 160-micron plate (to avoid irregular cuts), and treatment is accomplished with LASIK.

The laser is decentered and focused on the new ablation center, located exactly at the mirror point previously determined. Our laser (Apollo Vision, Inc, Pa, USA) enables us to do this very easily just by moving the mirror. Once this is done, the ablation is made at the new center using patient self-fixation. Closing the flap completes the surgery.

Figure 34A-2 shows the preoperative decentered topography using the TMS1 topographer and the perfectly centered result obtained after treatment. A comparison of the simulated topography (see Figure 34A-1) and the result (see Figure 34A-2) reveals that they are both practically the same. This demonstrates the effectiveness of topographic simulation in decentered ablation treatments.

LASIK Central Islands: Spontaneous Evolution

Heriberto Marotta, MD

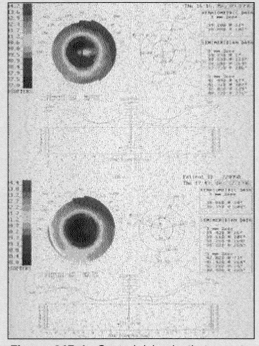

Figure 34B-1. Central islands that spontaneously resolved within a period of 6 months to 1 year.

Central islands are the most frequently observed topographic abnormalities after PRK and, contrary to past beliefs, they are also seen following LASIK. They are more frequent with broad beam homogeneous lasers and with optical zones above 6.0 mm, excimer lasers with flat energy beam profiles, single zone techniques, high myopia, and ablations performed on moist stromal beds. They appear as topographic elevations in the center of the ablated zone—as if the effected tissue had not been treated—showing an elevation of 1 to 3 D and a width of 1.0 to 3.0 mm diameter. They are accompanied by symptoms such as blurred vision, ghost images, halos, loss of best-corrected visual acuity, and undercorrection.

There are several theories to explain this complication: the vortex plume theory, laser optic degradation, the theory of acoustic shockwave (Machat) of differential hydration (Lin), and the multifactorial theory.

The vortex plume theory proposes that the detritus column, which is centrally aligned, might block the ablation of successive laser pulses. Accordingly, those lasers, which employ aspiration, should avoid this complication, and this has not happened.

Neuhann supports the idea that a low pressure center could be created behind the plume, which encases a small percentage of the ablation by products, leading to deposition, shielding, and formation of steep central islands.

Others have proposed a degradation of optics as a cause of the topographic alterations described, as well as keyhole patterns.

The acoustic shockwave theory states that each pulse generates a wave that leads to hydration toward the center of the cornea, which causes blocking, and a reduction of the photoablation in the central zone.

Shimmick and Col, using optic profilometry, have shown that in steep central islands there is not only a central underablation but a peripheral over ablation, which is more than the expected ablation rates caused by the spatial variance of the tissue ablated with a uniform laser beam.

As in all complications, prevention is most important and is obtained by means of a programmed anticentral island pretreatment, adding additional central pulses to the refractive treatment of 1 micron per diopter to treat at a 2.5 mm diameter in cases with single-zone treatment, and of 0.6 microns per diopter in those with multizone treatment.

Surgeons who dry the central stroma with a sponge or spatula practice another form of prevention.

The evolution of these islands should be observed, as they tend to resolve spontaneously within a period of 6 months to 1 year, as in the case presented in the Figure 34B-1. According to Lin's work in PRK, only 2% remain after 1 year.

Though the causes are still not established, it may be assumed that there are two types of central islands.

Type 1: Due to a retention of liquid in the interface, which may be treated by mechanical compression (as described by Avalos and Caro).

Type 2: Due to remaining residual tissue not sufficiently ablated in the central zone, which can be retreated with the excimer laser, taking precautions not to induce a hyperopic shift.

In order to treat the central island, the height of the elevation, as well as the diameter and location, must be calculated, using this information, it is possible to program the pulses needed and the diameter of the ablation. Munnerlyn's formula can be used. A PTK or PRK treatment must be applied to the originally ablated stromal surface. The flap should be lifted, the island treated, and the flap replaced very carefully. Topography-assisted excimer lasers would be useful in the future for these enhancements.

Correction of Decentered Ablation

Paolo Vinciguerra, MD

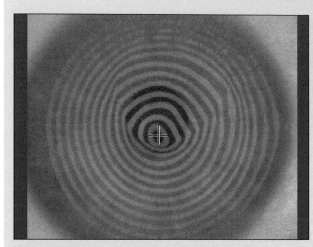

Figure 34C-1. Keratoscopy of a −16 D decentrated treatment.

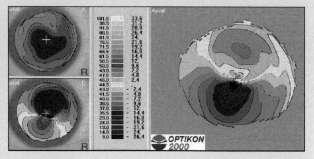

Figure 34C-2. Preoperative topography of the patient in Figure 34C-3.

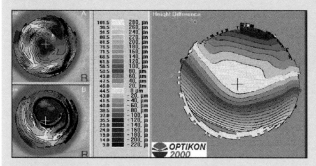

Figure 34C-3. Postoperative topography of the patient in Figure 34C-2.

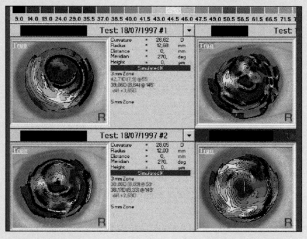

Figure 34C-4. Intraoperative exam of the patient in Figures 34C-2 and 34C-3; notice the progressive improvement.

A decentered ablation, occurring when the center of the ablation and the visual axis are not concentric, is difficult for the refractive surgeon to manage.

The cause of a decentered ablation may be related to the patient, the excimer laser, or the surgeon. Most causes are related to the excimer laser ablation and may occur both during PRK and LASIK.

Decentration symptoms significantly impair the patient's visual quality, and their importance depends on factors like decentration amount, optical zone size, and dioptric homogeneity within the ablated area.

Our procedure for the correction of decentration is based on the use of a series of metal diaphragms properly placed on a mask to protect the previous decentered ablation and to ablate any surrounding corneal areas in order to obtain a new, larger, and centered optical zone with the dioptric power originally anticipated.

Accurate measurements and calculations must be made before performing this technique.

By evaluating the tangential map, it is possible to calculate the decentration amount (distance between the visual axis and the ablation center) in millimeters and axis (corresponding to the meridian of the ablation center). These parameters are essential in planning the new ablation position and axis.

The ablation depth is established by multiplying the preoperative ametropia in diopters by a constant calculated with variable algorithms from the decentration amount (eg, 0.85 for a 1.0 mm amount); this value corresponds to the ablation depth in microns for each single diaphragm applied. A final PTK must be performed to smooth such irregularities and the transition between the old and the new ablation.

When the slit lamp and keratoscopy intraoperative exams show a regular and dioptrically homogeneous corneal surface, the PTK is suspended and the procedure ends.

Treatment of LASIK Decentrations

Daniel A. Lebuisson, MD and Cathy Albou-Ganem, MD

LASIK to correct refractive errors has gained worldwide acceptance, but despite a high level of success, significant visual complications can occur, especially early in the learning curve. Ablation decentration is one of the more frequent surgical problems. Surgeon inexperience is often the reason for such an event. Occasionaly, though, topographic decentration is not due to surgical error but results from the patient's eye characteristics: pupil malposition, nasal trans pupillary fixation, improper use of the fixation ring, or blurred vision. There is no absolute correlation between the applanation video map and the new true optic zone. A knowledge of postoperative topography patterns guides the surgeon's evaluation. Some patterns improve substantially from 1 day to 3 months postoperatively.

Obtaining homogeneity of the map is important before diagnosing decentration. The reproducibility of different maps has been questioned and the literature on categorization using postoperative patterns is very poor. We advise analyzing corneal decentration at least three times at 1-week intervals and to use two videotopographic devices before secondary surgery.

Any attempt to treat a decentration must be carefully preceded by a comprehensive refractive evaluation based on subjective and objective visual acuity, pachymetry, corneal topography, pupillometry (with a pupillometer). Experienced surgeons know that decentration can be well tolerated by the patient and does not, in all cases, require surgical correction, except in the case of undercorrection. In our practice, in a group of 800 cases including our first cases (1995/1996), the frequency of decentration over 1.0 mm is 0.1% and 0.6% over 0.5 mm. Only four patients who underwent LASIK were reoperated for decentration in a series of 1500 cases.

Decentration can induce side effects and complications. Irregular astigmatism, nonuniform refractive index, glare, halos, ghosting, diffraction, undercorrection, night visual disturbances, loss of the best-corrected visual acuity greater than two lines. In 87% of cases in our experience, there were two or more of these symptoms in the same eye. A decentration creates a pupil mismatch. Correction of this complication is difficult. In the near future the corneotopographic link with excimer laser delivery will give the surgeon an opportunity to treat with a topographically guided system. An aspheric algorithm can help achieve a subsequently smoother optical surface.

Decentration has been reported to occur more frequently after LASIK than after PRK. Although several studies demonstrate a mean ablation zone decentration of less than 0.7 mm, with a majority reporting a decentration of 0.3 to 0.6 mm, one study reports up to 32% greater than 1.0 mm decentration in treated eyes. Decentration is compatible with good visual acuity but rarely with comfortable vision. A 1.0-mm decentration with an optic zone of 4.0 mm results in one-third of light rays falling on the retina and passing through the untreated cornea. Before a diagnosis of decentration, it is important to be certain of the quality of the corneal flap. In undercorrection or loss of lines, an imperfect flap can induce refractive errors and even simulate decentration. Treatment can be performed as soon as the first week postoperatively by lifting the flap. This is very easy during such a short postoperative period. Improvement is usually rapid and the only complication is the risk of epithelial ingrowth, which is a potential undesired effect of every reintervention in corneolamellar surgery.

Surgical indications for decentration after LASIK are few, and its frequency is proportional to poor technique during the first procedure. Prevention is key. The main reason for reoperation is a loss of BCVA, but it is not easy to be certain that reoperation will increase the results if there is no undercorrection. The difficulty of surgery and the uncertainty of the indication explain why so few decentrations are surgically corrected.

THERE IS NO EASY SOLUTION TO TREAT DECENTRATION

Two different situations are recognized: decentration with major refractive errors and decentration with small refractive errors but rather important side effects. For the first situation, another operation is performed depending on the time since surgery. If decentration is still a problem during the first few days, new surgery in the same cornea layer is indicated. If the decentration is noticed many months after the new surgery, another LASIK procedure using a deeper flap thickness is performed. In the second case, a new photoablation directed to improve the refractive error as much as possible is enough to reduce side effects. In both cases, ultrasonic pachymetry indicates the potential for a new central ablation keeping in mind that 250 µm is the recommended residual corneal bed.

Case analysis is made with a corneotopographic map and by reviewing pre- and postoperative maps to get a

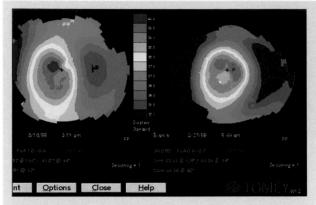

Figure 34E-1. Recentration of a LASIK treatment of hypermetropic astigmatism (new ring of +1 [+1 x +1]).

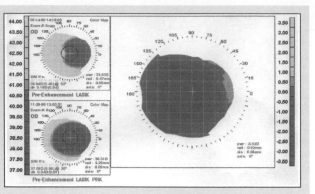

Figure 34E-2. Recentration LASIK post-decentered PRK.

sophisticated idea of the iatrogenic error. The decentration can be vertical, which is strongly suggestive of head displacement during laser delivery. A horizontal decentration is usually due to poor beam alignment. Pupil position is assumed to be central, but in some cases of high refractive error a nasal displacement is present and the laser must not be exactly centrated but very slightly moved to the temporal side of the central virtual pupil center. The light foveolar reflex is an important guide to fixation and there is a skill to learn with each laser model to achieve proper centering technique.

DECENTRATION TREATMENT TECHNIQUE

In myopia, the purpose of treatment is to correct residual undercorrection and decrease most of side effects. This depends on the particular excimer model. One of the most appropriate lasers is the one using a 2.0 mm flying spot. With this physical property the optic zone can be either small or larger in diameter, making a rather precise ablation.

Several techniques can be used:

1. New photoablation as large as possible, protecting the decentered zone. Fixation is made symmetrical to the decentration. The patient is asked to not fixate but to only allow his or her eye be moved by very thin forceps. There are two ways to protect the decentered zone: with a mask or a viscous solution. The mask can be made with a contact lens or Merocel sponge. The viscous solution is a viscous gel of methylcellulosis 1%, or diluted hyaluronate. The new ablation treats the spherical error. The power of the new photoablation is based on the topographic difference between the steepest and flattest meridian.

Treatment of an iatrogenic astigmatism should not be performed before this spherical treatment. In 27 of 41 cases such a technic is sufficient to obtain a recentered ablation zone (< 0.5 mm) and an uncorrected visual acuity greater than 20/40 without loss of more than two lines in all patients.

2. Another method consists of creating a new ablation zone of 2.0 mm diameter just opposite the decentered zone. The fixation is made symmetrical to the decentration. The patient is asked to not fixate but to only let his or her eye be moved by a very thin forceps. This technique works well with low refractive errors.

With both methods, we have to perform a new ablation that is asymmetric but complementary to the first ablation so that an area of uniform ablation is obtained. In all cases, the importance of the new ablation is difficult to calculate. Vinciguerra, with his own laser, multiplies the preoperative refractive error by a constant equal to 0.85 of the decentration in 1.0 mm (for an optic zone of 6.5 mm) The value works for a simple diaphragm and must be divided by the number of laser scans.

A final phototherapeutic keratectomy is performed to eliminate any irregularity of the photoablated surface.

Regardless of the method used, retreatment for decentration may be difficult, ineffective, and limited by the flap.

3. The Pallikaris technique creates relaxed corneal incisions in steep zones. This seems to give good results in experienced hands, but the paucity of peer review publications describing the technique does not create an incentive to adopt the procedure.

DECENTRATION RECENTRATION (RISK OF OVERCORRECTION IN THE CENTRAL ZONE)

Contact Lenses

Fitting contact lenses can be as useful as a complementary treatment of postoperative ablation decentration. Experience has shown that rigid gas-permeable lenses can usually be fit successfully, although postoperative keratometry readings are steeper than the true curvature.

After LASIK, the difference between soft and rigid contact lenses is reduced despite a better aptitude to vault in gas permeable contact lenses. The mid-periphery is normal without a steepened knee, as in incisional surgery. The central flattening post myopic LASIK is one of the easiest adaptations following refractive surgery. The epithelium is healed in a few weeks, there is no abnormal superficial scarring after PRK, there is no neo-vascularization risk as after radial keratotomy, and the microkeratome cut creates a plano-powered resection. In cases of decentration, all contact lenses are fit by the trial lens method. We feel, as does Al-Chuan Chou, that the postoperative keratometry measurement gives a reasonable idea of the base curve for the first trial. Of course, in corneal lamellar surgery the keratometry underestimates the central corneal flattening, but with decentration this problem is partially erased. A large diameter is required to facilitate centering for rigid lenses. With these lenses, a convex tear layer with plus refractive power must be compensated. Soft contact lenses are not the better choice for decentration because they have a tendency to move with lids movements as well as poor visual correction of optical aberrations.

Lens power calculation after decentered excimer ablation is a potential problem during the patient's future. Excentric ablation is encountered in 0.5% to 6% of the first 100 cases of beginning surgeons. Most patients have myopia and some individuals present scleral anomalies, staphyloma, and macular displacement. The calculation of an adequate intraocular lens may be problematic.

We know very little about IOL determination after refractive surgery. Most surgeons find a tendency to obtain hypermetropic refraction in pseudophakic patients who underwent refractive surgery. Knowledge of normal keratometry is very useful in achieving a better refractive outcome. Usually the change in refraction is subtracted from the preoperative corneal power. A hard contact lens trial is of great help before any myopic lens modification. The dioptric difference in the spectacle refraction before and after surgery is calculated and referred to the corneal vertex by using standardized tables; however, decentration can increase the risk of error. There is no firm recommendation in such cases. A cataract can attenuate the visual disturbance caused by decentration and complicate IOL calculation. A retreatment for recentration seems logical before cataract surgery. Once the cataract is present the only possible method is to estimate the lens power by the subtraction method, which necessitates knowing the preoperative corneal power. Patients must be advised that additional surgery may be necessary occur in the postoperative following months.

BIBLIOGRAPHY

Abbas UL, Hersh PS. Early corneal topographic patterns after excimer laser photorefractive keratectomy for myopia. *Journal of Refractive Surgery.* 1999;15:124-131.

Ai-Chuan C, Swinger CA, Cogger SK. Fitting contact lenses after myopic keratomileusis. *J Cataract Refract Surg.* 1999;25:508-513.

Astin CLK, Gartry DS, McSteele AD. Contact lens fitting after photorefractive keratectomy. *Br J Ophthalmol.* 1006;80:597-603.

Durrie DS, Aziz AA. Lift-flap retreatment after laser in situ keratomileusis. *Journal of Refractive Surgery.* 1999;15:150-153.

Gimbel HV, Anderson Penno EE. *LASIK Complications.* Thorofare, NJ: SLACK Incorporated; 1998.

Holladay JT. Cataract surgery in patients with previous keratorefractive surgery. *Ophthalmic Practice.* 1997;15:238-244.

Lyle WA, Jin GJC. Intraocular lens power prediction in patients who undergo cataract surgery following previous radial keratotomy. *Arch Ophthalmol.* 1997;115;457-461.

MCGhee CNJ, Ellerton CR. Complications of excimer laser photorefractive surgery. In: *Excimer Lasers in Ophthalmology.* London: Marin Dunitz; 1997.

Mulhern MG, Foley-Nolan A, O'Keefe M, Condon P. Topographical analysis of ablation centration after excimer laser photorefractive keratectomy and laser in situ keratomileusis for high myopia. *J Cataract Refract Surg.* 1997;23:488-494.

Perez-Santonja JJ, Ayala MJ, Sakla HF, Ruiz-Moreno JM, Alió JL. Retreatment after laser in situ keratomileusis. *Ophthalmology.* 1999;106:21-27.

Speicher L, Göttinger W. Intraocular lens power calculation after decentered photorefractive keratectomy. *J Cataract Refract Surg.* 1999;25:140-143.

Stulting RD, Carr JD, Thompson KP, Waring III G, Wiley WM, Walker JG. Complications of laser in situ keratomileusis for the correction of myopia. *Ophthalmology.* 1999;106:13-20.

Treating Excentric Ablations

Oscar D. Ghilino, MD

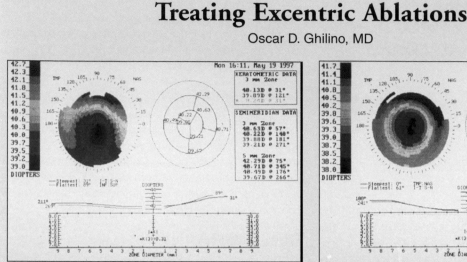

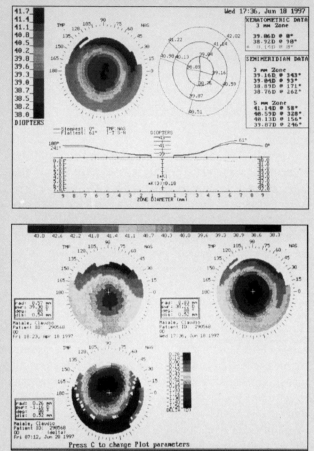

Decentration in LASIK is one of the most difficult complications with which we must deal.

A very careful ophthalmological and refractive examination is required before reoperating a decentered LASIK to determine the way in which the correction will be performed and if this problem should be corrected with a new lamellar refractive procedure.

A clear topographic analysis to determine the changes induced in the cornea and dioptric and elevation map will be very helpful to determine the way in which we should treat each particular case.

Pachymetry maps are also of great help and tell us whether we have enough residual cornea to make the reoperation, keeping in mind that we have to leave a total corneal thickness of 400 microns and a stromal bed of not less than 250 microns to prevent ectasia.

All decentrations promote irregular astigmatism, so we must determine whether we have decentration plus undercorrection or overcorrection.

For treating decentrations, we have to keep in mind that to correct a certain amount of myopia we have to remove a certain amount of stromal thickness and a certain width of optical zone to make a change in the corneal curvature based on Jose Ignacio Barraquer's law of thickness.

If we have an inferior decentration, we will have to ablate the cornea in the superior side, taking into account that as the optical zone will be enlarged, the resultant flattening will be less for the same thickness of ablation.

That is to say that if you ablate for myopia, 30 microns with an optical zone of 4.0 mm will induce more flattening and correction than the same thickness of ablation with an optical zone of 6.0 mm. Then, if we have, for example, a patient who was treated for -4 with an optical zone of 5.0 mm and it was displaced inferior, nasal, tem-

poral, or superior. When we add another ablation for 4 D in the opposite side, we will induce a change of the corneal curvature that will be the result of the whole optical zone and the whole depth of ablation. This allows us to enlarge the optical zone, recenter the ablation, and correct the refractive error; all these things are easy to postulate but not so easy to put into practice.

An aid in calculating the amount of ablation and the place where we have to put them over the cornea is the topographic simulation that permits us to simulate different approaches and how they look in the topography up to the time we obtain the better simulated result.

Presently, this treatment depends on the experience and skill of the surgeon, who must calculate the diameter, depth, number, and location of the areas to be ablated. We have to also take into account that the decentration is due to a decentrated ablation or if it depends on an incomplete flap in which the stromal bed was partially ablated and the inner surface of the flap was accidentally ablated.

In the case of a decentered ablation, we have to lift the flap and proceed with the additional ablations, always taking into account to leave enough stromal bed.

Other ways of treating the decentration have been proposed, such as making a new ablation and protecting the decentered area with different substances like methylcellulose, contact lens, etc, ablating the remaining areas. Another treatment consists of covering the surface of the cornea with a substance that reshapes its surface (biomask) with the ideal curvature. Afterward, ablate with PTK up to the corneal stroma to reshape its surface to the same shape of the biomask.

An important advance to treating decentration will be the use of topography-assisted excimer lasers that will automatically perform all the necessary calculations and simulations.

DIFFUSE INTERLAMELLAR KERATITIS: SANDS OF THE SAHARA SYNDROME

John F. Doane, MD

There has probably been no single entity that has caused more concern and speculation with the LASIK procedure than the clinical phenomenon of diffuse interlamellar keratitis (Figure 35-1). The major concerns are well warranted since the individual surgeon has been left to deal with a process that has been, until now, not that well understood. The surgeon and staff, without completely understanding the etiology let alone preventative steps, has had to accept very unwillingly the loss of control and potential for significant visual loss from this process. This entity was first described by Bobby Maddox of Texas in late 1996. The term *Sands of the Sahara syndrome* was coined by Kerry Assil of California because the clinical appearance resembled the shifting surface of desert sand.

The entity has received many different names including: diffuse lamellar keratitis, nonspecific diffuse intralamellar keratitis, diffuse intralamellar keratitis, nonspecific diffuse interlamellar keratitis, diffuse interlamellar keratitis, and lamellar keratitis. The author feels the most accurate anatomical name is diffuse interlamellar keratitis, since the process is between lamella and not within a lamella of corneal stroma per se.

DIFFUSE INTERLAMELLAR KERATITIS: THE CLINICAL ENTITY

Diffuse interlamellar keratitis (DIK) is typically noted 2 to 5 days postoperatively. The patient notices a progressive decrease in visual acuity. Slit lamp examination reveals a white cell infiltrate that is typically diffusely distributed across the interface. The condition, on occasion can involve only a sector or periphery of the interface. If bilateral simultaneous surgery is done, the condition can be uni- or bilateral. If unilateral, it typically affects the first eye, but there have been reports of only the second eye being affected. The white cells will delineate or highlight the ablation steps and chatter marks of the microkeratome. The flap and subkeratectomy stroma are not affected early in the process. Notably, the eyes are otherwise quiet. There is no conjunctival injection and no anterior chamber inflammation.

Jeff Machat has developed a three-tiered grading system to categorize the degree of inflammatory process. Grade 1 represents mild cases that usually resolve spontaneously over the first month. The clinical appearance is similar to trace or very mild photorefractive keratectomy (PRK) reticular haze with both vision and refraction unaffected. Grade 2 appearance could be compared to mild to moderate PRK haze that is more dense centrally (Figure 35-2). Best-corrected vision is usually reduced by one to two lines. The refractive error is slightly hyperopic. Patients are typically asymptomatic early but symptoms will progress unless aggressively treated.

Grade 3 results in a dense central infiltrate that can often be confused with a microbial infection and resembles grade 4 PRK haze. The patient will complain of decreased vision but will be surprisingly comfortable. The eye is otherwise quiet with no conjunctival discharge or anterior chamber reaction, although there have been reports of anterior chamber cell and endothelial keratic precipitates. The central flap may have striae over its surface but appears uninvolved as far as inflammatory cells. The stromal bed may appear to be minimally involved with inflammatory infiltrate. Best-corrected vision is usually decreased several lines from preoperative values and a few diopters of hyperopic astigmatism may be present upon refraction.

DIK: ETIOLOGIES

Historically, DIK has been termed nonspecific because no definitive causative factor has been defined. From a clinicians standpoint, it is important to define if

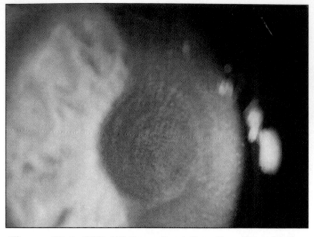

Figure 35-1. DIK. White cells delineating the ablation steps and chatter marks of the microkeratome (photo courtesy of Stephen G. Slade, MD).

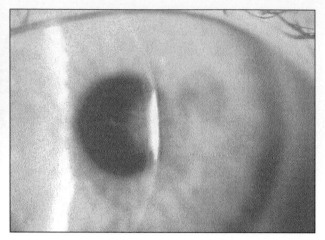

Figure 35-2. Clinical example of Grade 2 DIK (photo courtesy of Stephen G. Slade, MD).

the entity is an isolated sporadic case or if there are serial cases from several patients on the same operating day. Before addressing this important clinical point, it is important to define what DIK is, not by discussing several entities that could be confused with DIK.

EPITHELIAL TOXICITY

During the early postoperative period it is important to define the level of the pathology. Does it involve the corneal epithelium or does it reside in the interface? Figure 35-3 demonstrates epithelial toxicity at the 1-day visit from topical anesthetics and/or ink from epithelial marking for flap repositioning. It is very important, for obvious reasons, to make certain that a fine slit is achieved at the slit lamp to define the pathology at 160 microns or one-fifth of the corneal thickness. If there is fair certainty that the process is epitheliopathy, fluorescein staining will confirm this suspicion.

FLAP EPITHELIAL ABRASION

If a significant epithelial abrasion occurs on the flap, it is not uncommon for the patient to present with a classic "shifting sands" appearance in the interface. As the epithelial defect heals, the "sands" appearance resolves without any adverse effects. Two explanations for this appearance could be swelling of the cut ends of collagen fibrils or white blood cells layering in the interface as a healing response to the defect. Management consists of antimicrobial coverage and artificial tear application.

PERIPHERAL CORNEAL STROMAL COAGULATION VIA EXCIMER LASER BEAM

On rare occasions, I have noted a white ring opacity at the outer limits of the laser ablation. The ring is approximately 0.5 mm in width with somewhat feathered edges. I have postulated that the outer dimensions of the laser ablation does not achieve threshold fluence to effectively break molecular bonds (photoablate). Instead, the tissue is coagulated and a peripheral ring scar remains. This appearance can be noted as early as 24 hours after LASIK and will remain a chronic finding on slit lamp examination.

ENDOGENOUS MATERIAL

Meibomian Secretions

Probably the most frequent material deposited in the interface that could cause some confusion is the propensity for meibomian secretions to find their way onto the stromal surfaces. This can be minimized by conjunctival cul-de-sac irrigation with eye wash solution before initiating the procedure or interface irrigation with balanced salt solution (BSS) if foreign material is noted in the interface after flap repositioning.

Red Blood Cells

During the keratectomy, vessels from the peripheral

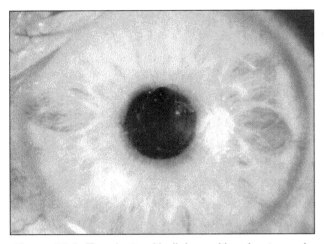

Figure 35-3. Transient epithelial opacities due to marking pin toxicity (photo courtesy of Stephen G. Slade, MD).

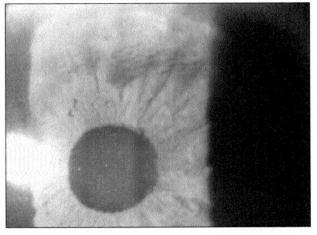

Figure 35-4. Red blood cells layered in the lamellar interface at 24-hour exam (photo courtesy of Stephen G. Slade, MD).

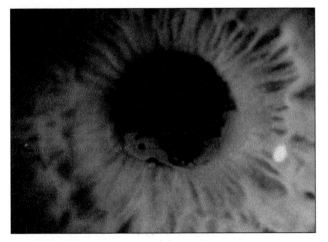

Figure 35-5. Marked inferior epithelial ingrowth. Note the cystic component and leading edge white line superior to the cystic component (photo courtesy of Stephen G. Slade, MD).

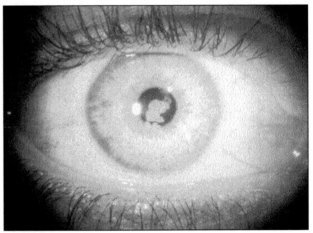

Figure 35-6. Central cystic epithelial ingrowth (photo courtesy of Stephen G. Slade, MD).

corneal vascular arcade can be incised and provide a source of red blood cells in the lamellar interface. Despite interface irrigation, some red cells may be evident at the 24-hour visit (Figure 35-4).

With time, these cells may lyse, leaving a white cast that could be confused for a white blood cell infiltrate. If the red blood cells are documented for location and extent at the 24-hour visit this can be used to ally fears about DIK if questions arise at later visits. Additionally, this situation would not demonstrate a progressive increase in opacity of the interface, as seen in DIK.

Epithelium

Epithelial ingrowth could also be confused with lamellar keratitis if appropriate clinical clues are not taken into account. The cystic appearance of epithelium in the interface could be confused with loculations of inflammatory cells. Unless the flap is melting, most eyes with epithelium in the lamellar interface, like eyes with DIK, are otherwise quiet with no anterior chamber reaction or conjunctival injection. Figures 35-5 through 35-9 depict several variants of epithelial ingrowth into the interface. It is important to delineate the depth of the pathology with oblique illumination of the slit beam. With epithelial ingrowth, it will be quite apparent that the process is in fact in the interface, as noted in Figure 35-7, and not on the corneal surface.

EXOGENOUS TOXINS

A host of exogenous toxins may be seen in the interface that should not be confused with an interface

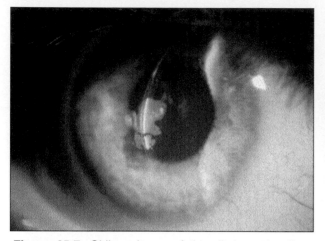

Figure 35-7. Oblique beam of the slit lamp localizes pathology to the lamellar interface (photo courtesy of Stephen G. Slade, MD).

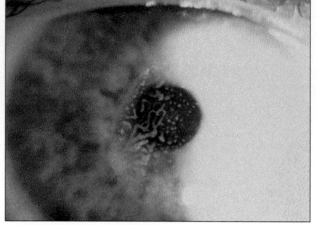

Figure 35-8. Central whorls of epithelial cysts (photo courtesy of Stephen G. Slade, MD).

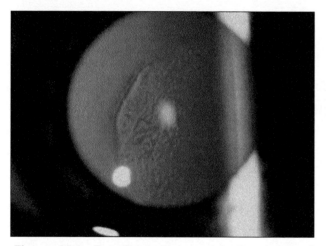

Figure 35-9. Retroillumination reveals the extent of ingrowth (photo courtesy of Stephen G. Slade, MD).

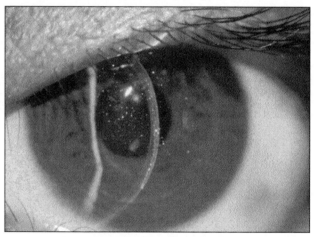

Figure 35-10. Oblique slit revealing talc particles at the depth of the interface.

inflammatory process. Virtually all are avoidable with proper instrument cleaning and a sterilization protocol.

Talc

If powdered gloves are used, it is very likely that talc will find its way into the interface. Once in contact with the raw stroma, it is extremely difficult to remove. From a visual standpoint, it is highly unlikely that talc will ever be implicated as the cause for unwanted visual symptoms during photopic or scotopic conditions. Figures 35-10 and 35-11 demonstrate typical appearances of talc contamination of the lamellar interface.

Oil

Microkeratome heads do not require lubricating oils to run properly. There have been reported cases of inter-face contamination with oils (Figure 35-12) that have been applied to microkeratomes for the intended purpose of making the microkeratome run smoother. It is assured that if the microkeratome has oils on its surface, they will find their way into the interface. Once in the interface, oil is virtually impossible to remove. Fortunately, it is highly unlikely to cause any loss of acuity or unwanted visual symptoms.

Instrument Milk

Instrument milk that is used to remove residue from surgical instrument surfaces has been applied to the microkeratome and can leave a similar appearance as seen in Figure 35-13. This is likely a toxicity reaction to the corneal collagen fibrils with white cell layering in the interface. This appearance is very similar to DIK.

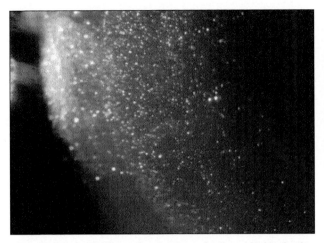

Figure 35-11. Diffuse distribution of talc particles in the interface.

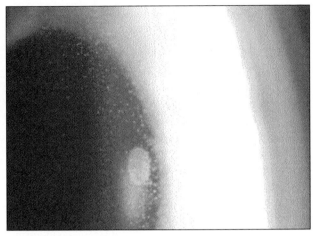

Figure 35-12. Oil from a microkeratome coating the stromal interface.

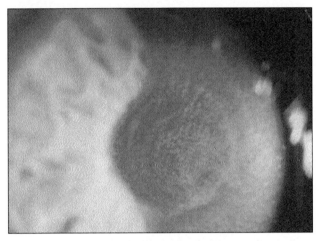

Figure 35-13. Appearance of the interface after instrument milk was placed on a microkeratome.

Nonsteroidal Anti-Inflammatory Drugs

Some surgeons have speculated that nonsteroidal anti-inflammatory drugs (NSAIDs) might play a role in DIK. This has been extrapolated from NSAID association with sterile subepithelial infiltrates with bandage contact lens use after PRK. There have been known cases of DIK in which no NSAID was administered and, likewise, the overwhelming majority of patients that have administered NSAIDs after LASIK do not present signs or symptoms of DIK.

Microkeratome Blades

Many have speculated that some aspect of blade preparation is responsible for DIK. Specifically, speculation has been that some chemical/toxin left on the blade surface during manufacture or sterilization incites an intense inflammatory reaction in the early postoperative period. To date, no specific compound has been identi-

fied. The fact that nonspecific DIK has not occurred with every surgeon who received blades from a specific lot takes away from this theory, making it merely speculation. Additionally, there have been reports of DIK occurring after LASIK-lifting enhancement when no blade or microkeratome has been in use.

BACTERIAL EXOTOXIN AND ENDOTOXIN ETIOLOGY OF DIK

It is my feeling that classical cases of DIK are likely due to bacterial exotoxins from eyelid colonization of bacteria in conditions such as staph marginal keratitis and endotoxins liberated from improperly cleaned microkeratome instrumentation.

I believe, in general, that DIK can occur in either isolated single occurrences (likely an endogenous exotoxin load from blepharitis) or consecutive serial cases (multiple cases on the same day from use of the same microkeratome) in which the endotoxin (bacterial cell wall lipopolysaccharide) contaminates the lamellar interface.

Bacterial Exotoxins

Bacterial exotoxins present in the tear film of patients with staphylococcal colonization of the eyelids can make its way into the lamellar interface and typically present as a focal white cell infiltrate within 24 to 48 hours after treatment at the flap periphery next to the gutter/eyelid intersection (classical 10, 2, 4, and 8 o'clock positions). These patients should be treated with topical corticosteroids to resolve the interlamellar inflammatory infiltrate and undergo standard staphylococcal marginal infiltrate management consisting of hot moist eyelid packs, eyelid scrubs, and antibacterial ointment application to the eyelid margin twice per day. Ideally, these potential cases should be noted and managed prior to LASIK treatment.

Bacterial Endotoxin Toxicity Scenario

There is a possibility that DIK can occur with any technique that uses a nondisposable instrument. Even if one uses a disposable keratome but still uses ancillary metal instruments, DIK is possible if certain cleaning, sterilizing, and drying practices are not maintained.

The first presumption is that the microkeratome, irrigating cannulas, or cleaning bath becomes contaminated from the patient, surgical environment, or possibly even the distilled water source with one of the ubiquitous gram-negative bacteria such as pseudomonas aeruginosa. Next, the instruments are cleaned and left wet and unsterile overnight. The bacteria, feeding upon residual trace protein and metabolites from cleaning, which is generally imperfect, subdivides at a rate of once every 20 to 40 minutes. In just 12 hours, the bacteria count is multiplied by roughly 16 million.

Let us then assume that the instrument is autoclaved in the morning, just prior to the first surgery of the day. In their death, all the accumulated bacteria release lipopolysaccharide (LPS) from their shells. This LPS is in no way detoxified by the autoclave. It coats the instrument(s), in particular the corneal chute of whatever microkeratome is being used. The instrument(s) are now highly contaminated with this LPS. In each keratectomy, the underside of the corneal flap is passed across this coating of LPS (Figure 35-14). LPS is well known to incite an extremely vigorous inflammatory reaction that will digest the stromal collagen in a relatively short time period.

DIAGNOSIS OF BACTERIAL ENDOTOXIN ETIOLOGY

Definitive diagnosis of a bacterial endotoxin as the cause of DIK is difficult and probably unlikely in almost all cases. In practice, there is nothing to culture since no live bacteria exist. Therefore, lifting and culturing the flap will not be of any utility. The endotoxin is virtually impossible to identify in vivo for the active practitioner let alone a dedicated bacteriologist. LAL assays are available to identify endotoxins on the surface of instruments, but would only be used after the fact or for identification before a particular instrument is to be used. Nevertheless, if a case of endotoxin-related DIK is encountered, it is recommended that all surgical instruments involved be laboratory tested for endotoxins. As

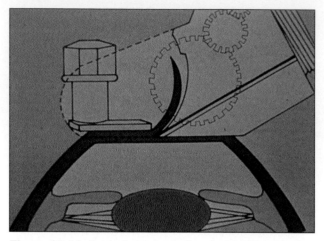

Figure 35-14. Posterior aspect of a corneal flap passing across an endotoxin-contaminated surface of a microkeratome's corneal chute.

mentioned above, LAL assay strips could be used. Special attention should be paid to the corneal chute of the microkeratome and to the interior of the cannula. The source of the endotoxin should then be deduced and eliminated by change of procedure.

MANAGEMENT OF BACTERIAL ENDOTOXIN DIK

The first key in management of endotoxin-related DIK is prompt identification and treatment. It is important to rule out active bacterial infection, epithelial ingrowth, and other causes of a DIK presentation (as previously noted). The mainstay of treatment is prompt and aggressive topical corticosteroid application. Prednisolone acetate or phosphate every hour is recommended during the first 24 to 48 hours with tapering depending on the clinical resolution. In rare circumstances flap lifting with irrigation in an effort to dilute toxin is necessary. It is not known if this technique actually removes an endotoxin. It may be that this act dilutes collagenases and minimizes tissue melting in aggressive cases. Some have advocated phototherapeutic keratectomy (PTK)-like ablation in grade 3 cases. It is likely that this will lead to some hyperopic shift. After the inflammatory process has abated and the clinical picture has stabilized, it is important to identify hyperopic shift and/or irregular astigmatism due to tissue melting. Hyperopic refractive errors can be treated with repeat LASIK. Irregular astigmatism can be treated with rigid contact lenses or with topography/wavefront analysis-assisted ablation techniques.

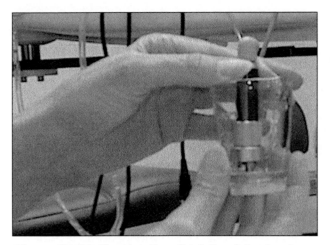

Figure 35-15. Running the distal tip of the keratome motor in anhydrous alcohol.

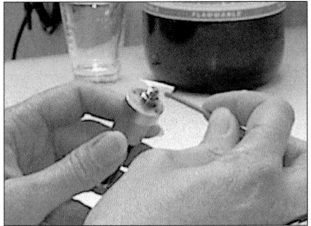

Figure 35-16. Drying the motor tip with a sponge.

ENDOTOXIN RELATED DIK AVOIDANCE: EQUIPMENT CLEANING PROTOCOL

The ultimate key to any complication is avoidance, so in this section, proper microkeratome hygiene etiquette will be reviewed in a step-by-step fashion.

1. At the end of the surgical day, place instruments in distilled water (room temperature) with a small amount of Palmolive soap. Scrub each instrument meticulously with a medium bristle toothbrush in and above the Palmolive bath. If there are any gears or moving parts on the microkeratome head, they should be rotated under the surface of the soap bath. Cannulated instruments should be flushed with distilled water followed by forced air from a syringe.

2. Remove the soap residue. One can dip and soak instruments directly in a separate bowl of distilled water or run under warm tap water and then move instruments to a distilled water bath soak for 10 to 15 seconds with gentle mixing of water.

3. Place instruments in the sterilizer. I use a STATIM sterilizer with a 5-minute cycle.

4. Remove the instrument tray from the sterilizer. Take the tray insert with instruments out of the tray. Manually dry the inside and outside of the tray and lid with a towel. Dry the inside and outside of the base and lid of the sterilization cassette with a towel and leave it disassembled and open to air. Use a hand held (hair) blow dryer to completely dry all surfaces of the keratome and instruments. Dry the back surface of the instrument tray insert and make certain all fluid col-

lecting around the "knobby fingers" of the top surface of the tray insert are free of standing fluid. I use a blow dryer and towel for this final step.

5. For an automated motorized advancement microkeratome, the motor external surface can be swabbed with an isopropyl alcohol swab. The external gear mechanism (one-fourth to five-eighths of an inch) should be advanced and reversed with the footswitch while submerged in anhydrous ethanol, which I prefer, or acetone. The pinion for blade oscillation should be depressed to express all fluid. A dry Merocel sponge can also be used to do this. The external threading should be dried. The motor should be stored upside down while not in use. The concern with this step is to prevent growth of bacteria on the driveshaft and inoculating the gear box with bacteria (between cases the geared pinion of the motor can be cleaned with alcohol and dried) (Figures 35-15 and 35-16).

For nonautomated advancement mechanisms, the physician should train his or her technical personnel on an appropriate cleaning ritual.

ADDITIONAL RECOMMENDATIONS

I would express caution to any facility or surgeon utilizing "traveling units" or obtaining "loaner" or demonstration units from any manufacturer to be aware of possible endotoxin load on the device that may not have been cleaned, sterilized, and stored in an appropriate fashion. If one of these units is planned for use, it would be prudent and behooves the surgical team to decontaminate the unit by soaking it in anhydrous ethanol for 5 to

10 minutes and then perform the previously mentioned sterilization routine.

It is also possible that the sterilization unit or even the distilled water used in sterilization could be contaminated with live gram negative bacteria that could, upon an active sterilization cycle, be the source of endotoxin. Sterilizer manufacturers can build systems to anticipate this scenario by having proper micropore filters in place to strain bacteria from the water as well as "charged" filters to actively absorb endotoxin.

The source of the problem, in the above theory, is failure to focus on the endotoxin problem created by large counts of certain dead bacteria. In the case of keratectomies, there are generally no problems attributable to live bacteria. The endotoxin-related DIK problem comes from liberation of lipopolysaccharide in the walls of certain dead bacteria. Overall, I believe endotoxin-related DIK is rare, yet, with an adherence to proper cleaning technique, should be totally avoidable. It is hopeful that ongoing research will provide additional substantiation of the endotoxin theory and additional preventative measures.

REFERENCES

1. Machat JJ. LASIK complications. In: Machat JJ, Slade SG, Probst LE, eds. *The Art of LASIK, Second Edition.* Thorofare, NJ: SLACK Incorporated; 1999.
2. Sterile interface inflammation after laser in situ keratomileusis: experience and opinions. *Journal of Refractive Surgery.* 1998;14:661-6.

Infections and Keratitis

Dimitrios S. Siganos, MD and Charalambos S. Siganos, MD

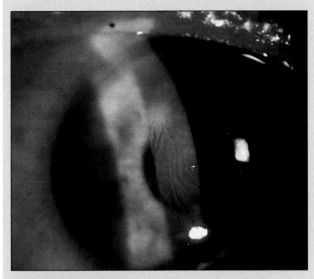

Figure 35A-1. Serratia keratitis following LASIK.

Keratitis following LASIK is not common; however, it should be considered a medical emergency. It usually appears between the second and sixth days following LASIK, and early recognition and prompt management are essential for restoration of the patient's vision with or without minimal sequelae. There are not many reports of keratitis following LASIK. Keratitis may be bacterial, viral, or related to toxins, dust, or other particles (eg, debris from the microkeratome blade, meibomian gland secretions, etc). Symptoms are pain, photophobia, redness, blepharospasm, and lacrimation. Signs depend on the causative agent. An interesting entity is that described by Smith and Maloney as a diffuse lamellar keratitis,[1] something that the authors believe is a new syndrome in lamellar refractive surgery. The infiltrate has the following characteristics:

1. It is confined to the interface, extending neither anteriorly into the flap nor posteriorly into the stroma.
2. It is diffuse and scattered through a large area.
3. There are multiple faint foci.
4. The infiltrates may be more concentrated around surgical debris.
5. There is little or no anterior chamber reaction.
6. There is no overlying epithelial defect.
7. The conjunctiva has relatively no inflammation, and there is little or no ciliary flush.

No surgical intervention was considered necessary and the authors managed this noninfectious keratitis using combined eye drops of ciprofloxacin and fluorometholone. In one of 12 cases, only fluorometholone was used without any antibacterial agents and the results were similar—all infiltrates resolving without sequelae.

Bacterial keratitis following LASIK has similar symptoms but with the following characteristics:

1. A single or dominant focus.
2. Extension anteriorly into the flap and posteriorly into the stroma.
3. Increasing opacity over time.
4. Stromal loss.
5. A significant anterior chamber reaction.
6. An epithelial defect if the infection develops on the surface or if an interface infection extends anteriorly.
7. Conjunctival inflammation with ciliary flush and discharge.

Bacteria blamed for this infection are nocardia,[2] mycobacterium chelonae, staphylococcus aureus and epidermidis,[3] streptococcus viridans, and serratia (unpublished data, Figure 35A-1). Viruses identified were adenovirus (unpublished data) and herpes simplex.

Early culture before initiating an antibacterial regimen is essential and surgical intervention in the form of raising the flap with proper washing and scrubbing with fortified antibiotic drops of tobramycin and ciprofloxacin before getting the culture results, as well as close follow-up, are essential. Continuation, alteration, and cessation of therapy depend on the clinical response.

Inflammatory reaction of the cornea caused by dust from surgical gloves, debris from the microkeratome blade, or meibomian gland secretions requires early washing of the interface and dexamethasone. Inflammation usually subsides within 5 to 15 days.

REFERENCES

1. Smith RJ, Maloney RK. Diffuse lamellar keratitis. A new syndrome in lamellar refractive surgery. *Ophthalmology.* 1998;105(9):1721-6.
2. Perez-Santonja JJ, Sakla HF, Abad JL, Zorraquino A, Esteban J, Alió JL. Nocardial keratitis after laser in situ keratomileusis. *Journal of Refractive Surgery.* 1997;13:314-317.
3. Detorakis ET, Siganos DS, Houlakis VM, Kozobolis VP, Pallikaris IG. Microbiological examination of bandage soft contact lenses used in laser refractive surgery. *Journal of Refractive Surgery.* 1998;14(6):631-5.

SANDS OF THE SAHARA

Eric J. Linebarger, MD, David R. Hardten, MD,
and Richard L. Lindstrom, MD

INTRODUCTION

Increasing popularity of the laser-assisted in situ keratomileusis (LASIK) procedure has created a veritable paradise for both physician and patient alike. With the volume of procedures growing exponentially, there is an expanding role for ophthalmologists and other eye care providers to be aware of an uncommon postoperative condition known as diffuse lamellar keratitis, which has the potential to derail an otherwise ideal outcome.

HISTORY AND EPIDEMIOLOGY

The first anecdotal reports of a mysterious post-LASIK inflammatory syndrome began to surface in the mid to late 1990s, in parallel with the rise in popularity and acceptance of the procedure. Maloney and Smith were the first to report on this unusual syndrome at the October 1997 American Academy of Ophthalmology meeting in Chicago. Their findings were later published in the March 1998 issue of *Ophthalmology*.[1] In their report, they described a peculiar, noninfectious, inflammatory reaction occurring in the lamellar interface shortly after LASIK. They documented 13 eyes with such a condition, characterized by a white, granular, diffuse, culture negative, lamellar keratitis occurring in the first week following surgery. In some eyes, the inflammation seemed to disappear almost spontaneously, while in other eyes, the condition worsened, followed by scarring and an adverse visual outcome. They termed the condition diffuse lamellar keratitis (DLK).

Further reports of this mysterious post-LASIK interface keratitis were presented at the 1998 American Society of Cataract and Refractive Surgeons meeting in San Diego by a variety of ophthalmologists, each noting a condition similar to that previously described by Smith and Maloney.[2,3] The condition would eventually come to be known by a variety of names, including Shifting Sands phenomenon or Sands of the Sahara syndrome, alluding to the white, granular appearance with waves of increased density.

Since the first documented case reports of this mysterious condition, a considerable amount of speculation has been focused on possible etiologies (Table 36-1). Anecdotal reports of case clusters seemed to point toward a contaminant in the lamellar interface introduced at the time of surgery. Indeed, Kaufman and others have used scanning, confocal, and electron microscopy along with liquid chromatography to document the presence of oil, wax, metallic, and other foreign particles in the LASIK interface.[4,5] Additional information has surfaced regarding the role of antigenic bacterial cell wall breakdown products in sterilization units that may lead to deposition of endotoxin into the interface, causing a sterile inflammatory response. Still other cases appear to be associated with epithelial defects at the time of surgery, or even delayed epithelial abrasions occurring weeks or months later. This cumulative evidence suggests that no one agent is completely responsible for the syndrome, and that a multifactorial etiology is likely.

While difficult to accurately document, the author's own experience suggests the incidence of severe vision-threatening DLK cases may be in the range of one in 5000, while very mild cases may be as frequent as one in 50. Despite efforts to eliminate potential causes of DLK, a growing number of cases are continuing to be reported in parallel with the expanding volume of LASIK procedures performed worldwide.

TREATMENT STRATEGY

The authors' experience in a high-volume LASIK practice has provided significant insight into this elusive condition, along with a strategy to successfully identify and manage this uncommon, yet potentially sight-threat-

Table 36-1
DLK: POTENTIAL SOURCES
√ Oil
√ Wax
√ Metallic fragments
√ Silicates
√ Betadine
√ Bacterial endotoxins
√ Epithelial defects
√ NSAID drops
√ Laser/contaminant interaction
√ Others?

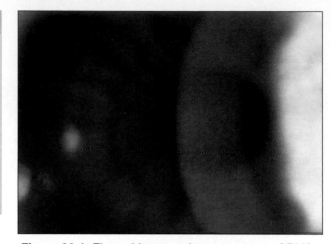

Figure 36-1. Fine, white, granular appearance of DLK.

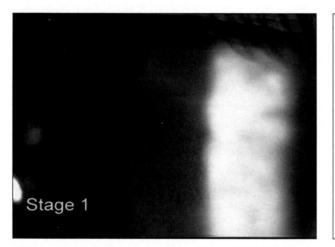

Figure 36-2a. Peripheral pattern of stage 1 DLK (photo).

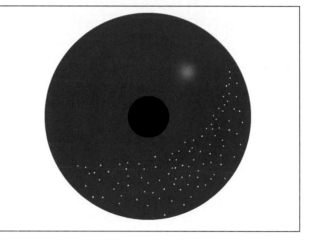

Figure 36-2b. Peripheral pattern of stage 1 DLK (diagram).

ening, complication. Our treatment strategy is three-fold, and includes:

1. Identifying cells in the lamellar interface
2. Staging their location and severity
3. Intervening at the appropriate point in time

Identification

Careful inspection by slit lamp examination on postoperative day 1 is crucial in identifying DLK, as the cellular reaction will almost always be present in the first 24 hours. A fine, white, granular reaction in the lamellar interface, frequently more prominent in the flap periphery, will be seen on day 1 (Figure 36-1). These cells should be carefully distinguished from epithelial surface abnormalities, such as punctate epithelial keratitis, epithelial edema, and tear film debris. The judicious use of fluorescein, as well as careful attention at the slit lamp, should eliminate any confusion. These cells should also be distinguished from meibomian gland

debris that occasionally finds its way into the lamellar interface. Meibomian gland secretions will have a glistening, oily appearance, unlike the flat, white, and granular appearance of DLK.

Staging

Once identified, a staging of severity and location can be made. We have found the following system helpful:

Stage 1. Stage 1 is defined by the presence of white, granular cells in the periphery of the lamellar flap, with sparing of the visual axis. This is the most common presentation of DLK at day 1, and with careful inspection, may be present in as many as one in 25 to 50 cases (Figures 36-2a and 36-2b).

Stage 2. Stage 2 is defined by the presence of white, granular cells in the center of the flap, involving the visual axis and/or in the flap periphery. This appearance, occasionally present at day 1, is more frequently seen on

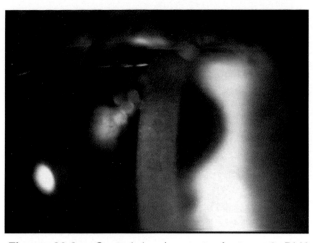

Figure 36-3a. Central involvement of stage 2 DLK (photo).

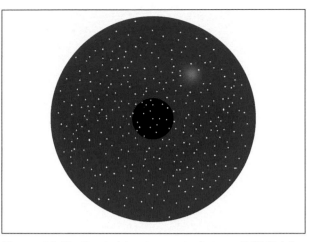

Figure 36-3b. Central involvement of stage 2 DLK (diagram).

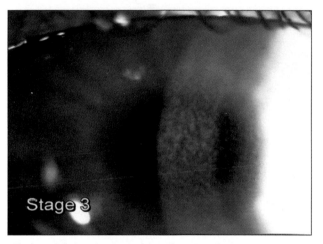

Figure 36-4a. Aggregation of more dense, white, and clumped cells in the visual axis of stage 3 DLK (photo).

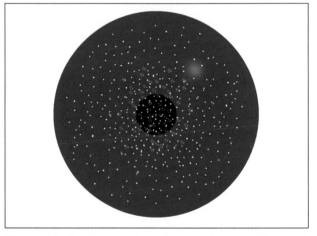

Figure 36-4b. Aggregation of more dense, white, and clumped cells in the visual axis of stage 3 DLK (diagram).

day 2 or 3, and is the result of central migration of cells in stage 1 DLK, giving it the so called "shifting sands" appearance. This occurs in approximately 1 in 200 cases (Figures 36-3a and 36-3b).

Stage 3. Stage 3 DLK is the aggregation of more dense, white, clumped cells in the central visual axis, with relative clearing in the periphery. This is often, but not always, associated with a subtle decline in visual acuity by one or two lines and a subjective description of haze by the patient. The cellular reaction collects in the center of the ablation and may settle with gravity slightly inferior to the visual axis. The frequency of stage 3 DLK may be as high as 1 in 500 cases (Figures 36-4a and 36-4b).

Identification of this more intense, central reaction of cells is paramount to preventing an unwanted outcome, for if left untreated, a significant portion of these eyes will go on to develop permanent scarring if left untreat-

ed. We have found that lifting the LASIK flap promptly following the appearance of stage 3, or when "threshold" DLK is present, can effectively blunt the inflammatory response and prevent permanent scarring from occurring. No eyes in our series have had any loss of best-corrected visual acuity (BCVA) when the interface is irrigated promptly following the identification of stage 3.

Stage 4. Stage 4 DLK is the rare end result of a severe lamellar keratitis with stromal melting, permanent scarring, and associated visual morbidity. The aggregation of inflammatory cells and release of collagenases result in fluid collection in the central lamellae, with overlying bullae formation and stromal volume loss. A hyperopic shift due to central tissue loss, along with the appearance of corrugated "mud cracks," are an ominous sign. Lifting and irrigating at this point is of little benefit and may actually result in additional stromal volume loss if aggressive tissue manipulation is performed. Proper

Figure 36-5a. Waves of increased density and permanent scarring associated with stage 4 DLK (photo).

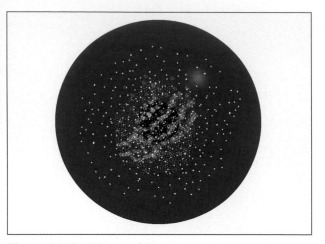

Figure 36-5b. Waves of increased density and permanent scarring associated with stage 4 DLK (diagram).

identification, grading, and appropriate intervention can prevent this from occurring. The incidence of severe stage 4 DLK is approximately one in 5000 (Figures 36-5a and 36-5b).

Intervention

A brief look at the timeline of DLK will illustrate the most appropriate time to intervene in the process (Figure 36-6). While the severity or stage of inflammation may differ from case to case, the time course of the disease is fairly consistent. Our experience has shown that cellular reaction is nearly always present at postoperative day 1 and peaks at approximately postoperative day 5. DLK can be best thought of as a "threshold" disease, meaning after a certain level of inflammation is reached, permanent scarring is likely to occur.

Stage 1 DLK, represented in Figure 36-6 in blue, will follow a self-limited course, resolving in 1 week to 10 days, as will stage 2 DLK, represented in green. Our management of both stage 1 and stage 2 DLK consists of topical steroid drops (flouromethalone 1%) administered every hour and steroid ointment administered at bedtime, although no randomized study has conclusively demonstrated this to be of benefit. Prompt follow-up in 24 to 48 hours will identify the minority of cases that will progress to stage 3.

Once stage 3 DLK is identified, management involves lifting the flap and debulking the inflammatory reaction by careful irrigation of the bed and undersurface of the cap. This should be performed as soon as stage 3 is identified, usually at postoperative day 2 or 3, in order to blunt the inflammatory response and prevent permanent scarring. As seen in Figure 36-7a, lifting all flaps at day 1 would miss the peak inflammatory reaction and result in unnecessary treatment of the majority of grade

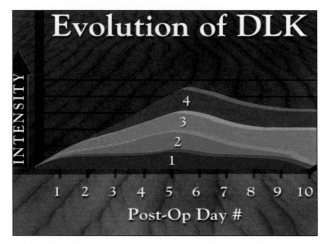

Figure 36-6. Timeline of DLK, with stage 1 (blue), stage 2 (green), stage 3 (orange), and stage 4 (red).

1 and grade 2 cases that are self-limited. However, Figure 36-7b shows that waiting until day 5 or 6 will risk the development of stage 4 DLK, with permanent scarring. Thus, we have found that lifting grade 3 DLK, usually at 48 to 72 hours after the initial procedure, is effective (Figure 36-7c).

The lifting procedure comprises of delineating the edges of the flap with a blunt spatula and lifting and retracting the flap peripherally to its hinge (Figure 36-8a). This can be accomplished with relative ease in the first 72 hours after surgery. Once the flap is retracted, the bed and undersurface of the cap are gently, but thoroughly, rinsed with balanced salt solution (BSS) from a blunt-tipped cannula (Figure 36-8b). The bed and cap are gently cleansed with a lightly moistened Merocel sponge. Bladed instruments and aggressive debriding is to be avoided. The flap is then carefully reflected, floated back into position, and allowed to dry in place. The

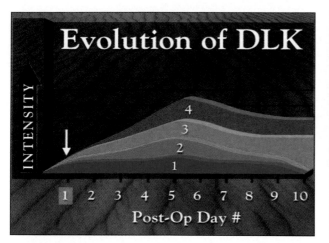

Figure 36-7a. Lifting of all flaps at day 1 misses the peak inflammatory response and results in unnecessary treatment of most stage 1 and 2 self-limited cases.

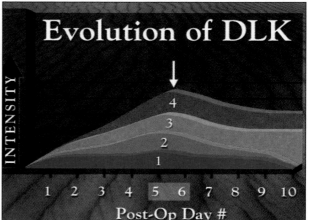

Figure 36-7b. Waiting until day 6 to lift the flap risks the development of stage 4, with permanent scarring.

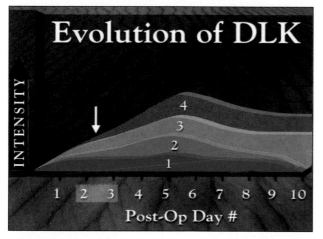

Figure 36-7c. Ideal time for lifting and irrigation of stage 3 DLK on day 2 to 3.

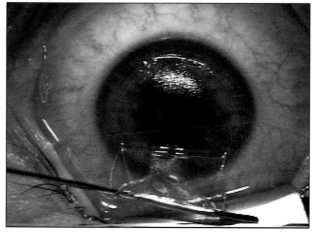

Figure 36-8a. Lifting the LASIK flap.

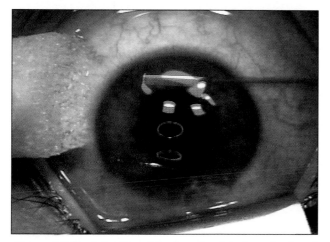

Figure 36-8b. Irrigation of the lamellar interface (bed and undersurface of cap).

patient is then maintained on continued intensive topical steroid administration for the next several days. This is tapered in concert with clearing and resolution of the cellular reaction.

CONCLUSION

In summary, management of DLK is a three-step approach:

1. Identification of granular white cells in the lamellar interface at day 1.
2. Staging the reaction, depending on the location and intensity of the cells.
3. Intervention, which comprises intensifying topical steroids for stage 1 and 2, with follow-up in 24 to 48 hours, and lifting and irrigation of the more severe stage 3 DLK, by postoperative day 2 or 3.

The proper identification and treatment of this mysterious condition will help keep LASIK an ideal treatment for physician and patient alike.

REFERENCES

1. Smith RJ, Maloney RK. Diffuse lamellar keratitis: a new syndrome in refractive surgery. *Ophthalmology.* 1998;105:1721-1726.
2. Maddox R, Hatsis A. Sands of the Sahara syndrome (poster). Presented at the American Society of Cataract and Refractive Surgeons annual meeting. San Diego, Calif; April 1998.
3. Gunn JL, Forstot SL, Hatsis A, et al. Sands of the Sahara: post-LASIK interface inflammation-reality or mirage? Presented at the American Society of Cataract and Refractive Surgeons annual meeting. San Diego, Calif; April 1998.
4. Kaufman SC, Maitchouk DY, Chiou AG, Beuerman RW. Interface inflammation after laser in-situ keratomileusis-sands of the Sahara syndrome. *J Cataract Refract Surg.* 1998;24:1589-1593.
5. Kaufman SC. Post-LASIK interface keratitis, sands of the Sahara syndrome, and microkeratome blades (letter). *J Cataract Refract Surg.* 1999;25:604-605.

Sands of the Sahara

Peter Stewart, MD

Synonyms include:
- DLK (diffuse lamellar keratitis)
- IK (interface keratitis)
- DIK (diffuse interface keratitis)

Interface keratitis is a noninfective inflammation of the LASIK interface of variable severity with an onset 1 to 5 days postoperatively. It is currently of unproven etiology, though bacterial toxins from instrument contamination are currently suspected.

DIAGNOSIS

If not diagnosed at slit lamp examination, symptoms are reported as decrease in quality of vision associated with a mild to moderate injection of the globe occurring up to 5 days postoperatively and photophobia.

Slit lamp examination in the early stages is characterized by a dusting of creamy colored leucocytes in the interface. They initially appear peripherally but later become diffuse. The cells can be seen occupying the linear potential spaces created by the oscillating keratome blade or arranged circularly in the steps of the broad-beam laser ablation profile. Hence, the reference to "sands" began in early reports of these cases. The eye is characteristically only mildly inflamed.

More severe cases that progress are characterized by migration of the inflammatory activity centrally with associated edema, cellular activity in clumps, criss-cross folds and fibrous-appearing opacity largely confined to the central 4.0 mm or so of the flap surface.

Differential diagnoses include:
1. Bacterial interface infection that is likely to be associated with focal areas of infiltrate, purulent discharge, pain, and marked inflammation.
2. A variant of staph-hypersensitivity marginal keratitis where, frequently 1 day postoperatively, multiple oval areas of infiltrate appear just within the periphery of the flap. The eye is injected, but not purulent, and there is an associated meibomianitis usually associated with active seborrhoeic blepharitis. This condition responds dramatically to intensive topical steroids within 24 hours.

NATURAL HISTORY

The spectrum of severity is the most striking feature of Sands of the Sahara. This accounts for the variability of incidence from 1:200 to 1:1000. Clinics commonly report cases of interface keratitis occurring in clusters. Milder cases characterized by peripheral patches of "sands" will resolve within days with no central involvement on the usual postoperative regimen of topical steroids four times per day.

More severe cases progress to central infiltration edema, folds, or scarring that resolves over weeks to months with topical steroid therapy to a stage of optical clarity centrally on slit lamp examination. However, stromal lysis results in flattening/hyperopic change as well as induced astigmatism and loss of BCVA.

For up to 18 months, there can be gradual spontaneous improvement in BCVA, such that enhancement can be considered. Very severe cases can result in flap melting and permanent severe loss of BCVA.

ETIOLOGY

The leucocytes are presumably attracted from the limbal vasculature to the interface preferentially because of the presence of endogenous or exogenous chemotactic factors present there.

Chemotactic Factors

Injured tissues alone can be chemotactic, but extra stimuli can be supplied by the presence of foreign materials (organic or inorganic).

Organic sources are toxins from contaminant bacteria or those associated with preoperative meibomianitis. Demodex fragments have been identified from the interface in one of the author's cases. Meibomian microdroplets, keratin/squames, red blood cells, and Betadine have all been considered but largely discounted as potent etiological factors. Oil from the keratome gearbox has been incriminated early in the search for causation. Patients with connective tissue disease may be more likely to develop an inflammatory response to damaged stromal tissue. Bacterial toxins from pseudomonas aeruginosa, and acinetobacter lwoffi (both gram-negative).

TREATMENT

First, explain the condition and prognosis to the patient. Prompt initiation of hourly dexamethasone or prednisolone drops and ointment at bedtime is the most widely practiced treatment. Some use NSAID drops as an adjunct.

Clinical opinion to refrain from lifting and toileting

the interface surfaces is widely uniform, unless there is central involvement or obvious interface debris that could be toxic. Opinion is divided on lifting the flap when a central infiltrate is observed. If performed, it should only be done in the acute phase; and when irrigating and cleaning, care should be taken not to scour the stromal material with metal tools—the stroma can be soft and the corneal profile degraded by such vigorous cleaning.

Intensive topical steroid therapy should be tapered over weeks. Intraocular pressure should be assessed by day 10.

Late Treatment

As stated, resolution leads to eventual central optical clarity in nearly all cases. As BCVA improves, consideration can be given to enhancement after 1 year. Any LASIK procedure should be undertaken with a recut, not an attempted flap lift. Preoperative topical steroids and NSAIDs should be used in case endogenous predisposition to keratitis exists. Similarly, topical steroid should be administered every two hours during the first 24 hours after the procedure.

Prevention of the complication in this elective refractive procedure should be paramount. In the light of current theories on etiology, the following measures could be practiced:

1. Pretreatment of patients with blepharitis, meibomianitis, and infected eyes.

2. Meticulous cleaning of keratome heads and instruments should be undertaken, followed by sterilization and drying. This is to prevent overnight bacterial growth and to remove bacterial toxin formation.

3. Prior to commencement of a list, these instruments should be Alco-wiped prior to sterilization.

4. Consideration should be given to use of topical steroids administered every two hours during the first 24 hours postoperatively to abort or reduce the severity of toxic interface keratitis.

5. Using a similar rationale, preoperative NSAIDs could be employed to blunt the potential inflammatory response.

6. Patients with a history of corneal herpes simplex or autoimmune disease should not be considered for surgery.

7. A surgical technique to remove as much stromal debris and foreign material from the interface as possible should be routinely utilized. This will involve not only irrigation, but Merocel sponging as well as isolating the interface from cul-de-sac fluid. The author has experienced only one case of central interface keratitis in 5000 cases and has a rigorous interface cleaning surgical protocol.

BIBLIOGRAPHY

Alaa El Danasoury M. Prospective bilateral study of night glare after laser in situ keratomileusis with single zone and transition zone ablation. *J Refract Surg.* 1998; 14: 512-516.

Amm M, Dunker GW, Shhröder E. Excimer laser correction of high astigmatism after keratoplasty. *J Cataract Refract Surgery.* 1996;22:313-317.

Arbelaez MC, Pérez-Santonja JJ, Ismail MM, Alió JL, Chansue E, Güell JL, Tsai RJF, Gimbel HV. Automated lamellar keratoplasty (ALK) and laser in situ keratomileusis (LASIK). In: Serdarevic ON, ed. *Refractive Surgery. Current Techniques and Management.* New York: Igaku-Shoin; 1997.

Arenas-Archila E, Sanchez Thorin JC, Naranjo Uribe JP, Hernandez Lozano A. Myopic keratomileusis in situ: a preliminary report. *J Cataract Refract Surg.* 1991;17:424-435.

Argento C. LASIK and Central Islands. Presented at Pre-AAO Conference: Chicago, October 24-26, 1996.

Argento CJ, Cosentino MJ. Laser in situ keratomileusis for hyperopia. *J Cataract Refract Surg.* 1998;24:1050-1058.

Argento C, Cosentino M, Biondini A. Hyperopic LASIK. Presented at the Centennial American Academy of Ophthalmology. October 1996.

Argento C, Cosentino MJ, Moussalli MA. Intraocular pressure measurement following hyperopic LASIK. *J Cataract Refract Surg.* 1998;24: 45(letter).

Arshinoff S, D'Addario D, Sadler C, et al. Use of topical nonsteroidal anti-inflammatory drugs in excimer laser photorefractive keratectomy. J Cataract Refract Surg. 1994;20:216-222.

Avalos G. Personal technique in moderate and severe myopia. Buratto L, Brint S, Ferrari M. LASIK techniques. In: *LASIK Principles and Techniques.* Buratto L, Brint S, eds. Thorofare, NJ: SLACK Incorporated; 1998; 195-202.

Balazsi GA. Comparison of PRK and LASIK to Corrrect Low and Moderate Myopia. Presented at Pre-AAO Conference. Chicago; October 24-26, 1996.

Barraquer C. Laser in situ keratomileusis. LASIK techniques. In: Buratto L, Brint S, eds. *LASIK Principles and Techniques.* Thorofare, NJ: SLACK Incorporated; 1998; 215-224.

Barraquer C. The microkeratome. In: Buratto L, Brint S, eds. *LASIK Principles and Techniques.* Thorofare, NJ: SLACK Incorporated;1998; 167-174.

Barraquer C, Gutierez A, Espinoza A. Myopic keratomileusis: short-term results. *Refract Corn Surg.* 1989;5:307-313.

Barraquer JI. Keratomileusis for myopia and aphakia. *Ophthalmology.* 1981;88:701-708.

Barraquer RI, Kargachin M, Alvarez de Toledo JP. Personal technique for the correction of myopic ametropia. In: Buratto L, Brint S, eds. *LASIK Principles and Techniques.* Thorofare, NJ: SLACK Incorporated; 1998; 229-246.

Barraquer Moner JI, Barraquer Granados JI. Intrastromal keratomileusis: complications associated with the microkeratome. In: Buratto L, Brint S, eds. *LASIK Principles and Techniques.* Thorofare, NJ: SLACK Incorporated; 1998; 365-370.

Bas AM, Onnis R. Excimer Laser in situ Keratomileusis for myopia. *J Refract Surg.* 1995;11(suppl):229-233.

Bende T, Seiler T, Wollensak J. Side effects in excimer corneal surgery. *Graefes Arch Clin Exp Ophthalmol.* 1988;226:277-288.

Bianchi C. I coloranti vitali in oftalmologia. *Contattologia medica e chirurgia refrattiva.* 1988; 9:101-117.

Boxer Wachler BS, Krueger RR. Normalized contrast sensitivity values. *J Refract Surg.* 1998; 14: 463-466.

Brint SF. Treatment of Pain and Photophobia After PRK. Presented at PRE-AAO Conference. Chicago; October 24-26, 1996.

Brint SF, Ostrich DM, Fischer C, et al. Six-month results of the multicenter phase I study of excimer laser myopic keratomileusis. *J Cataract Refract Surg.* 1994;20:610-615.

Buratto L. Intrastromal photoablation with excimer laser for the treatment of high myopia. Presented at the First Italian Meeting on Excimer Laser. Mestre (Venice); January 1990.

Buratto L. Down-Up LASIK. Presented at Pre-AAO Conference. Chicago; October 24-26, 1996.

Buratto L. A new device for a LASIK Surgeon in Training. Presented at Pre-AAO Conference. Chicago; October 24-26, 1996.

Buratto L. Personal LASIK technique with nasal hinge. In: Buratto L, Brint S, eds. *LASIK Principles and Techniques.* Thorofare, NJ: SLACK Incorporated; 1998; 203-214.

Buratto L. Down-Up LASIK. Presented at the IOMSG Congress. Tangensee; September 2, 1996.

Buratto L. Down Up LASIK. Presented at ISRK Pre-AAO Conference: Chicago; October 24-26, 1996.

Buratto L. Down-up LASIK is latest chapter in development of lamellar refractive surgery. *Ocular Surgery News.* Nov. 1996:22-23.

Buratto L. Down-Up LASIK with the Chiron Hansatome. In: Machat JJ, Slade SG, Probst LE. *The Art of LASIK. 2nd ed.* Thorofare, NJ: SLACK Incorporated; 1999; 95-108

Buratto L. Down-up LASIK. In: Buratto L, Brint S, eds. *LASIK Principles and Techniques.* Thorofare, NJ: SLACK Incorporated; 1998; 289-302.

Buratto L, Brint S, Ferrari M. Surgical Instruments. In: Buratto L, Brint S, eds. *LASIK Principles and Techniques.* Thorofare, NJ: SLACK Incorporated; 1998; 35-68.

Buratto L, Brint S, Ferrari M. LASIK techniques. In: Buratto L, Brint S, eds. *LASIK Principles and Techniques.* Thorofare, NJ: SLACK Incorporated; 1998; 259-268.

Buratto L, Brint S, Ferrari M. Keratomileusis. In: Buratto L, Brint S, eds. *LASIK Principles and Techniques.* Thorofare, NJ: SLACK Incorporated; 1998; 9-22.

Buratto L, Brint S, Ferrari M. Preoperative considerations. In: Buratto L, Brint S, eds. *LASIK Principles and Techniques.* Thorofare, NJ: SLACK Incorporated; 1998; 23-34.

Buratto L, Brint S, Ferrari M. Flap repositioning and postoperative management. In: Buratto L, Brint S, eds. *LASIK Principles and Techniques.* Thorofare, NJ: SLACK Incorporated; 1998; 133-139.

Buratto L, Brint S, Ferrari M. LASIK techniques. In: Buratto L, Brint S, eds. *LASIK Principles and Techniques.* Thorofare, NJ: SLACK Incorporated; 1998; 73-102.

Buratto L, Brint S, Ferrari M. LASIK complications. In: Machat JJ, Slade SG, Probst LE. *The Art of LASIK. 2nd ed.* Thorofare, NJ: SLACK Incorporated; 1999; 339-358

Buratto L, Brint S, Ferrari M. Complications. In: Buratto L, Brint S, eds. *LASIK Principles and Techniques.* Thorofare, NJ: SLACK Incorporated; 1998; 113-132.

Buratto L, Ferrari M. Homoplastic Keratomileusis: Clinical Results. Presented at First International Meeting about Myopic Keratomileusis. Mestre(Venice); June 1990.

Buratto L, Ferrari M. Excimer laser intrastromal keratomileusis: case reports. *J Cataract Refract Surg.* 1992;18:37-41.

Buratto L, Ferrari M. Intrastromal keratomileusis with excimer laser (Buratto's technique): long term clinical results. Presented at the International Meeting on Cataract and Refractive Surgery, San Diego; April 1992.

Buratto L, Ferrari M. The excimer laser in myopic keratomileusis. Presented at the First Internationl Congress on the Myopic Keratomileusis. Mestre (Venice); June 1990.

Buratto L, Ferrari F. Photorefractive keratectomy or keratomileusis with excimer laser in surgical correction of the severe myopia: which technique is better? *Eur J Implant Refract Surg.* 1993;5:183-186.

Buratto L, Ferrari M. LASIK: indications, technique, results, limits and complications. *Current Opionion in Ophthalmol.* 1997 (in press).

Buratto L, Ferrari M. Prevention and Management of Complications of Lamellar Refractive Surgery. In: Serdarevic ON, ed. *Refractive Surgery, Current Techniques and Management.* New York: Isaku-Shoin; 1997:151-163.

Buratto L, Ferrari M, Genisi C. Intrastromal keratomileusis by excimer laser (193 nm): clinical results with 1 year follow up. Presented at the First Annual Congress of the Summit International Laser User Group. Geneve; September 1991.

Buratto L, Ferrari M, Genisi C. Myopic keratomileusis with the excimer laser: one-year follow-up. *Refract Corneal Surg.* 1993;9:12-19.

Buratto L, Ferrari M, Rama P. Excimer laser intrastromal keratomileusis. *Am J Ophthalmol.* 1992;112:291-295.

Buratto L, Genisi C, Ferrari M. Intrastromal keratomileusis with excimer laser (Buratto's technique): short term clinical results. Presented at the Second Annual Congress of the Summit International Laser User Group. Montreux; September 1992.

Cantera E. Corneal topography in LASIK. In: Buratto L, Brint S, eds. *LASIK Principles and Techniques.* Thorofare, NJ: SLACK Incorporated; 1998; 157-166.

Casebeer JC. Systematized approach to LASIK. In: Buratto L, Brint S, eds. *LASIK Principles and Techniques.* Thorofare, NJ: SLACK Incorporated; 1998; 225-228.

Casebeer JC, Ruiz L, Slade SG, eds. *Lamellar Refractive Surgery.* Thorofare, NJ: SLACK Incorporated; 1996.

Casebeer JC, Slade SG, Dybbs A, Mahanti RL. Intraoperative Pachimetry

During Automated Lamellar Keratoplasty. *Refract Corneal Surg.* 1994;10:41-44.

Castellanos A. One Year Results of LASIK for High Myopia Using a Multizone Program. Presented at Pre-AAO Conference. Chicago, October 24-26, 1996.

Chayet AS, Assil KK, Montes M, Espinosa-Lagana M, Castellanos A, Tsioulias G. Regression and its mechanisms after laser in situ keratomileusis in moderate and high myopia. *Ophthalmology.* 1998; 105:1194-1199.

Cherry PM, Tutton MK, Adhikary HB, et al. The treatment of pain following photorefractive keratectomy. *J Refract Corneal Surg.* 1994;10(suppl):S222-S225.

Chu YR. The Efficacy, Predictability and Safety of LASIK in the Treatment of Low Myopia. Presented at PRE-AAO Conference. Chicago; October 24-26, 1996.

Crews KR, Mifflin MD, Olson RJ. Complications of automated lamellar keratectomy. *Arch Ophtalmology.* 1994;112:1514-5.

Ditzen K, Huschka H, Pieger S. LASIK for hyperopia. In: Buratto L, Brint S, eds. *LASIK Principles and Techniques.* Thorofare, NJ: SLACK Incorporated; 1998; 269-276.

Doane JF, Cavanaugh TB. Optical Zone Centration for keratorefractive surgery. *Ophthalmology.* 1994;101:215-216.

Doane JF, Slade SG. Microkeratomes. In: Machat JJ, Slade SG, Probst LE. *The Art of LASIK. 2nd ed.* Thorofare, NJ: SLACK Incorporated; 1999; 79-94.

Durrie DS, Aziz AA. Lift-flap retreatment after laser in situ keratomileusis. *J Refract Surg.* 1999;15:150-153.

Durrie DS, Lesher MP, Hunkeler TD. Treatment of overcorrection after myopic photorefractive keratectomy .*J Refract Corneal Surg.* 1994;10:295.

Edmison DR. Haze After PRK. Presented at Pre-AAO Conference. Chicago; October 24-26, 1996.

Emara B, Probst LE, Tingey DP, Kennedy DW, Willms LJ, Machat J. Correlation of intraocular pressure and central corneal thickness in normal myopic eyes and after laser in situ keratomileusis. *J Cataract refract Surg.* 1998;24:1320-1325.

Emara B, Probst LE, Tingey DP, Kennedy DW, Willms LJ, Machat JJ. Intraocular pressure and central corneal thickness following LASIK. In: Machat JJ, Slade SG, Probst LE. *The Art of LASIK. 2nd ed.* Thorofare, NJ: SLACK Incorporated; 1999; 445-450.

Epstein D, Tengroth B, Fagerholm P, Hamberg-Nystrom. *Reoperations in Corneal Laser Surgery.* St. Louis, Mo: Mosby-Year Book Inc; 1995.

Evans DW. Comparison of Contrast Sensitivity and Contrast Acuity in Lasik and PRK. Presented at Pre-AAO Conference. Chicago; October 24-26, 1996.

Farah SG, Azar DT, Gurdal C, Wong J. Laser in situ keratomileusis: literature review of a developing technique. *J Cataracxt Refract Surg.* 1998;24:989-1006.

Faucher A, Grégoire J, Blondeau P. Accuracy of Goldmann tonometry after refractive surgery. *J Cataract Refrac Surg.* 1997;23:832-838.

Ferrari M. Use of topical nonsteroidal anti-inflammatory drugs after photo refractive keratectomy. *J Refract Corneal Surg.* 1994;10(suppl):S287-S289.

Fiander D. LASIK complications in the first 1000 cases. Presented at Pre-AAO Conference: Chicago; October 24-26, 1996.

Fiander DC, Tayfour F. Excimer Laser in situ keratomileusis in 124 myopic eyes. *J Refract Surg.* 1995;11(suppl):S234-S238.

Fournier AV, Podtetenev M, Lemire J, et al. Intraocular pressure change measured by Goldmann tonometry after laser in situ keratomileusis. *J Cataract Refract Surg.* 1998;24:905-910.

Fukasaku H. Delayed Wound Healing in LASIK. Presented at Pre-AAO Conference. Chicago; October 24-26, 1996.

Gartry D, Kerr Muir MG, Marshall J. The effect of topical corticosteroids on refractive outcome and corneal haze after photorefractive keratectomy. A prospective, randomized, double-blind trial. *Arch Ophthalmol.* 1992;110:944-952.

Gartry D, Kerr Muir MG, Marshall J. Excimer laser photorefractive keratectomy. *Ophthalmology.* 1992;99:1209-1219.

Gimbel HV. Flap complications of lamellar refractive surgery. Editorial. *Am J Ophthalmol.* 1999;127:202-204.

Gimbel HV, Anderson Penno EE. *LASIK Complications. Prevention and Management.* Thorofare, NJ: Slack Incorporated; 1999.

Gimbel H, Surenda B, Kaye G, Ferensowicz M. Experience During the learning curve of laser in situ keratomileusis. *J Cataract Refract Surg.* 1996;22:542-550.

Gomes M. Laser in situ keratomileusis for myopia using manual dissection. *J Refract Surg.* 1995;11(suppl):S239-S243.

Gomes M. Keratomileusis in situ using manual dissection of corneal flap for high myopia. *J Refract Corneal Surg.* 1994;10:255-257.

Guell J. How to retreat after LASIK: undercorrection, overcorrection and epithelial ingrowth. Presented at Pre-AAO Conference. Chicago; October 24-26, 1996.

Guell J. Keratomileusis following other procedures. In: Buratto L, Brint S, eds. *LASIK Principles and Techniques.* Thorofare, NJ: SLACK Incorporated; 1998; 351-358.

Güell JL, Muller A. Laser in situ keratomileusis (LASIK) for myopia from -7 to -18 Diopters. *J Refract Surg.* 1996;12:222-228.

Guell JL, Muller A de, Gris O, Manero F, Vasquez M. LASIK after corneal and intraocular surgery. In: Machat JJ, Slade SG, Probst LE. *The Art of LASIK. 2nd ed.* Thorofare, NJ: SLACK Incorporated. 1999; 329-338.

Guimaraes R. LASIK using the clear corneal molder microkeratome. Presented at Pre-AAO Conference. Chicago; October 24-26, 1996.

Gutierrez AM. Reoperations with excimer laser. In: Buratto L, Brint S, eds. *LASIK Principles and Techniques.* Thorofare, NJ: SLACK Incorporated; 1998; 339-350.

Haight D. Slipped flap, irregular astigmatism and undercorrection after automated lamellar keratoplasty (Consultations). *J Refract Surg.* 1996;12:645-648.

Haimovici R, Culbertson WW. Optical lamellar keratoplasty using the Barraquer microkeratome. *Refract Corneal Surg.* 1991;7:42-45.

Handzel A. LASIK complications: how to avoid them? Presented at Pre-AAO Conference. Chicago; October 24-26, 1996.

Hanna KD, David T, Besson J, Pouliquen Y. Lamellar keratoplasty with the Barraquer microkeratome. *Refract Corneal Surg.* 1991;7:177-181.

Haw WW, Manche EE. Sterile peripheral keratitis following laser in situ keratomileusis. *J Refract Surg.* 1999;15:61-63.

Hersh PS, Shah SI, Durrie D. Monocular Diplopia Following Excimer Laser Photorefractive Keratectomy After Radial Keratotomy. *Ophthalmic Surg Lasers.* 1996;27(4):315-7.

Hoffman RF, Bechara SJ. An Indipendent Evaluation of second generation suction microkeratomes. *Refract Corneal Surg.* 1992;8:348-354.

Hoffman CJ, Rapuano CJ, Cohen EJ, Laibson PR. Displacement of Corneal Lenticle After Automated Lamellar Keratoplasty (Letter). *Am J Ophthal.* 1994;118:109-111.

Hoyos JE, Cigales M. Contact lens-induced and pachymetric modifications. In: Buratto L, Brint S, eds. *LASIK Principles and Techniques.* Thorofare, NJ: SLACK Incorporated; 1998; 151-156.

Ibrahim O, Waring GO, Salah T, Maghraby AE. Automated in situ keratomileusis for myopia. *J Refract Surg.* 1995;11:431-441.

Jones SS, Azar RG, Cristol SM, et al. Effects of laser in situ keratomileusis (LASIK) on the corneal endothelium. *Am J Ophthalmol.* 1998;125:465-471.

Kelley C. Diclofenac Sodium Used in Treating pain and Photophobia. Presented at Pre-AAO Conference. Chicago; October 24-26, 1996.

Keuch RJ, Bleckmann H. Comparison of three microkeratomes used for keratomileusis in situ in a swine model. *J Cataract Refract Surg.* 1999;25:24-31.

Kim K, Jeon S, Edelhauser HF. Corneal endothelial permeability after deep excimer laser ablation. *Invest Ophthalmol Vis Sci.* 1996;37:S84.

Kirkness CM, Ficker LA, Steele AD, Rice NS. Refractive surgery for graft-induced astigmatism after penetrating keratoplasty for keratoconus. *Ophthalmology.* 1991;98:1786-92.

Knorz MC. Assembly of the microkeratome and personal LASIK technique. In: Buratto L, Brint S, eds. *LASIK Principles and Techniques.* Thorofare, NJ: SLACK Incorporated; 1998; 175-184.

Knorz MC. Topography-assisted LASIK: reshaping the future. In: Buratto L, Brint S, eds. *LASIK Principles and Techniques.* Thorofare, NJ: SLACK Incorporated; 1998; 303-306.

Knorz MC, Liermann A, Seiberth V, et al. Laser in situ keratomileusis to correct myopia of -6.00 To -29.00 diopters. *J Refract Surg.* 1996;12:575-684.

Kremer FB, Dufek M. Excimer laser in situ keratomileusis. J Refract Surg. 1995;11:5244-5247.

Kremer FB. LASIK to Treat Primary Myopia with and without Astigmatism. Presented at PRE-AAO Conference. Chicago, October

24-33, 1996.

Kritzinger M, Probst LE. LASIK after penetrating keratoplasty. In: Machat JJ, Slade SG, Probst LE. *The Art of LASIK. 2nd ed.* Thorofare, NJ: SLACK Incorporated. 1999; 325-328.

Krumeich JH. Indications, techniques, and complications of myopic keratomileusis. *Intl Ophthalmol Clin.* 1983;23:75-92

Krumeich J. Indications, techniques and complications of myopic keratomileusis. In: Binder PS, ed. Refractive Corneal Surgery: the Correction of Aphakia, Hyperopia and Myopia. *Intl Ophthalmol Clinics.* Boston, Mass: Little, Brown and Co; 1983:75-92.

Lee DY. LASIK with a Turbokeratome—Visx Excimer Laser. Presented at Pre-AAO Conference. Chicago; October 24-26, 1996.

Lin RT, Maloney RK. Flap complications associated with lamellar refractive surgery. *Am J Ophthalmol.* 1999;127:129-136.

LiVecchi JT. The SCMD microkeratome. In: Buratto L, Brint S, eds. *LASIK Principles and Techniques.* Thorofare, NJ: SLACK Incorporated; 1998; 277-288.

Lohmann CP, Fitzke F, O'Brart D, et al. Corneal light scattering and visual performance in myopic individuals with spectacles, contact lenses, or excimer laser photorefractive keratectomy. *Am J Ophthalmol.* 1993;115:444-453.

Lohmann CP, Gartry D, Kerr Muir M, et al. Corneal haze after excimer laser refractive surgery. Objective measurements and functional implications. *Eur J Ophthalmol.* 1991;1:73-80.

Lugo M, Donnenfeld EO, Arentsen JJ. Corneal wedge resection for high astigmatism following penetrating keratoplasty. *Ophthalmic Surg.* 1987;18:650-653.

Machat JJ. Multizone PRK versus multizone LASIK for high myopia: principles and results. ISRS Mid-Summer Symposium and Exhibition. Minneapolis, Minn; July 29, 1995.

Machat JJ, ed. *Excimer Laser Refractive Surgery: Practice and Principles.* Thorofare, NJ: SLACK Incorporated; 1996.

Machat JJ. LASIK retreatment technique and results. In: *Excimer Laser Refractive Surgery: Practice and Principles.* Machat JJ, ed. Thorofare, NJ: SLACK Incorporated; 1996.

Machat JJ. Preoperative myopic and hyperopic LASIK evaluation. In: Machat JJ, Slade SG, Probst LE. *The Art of LASIK. 2nd ed.* Thorofare, NJ: SLACK Incorporated; 1999; 127-140.

Machat JJ. Postoperative LASIK management. In: Machat JJ, Slade SG, Probst LE. *The Art of LASIK. 2nd ed.* Thorofare, NJ: SLACK Incorporated; 1999; 241 262.

Maddox R, Hatsis A. Shifting sands of the Sahara. Interface inflammation following LASIK. In: Gimbel HV, Anderson Penno EE. *LASIK Complications. Prevention and Management.* Thorofare, NJ: SLACK Incorporated; 1999; 30-36.

Maguire LJ, Klyce SD, et al. Visual distortion after myopic keratomileusis: computer analysis of keratoscopy photography. *Ophthalmic Surgery.* 1987;18:352-356.

Maldonado-Bas A, Onnis R. Excimer laser in situ keratomileusis for myopia. *J Refract Surg.* 1995;11:S229-S233.

Maloney RK. Corneal topography and optical zone location in photorefractive keratectomy. *Refract Corneal Surg.* 1990;6:363-371.

Maloney R. Epithelial ingrowth after lamellar refractive surgery. Presented at Pre-AAO Conference. Chicago; October 24-26, 1996.

Manche EE, Maloney RK, Smith RJ. Treatment of topographic central islands following refractive surgery. *J Cataract Refract Surg.* 1998; 24: 464-470.

Marques EF, Leite EB, Cunha-Vaz JG. Corticosteroids for the reversal of myopic regression after photorefractive keratectomy. *J Refract Surg.* 1995;11(suppl):S302-S308.

Matta CS, Piebenga LW, Deitz MR, Tauber J. Excimer retreatment for myopic photorefractive keratectomy failures-six to 18 month follow up. *Ophthalmolgy.* 1996;103:444-451.

Montes M. Bandage contact leases after LASIK. Presented at Pre-AAO Conference. Chicago; October 24-26, 1996.

Moore CR. LASIK Pitfalls for the Beginning Surgeon. Presented at Pre-AAO Conference. Chicago; October 24-26, 1996.

Mortensen J, Carlsson K, Öhrström A. Excimer laser surgery for keratoconus. *J Cataract Refract Surg.* 1998;24:893-898.

Naranjo-Tackman R. The learning curve in LASIK: review of complications in the initial cases. Presented at Pre-AAO Conference. Chicago; October 24-26, 1996.

Pallikaris IG. Quality of vision in refractive surgery. *J Refract Surg.* 1998;

14: 551-558

Pallikaris IG, Papatzanaki Me, Siganos DE, et al. A corneal flap technique for laser in situ keratomileusis: human study. *Arch Ophthalmol.* 1991;109:1699-1702.

Pallikaris IG, Papatzanaki ME, Stathmi EZ, et al. Laser in situ keratomileusis. *Lasers Surg Med.* 1990;10:463-468.

Pallikaris IG, Siganos DS. Excimer laser in situ keratomileusis (LASIK) versus photorefractive keratectomy for the correction of high myopia. *J Refract Corneal Surg.* 1994;10:498-510.

Pande M, Hillman JS. Optical zone centration in keratorefractive surgery, entrance pupil center, visual axis, coaxially sighted corneal reflex, or geometric corneal center? *Ophthalmology.* 1993;1100:1230-1237.

Pepose JS, Laycock KA, Miller JK, et al. Reactivation of latent herpes virus by excimer laser photokeratectomy. *Am J Ophthalmol.* 1992;144:45-50.

Pérez-Santonja JJ, Alió J. LASIK for the correction of moderate and high myopia. In: Buratto L, Brint S, eds. *LASIK Principles and Techniques.* Thorofare, NJ: SLACK Incorporated; 1998; 185-194.

Pérez-Santonja JJ; Bellot J; Claramonte P; Ismail MM; Alió JL. Laser in situ keratomileusis (LASIK) for the correction of high myopia. *J Cataract Refract Surg.* 1997;23:1-14.

Pérez-Santonja JJ, Sakla HF, Alió JL. Contrast sensitivity after laser in situ keratomileusis. *J Cataract Refract Surg.* 1998;24:183-189.

Peters DJ, Lim DTC. Central islands: which machines cause the least of these complications and why? *Ophthalmic Pract.* 1995;13(4):139-141.

Price FW. Keratomileusis. *Ophthalmol Clin N Am.* 1992;5:673-681.

Price FW. Central islands of corneal steepening after automated lamellar keratoplasty for myopia. *J Refract Surg.* 1996;12:36-41.

Price FW, Whitson WE, Gonzales JS, Celedon RG, Smith. Automated lamellar keratomileusis in situ for myopia. *J Refract Surg.* 1996;12:29-35.

Probst LE, Treatment of epithelial ingrowth and flap melts following LASIK. In: Machat JJ, Slade SG, Probst LE. *The Art of LASIK. 2nd ed.* Thorofare, NJ: SLACK Incorporated; 1999; 435-440.

Probst LE. LASIK instrumentation. In: Machat JJ, Slade SG, Probst LE. *The Art of LASIK. 2nd ed.* Thorofare, NJ: SLACK Incorporated; 1999; 73-79.

Probst LE, Machat J. Removal of flap striae following laser in situ keratomileusis. *J Cataract Refract Surg.* 1998;24:153-155.

Probst LE, Machat JJ. Epithelial ingrowth following LASIK. In: Machat JJ, Slade SG, Probst LE. *The Art of LASIK. 2nd ed.* Thorofare, NJ: SLACK Incorporated; 1999; 427-434

Probst LE, Machat JJ. Removal of flap striae following LASIK. In: Machat JJ, Slade SG, Probst LE. *The Art of LASIK. 2nd ed.* Thorofare, NJ: SLACK Incorporated; 1999; 441-444.

Probst LE, Machat JJ. LASIK enhancement Techniques and results. In: Machat JJ, Slade SG, Probst LE. *The Art of LASIK. 2nd ed.* Thorofare, NJ: SLACK Incorporated; 1999; 225-240.

Probst LE, Machat JJ. LASIK enhancement techniques and results. In: Buratto L, Brint S, eds. *LASIK Principles and Techniques.* Thorofare, NJ: SLACK Incorporated; 1998; 325-338.

Reviglio V, Rodriguez ML, Picotti GS, Paradello M, Luna JD, Juárez CP. Mycobacterium chelonae keratitis following laser in situ keratomileusis. *J Refract Surg.* 1998;14:357-360.

Rispoli E, Guizzi M. Sulla sensibilità al contrasto. *Ottica Fisiopatologica.* 1999;3:189-197.

Roholt PC. Automated Lamellar Keratoplasty After Penetrating Keratoplasty. ASCRS: Best Papers of Sessions Symposium of Cataract IOL and Refractive Surgery. San Diego; April 1995: 36-37.

Roy FF. Regression in LASIK: Pathophysiology. Presented at Pre-AAO Conference. Chicago; October 24-26, 1996.

Rozakis GW. Keratomes. In: Rozakis GW, ed. *Refractive Lamellar Keratoplasty.* Thorofare, NJ: SLACK Incorporated; 1994; 19-32.

Rozakis GW. The first keratectomy. In: Rozakis GW, ed. *Refractive Lamellar Keratoplasty.* Thorofare, NJ, SLACK Incorporated; 1994; 45-55.

Salah T, Waring GO III, El-Maghraby A. Excimer laser keratomileusis in the corneal bed under a hinged flap: results in Saudi Arabia at the El-Maghraby Eye Hospital. In: Salz JI, McDonnell PJ, McDonald MB ed. *Corneal Laser Surgery.* St Louis, Mo: Mosby-Year Book. 1995.

Salah T, Waring G, El Maghraby A, Moadel K, et al. Excimer Laser in Situ Keratomileusis under a Corneal Flap for Myopia of 2 To 20 Diopters. Am J Ophthalmol. 1996;121:143-55.

Schuler A, Jessen K, Hoffmann F. Accuracy of microkeratome keratectomies in pig eyes. *Invest Ophthalmol Vis Sci.* 1990;31:2022-2030.

Seiler T. Central islands after LASIK. Presented at Pre-AAO Conference. Chicago; October 24-26, 1996.

Seiler T, Schmidt-Petersen H. The Schwind microkeratome in clinical practice. In: Buratto L, Brint S, eds. *LASIK Principles and Techniques.* Thorofare, NJ: SLACK Incorporated; 1998; 307-310.

Seiler T, Wollensak J. Komplikationen der laser keratomileusis mit dem excimer laser (193 nm). *Klin Monatsbl Augenheilkd.* 1992;200:648-653.

Shu-Wen Chang, Benson A, Azar DT. Corneal light scattering with stromal reformation after laser in situ keratomileusis and photorefractive keratectomy. *J Cataract Refract Surg.* 1998;24:1064-1069.

Siganos DS, Pallikaris IG. Laser in situ keratomileusis in partially sighted eyes. *Invest Ophthalmol Vis Sci.* 1993;34(4):800.

Slade SG. Treatment of astigmatism. In: Buratto L, Brint S, eds. *LASIK Principles and Techniques.* Thorofare, NJ: SLACK Incorporated; 1998; 247-258.

Slade SG. Abnormal induced topography. Central islands. In: Machat JJ ed. *Excimer Laser Refractive Surgery. Practice and Principles.* Thorofare, NJ: SLACK Incorporated; 1996; 399.

Slade SG, Brint SF. Excimer laser myopic keratomileusis. In: Rozakis GW, ed. *Refractive Lamellar Keratoplasty.* Thorofare, NJ: SLACK Incorporated; 1994:125-137.

Slade SG, Doane JF, Hohla C. Topography-assisted excimer laser techniques. In: Machat JJ, Slade SG, Probst LE. *The Art of LASIK. 2nd ed.* Thorofare, NJ: SLACK Incorporated; 1999; 461-468.

Slade SG, et al. Keratomileusis in situ: a prospective evalutation. Poster presentation of the AAO Meeting; 1993.

Smith RG. SCMD keratome unit. *Refract Corneal Surg.* 1990;6:207.

Smith RJ, Maloney RK. Diffuse lamellar keratitis. A new syndrome in lamellar refractive surgery. *Ophthalmology.* 1998;105:1721-1726.

Solomon K. The Wound Healing Responce Following LASIK and PRK. Presented at Pre-AAO Conference. Chicago; October 24-26, 1996.

Stein R, Stein HA, Cheskes A, et al. Photorefractive keratectomy and postoperative pain. *Am J Ophthalmol.* 1994;117:403-404.

Stonecipher KG, Parmley VC, Rowsey JJ, Fowler WC, Nguyen H. Refractive corneal surgery with the Draeger rotary microkeratome in human cadaver eyes. *J Refract Corneal Surg.* 1994;10:49-55.

Stulting RD, Carr JD, Thompson KP, Waring III GO, Wiley WM, Walker JG. Complications of laser in situ keratomileusis for the correction of myopia. *Ophthalmology.* 1999;106:13-20.

Suarez E, Cardenas JJ. Intraoperative complications of LASIK. Buratto L. Personal LASIK technique with nasal hinge. In: Buratto L, Brint S, eds. *LASIK Principles and Techniques.* Thorofare, NJ: SLACK Incorporated; 1998; 371-380.

Swinger CA, Barker BA. Prospective evaluation of myopia keratomileusis. *Ophthalmology.* 1984;91:785-792.

Tamburelli C. Preoperative evaluation by ultrasonography in myopic LASIK. In: Buratto L, Brint S, eds. *LASIK Principles and Techniques.* Thorofare, NJ: SLACK Incorporated; 1998; 143-150.

Thompson K. Repeated Surgery for Residual Myopia following Lasik. Presented at Pre-AAO Conference. Chicago; October 24-26, 1996.

Trokel SL. Evolution of excimer laser corneal surgery. *J Cataract Refract Surg.* 1989;15:373-383.

Tuunanen TH, Ruusuvaara PJ, Uusitalo RJ, Tervo TM. Photoastigmatism keratectomy for correction of astigmatism in corneal grafts. *Cornea.* 1997;16(1):48-53.

Uozato H, Guyton DL. Centering corneal surgical procedures. *Am J Ophthalmol.* 1987;103:264-275.

Villasenor RA. Homoplastic keratomileusis for myopia. *Refract Corneal Surg.* 1985;25:515-525.

Vinciguerra P, Azzolini M, Airaghi P, Radice P, De Molfetta V. Effect of decreasing surface and interface irregularities after photorefractive keratectomy and laser in situ keratomileusis on optical and functional outcomes. *J Refract Surg.* 1998;14:S199-S203.

Vinciguerra P, Azzolini M, Airaghi P, Radice P, Sborgia M, De Molfetta V. A method for examining surface and interface irregularities after photorefractive keratectomy and laser in situ keratomileusis: predictor of optical and functional outcomes. *J Refract Surg.* 1998;14: S204-S206.

Vinciguerra P, Azzolini M, Prussiani A, Sher N, Genisi C, Nizzola GM. Photoablative treatment of LASIK complications. In: Gimbel HV, Anderson Penno EE. *LASIK Complications. Prevention and Management.* Thorofare, NJ: SLACK incorporated; 1999; 101-111.

Vrabec MP, Durrie DS, Chase DS. Recurrence of herpes simplex after excimer laser keratectomy. *Am J Ophthalmol.* 1992;116:101-102.

Waring GO III, Seiler T. Laser corneal surgery: fundamentals and background. In: Brightbill FS, ed. *Corneal Surgery, Theory, Technique and Tissue.* St Louis, Mo: Mosby-Year Book, Inc; 1993; 480-511.

Yee RW. Comparison of Chiron and SCMD Microkeratome on Porcine Eyes Using Scanning Electron Microscopy. Presented at Pre-AAO Conference. Chicago; October 24-26, 1996.